Choices

REALISTIC ALTERNATIVES IN CANCER TREATMENT

Revised Edition

MARION MORRA & EVE POTTS

AVON
PUBLISHERS OF BARD, CAMELOT, DISCUS AND FLARE BOOKS

This book was current to the best of the authors' knowledge at publication, but before acting on information herein the consumer should, of course, verify information with the appropriate physician or agency.

CHOICES: REALISTIC ALTERNATIVES IN CANCER TREATMENT is an original publication of Avon Books. This work has never before appeared in book form.

AVON BOOKS
A division of
The Hearst Corporation
1790 Broadway
New York, New York 10019

First Avon Trade Printing: April 1980
First Revised Edition: March 1987

AVON TRADEMARK REG. U.S. PAT. OFF. AND IN OTHER COUNTRIES, MARCA REGISTRADA, HECHO EN U.S.A.

Printed in the U.S.A.

OPM 10 9 8 7 6 5 4 3 2 1

To our wonderful supportive family
who made it possible for us to write this book
and to the many cancer patients and their families
who inspired us with their courage and their need for
information

Preface

Learning that you, or someone you love, has cancer is frightening. One of the best weapons to help you deal with this diagnosis is accurate information. The fears of the unknown and the misconceptions about cancer and cancer treatment are replaced with well-researched, easily understood information. This book is practical and sensible. It provides valuable guidance on diagnosis and treatment of cancer in an accurate, up-to-date way.

This second edition of *CHOICES* adheres to the original objectives of the first edition: to present specific, current facts so that patients and their families may understand their illness, ask appropriate questions, receive clarification and, hopefully, cope with problems more effectively. In addition, many changes have been made to reflect the revolutionary progress that has occurred in cancer therapy since the first edition was printed in 1980.

The quality of information which doctors, nurses and other health professionals present to their patients and the amount of time they can spend with them and their families varies greatly. This book is meant to be a resource so that those involved can absorb the material at their own speed. It fills the gap between the material available in medical textbooks—which often is difficult for the lay person to understand—and the information presently printed in the press—which many times is premature and incomplete. This book deals with the latest information and will serve as a guide to the most modern diagnoses and treatments available in this rapidly changing field.

Joseph M. Bertino, M.D.
Co-Program Director, Developmental
Therapeutics and Clinical Investigation
Memorial Sloan-Kettering Cancer Center
New York, New York

M.K. Tish Knobf, R.N., M.S.N.
Oncology Clinical Nurse Specialist,
Section of Medical Oncology
Yale University School of Medicine
Yale Comprehensive Cancer Center
New Haven, Connecticut

To the Cancer Patient

There are so many practical things you need to know when the diagnosis is cancer—yet most of us are so gripped with fear of the verdict that practical considerations are often lost in emotional chaos. This book is designed to unlock some of the fears.

It is important for you to know that cancer is a different disease today than it was even ten years ago. Though no miracle cure has been found, it is a fact that many advances have been made in treatments. Cancer is no longer considered an incurable disease. Recoveries are being made. The future now exists for many cancer patients who would not have had a future ten years ago. Because the explosion of information has been so rapid, much of it has been slow in sifting down to the consumer.

What we have tried to do in this book is to cover every facet of cancer care, making it possible for you and your family to have enough information to ask intelligent questions that will give you the answers you need to know so that you can be a partner with your health-care team in making decisions. We have tried to limit the use of medical jargon and to translate information into understandable terms. The book is designed to be used as a reference. Make use of the index. Take notes when your doctor gives you information, so you can check things out in the book and get a better understanding of what is happening. Naturally, the book is not designed to take the place of your doctor but to supplement what he tells you and to guide you in asking the questions you need to know in order to get the best care.

The fact that you have cancer is irreversible and unchangeable. The way you and your family handle that fact makes the real difference in what happens to you.

If we can leave you with just one piece of good advice it would be: *Ask, ask, ask, and ask again.* Don't take anything for granted and don't be put off by medical jargon or a doctor who doesn't want to talk. Remember—you are a consumer and are entitled to answers to your questions.

Introduction to the Revised Edition

Many things have changed in the seven years since the first edition of *CHOICES* was written. There have been dramatic advances in the treatment of many kinds of cancer. We have included all the newest techniques and terminology to make this edition the most complete and up-to-date information currently available to the general public. We feel certain that this new *CHOICES* will make the same kind of impact as its predecessor which was the first comprehensive handbook designed to cover all the down-to-earth questions that people had about cancer. It is used as a major reference by thousands of patients and families as well as by cancer centers and hospitals throughout the world.

Our continuing work with patients, doctors and other health professionals, the workshops and conferences we have given and attended and expanded information available to the medical profession in the many areas of continuing cancer research have increased our own awareness of issues, problems and concerns. Our own family bouts with cancer have given us further personal insights into the special needs of others. These experiences are responsible for the addition of many new sections in this revised *CHOICES*, covering such important issues as how to deal with the emotional and sexual side effects of cancer, how to cope with cancer if it metastasizes, new ways of dealing with the side effects of radiation and chemotherapy and the latest information on standard and experimental treatments. Each of the charts that deal with the stages and treatments available for each kind of cancer have been updated and simplified using material available to top cancer specialists through the resources of the National Cancer Institute.

While every cancer case is different, every type of cancer is different and the course of every cancer illness is different from every other, this book helps to describe the common developments and problems in general, easy-to-understand terms that can be applied by you in helping to make the course of your own illness go more smoothly. The one common factor we have found in talking with cancer patients and their families is that those who are knowledgeable about their own health are those who seem best able to cope.

We hope this totally new edition will help you take greater control over your own health care. Of course, it is not meant to replace the care and advice of your doctor, but rather to supplement and explain in understandable language what is happening to you, giving you the ability to deal with your health caretakers in a more intelligent fashion, rather than with the feeling of being at the mercy of an indifferent system. We hope it will give you the power to take a far more active role in your recovery.

Contents

Preface   v

To the Cancer Patient   vi

Introduction to the Revised Edition   vii

List of Illustrations   xiii

Acknowledgments   xv

1 Facing the Diagnosis   1
    Coping with the diagnosis • Judging your attitude

2 Deciding on Your Doctor and Hospital   8
    Judging your doctor • What is an oncologist? • Judging your hospital • What is a comprehensive cancer center?

3 Understanding What Cancer Is   38
    Tumors, cysts, polyps, dysplasia • Understanding how cancer grows and behaves • Different kinds of cancer • Metastasis—what it means • Myths and facts • Basic warning signs • How cancers are staged and classified

4 Diagnostic Tests   59
    Questions to ask about different tests • Asking for another opinion • The difference between a referral and a consultation • Getting a second opinion on a pathology report • Questions to ask before having x-rays • All the "oscopy" tests—cytoscopy, bronchoscopy, endoscopy, etc. • Radioactive scans, metastatic workups, ultrasound, CT scans, MRI • Different kinds of biopsies • Frozen section versus permanent section biopsies • Tests used to determine if cancer has metastasized

CONTENTS

5 Treatment   112

Questions to ask about treatment • Types of treatment • How to get treatment with the newer experimental or investigational drugs

6 Surgery   119

General types • Questions to ask before the operation • Questions to ask the anesthesiologist • Questions to ask when you are in the hospital • Questions to ask before leaving the hospital • Different kinds of surgeons • Choosing your surgeon • All about anesthesia • Knowing your blood type • What happens before and after the operation

7 Radiation   153

Questions to ask about radiation therapy • Terminology • Different kinds of radiation therapy • How radiation is given • Side effects of radiation treatment • Radiation implants

8 Chemotherapy   200

Questions to ask about chemotherapy • How chemotherapy is given • Major chemotherapy drugs • Side effects of chemotherapy • What to do about side effects • What to do about hair loss • Bone marrow depression, low blood count, anemia • How drugs are evaluated

9 Investigational Treatments   262

Questions to ask before trying new treatments • What is immunotherapy? • Biological response modifiers • AIDS • New methods • Interferon, hypothermia, vitamins • How testing is done

10 Unproven Methods of Cancer Treatment   293

Questions to ask yourself before using unproven methods • Difference between experimental and unproven methods • Diet • Bahamas clinic • Laetrile

11 Breast Cancer   303

Symptoms • Early detection • Questions to ask if you have a lump • Questions to ask yourself • Steps to take if biopsy suggested • Steps to take if biopsy shows malignancy • Tests • Questions to ask before agreeing to a breast operation • Kind of doctor to see • How to examine your breasts • Mammography, Xeroradiography and thermography • Biopsies for breast cancer • Two-step procedure versus one-stop procedure •

CONTENTS

Breast Cancer *(continued)*
Understanding the doctor's terms • Stages and types of
breast cancer • Choices of treatment for breast cancer •
Lymph-node surgery • Treatment choices •
Mastectomy surgery • Questions to ask following
mastectomy • Exercises • Choosing a prosthesis •
Follow-up care • Questions to ask before breast
reconstruction

12 **Lung Cancer**   381
Symptoms • Questions to ask the doctor • Kind of
doctor to see • Kinds of lung cancer • Tests •
Diagnosing lung cancer • Stages • Treatment choices •
Lung surgery • After the operation

13 **Skin Cancers**   411
Symptoms • Tests • Questions to ask the doctor • Kind
of doctor to see • Different kinds of skin cancer •
Treatment choices • Difference between moles and
melanoma • Stages of melanoma • Treatment choices
for melanoma • Skin grafts • Mycosis fungoides

14 **Adult Leukemia, Lymphoma, and Sarcoma**   442
Leukemia • Symptoms • Questions to ask if you have
leukemia • Kind of doctor to see • Treatment choices •
Hodgkin's disease and non-Hodgkin's lymphoma •
Questions to ask • Malignant lymphomas • Myeloma •
Sarcomas • Bone cancers • Stages and types •
Treatment choices

15 **Gastrointestinal Cancers**   499
Symptoms • Abdominal cancer • Colon-rectal cancer •
Colostomies • Bladder cancer • Kidney cancer •
Stomach cancer • Liver cancer • Pancreatic cancer

16 **Cancer of the Female Reproductive Organs**   546
Questions to ask the doctor • Kind of doctor to see •
Symptoms • Kinds of operations • Cancer of the vulva
• Cancer of the vagina • Cancer of the cervix • Pap
tests • Conization • Cryosurgery • Cancer of the
endometrium or uterus • Hysterectomy • Cancer of the
fallopian tubes • Cancer of the ovary • Estrogen, oral
contraceptives • DES

17 **Cancer of the Male Reproductive Organs**   603
Symptoms • Kinds of operations and treatments •
Questions to ask the doctor • Cancer of the prostate •
Cancer of the testicle • Cancer of the penis

CONTENTS

18 Cancers of the Head and Neck   634
> Questions to ask • Kind of doctor to see • Symptoms •
> Oral cancer • Cancer of the nasal area • Thyroid cancer
> • Cancer of the larynx • Laryngectomy • Cancer of the
> esophagus

19 Cancer of the Brain and Spinal Cord   692
> Symptoms • Tests • Questions to ask • Kind of doctor
> to see • Types of cancers • Brain tumors • Spinal cord
> tumors • Treatment choices

20 Childhood Cancer   709
> Types of cancers • Symptoms • Kind of doctor to see •
> Questions to ask the doctor • Leukemia (ALL) •
> Non-Hodgkin's lymphoma • Bone tumors (osteogenic
> sarcoma, Ewing's sarcoma) • Neuroblastoma • Brain
> tumors • Retinoblastoma • Wilms' tumor • Emotional
> and financial aspects

21 Coping When Cancer Spreads or Comes Back   743
> Metastasis • Treatments for pain • Things to tell the
> doctor about pain • Acupuncture, hypnosis, biofeedback,
> relaxation exercises • Brompton cocktail, heroin,
> marijuana, nerve blocks • Surgical pain control

22 Living with Cancer   772
> Diet and nutrition • Recuperating at home • Questions
> on sex • Thinking about dying • Hospices • Caring for
> the patient at home • Health insurance, financial help,
> wills, donating the body

23 Where to Get Help   831
> Cancer Information Service • American Cancer Society
> • Specialized organizations for patient help • Camps for
> children • National Cancer Institute • Comprehensive
> Cancer Center locations • Clinical and non-clinical
> Cancer Center locations • National Cancer Institute
> clinical cooperative groups • Clinical cooperative groups
> in Canada and Europe • National Cancer Institute
> clinical treatment programs • Cancer programs approved
> by the American College of Surgeons

References   924

Index   927

List of Illustrations

How cancer grows	39
Incisional biopsy	105
Excisional biopsy	105
Breast	312
Breast self-examination	317–318
Breast self-examination (lying down)	320
Tumor sizes	342
Examples of breast operation scars	351
Lungs	384
Cross-section of skin	421
Lymph system	475
Colon-rectal area	505
Front view, major internal organs	521
Rear view, major internal organs	522
Female reproductive organs	549
Male reproductive organs	612
Head and neck	638
Brain	697

The publisher gratefully acknowledges the generous participation of the following companies who have contributed time and materials in their respective areas to the manufacturing of this edition. They have enabled Avon Books to make a donation to the American Cancer Society for every copy of CHOICES sold.

HORIZON PAPER COMPANY

WESTCHESTER BOOK COMPOSITION, INC.

OFFSET PAPERBACK MANUFACTURERS, INC.

FOLEY'S GRAPHIC CENTER

PHOTOTYPE COLOR GRAPHICS

Acknowledgments

To list all of the people, books and sources such as magazine articles, original scientific writings, pamphlets, oncology seminars, and medical textbooks which made it possible for us to write this book would be an almost impossible task. We do want to thank publicly all those from whom we learned, especially the writings of the National Cancer Institute and the American Cancer Society and the many doctors, patients, and families kind enough to share their experiences, problems, and questions with us. We gained special insight from Shirley Mead and Betty Sheffer, two good friends who died of cancer, who made us most aware of the need for real answers to patients' questions.

Two of our colleagues deserve extra-special thanks—Tish Knobf, one of the country's most experienced cancer nurses, and Joe Bertino, a world-renowned cancer researcher as well as an experienced and sensitive oncologist, who gave us many hours of their scarcest commodity, time. We thank them for their invaluable, continuing, and personal involvement in helping us to avoid medical pitfalls in our writing.

We thank the members of our family for their encouragement and their assistance from beginning to end—especially Bob Potts and Abby, Amy, Matt, and Mark, for putting up with late dinners, early mornings, and short tempers; Mollie Donovan, our other sister, for help in layout, art, and typing and for encouragement; and Ann and Gil Maurer, for their guidance. We thank our mother, who brought us up to believe that we could accomplish any task we felt we wanted to do, and our father, who did not live to see this book completed, but who would have been very proud.

Though it is through the help of many, many people that this book came to be, we alone take responsibility for any possible errors or misinterpretations.

chapter 1

Facing the Diagnosis

Cancer is a major illness, but it is not necessarily fatal, contrary to what many people believe. Nearly two million Americans are alive and considered cured of cancer 5 years or more after their initial diagnosis and treatment. Overall, one in three people with cancer is considered cured. For some forms of the disease, nine out of ten people diagnosed can be considered cured. Many others will live a long time before dying of the disease. Yet the diagnosis of cancer is the most dreaded of any medical problem. And the normal reaction is: *How long will I live?* The answer, of course, is that no one really knows. And the answer is exactly the same for all of us—*whether or not we have cancer.*

There is hope for every patient. Some patients with cancer are cured at once, by surgery, chemotherapy and radiotherapy. Some are never cured, but their disease is controlled so that they can expect to live for many years. Some treatments—such as those that reduce hair loss and nausea or remove a limb or a breast—seem to some to be worse than the illness itself. Some treatments prolong life for no more than a few months. But the fact is that with the proper attention, no patient needs to suffer. You can have cancer and still enjoy life.

Prepare for a host of nagging feelings. You will probably experience all of them to a greater or lesser degree. Check off those that match your own most intensely.

- I don't want to die.
- I can't believe this is happening to me.
- I feel as though I've been thrown off a cliff.
- This is the loneliest experience of my life.
- No one else can know how I feel.
- Maybe it will all go away.
- It couldn't be cancer because no one in my family ever had cancer.
- If it really is cancer, what will it mean to my life?
- I don't know how to tell my family.
- What if the doctor says I have to go to the hospital right away?
- People will treat me differently if they find out I have cancer.
- I'm afraid.
- I'm going to be in a lot of pain.
- This is a challenge to be met and I know I can beat it.
- Why me? Why couldn't it be someone else?
- I don't want to lose my breast (or lung or leg).

Coping with the Diagnosis of Cancer

Once you suspect you have cancer, you can live in fear. Or you can learn to live with the facts and you can begin to do positive things. Knowing the facts and facing them takes a lot of the scare away.

Here are a few basics for starters. Check them and see how many actually coincide with your own thinking.

- The fact that you may have cancer cannot be changed. The time that is most important in decision-making is right now—at the very beginning—when numerous alternatives are open to you.
- Demand to know all the alternatives. If you make a decision to go ahead with surgery without sufficient testing or a second opinion, you limit the possibility for other alternatives right from the very start. Often, unless you remain calm and in control, a decision is made for you by circumstances that will take it out of your control.

Learning all you can about your case and the alternatives means you can control the way your illness is handled.

- Call the Cancer Information Service, toll-free at 1-800-4-CANCER for the latest up-to-date information and facts on your type of cancer.

- Do your homework. Ask your friends and family to help you search the library for any available articles on your specific illness. If a medical library is available to you, look for help there. So much new research is being done in so many places that you may find a clue to a treatment even your doctor hasn't heard of. Check with the nearest cancer center. Call your nearest American Cancer Society office; its staff will have a great deal of information and expertise on the illness.

- Make sure you have the *right* doctor. The kind of treatment you get depends on how much your doctor knows about your specific disease.

- As a cancer patient, you must be an activist. You must become a partner with your doctors in the fight so that you can live your life in the way that is best for you.

- You can't cope with cancer by denying you have it. You can cope with it by learning as much as you can about what is happening to you.

- Hope is not the same as denying. Denying you have cancer closes your mind and your resources to all the possibilities that exist for you. You shut off your inner abilities to deal with what is real. Denial closes the doors. Hope opens the channels for action.

- None of us knows how long he or she will live. A patient with breast cancer, diagnosed early, who is receiving adequate treatment may live longer than a patient with heart disease.

- Without any doubt, the very worst time you will experience is at the beginning, when the diagnosis is first presented to you. At that moment, cancer becomes an inescapable fact for you. That is the time when you must mobilize yourself and your resources to plan your future intelligently.

- If at all possible, a second opinion is an absolute must at the start before submitting to *any* cancer treatment of *any* kind. This is not to suggest that the diagnosis you were given is not correct or that the suggested treatment might not be the best. It is only to say that you deserve the right to have the doctor's diagnosis reconfirmed and alternative treatments explored and explained to you.

- In some cases, a second pathological opinion is a good idea. The pathology report is the basis on which all future decisions will be made, and although some cancers are pathologically diagnosed without any question, you need to check and ask about it.
- Ask your doctor to check the computerized Physician Data Query (PDQ) information for the very latest data on what is being recommended for your type and stage of cancer. He can also direct you to oncologists who specialize in your kind of cancer with whom you may wish to consult.
- You, as a cancer patient, are a consumer. As a consumer you have the right to ask questions just as you would as a consumer of any other product. However, you need to learn what questions to ask, what the terminology means, what possibilities exist. You have to set your mind to facing the fact that you have cancer—but you must also realize that if you have all the information at hand, you will greatly increase your chances for different treatment that might lead to a cure.
- One of the most important things to remember is that there are cancer specialists (called oncologists) who see many cancer patients every day. If you have cancer, your primary care should be under the direction of a specialist who spends most of his time dealing with cancer.
- Choose your plan of action and take time to make sure your decisions are informed ones. Carefully take notes whenever talking with the doctor, radiologist, physical therapist or nurse.
- Bring a list of questions with you, take notes when you are there, review them when you get home, and save them for future reference.
- Try always to have a family member or good friend with you when discussing your case with the doctor. People hear different things being said. It is important to have

someone who is informed talk over the information with you.

- Expect some degree of depression. Cancer is a serious illness. Expect "down" days. Plan ways of coping with them. Call a friend. Take a walk down a favorite beach or pathway. Make a trip to a museum or wherever you feel happy.

- You need to do some thinking about whether quality or quantity of life—how good or how long—is more important to you. You may be faced with some decisions along the way where the answer to this question will determine which way to go.

- Don't be a martyr. Try to deal with your feelings honestly. Don't try to hide your illness and prognosis from your family and your friends. Try to face the facts openly. Accept and welcome the help of others. Only by tapping every resource will you be able to deal with your illness in an informed manner.

- Once you and your doctors have embarked on a course of treatment, your own unique style of coping will help to make you feel in control. You will be able to face your problems if you know what is being done to you, how it will be done, and what the prognosis is. You will undoubtedly find your optimism tempered with anxiety— and this is normal. You may be surprised that along the way you will experience a feeling of relief, or a feeling of calmness about what is happening, and even an increased zest for living. Many patients tell of a greater appreciation for the simple things in life once the initial decision on the course of treatment is made.

- Remember, your doctor will continue to work with you to control your disease. If the first treatment fails, there are others available that can be used.

Judging Your Own Attitude Toward Cancer

YOUR TRUE OR FALSE ANSWER	THE REAL ANSWER
_____ You will die if you have cancer.	False. Cancer, if discovered at an early stage, is curable in many instances.
_____ Smoking can cause lung cancer.	True. Heavy cigarette smokers get lung cancer 23 times more often than non-smokers.
_____ A lump in the breast means you have cancer.	False. Eighty percent of all lumps are not cancer.
_____ Some cancers can be prevented.	True. Preventive steps, such as not smoking or not being overexposed to the sun, have proved to reduce the chances of getting some types of cancer.
_____ Cancer is contagious.	False.
_____ Cancer is hereditary.	False. However, the tendency toward breast and colon cancer, for example, seems to run in families.
_____ Cancer is more frequent in men and women over 35.	True. It is primarily a disease of middle age and old age—rare in children and young adults.
_____ Cancer can develop in any part of the body.	True. All parts of the body are susceptible—the nervous system, bone, lymph, skin, etc.
_____ Half of cancer patients are cured.	True. Of more than half a million newly diagnosed cancer cases each year, one-half can be permanently cured, and many more lead normal lives for many years.
_____ The outlook for cancer therapy is hopeful.	True. The rate of cure is now one in two as compared with one in four in 1950 and one in three in the 1970s.

Judging Your Own Attitude Toward Cancer (continued)

YOUR TRUE OR FALSE ANSWER	THE REAL ANSWER
———— The doctor can tell how long you have to live.	False. Every case is different, and doctors' estimates on how long a patient will live are many times guesswork and often do a great disservice to the patient.
———— There are no untreatable cancers.	True. There are always treatments that can be prescribed to make a patient more comfortable, although treatments are not always available to effect a cure.
———— Putting off seeing a doctor can forfeit the possibility of a cure.	True. Of those who die of cancer each year, 100,000 will die needlessly because of late diagnosis and inadequate treatment.
———— More people are having cancer diagnosed than ever before.	True. This is because more people are living to an age when cancer occurs more frequently, and because diagnosis is better, so more cases are being found.
———— You should try to get a second or even a third opinion before having anything done.	True. A very wise idea, and any doctor who advises against another opinion is probably a doctor you shouldn't be using.

chapter 2

Deciding on Your Doctor and Hospital

Let's backtrack a bit and return to the basic question of who your doctor is at the moment. So much has been said and written about how to find a good doctor, yet so often in the cancer area the decision must be made on the spur of the moment. Most patients do not go through logical steps in making this important choice.

And once a doctor starts on a case, most people find it difficult to change doctors, or even to bring up the subject of a second opinion. Remember, you are not alone in this problem. Most people find it difficult to challenge a doctor. On the other hand, most people even have a hard time changing hairdressers or standing up to their auto mechanics. It has only been in very recent times that people have felt they have the right to ask questions about their medical care.

Don't feel you are limited to the doctor you have right now. Use the checklist to help you determine if you are in partnership with the right doctor. This is one of the most important decisions you are going to make in handling your illness. (The right hospital is another important factor and will be discussed next.)

You might think that some of the questions that follow are irrelevant in your particular case—that they relate more to finding a good general doctor than an oncologist. But they are important for you to get an overall understanding

Judging Your Doctor

FILL IN HERE	SCORING	REASON FOR SCORE
+ −	+ −	

Kind of Practice

		+	−	
__ __	Multi-specialty group	5		Generally, a doctor who practices with a group that specializes in a variety of disciplines is better for your family doctor. Specialists who practice in a group or in a hospital are subject to constant review by peers.
__ __	Hospital-based office	5		
__ __	One-specialty group	5		
__ __	Loose association with others	2		
__ __	With partner	1		
__ __	Alone		1	

Hospital Affiliation

		+	−	
__ __	University or medical school hospital (part- or full-time staff member)	5		Same reasoning as above holds true here. You can be sure that a doctor who is part- or full-time staff member at a university or medical school hospital or a larger community hospital has probably shown his merit and is respected by his colleagues. The doctor who practices in a small for-profit hospital might be just as qualified but should be more closely checked for other credentials.
__ __	On teaching staff of medical school	5		
__ __	Staff member, community hospital with 200 or more beds	4		
__ __	Staff member, community hospital with fewer than 200 beds	3		
__ __	Part owner, staff of small private hospital (proprietary hospital)	1		
__ __	No hospital affiliation (ask doctor for reason, then score either −1 or +1)	1	1	

Judging Your Doctor (continued)

YOUR TRUE
OR FALSE
ANSWER   THE REAL ANSWER

Boards

___ ___ Board-certified in his specialty and specialist in oncology   10

___ ___ Board-certified and/or fellow of the board   5

___ ___ Board-certified   4

___ ___ Board-eligible   3

___ ___ No longer eligible   1

The fact that a doctor has been
certified in his specialty means
that beyond training in his field
he has subjected himself to the
scrutiny of his peers in written
and oral examinations. A fellowship is an extra flag of distinction. Oncology specialty means
that the bulk of patients are cancer patients, but since this is a
new specialty, many of the older
and more experienced cancer
doctors have not taken the boards
in the field.

Manner

___ ___ Explains procedures, asks
and answers questions,
keeps complete records,
has laboratory tools in office or available nearby (x-
ray, urine and blood-
chemistry lab, etc.), takes
full history at first visit   5

___ ___ Seems interested but has
never taken full history or
given complete examina-
tion; lab tests done at different location   2

___ ___ Difficult to communicate
with, uses unfamiliar
terms, doesn't seem able
to communicate in plain
language, forgets facts because doesn't take notes   1

___ ___ Always in a hurry, doesn't
care about problem, seems
overly concerned about
money   5

Your own personal observations
about how the doctor's skills
measure up are an important part
of the evaluation. Think back
over his care of you before scoring this one.

Judging Your Doctor (continued)

YOUR TRUE
OR FALSE
ANSWER   THE REAL ANSWER

How Office Is Run

__ __ Personable, warm, efficient office personnel; office looks cheerful, comfortable, neat; appointments kept on time or explanations given   5

__ __ Clinical, impersonal atmosphere—both office and personnel; office always jammed; waiting the rule rather than the exception   3

__ __ Concerned office staff—nurse seems more interested than doctor—but haphazardly run appointment schedule in attempt to keep everyone happy   2

__ __ Messy, dingy office, inefficient personnel; record-keeping haphazard; overemphasis on paying   1

The manner in which the doctor's office is run tells you a great deal about the doctor's own standards and probably reflects upon the way he conducts the professional side of his life. Taken alone, this part of the scoring is not as vital as the doctor's credentials, but added to the other material it stands as an important guideline to the kind of medical care you will receive.

Personality

__ __ Warm, concerned, listens, interested, willing to explain and answer questions   5

__ __ Very professional but impersonal, cold and stiff   4

__ __ Seems overly busy, average personality   3

__ __ Doesn't relate well   1

How well you relate to your doctor has a bearing on the kind of treatment you will get and how well you will respond. Therefore, it is important that he be someone for whom you have thorough respect and who sees you as a person as well as a patient.

Judging Your Doctor (continued)

FILL IN HERE		SCORING	REASON FOR SCORE
+	−	+ −	

Other

__	__	Willing to make house calls or has 24-hour telephone accessibility to someone who knows you or has your records 5	These extra-point items are all pluses for a doctor since they give an indication of his compassion for his patients.
__	__	Willing to discuss fees 5	
__	__	Takes Medicare and Medicaid patients 5	

of how the medical profession operates and will help you make some of those doctor decisions which will face you.

How do I choose a family doctor?

Today people commonly move from one area to another, and most of us do not have what is lovingly called a "family doctor." Ideally, your family doctor should be one who is either in general practice or in family practice or whose specialty is internal medicine (known as an internist or as a gastroenterologist or "G.I. man"). Your gynecologist/obstetrician and your pediatrician are usually not considered family doctors because of the nature of their specialties. Many younger doctors are turning to the specialty of family practice. This is a new or a renewed specialty which requires a three-year residency as well as a reexamination every three years to remain board-certified. Thus the new family practitioner is more highly trained than the old general practitioner.

How do I check out my doctor's credentials?

This is a relatively easy thing to do—and worth the half-hour it will take, especially when you consider that you will be spending hundreds of dollars for his expertise and putting your physical and psychological well-being in his hands. Go to the reference room at your local library and ask for a copy of either the Directory of Medical Specialists or the American Medical Directory. If possible, use the Directory of Medical Specialists, since it lists only those doctors who are "board-certified"—that is, those who have passed tests in their particular specialty, under the watchful eyes of their fellow doctors. The listings of doctors in the American Medical Directory, though it lists credentials, include any doctor who belongs to the American Medical Association, whether or not he has received board certification. If your library does not have either of these books, try calling your state or local department of health or medical society and ask them for the information.

What does board certification mean?

The specialty boards are private, voluntary, nonprofit, autonomous organizations founded to conduct examinations, issue certificates of qualifications, and improve and broaden opportunities for graduate education and training. Once a doctor finishes his required residency in his specialty, he becomes eligible to be certified by the board. This requires him to take a rigorous written and oral examination before other doctors who practice in his specialty. Many doctors are not "certified" on their first examinations by the board. Some boards require recertification after a specified number of years. An *F* after a doctor's name means he has been elected to a fellowship in the "college" of his specialty and is qualified to teach others. It is another step up the ladder and earns him an especially esteemed place among his colleagues.

Are there good doctors who are not board-certified?

Board certification and fellowships are designed to indicate a high level of competence, but there are many reasons why doctors who are equally competent may not be board-certified. In the field of cancer, especially, there are many doctors who treat only cancer patients, yet are not board-certified in oncology. This is because the boards in oncology are new and were not available to the older doctors when they started in practice. Some doctors in medical centers who combine research with patient care do not take boards. The main thing to remember is that if you are choosing a doctor without any personal recommendations from other physicians or health professionals, stick to those who are board-certified. You will have a guarantee from other physicians in his specialty that you have chosen a qualified person.

What is the difference between a board-certified doctor and one who is board-eligible?

The physician who passes the examination of a given specialty is known as a diplomate of the board and is said to be board-certified. A physician who has completed a formal training program in the specialty but has either chosen not to take the exams or has not completed the exams is called board-eligible (newly trained doctors are board-eligible between the time they finish their residency and the time they take their boards and get the results). There are well-trained specialists who for good, legitimate reasons are board-eligible, but these are exceptions. It is better to have passed the exams than not to have passed them.

Don't physicians have to be recertified periodically once they have passed their boards?

There are only two specialty societies at the present time which have taken definite steps to require periodic recertification—family practice and surgery. In general, most physicians are diligent in keeping up with the latest knowledge. However, there are obviously some doctors in practice who are not as up-to-date as others.

How do I use the medical directories to check out a doctor?

The book will tell you the year the doctor was born, the medical school he attended, the year he was licensed to practice, if and when he was certified in his specialty, both his primary and secondary specialties, and his type of practice. The Directory of Medical Specialists has more detailed information as to where he trained, what societies he belongs to, his appointment to medical schools, and his hospital accreditations. Each book has its own method of coding, which is carefully explained in the foreword. (Bring your glasses or magnifying glass with you, as the type is small and hard to read.) There is nothing mysterious or difficult about getting this information—it takes only a few minutes and it is important to you in getting the very best and most advanced treatment possible. Take the time to search it out.

The listings in both books are geographical, so this is a good time to find out and jot down the names and credentials of other specialists in your area—such as surgeons, anesthesiologists, gynecologists, urologists, etc. Each specialty in the Directory of Medical Specialists is listed separately by geographic areas. If no one in your town is listed, look for names of doctors in nearby towns.

What kinds of things are important to look for in analyzing the listings in the book?

There are several questions you should ask yourself:

- Does he have a teaching appointment at a medical-school-affiliated hospital? This indicates that he is up-to-date and respected by his peers.
- What kind of hospital is he affiliated with? Is it a medical-school-affiliated hospital? Requirements for this sort of hospital are rigid and must be earned through teaching appointments.
- If he is a surgeon, does he have privileges at three or more hospitals? This sounds impressive but it takes so much of the doctor's time that you might be better served by someone who concentrates his efforts on one or two hospitals. The quality of the hospital he is associated with is more important than the number.
- How large is the hospital? If you don't live in an area with a university hospital center, the larger the hospital (200 beds or more) the more equipment and facilities it will have.
- Is it a privately owned (proprietary) hospital? If so, the doctors who practice may be part owners—and though that is not a reflection on their abilities, it can mean that standards may not be as high as in community hospitals.
- What societies does the doctor belong to? He should belong to one or more, for these help keep him up-to-date on the latest information being developed by others in his specialty.

Does my doctor belong to a multi-specialty group?

This is important if you are looking for a family doctor but not as essential for a specialist. If you are looking for a family doctor, find a group with a family practitioner, a pediatrician, an internist, a general surgeon, a gynecologist, and possibly a radiologist. Groups vary by size and category— but they offer the best overall coverage for a patient as well as the most convenient kind of setup, since all services can usually be provided within one building. Blood counts, electrocardiogram, urinalysis, and x-rays can all be done without having the patient run from one end of town to the other. You can find such a group by writing to the American Group Practice Association (P.O. Box 948, Alexandria, Va. 22313) for information on whether there is such a group near you.

Can any doctor be a specialist?

After earning his M.D. degree (4 years of study after college) plus 1 year of internship, a physician can be licensed to practice if he can pass certain requirements. There are still a few states which do not even require an internship for a doctor to become eligible for licensing. Once licensed, a physician can call himself anything he wants. Even if a physician has no training beyond internship, he can call himself a psychiatrist or an internist, and he can legally perform operations as a surgeon. That is why it is important to determine whether or not the physician has had additional training, is board-certified, and is practicing in a legitimate hospital. The best way to do this is to check his credentials in the Directory of Medical Specialists.

If my doctor has no hospital affiliation does that mean he is not a good doctor?

Not necessarily, though that once was the case. Some perfectly good family doctors confine themselves to an office practice and when the patient needs hospitalization, they recommend the specialist they feel has the proper skills. If, however, the doctor was once affiliated with a hospital and no longer has that affiliation, make sure you ask some questions.

If the doctor is in solo practice, is that a good sign?

This really depends upon the area in which the doctor is practicing. Many doctors practice in rural areas and may have no choice but to be in solo practice. However, in general the doctor who works with other doctors is usually a better bet than one who works alone. Solo practice limits the exchange of ideas and cuts off the possibility of someone else evaluating the doctor's practices. Some solo doctors practice in the same building with other doctors and cover for each other. This is better than a doctor who is off by himself in an office with no contact with other medical professionals. (You should check what the arrangements for covering are. If the covering doctor does not have access to your medical records, he is very limited in how he can treat you in your doctor's absence.) Your doctor may be part of a group that consists of several other doctors who practice the same specialty, such as a group of internists, each with a different area of expertise. This gives them and you the advantage of other opinions on a specific case.

What is an HMO?

The letters HMO stand for *h*ealth *m*aintenance *o*rganization, which delivers comprehensive health care to members. The members pay a set fee each month. Check-ups and physicals, doctor's office visits, surgery, hospital services, emergency care and other health care are covered. In most HMOs you are required to go to a set location and use the doctors they have selected for you.

Are there any HMOs where you can go to a doctor in private practice for your care?

Some HMOs are "independent practice associations"—physicians in individual practice or in group practice contract to serve HMO members. The patient chooses from a list of private, community-based primary doctors. This primary doctor serves as the patient's personal advisor on all health matters and refers to a wide range of specialists such as surgeons, cardiologists or oncologists when the patient needs them.

What are the major specialties?

The Directory of Medical Specialists lists some twenty-two specialties. Among those which pertain to what might be needed for cancer treatment are

- *Dermatologists*: doctors who treat skin diseases and conditions, including skin cancer
- *Family practice*: doctors specializing in the continuing and total care of the family
- *Internists*: doctors who treat a wide range of medical problems. Subspecialists who are internists take an additional 1 or more years of "fellowship":
  - Endocrinology: diseases of organs which secrete hormones into the bloodstream, such as the pancreas, thyroid, etc.
  - Gastroenterology (GI): diseases of the GI tract (mouth to anus, including stomach, liver, pancreas, intestines)
  - Hematology: diseases of the blood and blood-making tissues
  - Infectious disease: difficult cases of infection
  - Nephrology: disease of the kidneys, the rest of the urinary system, and related disorders of metabolism
  - Neurology: diseases of the nervous system (brain, spinal cord and nerves)
  - Oncology: diseases of abnormal tissue growth (cancer)
  - Pulmonary disease: disease of the lung
- *Otolaryngologists (ENT)*: doctors who specialize in the ear, nose, and throat, air tubes to the lungs, and neck region
- *Pediatricians*: doctors who take care of children up to age 16. Subspecialties are similar to internists: pediatric cardiology, pediatric endocrinology, pediatric hematology
- *Psychiatrists*: medical doctors who treat emotional and mental disorders. Board-certified psychiatrists have 3 or more years of residency training after obtaining an M.D. (Clinical psychologists deal with nonclinical matters such as education and have no formal medical training. They

obtain a Ph.D. instead of an M.D. but have post-M.D. training similar to that of the psychiatrist.)

- *Surgeons*: doctors who treat by cutting out or operating. Subspecialties that require 4 or more years of special training:
  - General surgery: operations within the abdominal cavity and chest cavity
  - Neurological surgery: operations involving the skull, brain
  - Obstetrics and gynecology: operations on the female reproductive organs, childbirth
  - Ophthalmology: operations of the eye and optical structures
  - Orthopedic surgery: surgical treatment of injury and diseases of bones and joints
  - Plastic surgery: operations involving skin grafts, facial injuries, and tendon and nerve repair
  - Proctology: study and treatment of colon and rectal conditions
  - Thoracic surgery: operations in area of chest, including lungs, heart, and blood vessels
  - Urology: treatment of the urinary system (kidneys, bladder, and prostate)
- *Pathologists*: doctors who study, grossly and microscopically, abnormal conditions of all tissues and interpret blood tests and tissue specimens to determine origin, nature, causes and development of disease
- *Radiologists*: diagnostic radiologists perform and interpret x-ray studies; therapeutic radiologists or radiation oncologists treat cancer with x-rays

Is it better to use a younger doctor or an older doctor?

It is generally thought that the younger doctor is probably more up-to-date and the older doctor has more experience. This may be true in private practice, but in the medical academic area, the older doctor is probably both more up-to-date and more experienced. Teaching in a medical school means he must stay up-to-date and be ready to explain to the students why he is using a particular procedure or treatment.

Are psychiatrists interested in treating cancer patients?

Generally, no. Cancer patients are not usually mentally ill. Sometimes, however, both the patient and other family members need to talk with someone. For some, a small amount of psychotherapy is needed. A psychologist (rather than a psychiatrist) or someone who has had training in social work may fill this role. Many times nurses, clergymen, friends, family members, or other patients can be of the most help. The main point is for persons to recognize that they are living through a stressful situation, and that they should accept and seek help from others.

What is an oncologist?

If you have cancer, *oncology* and *oncologist* are words you should be familiar with. The word *oncology* is from the Greek word *onkos*, meaning "bulk" or "mass," and relates to that part of medical science that treats tumors. It is only in the past 10 years that medical oncology has been listed as a subspecialty for internists in the Directory of Medical Specialists. The bulk of the practice of these physicians deals with cancer patients. You are indeed fortunate if you can arrange to have an internist who is a specialist in medical oncology as your doctor.

What is a surgical oncologist?

Although this is not listed as a specialty, some surgeons who are known in their professions as dealing primarily with cancer patients are referred to as surgical oncologists. Because they see many cancers, their treatment can be expected to be more up-to-date than that of a surgeon who deals with a broader spectrum of general cases. There are also surgeons who do diagnostic biopsies, laparotomies (operations to open the abdomen either to make an inspection of the contents or as a preliminary to further surgery), and splenectomies (removal of the spleen to see if it contains cancer cells). These specialists are important to cancer patients especially because of their expertise in diagnosing the problem.

What is a radiation therapist?·

A radiation therapist is a doctor who specializes in treating the cancer patient with radiotherapy. Sometimes this doctor is called a therapeutic radiologist, radiation therapist, or radiotherapist. You will also hear the term *diagnostic radiologist*. This is a specialist who performs and interprets x-rays used in diagnosing your illness.

What is a medical oncologist or a chemotherapist?

A medical oncologist is a doctor of internal medicine who specializes in the administration of a variety of drugs needed to treat specific cancers. He can also be referred to as a hematologist (one who specializes in blood diseases) or a chemotherapist (one who specializes in chemotherapeutic drugs). Most chemotherapeutic drugs are too risky to be administered by general physicians without special training. It is important, if you are living in a community that does not have an oncologist, to make sure that your doctor has consulted with a cancer center, a medical school, or an oncologist to determine which drugs are best for your case, the dose of drug to be given, and the side effects to be expected. This field of medicine is relatively new and changes constantly. At the present time, the newest, most experimental chemotherapeutic drugs are available only at the large cancer centers, specialized hospitals, or community hospitals affiliated with a cancer center. The use of chemotherapeutic drugs is a very specialized field. The drugs have many side effects and should be administered only by qualified personnel. In many areas, doctors, nurses, and pharmacists work as a team in this newly emerging field.

What is the difference between an anesthesiologist and an anesthetist?

An M.D. degree. An anesthetist is a person who administers anesthetics. An anesthesiologist is an M.D. whose specialty is the administering of anesthesia. This specialty has become an extremely important one in the last 30 years as anesthesia has become more sophisticated and diversified.

The anesthesiologist should be your choice to administer anesthesia during the operation. He will check your specific needs during the operation—oxygen requirements, heart action, blood pressure, pulse, and body functions. For any operation which requires the use of anesthesia, you should make certain that your anesthesia is administered under the supervision of a board-certified anesthesiologist.

What is the role of the nurse in cancer care?

You will find that the nurse is a very important part of the health team in cancer care. A growing number of nurses in this country are specializing in the cancer field. Some of these nurses work in medical centers with the physicians who are doing investigational work in the fields of chemotherapy and radiation therapy. Some work in the offices of oncologists. Others are ostomy nurses or enterostomal therapists who take care of the needs of patients who have had operations in the gastrointestinal areas. Some nurses give chemotherapeutic drugs under the doctors' supervision. Others are involved with teaching patients how to take care of themselves after leaving the hospital. Many of them take time to evaluate how the patient and his family are coping with the illness. Whether your long-term care is in the hospital, the outpatient clinic of a hospital, or in a doctor's office, get to know the nurses who are involved with your care. They can be your best allies.

Should I discuss finances with my doctor?

Absolutely. Cancer is a very expensive illness, and you should know what kinds of costs will be involved. You should never be afraid to ask the doctor about his fees, what the laboratory tests will cost, how much the hospital bill will be, or what x-rays and drugs cost. The earlier you have this kind of discussion, the better off you will be. If the doctor does not know all the answers, he can direct you to someone else who will. If the doctor refuses to discuss costs with you, you should think about getting yourself another doctor.

Is it a good idea to go to a research or a teaching hospital?

Naturally, this is a personal decision, based on many factors. Certain demands are made on patients in these hospitals

Judging Your Hospital

SCORE	TYPE OF HOSPITAL	SCORING GUIDE	REASON FOR SCORE
_____	Comprehensive cancer center designated by National Cancer Institute (see Chapter 23)	50	If one of these facilities is nearby, by all means take advantage of it. Use its expertise for your care or have your case reviewed by the experts on the staff. This is where much of the newest work on cancer is taking place; consider yourself fortunate if one of these facilities is available to you.
_____	Clinical cancer center designated by National Cancer Institute (see Chapter 23)	40	
_____	Community hospital with a community clinical oncology program grant (see Chapter 23)	40	
_____	Approved hospital cancer program sponsored by American College of Surgeons (check Chapter 23 for listings)	20	Accredited hospitals have voluntarily been surveyed by the College of Surgeons and have set up a multidisciplinary cancer committee and fulfilled additional requirements.
_____	Directly affiliated with medical school which uses hospital for internship and residency programs	20	Provide excellent care, generally, since medical schools attract some of the top doctors as faculty members and range of services is extremely broad.
_____	Teaching hospital, residency and internship training, medical-school affiliation, but hospital located away from medical school	15	Have good facilities, usually not as wide-ranging as in hospitals directly connected with medical school.
_____	Residency and/or internship program, without medical-school affiliation	10	These programs are a sign of better-than-adequate care and put these hospitals a step above those which simply are accredited.

Judging Your Hospital (continued)

SCORE	TYPE OF HOSPITAL	SCORING GUIDE	REASON FOR SCORE
_____	Accredited by Joint Commission on Accreditation for Hospitals, but without approved internship and/or residency programs	5	Accreditation is a minimum standard ensuring adequate care.
_____	Not accredited	0	About one-quarter of hospitals in U.S. fall into this category. Unaccredited hospitals are not eligible for Medicaid payments.
_____	Government-supported (so-called public) hospital (VA, Public Health Service, county, city, or state)	0	Care in these varies from excellent to substandard. No score suggested.
_____	Proprietary or for-profit hospital, owned by individuals or stockholders, including doctors who practice there	0 or −10	Medical services frequently limited, although there are a few outstanding exceptions. If local reputation is excellent, do not score this category. Generally, however, this type of hospital is poorly equipped or has serious problems because of efforts to keep costs low and profits high. Score −10 if local reputation is unacceptable.

Number of Beds

SCORE	TYPE OF HOSPITAL	SCORING GUIDE	REASON FOR SCORE
_____	Over 500 beds	20	Larger hospitals generally offer more services. Of the more than 3,000 hospitals with fewer than 100 beds, only a handful are medical-school-affiliated, less than 1 percent offer residency programs. Be aware that there are a few outstanding exceptions in this category and score accordingly.
_____	100 to 500 beds	15	
_____	Under 100 beds	5	

Judging Your Hospital (continued)

SCORE	TYPE OF HOSPITAL	SCORING GUIDE	REASON FOR SCORE

Location of Hospital in Relation to Your Home

_____	Within 20 miles	25	Location is important. If your local hospital does not seem adequate to provide you with the services you will need, you should ask your doctor to refer you to a specialist who is affiliated with a hospital which is better suited to your needs. However, weigh carefully your own need for the emotional support of having visits from friends and relatives and the added burden of having to travel long distances for your care. Generally, you can arrange to be evaluated by one of the specialists, who can then advise your doctor how to treat your case. The specialist is important in making the diagnosis and planning the treatment. Your local doctor and hospital can usually carry out the treatment plan successfully.
_____	Within 100 miles	15	
_____	Within 200 miles	5	

General Hospital Services

_____	Postoperative recovery room	5	20 percent of our hospitals do not have a room where the patient is monitored by specially trained personnel during the crucial first hours following surgery.
_____	Intensive care unit	5	Referred to as the ICU, the facility is designed to give seriously ill patients carefully monitored attention 24 hours a day.

Judging Your Hospital (continued)

SCORE	TYPE OF HOSPITAL	SCORING GUIDE	REASON FOR SCORE
_____	Pathology lab	10	Importance of adequate pathology services cannot be overstressed in cancer diagnosis and care.
_____	Diagnostic laboratories	10	Well-equipped and well-staffed diagnostic facilities are an important factor in good patient care.
_____	Pharmacy	5	Well-trained personnel with up-to-date knowledge of drugs, side effects, etc. contribute to overall quality of hospital.
_____	Blood bank	5	Careful, accurate, and rapid service by specially trained personnel around the clock is a must for a well-equipped hospital.
_____	X-ray equipment, radiation therapy such as cobalt, linear accelerator, radium implants	5	A great deal of expensive machinery used in cancer diagnosis and treatment is available only at sophisticated treatment centers.
_____	Radioactive scanning equipment	5	Newer diagnostic equipment
_____	CT scanner	5	Newer diagnostic equipment
_____	Brain-wave equipment (EEG)	5	Highly specialized testing equipment
_____	Tumor registry, tumor committee	10	Indicates cancer is being treated regularly, statistics are kept on treatment, and group discussions are held.

Judging Your Hospital (continued)

SCORE	TYPE OF HOSPITAL	SCORING GUIDE	REASON FOR SCORE
_____	Respiratory therapy	5	Requires trained personnel. Necessary in many basic treatments. Should be available on a 24-hour basis.
_____	Physical therapy	5	Sounds like peripheral service but is important aspect of rehabilitation.
_____	Social services	5	Necessary to provide help with financial aid, post-hospital care, housing, homemaker service, etc. A sign of a "caring" hospital attitude.
_____	Anesthesiologists	10	Use of anesthesiologists (M.D.s) in operating room, rather than anesthetists, is an important dimension of good hospital practice.
_____	Nursing staff	10	Numbers depend upon patients and beds. Some hospitals practice team nursing. Reputation for caring attitude and prompt attention will determine score.
_____	Physician staff	10	24-hour-a-day staffing is an absolute must.

This hospital scoring checklist is designed to allow you to check your hospital on its ability to deliver cancer care. It is not meant to be used to judge your hospital on its adequacy for emergency care, general surgery, etc.

Over 250—Excellent
Over 180—Very good
Over 130—Good
Over 100—Adequate
Under 100—Poor

which might be disturbing to some and comforting to others. Physicians, nurses, psychologists, and social workers often interview patients. Members of the medical staff other than the patient's physician may drop by to examine the patient's condition. Of course, the patient always has the option of refusing to be examined by or treated by anyone other than his own doctor (except in emergencies where quick decisions are essential). Some people object to being treated by anyone except their own personal physician. If you feel this way, it is important for you to understand how these hospitals operate. However, the care in research and teaching hospitals can be very attentive, the staff is very competent, and the patient can be assured that the latest and most up-to-date treatment is available.

If I go to a research or teaching hospital will I become a guinea pig for a cancer-research project?

Many people are frightened at the thought of being used in a research project without their consent. Rest assured that each research project must first be approved by the hospital's research committee (usually called the human investigations committee), which has strict guidelines it follows in evaluating whether or not the project can be carried out at that hospital. Moreover, each patient participating in the research project must sign a consent form which explains both the potential value and the possible risks.

What questions should I ask before consenting to becoming a part of a research project?

Good questions to ask include
- What is the purpose of the study?
- What does the study involve? What kinds of tests and treatments? (Find out what is done and how it is done.)
- What is likely to happen in my case with, or without, this new research treatment? (What may the cancer do and what may this treatment do?)
- What are other choices and their advantages and disadvantages? (Are there standard treatments for my case and how does the study compare with them?)
- How could the study affect my daily life?

- What side effects could I expect from the study? (There can also be side effects from standard treatments and from the disease itself.)
- How long will the study last? (Will it require an extra time commitment on my part?)
- Will I have to be hospitalized? If so, how often and for how long?
- Will I have any costs? Will any of the treatment be free?
- If I am harmed as a result of the research, what treatment would I be entitled to?
- What type of long-term follow-up care is part of the study?

What is the National Cancer Institute?

The National Cancer Institute (NCI) is the federal government's principal agency for research on cancer prevention, diagnosis, treatment, and rehabilitation and for dissemination of information for the control of cancer. The Institute is one of eleven research institutes and four divisions that form the National Institutes of Health, located in Bethesda, Maryland. As an agency of the Department of Health and Human Services, the NCI receives annual appropriations from Congress. These funds support cancer research in the Institute's Bethesda headquarters and in about 1,000 laboratories and medical centers throughout the United States. The director of the NCI is Vincent DeVita, M.D. The address is National Cancer Institute, National Institutes of Health, Bethesda, Maryland 20205-3100.

What is a comprehensive cancer center and what services does such a center offer?

There are twenty comprehensive cancer centers in the United States, so designated by the National Cancer Institute. They vary from centers which treat only cancer patients to centers in medical schools or in community hospitals. All of them were well known for their expertise either in cancer research or patient care or both before being designated as comprehensive cancer centers. The centers are devoted to the diagnosis and multidisciplinary treatment of cancer patients, to basic clinical and pharmacological research, and to the training of personnel in cancer diagnosis, treatment, and research. In addition, most have facilities for rehabilitation, social services, convalescent and intermediate care, home-care support, and patient follow-up. They are responsible for maintaining a cancer registry and for giving public information. They are specifically geared to treating cancer with the most up-to-date methods. The list of comprehensive cancer centers appears in Chapter 23.

Should I go to a comprehensive cancer center for diagnosis and treatment of cancer?

If one of the twenty NCI-designated comprehensive cancer centers is nearby, by all means take advantage of it. Use its expertise for your care, or have your case reviewed by the experts on its staff. This is where much of the new work on cancer is taking place. However, if you are not close to a comprehensive center, you can ask your doctor to refer you for evaluation by one of the specialists, who can then advise your doctor on your treatment. Sometimes, the doctor can make a telephone call and talk to someone who is treating your kind of cancer; this is especially important if you have a rare type of cancer which your doctor does not see very often. Remember that there are also qualified cancer specialists at local hospitals who are up-to-date on standard, proven treatments. You need to weigh carefully your own needs for having the emotional support of family and friends against the added burden of having to travel long distances for your cancer treatment and care.

Are all comprehensive cancer centers funded and designated by the National Cancer Institute?

You need to be aware that there is now a for-profit group called the Comprehensive Cancer Care Corporation which is opening comprehensive cancer centers around the country. These centers are not the same as the NCI-designated comprehensive cancer centers which have been described above. The for-profit centers are usually free-standing, not affiliated with medical schools and do not participate in research. They do however make available standard care, including chemotherapy and radiation therapy and have oncologists on their staffs. Don't forget that you are a consumer and you need to carefully evaluate where you are getting your care. If your center is not listed in Chapter 23 as a comprehensive cancer center, then it is not a comprehensive cancer center designated by the National Cancer Institute.

What are clinical and laboratory centers?

Clinical and laboratory centers are medical centers which have support from the National Cancer Institute for programs to investigate promising new methods of cancer treatment or for research programs. Some of the leading medical centers in the country are clinical or laboratory centers; clinical centers treat patients and can offer many of the same services as a comprehensive cancer center. A listing of these centers is in Chapter 23.

What are cancer clinical cooperative groups?

These groups, under the sponsorship of the National Cancer Institute, include more than 4,000 cancer research physicians at institutions throughout the country. Each clinical cooperative group specializes in a particular type of cancer and conducts controlled studies to determine the best possible treatment for patients with those diseases. The approaches may include chemotherapy, radiotherapy, immunotherapy, and surgery alone or in various combinations. These groups allow many patients from different parts of the country to be given the same treatments so as to compare the new therapy with standard methods.

Who pays for the treatment given to patients in clinical cooperative groups?

Most costs of medical treatment in clinical cooperative groups are borne by the patient, although medical insurance usually pays for the doctor's visit. Sometimes the drugs are paid for by the clinical cooperative group. Drugs not yet commercially available and extra tests not required in usual treatment may be provided free of charge. In some specialized treatments, all costs are paid for. In Chapter 23 you will find the name of the chairman of each clinical cooperative group and the phone number for contact. The address listed is not an indication of where these groups are located. It is simply the information center for the specific type of study group. Your doctor or you may contact that person for information on what clinical trials are available in your area. You can get information about physicians located in your area by calling the Cancer Information Service toll-free at 1-800-4-CANCER.

What is PDQ?

PDQ, which stands for Physician Data Query, is a computerized service of the National Cancer Institute to inform doctors of the latest and best treatments for cancer patients. It provides the latest information on the state-of-the-art treatment for each type and stage of cancer. It also gives information on more than 1,000 active treatment studies under way in the country, as well as a directory of 10,000 doctors who devote a major portion of their practice to treating cancer and 2,000 institutions that have organized programs for cancer. The doctor can "look up" the latest information by simply dialing up the database from a home, hospital, or office computer.

How can a cancer patient get the same kind of information that is available to physicians from PDQ?

Because the information is written in medical language and needs interpretation, the PDQ database itself is not available to the public. However, by calling the Cancer Information Service's 1-800-4-CANCER, a toll-free number, you can get the latest information on cancer treatment. Trained counselors use many information resources including PDQ to help patients. They also have many different kinds of materials that can be sent to callers, including information on the latest treatments, investigational studies, and the names of physicians who are caring for cancer patients.

How can someone be treated at the National Institutes of Health Clinical Center?

The National Cancer Institute conducts clinical research programs at the National Institute of Health Clinical Center in Bethesda, MD. This combined research laboratory and hospital is operated by the federal government as part of the National Institutes of Health just outside the District of Columbia. At full capacity it can accommodate about 500 carefully selected patients. It is not a diagnostic clinic, and it does not accept patients with conditions doctors have been unable to diagnose. The clinical center provides nursing and medical care without charge for patients who have been diagnosed as having the particular kind or stage of cancer being studied in its clinical research programs. It is principally interested in long-term conditions, many of which have no specific treatment.

The following steps should be followed by those interested in being admitted to the National Institutes of Health Clinical Center:

- Discuss the matter with your doctor. To determine if you can be considered, the doctor must call or write the Office of the Director, The Clinical Center, National Institutes of Health, Bethesda, MD 20205. (Telephone: 301-496-4891.) Your physician must furnish the center with a full medical report.
- The medical report is studied by medical scientists to determine whether your condition is of a kind presently under study at the clinical center. The clinical center will reply to your doctor, who, in turn, will notify you.
- If you are accepted, correspondence between the clinical center and the doctor, and sometimes with you, will settle details as to when and how you will be admitted. When you are discharged, a full report on the results of studies and on treatment given is sent to the referring doctor.

How can I tell a good from a bad hospital?

Some people judge a hospital by the food it serves. This is *not* a criterion for choosing a hospital. The checklist on pages 23–27 lists the services important for consideration. It will help you sort out the pros and cons of your local hospital. You'll be interested to know that there are about 7,000 hospitals in the United States. Of these, about 500 are medical-school-affiliated and another 1,500 have intern/residency teaching programs. Approximately 1,600 hospitals continue to lack minimum accreditation. In the middle is a group of average hospitals which offer care ranging from superior to substandard. However, in surveys done among hospital professionals, only between 25 and 50 hospitals in the country are categorized as superior.

Why is the care in some big-city public hospitals considered comparable to that in many nonprofit private hospitals?

It is mainly because many of the top medical students choose the big public hospitals for their internship and residency training. The students know that these hospitals tend to get the widest range of cases and that the interns and residents are given more responsibility than in private hospitals.

Why is a teaching hospital considered to be superior to a hospital which does not have an intern/residency program?

Simply because there are more professionals on the job—more doctors checking up on the competence of other doctors. You will be seen on regular daily "rounds" by your doctor and other interns and residents. Doctors who receive appointments to these hospitals are usually tops in their fields. Teaching hospitals attract the finest medical minds in the country. (However, some people are annoyed by being "poked at" by countless interns and residents. If you should find this to be the case, you have a perfect right to state that you wish to be seen only by your own doctor.)

Is size an important factor in considering a hospital?

In our listing, we have given greater weight to a hospital with 500 or more beds than we have to one with between 100 and 500 beds or one with less than 100 beds. This is a general rule of thumb. There are some excellent small hospitals. There are some poor large hospitals. Size is not all—but the number of patients with serious illnesses seen by the staff is an important factor. In a larger hospital, in the course of a week a doctor will probably treat as many patients with a specific illness as the small-hospital doctor will see in a year. Hospital death rates have been estimated to be 40 percent higher in less-than-100-bed hospitals than in larger hospitals. The overall capabilities of a large hospital are greater than those of a small one. People sometimes complain that large hospitals are impersonal. This can be true—but it can also vary from department to department, from floor to floor, and from person to person.

What if the doctor sends me to a hospital I don't approve of?

You do have a right to go to the hospital of your choice— and that is why, in choosing a doctor, an important consideration is his hospital affiliation. Most doctors have admitting privileges at more than one hospital. Therefore, if you have a specific request for a hospital, be sure to discuss this with your doctor.

What kinds of nurses are involved with taking care of me in the hospital?

There are many changes taking place in the nursing profession, and the field is becoming more specialized. It may be useful to understand what the functions of the various nurses are. In most hospitals, particularly the larger ones, you will find, in order of authority

- Director of nursing (responsible for the entire nursing staff)
- Nursing supervisor (in charge of major nursing areas)
- Head nurse (responsible for a particular floor)
- Floor nurses or staff nurses (handle specific nursing problems)
- Licensed practical nurses (LPNs) (assist staff nurses with patient care)
- Nursing assistants (handle routine patient needs)
- Aides (handle routine patient needs)

The first four in the list are generally registered nurses who have completed a nursing training program, possess an associate's, bachelor's or master's degree and are licensed by the state to practice nursing. These nurses have fundamental knowledge of most diseases and know how to observe and manage patients. They handle patient care which requires special knowledge such as giving out medication, adjusting medical devices (such as tubes, drains, respirators, etc.), changing intravenous bottles, giving injections, and recognizing problems which need a doctor's care. These nurses are skilled practitioners in nursing management and care and, in the cancer field especially, are very important members of the health-care team.

What are the duties of the licensed practical nurse?

The licensed practical nurse (LPN) is usually a graduate of a one-year course. Although the LPN has some medical knowledge, she is usually not as expert as the registered nurse (RN). An LPN must take a state examination to practice nursing, but because her formal training is not as extensive, she cannot do all the things an RN can do. Normally, the LPN takes a patient's temperature, pulse rate, and respiration rate, delivers medication which the patient takes by mouth, and helps the patient with personal needs.

What are the jobs of the nursing aides and nursing assistants?

Nursing aides and nursing assistants are usually trained by the hospital to take care of very routine patient needs. They usually do not have medical education or training, and they are not licensed. Their tasks include feeding patients who need help, helping patients get out of bed to go to the bathroom, helping patients move on and off bedpans, giving patients baths, and generally assisting patients to feel comfortable.

Is it true that hospitals seem to "shut down" on weekends and holidays?

Most hospitals, like many other businesses, seem to operate with a skeleton staff on weekends and holidays—so if you have any choice, and are not facing an emergency situation, be aware that it is wise to try avoid holidays. If you are being operated on, try to check into the hospital on a Monday or Tuesday so that your tests and your surgery can be done before the end of the week.

Do I have a right to see my hospital records?

Though many nurses and doctors are extremely secretive about hospital records, you do have a right to see yours. You may not be able to understand much of what is in it because it is written in medical shorthand. Usually a nurse or a doctor will be present so that you will not misunderstand or misinterpret the information.

Can I refuse to be examined by a medical student?

This is a right that is yours—but many a helpful diagnosis
has been made by a medical student who was doing his job
as painstakingly as only a novice will. Usually, it will be to
your advantage to allow the services of the soon-to-be doctor. Of course, if you are feeling very ill and find the poking
and probing troublesome, you have a perfect right to refuse
such an examination.

Am I obligated to sign consent forms?

Consent forms are necessary before the doctor can go ahead
with any procedure that entails any element of risk—surgery, anesthesia, spinal taps, etc. However, do not sign a
blank consent form. Do not let the doctor get away with an
explanation that he is not certain what the surgical procedure will entail and so is asking you to sign a consent form
to be filled in later. Your doctor has an obligation to inform
you of the risks and consequences of any procedure and to
state the specific procedure for which you are being asked
to give your consent. (Specifications for surgery should include the specific area to be operated on and the specific
procedure the surgeon expects to perform.) Do not sign any
form unless *all* your questions have been addressed.

How can I guard against medication errors in the hospital?

You should ask and know what medications your doctor has
prescribed for you, what they are designed to do, and what
they look like. If you have any question at all about a medication, ask the nurse to check the order book to make certain the doctor's orders have been followed or to check back
with the doctor in case he has made an error. Many a medical disaster has been averted by a patient who asks, "Is
this a new pill?" Be alert to what medications you are taking
and why they are being given.

chapter 3

Understanding What Cancer Is

What is cancer?

Cancer is a group of diseases in which there is irregular growth of abnormal cells.

How do normal cells and abnormal cells differ?

Normal cells grow in an orderly, controlled pattern. As normal cells wear out and die, new ones are produced. Just enough new cells grow to replace the old ones. Abnormal cells grow in an uncontrolled pattern; they never stop reproducing themselves, and soon there are many more of them than of the healthy cells in the tissue surrounding them.

Do all normal cells look alike?

No. Each normal cell has a specialized structure designed to do a particular job in a particular organ. For example, those cells which form the skin tend to be flat. The class of cells which make up the nerves are long and slender. Within each class, all normal cells are quite uniform in size and almost identical in shape. Each class of cells presents different arrangements when they join each other. For instance, glandular cells form circles which build upon each other like the stones lining a well. Skin cells stretch out in sheetlike layers row on row like a brick wall. These joined cells form tissues which arrange themselves in orderly pat-

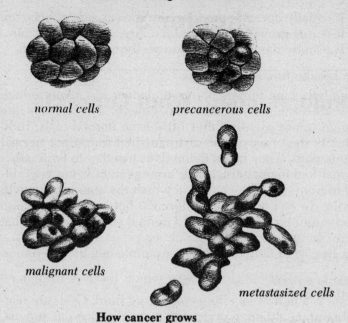

normal cells   *precancerous cells*

malignant cells

metastasized cells

How cancer grows

terns to form organs such as the breast, stomach, kidney, and so on.

Are all growths or tumors cancer?

No. A tumor can be either benign (noncancerous) or malignant (cancerous). The word *tumor* itself is usually defined as "an abnormal mass of new tissue, the growth of which exceeds and is uncoordinated with that of normal tissue." The characteristic of a tumor is cell division—growth—that serves no useful purpose.

What is a benign tumor?

A benign tumor is a growth that is not cancerous. It has four main characteristics:

- It has limited growth potential and does not usually grow rapidly. It does not destroy normal cells while it is growing.
- It remains localized—that is, it does not metastasize (spread to other places).

- It usually does not produce any serious side effects, unless it is growing in a confined area such as the brain.
- It usually has an orderly and well-organized growth.

Are benign tumors dangerous?

Usually benign tumors do not endanger life, even though they are examples of abnormal growth. The cells in the benign tumor usually differ little from normal cells; individually they may not be distinguished from their normal counterparts. They group themselves together to form rather normal-looking patterns; their arrangement is not very different from that of the tissue in which the abnormal growth begins. In fact, the chief difference between the makeup of a benign tumor and that of a normal structure is just that there are more cells in a tumor.

A lipoma or fatty tumor is an example of a benign tumor.

What is a cyst?

A cyst is a hollow swelling containing fluid. Cysts are usually benign, although cysts may form in cancerous tumors, either because the tumor is made up of tissue that secretes fluid or because the inside of the tumor breaks down and becomes fluid.

What is a polyp?

Polyps are growths in a mucous surface. They can occur in the nose, vocal cords, bladder, bowel, uterus, and other places where there is mucous membrane. Most polyps do not become malignant—but a small percentage are malignant from the start. Their removal is recommended by many doctors.

What do abnormal cells look like?

Abnormal or malignant cells vary in size and shape. They sometimes look almost like normal cells but most often are quite different-looking from the normal ones. The malignant cells do not organize themselves into normal patterns, although generally there is a tendency to reproduce the tissue in which they originate. For instance, skin-cancer cells tend to arrange themselves in the same sheetlike layers row on row as normal skin cells. But they do so imperfectly. Sometimes the cancer cells are so dissimilar from the normal structure that it is hard to identify the tissue from which the cancer started. The imperfection of the abnormal cell is the failure of the cancer cells to mature (or differentiate, as the physicians would say).

It has been said that cancer cells grow wild and uncontrolled. Is that true?

Not in the true sense of the terms. What the scientists are saying is that cancer cells are growing wild and uncontrolled in comparison with the normal cells around them. If a healthy normal cell is one that is slow-growing such as in the liver, then the cancerous liver cell is also slow-growing. There are also fast-growing and slow-growing tumors, which is why different tumors are treated with different kinds of drugs. The important fact is that the cancerous cells never stop reproducing and soon there are many more of them than of healthy cells in the tissue around them. Cancer cells do die, but their death rate is lower than their birth rate.

Why are malignant or cancerous cells so dangerous?

Mainly because they deprive normal cells of nourishment and space. In most types of cancer, the cells build up into a mass of cells that compresses, invades, and destroys surrounding tissues. This mass is often called a growth, a tumor, or a neoplasm (new growth).

Do benign tumors become cancerous or malignant tumors?

In most cases they do not. The tumor that begins as a benign tumor usually remains a benign tumor. However, there are lesions that are considered precancerous, such as a thickening of the lining of the mouth. These should be taken care of before malignancy occurs.

What is a malignant tumor?

A malignant tumor is made up of cancer cells. This tumor also has four main characteristics:

- It divides and keeps dividing relentlessly; it reproduces in excess of the tissue's or organ's normal needs; it has a higher rate of cell growth than the normal tissues from which the cells came.
- It assumes, to a varying degree, a different appearance from the cells from which it came; the cells fail to maintain the boundaries of the normal tissues and organs; the cells resemble immature rather than mature tissues; they are without specific structure and function.
- It loses, to a varying degree, the ability to perform the functions of the tissues from which it came; the cells either stop that function, function differently, or function incompletely.
- It has uncontrolled movement; it is capable of breaking away and spreading throughout the body; the tumor tends to invade and destroy distant areas by spreading away from the original site. This property varies from tumor to tumor.

Is it true that the more irregular the cells, the more malignant the cancer?

This is usually the case. As a general rule, the more abnormal (the doctors refer to it as undifferentiated) the cells look under the microscope, the more malignant the cancer. The greater the difference in their appearance from the normal cell, the more active the cancer is likely to be and the more uncontrollable its course. The term *differentiated* refers to malignant cells which resemble normal cells.

What is dysplasia?

Dysplasia refers to abnormal tissue development. It means that the cells or tissue are abnormal in their growth and organization for the location in which they are found. It does not mean necessarily that they are abnormal to the extent of being malignant, nor does it mean they have formed a tumor. Dysplasia occurs more often in tissues that "turn over" (or reproduce) frequently. Dysplasia may precede the development of some cancers by years or months. Not all dysplasia develops into cancer.

How many cells are in a cancerous tumor?

The number varies by the size of the tumor and the type of cell. First of all, you should understand that there is considerable variation in the size of cells making up the human body. The most numerous of the body cells are so small that it would take between 700 and 800 cells to cover the head of a pin. A 1-centimeter lump in the breast, which is a little larger than the size of a pea and is about the smallest lump which you can feel with your fingers, contains over a billion cells. This size tumor has undergone about thirty doublings since it first became an abnormal cell.

What is meant by doublings or by doubling time?

It is believed that cancer cells divide at a steady rate and the tumor steadily increases in size. One cell becomes two, two cells become four, four cells become eight. The body systematically continues the growth in this manner, with the number of cells doubling each time. The average length of time necessary for all the cells in a tumor to divide has been designated as the doubling time. With the passage of one doubling time, the number of cells in the mass is doubled and the weight of the mass is doubled. By the time a lump can be felt in the breast, for example, it has gone through at least thirty generations of doubling in size. The doubling time for breast cancer has been estimated to range from 6 to 540 days, depending upon the kind of cells and their rate of growth. That is why it is important that you see a doctor without delay as soon as you feel a lump.

Is it true that a two-step process is necessary for cancer to develop?

Scientists now believe that most cancer is caused in two steps, by two kinds of agents: initiators and promoters. Initiators start the damage to the cell, damage that can lead to cancer. Cigarette smoking, x-rays, and certain chemicals are considered initiators. Promoters stimulate the development of cancer but usually do not cause cancer. They change the cells already damaged by the initiator from normal cells to cancerous cells. Research has shown that alcohol promotes the development of cancer in the mouth, throat, and possibly liver, when combined with an initiator such as smoking. Alcohol is an example of a classic promoter: It alone does not cause cancer, but it is clearly associated with the development of cancer. Many chemicals in the environment can act as promoters. Phenobarbital, for example, is a strong promoter of cancer in liver cells. Cigarette tars contain not only carcinogens that initiate cells but also promoters that act on lung tissue. Even some mechanical processes, such as abrasions or other wounds, can act as promoters.

What are oncogenes?

Oncogenes, which are genes that can cause cancer, have become a hot topic in cancer research. The word comes from the Greek term *onco*, meaning tumor. Most cancer researchers believe that somehow, usually over a period of years, cancer-causing agents (carcinogens) repeatedly brought into the body, finally damage a critical piece of a cell's genetic code. The damage causes the cell to send out abnormal messages related to some aspect of cell growth. As new cells spring from old, the misled cell leads an onslaught of others that result in runaway growth. The altered ones—oncogenes—take charge. More than twenty cancer genes have been identified in experiments in animals or in normal cells grown in the laboratory.

How do oncogenes work?

The oncogenes start dominating the way the cells behave. They disrupt the usual schedule and direct the cell to continue to grow. Most researchers believe that at least two cancer genes must be created, by random error, before the process starts. Although the role of each cancer gene is not yet understood, scientists believe that the cancerous cell growth is set off through a series of steps within the cell. Some cancer genes apparently instruct the cell to overproduce a growth-factor protein or mistakenly produce an abnormal growth factor. Others may tell the cell to ignore signals to stop growing, perhaps by leaving growth-factor receptor switches on at various points along the cell's surface.

Where have oncogenes been found?

Scientists have found versions of oncogenes in several kinds of human cancer, including those of the breast, lung, bladder, and bowel. In addition, DNA sequences nearly identical to oncogenes have been discovered in normal tissue cells throughout the animal kingdom, including those of man. Researchers think that such "proto-oncogenes" have existed throughout evolution and play a useful role in normal cell division. What the researchers are investigating is how these seemingly harmless genes become altered and turned into cancer genes. They have found that by replacing the genetic "on-off" switch of one gene, called *c-myc*, they are able to control when and in what tissues it causes tumors in mice. This is a critical breakthrough in learning precisely how this gene and perhaps other cancer genes function. The gene *c-myc* plays a role in the human cancer known as Burkitt's lymphoma. Other researchers working with another strain of oncogene, the *ras* family of oncogenes, have found a single changed amino acid in the protein product as the site for an altered gene product which they feel is somehow critical in the development of cancer.

Can viruses cause cancer?

Researchers believe there is some relationship between viruses and cancers of the liver and cervix, Burkitt's lymphoma, nasopharyngeal cancer, and adult T-cell leukemia. However, although it is believed that these cancers may be stimulated by viruses, there is no evidence that they spread like typical viruses. Some other factor appears to be necessary to cause the disease to spread.

What is the HTLV virus that is in the news?

There are three HTLV viruses—HTLV-I, HTLV-II, and HTLV-III—all belonging to a family of retroviruses that have been identified in human tissues. The first, called human T-cell lymphotropic virus I, has been implicated in adult T-cell leukemia. It has infected many people in Japan, the Caribbean, South and Central America, Africa, and the southwestern United States. It is estimated that one of every hundred people infected with the virus will develop leukemia. HTLV-II has been isolated from a patient with hairy-cell leukemia, but the virus has not yet been linked to the cause of this disease. A major discovery is that HTLV-III is the cause of acquired immune deficiency syndrome (AIDS). Although there are some similarities between HTLV-III and the other HTLV viruses, researchers have concluded that the AIDS virus did not arise through a small change in known viruses but, rather, is a completely new virus. There is more information on AIDS in Chapter 9.

What is the HBLV virus?

HBLV stands for human B-lymphotropic virus, believed to be the first new human herpes virus to be found in about 20 years. It was discovered by scientists at the National Cancer Institute in patients who had cancers and other abnormalities in cells of their immune systems. It infects human immune defense cells called B-lymphocytes and apparently no other cells, which makes it different from other known herpes viruses. B-lymphocytes are the immune defense cells responsible for producing protective antibodies. However, the scientists note that the presence of a virus in a patient's tissues does not prove the virus caused the disease. There is no evidence of a link between the new HBLV virus and AIDS.

Is cancer one disease?

That question is still being studied. Some scientists believe that cancer may be one disease, but others feel it is many diseases that share some basic mechanism to start off. There are over 100 kinds of cancer, and each kind and site has its own distinguishing characteristics. Depending upon the location of the cancer in the body, the cause, symptoms, growth, kind of treatment, response to treatment, and possibility of cure are different. Cancer may behave very differently in different people. Generally, malignant tumors are divided into five main classifications, with many subdivisions in each group.

What are the five classifications of cancer?

The five classifications are as follows:

- *Carcinomas*: These are the most common cancers. The tumors arise from tissues which cover a surface or line internal organs and passageways of the body (epithelial tissue). Skin, intestinal, uterine, and lung cancers are all carcinomas. There are several different kinds of carcinomas, including squamous cell, basal cell, transitional cell, and glandular epithelial.
- *Sarcomas*: These tumors arise in the connective tissue and muscles. They attack the bone, muscle, cartilage, and lymph system. Types of sarcoma include fibrosarcoma, liposarcoma, myosarcoma, chondrosarcoma, and osteosarcoma.
- *Myelomas*: These tumors arise in the plasma cells which are in the bone marrow. The plasma cells produce some of the protein that circulates in the blood.
- *Lymphomas*: These tumors arise in the cells of the lymph system. Lymph is a waterlike fluid that drains from all the tissues of the body through clusters of small glands called nodes. The nodes are the size and shape of lima beans and are found in many places in the body, such as the neck, the groin, the armpits, and the spleen. These glands swell up when bacteria or tumor cells drain into them or when the cells of which they are composed become malignant. The lymph system normally acts as a filter of impurities in the body. Hodgkin's disease, for example, is a lymphoma.
- *Leukemia*: This is a cancer of the blood-forming tissues (bone marrow, lymph nodes, and spleen). It is characterized by the overproduction of white blood cells.

What does the doctor mean when he says I have a solid tumor?

A solid tumor means a tumor such as carcinoma and sarcoma which forms a mass of growth.

What is a disseminated tumor?

A disseminated tumor means a growth that is not confined to one area of the body; it has spread or has started to spread.

Major Classifications of Cancer

MEDICAL TERM	DEFINITION
Carcinoma	Originates from tissues that cover a surface or line a cavity of the body (epithelial tissue). This is the most common type of cancer.
Sarcoma	Originates from tissues which connect, support, or surround other tissues and organs. Can be either soft tissue or bone sarcomas.
Myeloma	Originates in the bone marrow in the blood cells that manufacture antibodies.
Lymphoma	Originates in lymph system—the circulatory network of vessels, spaces, and nodes carrying lymph, the almost colorless fluid that bathes the body's cells.
Leukemia	Involves the blood-forming tissues and blood cells.

Descriptions of behavior

Localized	Found only in the original or primary site; not spread to other parts of body.
Invasive	Cancer cells go beyond surface of tissues, invade tissues below but stay as one mass. A type of localized cancer.
Metastatic	Clumps of cells break off from original mass. Carried by lymphatic vessels or bloodstream to distant part of body. May also spread directly to another part of body.

What is the meaning of the term *in situ*?

This term is used to describe a noninvasive cancer. One of the most constant characteristics of cancer is the invasion of healthy tissues bordering the tumor. However, there appears to be a brief period before the invasion begins. Such growths are termed *in situ*, and the results of their removal are more positive than those for cancers which have already begun to invade neighboring tissues. The term also applies to another group of tumors—usually found on surfaces—which have other characteristics of malignancy but in which normal cells may be completely replaced by tumor cells before there is evidence of invasion of surrounding tissues.

What is meant by the term *regression*?

Regression indicates that the tumor is getting smaller. This does not necessarily mean that the tumor has gone away, but if a tumor regresses far enough, it could eventually disappear altogether.

What is meant by the term *remission*?

Remission can be partial or complete. If it is complete, it means that all symptoms and signs of the disease are gone, although cancer cells may remain in the body. The patient does not feel any of the former symptoms, and the doctors cannot find clinical signs of the tumor. A partial remission means that some of the signs and symptoms are gone.

Is a remission a cure?

A remission may or may not be a cure. Sometimes the disease can be in remission for anywhere from weeks to years, while undetected tumor cells in the body remain inactive. The cancer cells may begin to grow again until once more they produce symptoms.

Is cancer ever cured?

Yes. The term *cure* is used only after a patient's disease has been in remission for a long enough time to indicate that the cancer probably has been completely destroyed. Cure means that the treatment is successful and that all the cancer cells have been removed or destroyed. In terms of symptoms and test results, cure is almost the same as remission. For many kinds of cancer, 5 years of remission is considered a cure. This is because if cancer has spread to other areas it will usually become apparent and begin to cause problems within the 5-year period. The length of remission necessary for cure differs for various kinds of cancer. In some kinds of skin cancer, for example, a person is considered cured as soon as the spot of cancer is removed. On the other hand, certain tumors are not considered cured until 8 or 10 years have passed.

What is meant by the term *high risk*?

Risks in medical terms are arrived at by looking at the various characteristics of a group of people and by comparing that to how often something occurs. Being at "high risk" means that your chances of getting the disease are somewhat greater than those of the general population, but it certainly does *not* mean you will definitely get the disease.

What does the doctor mean when he says the cancer is localized?

When cancer is localized, it is found only in the original or primary site; it has not spread, or metastasized, to another part of the body.

What is invasive cancer?

Invasive cancer is when some of the cancer cells go beyond the surface of the tissues and "invade" the tissues around them. After invading, the cancer continues to grow, though for a time the cancer cells may remain as one mass. Sometimes the mass can be seen by the naked eye. As long as all the living cancer cells remain where the disease started, the cancer is still said to be localized.

Do all cancers spread the same way?

No. Cancer cells spread in several ways. Some cancers, like certain skin cancers, simply keep growing in the same location, becoming bigger and bigger until they invade normal neighboring tissue and destroy it. Other cancers keep growing in the original site but also spread, through the bloodstream and lymphatic system, to distant parts of the body.

What does the doctor mean when he says the cancer is about 2 centimeters in size?

Perhaps it will help if you can visualize the size of the cancer by comparing it with objects you know. For instance, a pea is slightly smaller than a centimeter; a marble or a dime is slightly larger than a centimeter. A cherry or a nickel would be about 2 centimeters. A ping-pong ball and a half dollar would be about 3 centimeters. A golf ball or a silver dollar would about equal 4 centimeters. A hen's egg would be about 5 centimeters; a baseball, about 7 centimeters; and a grapefruit, about 10 or 12 centimeters.

The doctor said my cancer has metastasized. What does that mean?

The process by which cancer spreads from where it began (that is, from the primary tumor) to distant parts of the body is called metastasis. Tiny clumps of cells break off from the tumor and are carried in the lymphatic vessels or the blood-stream to a distant part of the body. These "seeds" from the original cancer start growing in the new place. The new tumor is said to have metastasized to the new site, and such a tumor is often referred to as a metastatic tumor. The plural of *metastasis* is *metastases*. Sometimes you will hear the word *mets*, a shorthand term for *metastases*.

Where does cancer usually spread to?

Different types of cancer have different tendencies to spread to certain organs. Breast cancer, for instance, generally spreads or metastasizes from the breast (primary site) to four places in the body: liver, bone, lung, and brain. More rarely, it can spread to the spinal cord, to distant lymph nodes, and to other places such as the face, lips, urological and genital areas, and alimentary tract. The identification of metastases is the most decisive factor in the choice of treatment and the success of the treatment.

When a tumor metastasizes or spreads, is it called by the name of the organ to which it has spread?

No. If the original tumor is in the breast and it has spread to the bone, it is not then bone cancer. It is breast cancer in the bones. The type of cancer cells found in the bones will be the same type as the cancer cells found in the breast. These cells will grow, reproduce, and behave according to the pattern of metastatic breast cancer (breast cancer which has spread into other areas) and not like bone cancer. Because of this fact, metastatic cancer of any kind is generally treated in the way the original cancer responds best. In other words, cancer that starts in the breast and spreads to the bones is not treated the same way that cancer which starts in the bones would be treated, but is treated like breast cancer.

We hear so much about cancer these days—is it a new disease?

No. Cancer is more than a million years old. Evidence of cancer has been found in skeletons of prehistoric animals and in Etruscan, Peruvian, and Egyptian mummies. The reason you hear more about it today is that it is a general disease of older people, and as people live longer (since we have cured many of the ailments which used to cause people to die younger), more people are getting cancer.

At what age do persons usually get cancer?

Cancer is predominantly a disease of middle and old age. In the United States, 66 percent of cancer in men and 63 percent of cancer in women is diagnosed at age 55 or over. Persons at about the age of 70 account for a higher number of cases than any other age group. Overall, in new cases of cancer, men and women account for about the same number.

Don't young children sometimes get cancer?

Cancer is quite rare in children and in young adults. However, for children under 15, cancer is the second leading cause of death, accounting for one out of twenty-eight deaths. Leukemia is the most common form of childhood cancer, followed by tumors of the central nervous system.

What does the word *oncology* mean?

Oncology is from the Greek word *onkos*, meaning "bulk" or "mass," and refers to the study and treatment of a large variety of tumors. The doctors who specialize in cancer treatment are called oncologists. There are surgical oncologists, medical oncologists, radiation therapists, pediatric oncologists, and gynecological oncologists.

What is chrono-oncology?

Chrono-oncology is the study of ways in which time-oriented body rhythms affect the development, diagnosis, and treatment of cancer. According to experts, healthy tissue cells have a daily rhythm of division and activity; some cancer cells—but probably not all—also seem to have a pattern. Research seems to indicate that it might be possible to attack cancer cells with larger-than-usual doses of chemotherapy during the time of day when normal tissues most likely to be affected are most active. Research in chrono-oncology is being conducted at the University of Minnesota Medical Center and at the University of Wisconsin's McArdle Laboratory for Cancer Research.

Does cancer run in families?

Cancer is a common disease, and some "clustering" of cases in families will occur by chance alone. However, there is some limited information which suggests that there is some increased family risk of developing cancer of the same site for cancers of the female breast, stomach, large intestine, endometrium, prostate, lung, and possibly ovary. It is known, for example, that a woman whose mother and/or sisters have had breast cancer is at a risk approximately two times higher than average. Brain tumors and sarcomas also seem to occur more frequently than expected in brothers and sisters of children with these tumors. When an identical twin has childhood leukemia, the probability that the other twin will develop the disease within 2 years of the date of diagnosis of the first twin is about one in five, far greater than the rate for the general population. A rare cancer of the eye, bilateral retinoblastoma, also seems to run in families. The chances that a patient cured of this kind of cancer will have a child with it are high. Scientists still do not know whether family clustering of cancer cases is due to inherited characteristics or to other factors, such as diet or occupation, which may continue unchanged from one generation to the next.

Is a cancer patient likely to develop a second cancer?

Persons with cancers of the skin, mouth, colon, and rectum run an increased risk of a second cancer in the same organ. Patients with cancers of the breast, ovary, and, perhaps, lung run a slightly higher risk of developing the disease in the paired organ. There is some evidence that tumors of certain different sites often occur together. Such combinations include colon and breast, colon and endometrium, uterine cervix and rectum, and combinations of sites in the digestive tract, respiratory system, and female reproductive organs.

Is there a cancer "smell"?

Not as such. There are some open wounds which do have an odor, whether the person has cancer or some other disease. It is important, if the patient has such a wound, to change the dressing often and to dispose of the dressing when it is changed.

Can a person "catch" cancer?

There is no indication that cancer can be considered contagious in the popular sense of the word. You should not be afraid that you will "catch" cancer. People who care for cancer patients on a daily basis do not have a higher incidence of cancer than the general population. There is no evidence to suggest that living in the same household with a cancer patient over a long period of time, sharing his or her possessions, kissing, or having intercourse with a cancer patient, increases your chances of getting cancer.

Are there any basic warning signs of cancer?

There are seven basic symptoms of cancer as emphasized by the American Cancer Society:
  • Unusual bleeding or discharge
  • A lump that does not go away
  • A sore that does not heal within two weeks
  • Change in bowel or bladder habits
  • Persistent hoarseness or cough
  • Indigestion or difficulty in swallowing
  • Change in a wart or mole
Any of these symptoms signal you to see a doctor. They might mean you have cancer, but in most cases the doctor will find you do not. The most important thing is that the symptoms should be checked out by a doctor, for only a doctor can make a definite diagnosis.

Can I have cancer without any of these symptoms?

It is possible. But the symptoms seem so trivial to most people that they may be ignored. For example, coughs are so common that we do not get alarmed when we have one. Usually you can tell yourself that you have been smoking too much or blame your sinuses or say that everybody is coughing at the office. However, coughing can also be the first visible sign of lung cancer. Irregular vaginal bleeding can be due to a whole list of causes, which can lull you into not bothering to see a doctor. But irregular vaginal bleeding can also be the first sign of cancer of the uterus. What all this means is that any suspicious symptom that persists longer than two weeks should be investigated by a qualified physician.

What does the term *staging* mean?

Staging is the process doctors go through to tell how much cancer there is in the body and where it is located. It is necessary for the doctor to have this information to plan your treatment. Staging is also a way for doctors to communicate with each other about your specific case.

Why is staging needed?

The doctor needs to determine the amount of cancer in your body in order to give you the right treatment for your specific kind. The treatment for breast cancer at one stage of the disease, for example, is different from what it is at another stage. Your doctor also needs to anticipate the course your disease is likely to take. Staging also makes it possible to compare the results of the different treatments being used by different physicians in different parts of this country and around the world.

What is the doctor looking for when he stages cancer?

The doctor wants to know basic information about the original (primary) tumor—what size and type it is, where it is in the body, whether or not it has spread to other areas around the original site, and whether or not it has spread to other parts of the body away from the original site.

Are the answers to these questions important?

The answers to these preliminary questions are vital. Tumors must be staged at the beginning of the diagnosis to the fullest extent possible in order to give you the most effective treatment. For example, if the doctor finds that the cancer which began in your lung has already spread to other parts of your body, he may decide to treat you with chemotherapy and radiation rather than surgery, since an operation might offer little or no chance of cure for you and could seriously weaken your system.

How does the doctor decide on the stage of the disease?

There are four types of evidence used for classifying the extent of disease at different sites and at different time periods.

- *Clinical-diagnostic staging*: This is determining how much cancer there is by what the doctor can see and feel by any means other than looking at cells under the microscope. This includes examination of the tumor by x-rays and tests.
- *Surgical-evaluative staging*: This term is used to describe the extent of the disease as known after a major surgical exploration or biopsy or both.
- *Postsurgical treatment—pathologic staging*: This is determining the stage of the disease by examining the tumor directly, looking at cells under the microscope.
- *Retreatment staging:* This is determining the extent of the disease when additional or new treatments are being given for the same disease.

What do the letters TNM stand for in the TNM classification system?

Cancer is sometimes classified by the letters TNM.

T, plus the numbers 1 through 4, stands for the primary tumor. This is used to describe the size and/or level of invasion. The higher the number, the larger the size of the tumor and/or the depth or amount of involvement in the local area of the tumor. TX means the tumor cannot be assessed. T0 means there is no evidence of primary tumor. TIS means carcinoma in situ.

N, plus the numbers 1 through 4, indicates whether or not there is evidence that the tumor has spread to the regional lymph nodes, the size of the nodes involved, and the number of nodes involved. NX means the regional lymph nodes cannot be assessed clinically. N0 means regional lymph nodes are not demonstrably abnormal.

M, with a zero or plus sign, indicates the absence or presence of distant metastases (cancer which has spread to other parts of the body). A letter is sometimes added to the M to show the other areas involved. P, for instance, would indicate "pulmonary"—that the cancer has spread to the lungs. MX means the metastasis is not assessed. M0 means there are no known distant metastases.

Do these letters and numbers mean the same thing for every kind of cancer?

Each tumor type has its own classification system. Some sites of cancer do not as yet have an agreed-upon classification and staging. Some types of cancer, such as lymphomas, use a different system from the one just described.

A T1 in lung cancer and in breast cancer means about the same, although a T1 breast tumor is less than or equal to 2 centimeters in size and a T1 lung tumor is less than or equal to 3 centimeters in size. Also, the treatment for the two types of cancer would be different. The variation depends upon what the doctors know about each kind of tumor, how it spreads, what treatments are most effective at each stage, and what the prognosis is.

What does it mean when the doctor says I have Stage I disease?

This means your disease is curable in the highest degree. Staging numbers were originally used by doctors to indicate how far the disease had advanced—Stage I being the most curable, Stage IV the least curable. Staging is still used to define cancers, but more refined designations include the T, N, and M categories. Many hundreds of doctors and many national and international committees are working at trying to standardize cancer language so it can be interpreted accurately by all doctors.

What are examples of how to interpret the letter designations?

Here are a few examples of how to interpret a series of letters when you see them on your reports or when they are used as a reference by the doctor.

- *Stage I, T1, N0, M0.* This would tell you that clinical examination reveals a mass or tumor limited to the organ where it appears. The tumor is operable, with only local involvement. There is no nodal spread or signs of metastases.

- *Stage II, T2, N1, M0*: This indicates that there is evidence of local spread into surrounding tissue. The tumor is operable, but because of its location and size, there is uncertainty as to completeness of removal. There is evidence that there is spread to the lymph nodes but no signs of metastases.

Most parts of the body which are commonly affected by cancer have their own sets of designations, although some sites have not yet been classified by the medical profession. The T classifications are designed to pinpoint the size and location by individual area. The N (node) and M (metastases) designations follow a fairly standard pattern. Because many new advances in diagnosis have been made in the past few years, many of the classifications are in the process of evolving and new, changing criteria are being used. The material in this book, both in this chapter and in other parts of the book dealing with specific parts of the body, is meant to act as a guide to you in better understanding your disease. You can ask your doctor for further explanations, if the information is not detailed enough.

chapter 4

Diagnostic Tests

Accurate diagnosis depends upon a series of diagnostic tests. Inform yourself about tests being ordered. Make certain that all necessary diagnostic testing is done before any treatment begins. Diagnostic findings will be the basis for future treatment, and if diagnosis is not complete or is uncertain, your treatment may be inappropriate or less than satisfactory.

Questions You Should Ask Your Doctor When He Orders Tests

- What is the test for?
- What will the procedure be like?
- What will you learn from the test?
- Why is it important for me to have the test?
- Will I need to be hospitalized for the test? For how long?
- Can it be done on an outpatient basis instead? Why not?
- How much will the test cost?
- What risks are there in doing the testing?
- When will we get the results of the test?
- What decisions will I have to make if the test is positive?

Questions You Need to Ask Yourself When You Get Your Diagnosis and Before You Make Appointments for Surgery or Other Treatment

- Is this the doctor I want to handle my case?
- Am I comfortable with him?
- Is he someone who understands how I feel and is sensitive to my needs?
- Do I have enough information about my case to make a judgment?
- Who do I want with me when I receive my diagnosis?
- Should I have a second opinion?
- Should I go to a large medical center for more diagnostic work or for my treatment?
- Which hospital will I go to for my surgery and treatment?
- Have I had the appropriate tests to see if the cancer has spread before surgery is done?

Questions to Think About When You Are Facing a Diagnosis of Cancer

QUESTION	REMARKS
Do I want to know exactly what plans the doctor has for my treatment and what alternative treatments there might be for my type of cancer?	Many people want to participate in the decisions about the treatment of their illness. Knowledge about the treatment plan is important to you if you want to be a part of the decision of how and where you will receive treatment.
Do I want to ask the doctor for a second pathologist to do an independent report?	The pathology report is the basis on which all future decisions will be made. You should think about talking with your doctor about how the pathology report was done, whether he has talked with the pathologist, whether or not there is any question or doubt about the diagnosis. If there is, ask to have the pathology checked by the laboratory of a large hospital or medical center.

Questions to Think About When You Are Facing a Diagnosis of Cancer

QUESTION	REMARKS
Do I want to know specifically what kind of cancer I have and the stage it is in?	Some people do. They like to have all the facts so they can do research at the medical library to find out what treatments are being offered. Others do not. However, if you have a rare type of cancer, you should know it, because you need to decide whether you want to go to one of the cancer centers or medical schools specializing in your type of disease for consultation or treatment. Or you should at least ask your doctor to have a phone consultation with a physician doing research in the area.
Do I want my doctor to consult with the nearest cancer center or cooperative group about my case? Do I want to make some phone calls myself?	There are clinical cooperative groups across the country specializing in treating particular types of cancer. Controlled studies are being conducted to determine the best possible treatments. Your doctor needs the latest information to give you the best possible treatment.
Do I want to go to a cancer center or medical school for my treatment?	You need to weigh this decision most carefully. The cancer centers and other hospitals specializing in cancer treatment have on their staffs doctors who are especially trained in the various cancer disciplines. In the course of a week, they will probably be treating more patients with your illness than many local doctors see in a year. On the other hand, the practical question of geography and your emotional energy will have to be considered.

What are the kinds of tests used to help detect cancer?

The tests used to detect cancer depend upon the kind of cancer and the degree to which it has spread. They fall into the following categories:

- Clinical history and physical examination, including routine blood and urine analyses, heart exams, and chest x-ray

- X-ray examinations
- Optical instruments (endoscopy)
- Examination of sloughed-off cells (cytology)
- Radioactive scans
- Ultrasound
- CT scans (also called CAT or ACTA scans)
- MRI (magnetic resonance imaging)
- Monoclonal antibodies
- Biopsies

Do doctors do too many diagnostic tests?

Sometimes, but in the area of cancer, it seems that the problem is that too *few* diagnostic tests are done before operating rather than too many. Laboratory tests are a vital part of any diagnostic workup, but especially so in the treatment of cancer. It is of major importance for the doctor to determine if the cancer has spread to other areas from the primary site of the growth. If it has already spread from the primary site, in some cases an operation may not be advisable. Instead chemotherapy or radiation treatment may be used. The treatment for cancer which has spread, therefore, is different from the treatment for cancer which is located only in the primary site. A good, thorough workup is vital before any surgery at all is done for cancer.

Are the risks great in waiting to do the surgery while spending time to do the diagnostic tests?

There is very little conclusive evidence to show that there is harm in delaying a short time (such as two weeks) while you are having the diagnostic tests. Occasionally, of course, rapid treatment is necessary for some specific problems of cancer patients. It is also harmful to delay seeing the doctor if you have suspicious symptoms such as a lump in your breast or blood in your stool.

What are some of the things the doctor should tell me about the tests he is going to do or going to order?

The doctor should tell you what the test is for, what the procedure will be like, what he feels he will learn from the test, why it is important in light of your symptoms, what the risk of the test is, whether you need to be hospitalized, how much it will cost to do the test, and when you can get the results. If the doctor does not offer this information, ask for it.

What kind of risks are there in the tests done for cancer?

The risks depend upon the test and on the condition of the person on whom the test is being done. Certainly the more simple ones, such as blood counts, involve little or no risk. X-rays which involve small amounts of radiation are low-risk tests. However, some of the x-rays, as well as some of the procedures, do involve quite a bit of risk. Risks are discussed in this chapter, along with the procedures. You should ask the doctor to discuss the risk versus the benefit of the tests he recommends. Generally in the area of cancer, the benefits of the tests are worth the risks.

What is the best place to go for laboratory tests?

In general, the most reliable laboratories are in the hospitals. However, there are many independent labs (independent of doctors' offices or hospitals) which also do an excellent job. Many small independent laboratories do so few of some tests that the results may be questionable. The results are only as accurate as the person or laboratory doing them.

Is it all right for me to ask for information about testing, test results, and other procedures?

It certainly is. You are entitled to all information that the doctor has about your case.

How long does it take to establish a diagnosis?

Ask your doctor about the time it will take. It will depend upon several factors—and the slightest delay will seem like an eternity because you will be living with the fear of the unknown. A full evaluation can take from several days to several weeks—or may even have to be postponed because a decision cannot be made for any of a number of reasons. Don't be in a rush for that final diagnosis. Allow time for as many diagnostic procedures, additional consultations, and reviews as you can. This is the point in your treatment that is most important to you—because what happens at this point sets the stage for determining much of the future course of your disease.

It is at this point that you must evaluate the following:

- Is this the doctor I want to handle my case?
- Do I have enough information about my case to make a judgment?
- Am I comfortable with the doctor?
- Is he someone who understands how I feel and is sensitive to my needs?
- Whom do I want with me when I receive my diagnosis?
- Should I have a second opinion?
- Should I go to one of the large medical centers for more complete diagnosis and treatment?
- What hospital will I go to for my surgery and treatment?

Won't my doctor be offended if I ask for another opinion?

If he is, you should find yourself another doctor. The important thing to remember is that most doctors *welcome* a second opinion. Because the public has held doctors in reverence for so long, many people think that the doctor will be upset if they ask for a second opinion. But *a second opinion does not mean you are questioning your doctor's competence*. If you have cancer, a decision about how you proceed with treatment is probably the most important decision you will make in your life. You need the best advice you can get before proceeding with a course of treatment. You don't hesitate to check out various makes and models of cars when you are making a decision about buying one. Certainly you should not hesitate to check out all the possible angles when making a decision about your health.

Can I do this tactfully?

Yes. Often it is easier if you ask your husband, wife, sister, or whoever usually accompanies you to help you with this. He or she can simply explain to your doctor that before going any further you would like to have a confirming opinion. This is *not* an unusual or unreasonable request. It is a very *necessary* step for you to take. The doctor may explain that the x-rays and tests are conclusive as far as he is concerned. Don't let that put you off or pressure you to agree to go along with his treatment. A second opinion will strengthen his conclusions and set your mind at ease.

Who will recommend a specialist to me?

Usually your primary doctor will make the recommendation. Sometimes he will give you more than one name. You should ask questions about the specialist's credentials, such as:

- Why do you recommend this particular doctor?
- Is he a specialist in the operation (or field)? How often does he perform this particular operation (or service)?
- Is he board-certified?
- Is he on the staff of an accredited hospital?

There are some competent doctors who are not board-certified, but your doctor should be able to tell you why he has chosen the specific specialists he is recommending.

What do I tell the doctor who is doing the consulting?

Sometimes the doctor who refers you will make the appointment. If you are calling yourself, explain that you have already had a diagnosis and are coming to him for a consultation. Don't make the mistake of trying to let him think you haven't been to another doctor. Using him on a consulting basis means that you will get a straight answer, since he has nothing to gain from recommending one treatment over another.

How do I go about finding the right doctor for a second opinion?

- You can ask your own doctor to suggest the name of someone to see for a second opinion.
- You can make the appointment yourself, or you can ask the doctor to make the appointment for you.
- You should always discuss your plans for consultation with your doctor. He has your original x-rays and tests, which the other doctor will need in his deliberation. If your doctor is uncooperative, then you have other decisions to make about continuing your relationship with him.
- You can call the nearest cancer center (many of them

are affiliated with the 1-800-4-CANCER number) and
ask for names of doctors who are specialists in your kind
of cancer. If there isn't a cancer center close to you, you
can call the toll-free 1-800-4-CANCER and ask for names
of physicians in your area.
- You can call your nearest medical school and ask for
  suggestions.
- You can call the nearest unit of the American Cancer
  Society or state or local medical society.
- You can check the Directory of Medical Specialists at
  your library and call the specialist directly.
- You can check the Directory of Medical Specialists, get
  the names of two or three top-notch doctors in the area,
  and ask your doctor to suggest which one he thinks you
  should see.

**Is a medical school's outpatient clinic a good place to go
for a second opinion?**

Yes. This is probably one of the better places to turn for a
second opinion. Physicians who practice there are on the
faculty of the medical school and are usually using the latest
methods of treatment. Because most outpatient clinics are
divided into specialties, this is where some of the top specialists in the country are practicing. You can contact the
clinic by calling the medical school and explaining that you
are interested in contacting a doctor at the clinic who specializes in the area of your specific problem. Don't be afraid
to explain that you want to get a second opinion and what
your experience has been to date. Each clinic, of course,
has its own setup—but most have appointment secretaries
who are very knowledgeable about the clinic and the doctors in their service and will be most helpful in making
arrangements for a consultation.

What will such a consultation cost?

You will be amazed to find that some of the finest physicians
in the country charge no more—and sometimes less—than
doctors with far less experience and expertise. Part of the
reason is that medical-school-faculty clinic physicians are
often salaried and their fees returned to the medical school.

Does such a consultation mean I have to go to that institution for my treatment?

No. You have free choice in this matter—and the decision should be yours. Sometimes people shy away from getting expert advice from doctors at a large medical center because they feel this will mean that they will have to return to the medical center for their treatments. However, this is not the case. Many medical and cancer centers diagnose and recommend treatment for patients to be followed by doctors in local communities. If the medical center is a long distance from your home and you do not want to be bothered with the expense and inconvenience of returning there each time you need treatment, you can take advantage of a consultation and continue to be treated at your local hospital by your own doctor—but with the added experience and continuing advice of the specialist at the medical center.

Who pays for a second opinion?

Many insurance companies now pay for second opinions. Even if your particular insurance company does not, the cost should be less than for the first consultation, because all of the test results and x-rays are available to the second doctor.

What if the second opinion differs from the first doctor's advice?

Second opinions can sometimes be confusing. If the first doctor recommends a course of treatment different from the second, you are left more confused than when you started. You have three alternatives in this case: Ask the two doctors to discuss the case to see if they can resolve the conflict, ask for a third opinion and accept the majority decision (two out of three), or follow your own instincts about what is best for you.

What is the difference between a referral and a consultation?

If your doctor decides that your illness requires the attention of a specialist, he will recommend the names of one or several specialists for you to see. This is called a referral and differs from a consultation. A referral means that once you see the specialist you become his patient. For a consultation, a consultant is called in to advise you and your doctor but does not take over responsibility for treating you.

If I am unhappy with my doctor, should I ask him for a referral or a consultation?

When you are satisfied with your doctor but want to get a second opinion because you want confirmation of a diagnosis, you should ask for a consultation. However, if you are really unhappy with your doctor and the kind of treatment he has been giving you and if you really feel that someone else should be handling your case, what you want is not a consultation but a referral. Ask your doctor to refer you to the top specialist in the area dealing with your condition. Many times, this is a step that may be difficult for the patient to take and can be more easily handled by a family member or a friend. The important thing to remember is not to waste time trying to be patient about the treatment being received when in your own mind you know that things are not going as well as they should. Be bold and ask the doctor for a referral or take steps to find a new doctor on your own.

Can I take advantage of a comprehensive cancer center or research center while using my own local hospital?

Yes, you can, and it is wise to do so. You can make an appointment to be seen by the specialists at the cancer center or research center for a consultation. Your doctor can call for information on getting a consultation with a doctor on the staff to discuss a case, or you can call for information. As stated before, these centers are designed for treatment of cancer patients and most have up-to-date cancer information available.

What do I do if I want a second opinion and I am already hospitalized?

It is a little more difficult to arrange unless your doctor is agreeable to your having it. Explain to your doctor that before you go ahead with any treatment you would like to have another consultation. If there is a specialist on the hospital staff who is qualified, arranging a consultation will be easier than if the specialist is located at another hospital. However, don't allow difficulties to deter you from seeking a consultation that will give you further insight into what alternatives are open to you. Even when you are hospitalized, it is still your right to demand that your doctor find another physician—even one from another hospital—to give you an independent opinion. Some hospitals have patient advocate services which can be helpful in this kind of situation.

Is it a good idea to get a second opinion on a pathology report?

The kind of treatment you will get and the outlook for your future are often based on the pathology report. Pathologists are human—and pathology is not an exact science. The diagnosis of cancer sometimes requires more than just the examination of a very thin slice of tissue through a series of lenses which magnify the tissues several hundred times. Question the pathology report. Ask your doctor whether he has consulted personally with the pathologist. Many doctors do this as a routine matter. If the doctor has not already done so, indicate that you would like the opinion of a second pathologist to confirm the first report. In most large hospitals where several pathologists are employed, consultations are routine, assuring the patient that the report is the consensus of a number of trained pathologists.

How are clinical histories taken?

First, the physician or a trained medical assistant takes a family history, exploring the kinds of illnesses and diseases you have had, whether or not there has been a history of cancer in your family, and the kinds of medication or radiation administered to your mother during pregnancy and to yourself during your lifetime. He asks questions about your body's organs and any suspicious symptoms you may have noticed. You may be asked about your work area, whether or not you are exposed to carcinogens such as asbestos or vinyl chloride, and your smoking habits.

If I have no cancer symptoms and I go to a doctor for a complete cancer-detecting physical, what should that physical consist of?

There is certainly not full agreement on what a comprehensive cancer-detecting physical should consist of. Here are some of the items a complete checkup for detecting hidden cancer could involve:
- Complete medical and family history
- Complete blood count
- Complete urinalysis
- Digital rectal exam
- Proctosigmoidoscopy for persons over 50
- Pelvic exam and Pap test for women
- Chest x-ray
- Manual examination of the abdomen, thyroid gland
- Examination of the prostate gland in men and breasts in women (mammography according to age and risk guidelines)
- Check of all skin areas
- Mouth check using a mirror to see into throat and larynx
- Eye exam with a lighted instrument
- Test for occult blood in the stool

Why does the doctor always order basic blood and urine tests?

These simple tests, sometimes called CBC (complete blood count), SMA 12 (serum factors), and UA (urine analysis), give the doctor a great deal of basic information about your general health problems. They can usually be done in the doctor's office.

What does the complete blood count consist of?

The technician takes whole blood from your vein as well as a blood smear from your finger and uses the samples to check the hemoglobin, white blood cell count, and complete red and white cells in the blood and the platelets. The hematocrit test requires that the blood be spun in a centrifuge and measures (usually on an automatic counting machine with computer printout) the volume of red cells as a percent of the total volume. This test can help detect if anemia is present, though it cannot identify the type of anemia. The hemoglobin test measures the number of grams of red cell pigment in 100 cubic centimeters of blood. A low count is a sign of some type of anemia. The white cell count (listed as WBC) shows the number of white cells per cubic millimeter of blood. Usually an elevation of this count points to infection.

The microscopic examination and count of the blood smear helps to determine the type of infection, type of anemia, or blood-clotting conditions. The technician examines the smear to determine the proportions of various types and numbers of white cells (called differential), the size and shape of red cells, and the number of platelets present.

What does the urinalysis tell the doctor?

The degree of concentration of the urine (weight of urine relative to plain water), called specific gravity (SG), indicates urinary obstruction with kidney damage if the count is low or dehydration if the count is high. Using a simple plastic strip with a series of chemically sensitive patches, the doctor or his nurse or technician can also check the amount of acidity, protein, sugar, and ketones in the urine— to diagnose acidosis or alkalosis, kidney damage, diabetes, etc. The microscopic examination of centrifuged urine, called the urine sediment exam, checks for red cells, white cells, kidney cells, crystals, and microorganisms in the urine which might indicate kidney damage, urinary-tract infection, or gout.

Are blood tests used for detecting cancer?

At the present time there is no one blood test which conclusively tells if cancer is present, either for the initial diagnosis of cancer or for monitoring disease recurrence. The tests now available are not sufficiently accurate; they may be negative when no cancer is present and also when it is known that the person has cancer. Sometimes they are positive when cancer is not present. Therefore they are currently being used only along with other cancer detection exams.

Are monoclonal antibodies being used to detect cancer?

At present they are being used experimentally. Radioactive antibodies can be sent through the body to seek out specific cancer cells and to attach themselves only to those kinds of cells. The radioactive hot spots, where the antibodies have lodged, can be photographed with x-rays.

Has any progress been made in finding a blood test to detect cancer?

Progress has been made in identifying what are called biological markers—substances present in abnormal amounts in the blood or urine of a person with cancer. Such substances are produced either by the tumor itself or by the patient in response to the tumor tissue. Researchers are still hoping to develop a simple laboratory test, using a sample of blood or urine, to reveal the presence of cancer before other signs appear. Such a test has not yet been developed. However, some techniques presently used in cancer treatment are based on biological markers. For instance, the ability to determine estrogen and progesterone receptors helps doctors decide on treatments for breast cancer. The monitoring of carcinoembryonic antigen (CEA) is useful in determining whether or not colorectal cancer is shrinking or spreading during treatment. Unfortunately, neither of these indicators is useful in detecting the cancer itself. Markers can be produced by diseases other than cancer. They are not sensitive enough or levels remain normal in a certain percentage of cancer patients. Scientists hope that the use of monoclonal antibodies, along with an increased understanding of chromosome changes associated with cancer, will provide an increase in reliable tumor markers in the future.

Is the CEA (carcinoembryonic antigen) test now being used?

The CEA test detects changes in the body that often accompany cancers. This test is now being used but only in combination with other established procedures for both diagnosing and managing cancer. Although it may be useful as an early indication of recurrence in some patients previously treated for cancer, alone it is not a conclusive test either for initial diagnosis or for monitoring disease recurrence.

What is the blood stool test?

The blood stool test, also called the occult (hidden) blood test or the guaiac test, detects blood in the stool not visible to the naked eye. Many doctors give you this test to do at home following a regular physical examination. Do-it-yourself test kits can also be bought at most drugstores. To do the test, you are usually asked to follow a diet containing increased fiber and no meat for several days before and during the stool sampling period. You are also advised not to take aspirin or vitamin C pills during that time. A small amount of feces from three different stools is transferred with an applicator stick to a labeled card. A solution is added to each specimen on the card. If blood is present, the test paper turns from white to blue. If this happens, additional tests must be done to determine whether a precancerous or cancerous condition is present.

What routine is followed in doing an ECG (EKG) exam?

The electrocardiogram is an electrical record of the performance of the heart. When the heart muscle contracts and relaxes, changes are produced which can be picked up from the skin surface by electrodes applied to the various parts of the body. This test is part of most routine physical examinations when a patient is past 40, and is a part of most routine hospital examinations. The electrodes—round, cold metal discs—are smeared with a jellylike substance to heighten conductivity. They are attached to the wrists and ankles. Another disc is used by the operator to move in a series of prescribed positions on the chest. The wires or "leads" record the vertical peaks and horizontal lines made as the heartbeat travels from an upper chamber to the lower chamber of the heart. An inked stylus traces the pattern on graphed paper affixed to a drum that rolls through the electrocardiograph machine. From this tracing, the doctor has a graphic record of the patient's heartbeat.

What is a lumbar puncture?

A lumbar puncture is a diagnostic procedure sometimes referred to as a spinal tap, usually performed under local anesthesia. A thin needle is inserted in the space between the two lower vertebrae of the spine to remove fluid that normally is in this area. Lumbar punctures are used in cancer, for instance, to diagnose leukemia in the central nervous system. This examination indicates the pressure within the spinal fluid system and can show evidence of tumor, infection, or inflammation in the central nervous system. If spinal fluid is being removed, a headache following the procedure is not unusual.

When are x-rays used in diagnosis?

X-rays are an important part of the diagnostic workup. X-rays are used to detect and diagnose many forms of cancer, including cancer of the lung, digestive tract, and breast. They are also used to determine whether the cancer has spread to places such as the lung or the bone. Properly taken and read, x-rays are one of the doctor's most valuable diagnostic tools.

How are computers being used for x-rays?

Computers, which up to now have only been used in special diagnostic procedures such as CT scans, are starting to be used for routine x-rays. In what is called digital radiography, the technique uses computer monitors to view the image. Doctors can zoom in on a specific area of the x-ray, adjust the contrast in too-dark or too-light areas, and tell the difference between soft tissue and bone. Some systems stand alone, and others are used in conjunction with standard x-ray equipment. All work by converting x-ray images to digital signals, electronic data that can be stored and examined by a computer. Digital radiography is still in its early stages, but someday its use should reduce the number of x-rays that need to be taken again as well as lowering radiation levels for those systems using filmless methods.

What are the main kinds of x-rays?

There are two major types of diagnostic x-rays: plain films and contrast films.

What are plain films?

These are regular, standard x-rays you have always known. They are ordinary films of various parts of the body. A chest x-ray is an example of a plain film. For a tumor to be seen on a standard x-ray it must be big enough and it must be more dense than the surrounding normal tissues. Tumors are not always detectable on an x-ray.

What are contrast films?

A contrast film is used when some foreign substance is put into the body to contrast with normal body tissues. For example, a chemical dye or air or a radioactive material may be introduced into the body to allow some organ to be outlined on the x-ray. A barium-enema x-ray is an example of a contrast film.

What is an air-contrast x-ray?

An air-contrast x-ray is produced when air is introduced into a selected part of the body. The air is used to outline soft-tissue structures within the body. Since air does not absorb x-rays like the surrounding tissues, it provides a contrast on the film. Depending on the test, the air may be inhaled, swallowed, injected, or obtained from carbonated beverages. For example, a deep breath held during a chest x-ray fills the lungs with air. X-rays pass through the air readily, so the tissues surrounding the lungs will show up, and any areas where the lungs do not readily fill up with air will be cloudy on the x-rays.

What are the names of some of the different kinds of contrast-film tests using dye?

There are many of them, and their names normally correspond with the part of the body being tested.

- *Barium enema (BE)* outlines the colon (intestines) and rectum. Barium is given rectally by enema.

- *Barium swallow* outlines the upper digestive tract including the pharynx and esophagus. Barium is swallowed.
- *Bronchogram* outlines the bronchial tree. Dye is injected into the lung bronchi (air passages). High-risk procedure.
- *Cerebral angiogram* outlines the blood vessels in the neck and brain. Dye is injected into carotid and/or vertebral arteries in the neck. Also called an arteriogram. High-risk procedure.
- *Coronary angiogram* outlines the heart chambers, valves, and surrounding arteries in the veins. Dye is injected into the chambers of the heart. Also called an arteriogram. High-risk procedure.
- *Cholecystogram* outlines the biliary tract (gallbladder and bile ducts). Contrast medium is given as pills 12 hours before x-rays are taken.
- *Cystogram* outlines urinary bladder (cystourethogram outlines bladder and urethra). Dye is placed in bladder by means of urinary catheter.
- *GI series* outlines the stomach, duodenum, and remainder of the small intestine. The contrast medium is swallowed.
- *Hysterogram* outlines the stomach, duodenum, and remainder of the small intestine. The contrast medium is swallowed.
- *Hysterogram* outlines inside of uterus and the fallopian tubes (hysterosalpingogram outlines uterus and oviducts). Dye is injected through a vaginal catheter into uterus.
- *Intravenous pyelogram (IVP)* outlines the urinary tract (kidneys, ureters, and bladder). Dye is injected into the arm vein.
- *Lienography* outlines the spleen. Dye is injected.
- *Lymphangiogram* outlines the lymph nodes. Dye is injected into involved lymph system. Usually used for patients with Hodgkin's disease, lymphomas, or testicular cancer.
- *Myelogram* outlines the spinal cord and adjacent structures. Dye is injected by needle into the fluid surrounding the spinal cord.

- *Pneumoencephalogram (PEG)* outlines the chambers and surface of the brain. Air is injected and rises into the brain. High-risk procedure.
- *Pulmonary angiogram* outlines blood vessels (arteries and veins) in the lungs. Dye is injected into the pulmonary arteries as they leave the heart. High-risk procedure.
- *Venogram* outlines the venous system of the body. Dye is injected into vein.

Why are some of the contrast films noted as high-risk procedures?

Most of the contrast films involve little risk. The high-risk procedures are those in which a stroke might be induced, nerve damage may be caused, or other complications may occur when the dye is being introduced into the body. Those which involve more risk include the bronchogram, cerebral angiogram, coronary angiogram or arteriogram, pneumoencephalogram, and pulmonary angiogram. These tests demand skilled personnel. Also, some people are allergic to the dye, particularly that used in the intravenous pyelogram (IVP.)

Why is lymphangiography important in the diagnosis of cancer?

Lymphangiography is important to cancer diagnosis because one of the ways that cancer spreads is through the lymph nodes. Lymphangiography can be useful in the diagnosis and staging of persons with Hodgkin's disease and lymphomas and sometimes for other cancers. It is a procedure which is done in an outpatient setting or in a hospital. A blue dye is injected into the small lymph vessel after a cut is made in the big toe. The lymph system in the abdomen can then be looked at by means of x-rays. Since the lymph glands are very small, it usually takes 2 to 3 hours for the dye to reach the lymph nodes. Lymphangiography is used to localize and determine the extent of the tumors. The surgeon can use it as a guide to finding specific lymph nodes and determining the size of the tumor. The radiotherapist uses it to evaluate how a person is responding to therapy. Since the dye stays in the system for some 3 to 4

months, progress usually can be followed through x-rays
without repeating the procedure.

Do some of the parts of the body absorb more x-ray beams than others?

If you put a part of the human body in front of a beam of
x-rays, some of the rays will pass through, while others will
be absorbed and scattered inside the body. Bone, for example, which is more dense, will absorb x-rays more readily
than surrounding tissues. It is the shadows of these denser
parts of the body which show up on the developed film or
screen.

What kinds of contrast media are used for x-rays?

X-rays are absorbed by dense substances such as barium or
iodine. These contrast media can be swallowed, injected
into the bloodstream, or inserted with a plastic tube or catheter. Sometimes dye and air are both used in contrast films.
For example, often both barium and air are used for gastrointestinal examinations.

What kind of physician should read diagnostic x-rays?

Diagnostic x-rays should be interpreted by doctors who are
board-certified (or board-eligible) radiologists.

What kind of background does a radiologist have?

A board-certified radiologist (certification is by the American Board of Radiology) must be a graduate of an approved
medical school; must have four years of postgraduate training in the department of radiology, including training in
pathology, nuclear radiology, and therapeutic radiology; and
must have successfully completed written and oral examinations administered by the board.

What is the difference between a diagnostic radiologist and a therapeutic radiologist?

A diagnostic radiologist administers and interprets x-rays
used in diagnosing illness. A therapeutic radiologist (also
sometimes called a radiation therapist, a radiotherapist, or
a radiation oncologist) specializes in treating cancer with

radiotherapy. The American Board of Radiology gives separate certification to these two specialties.

How do I know where to go for my diagnostic x-rays?

This is a subject you should discuss with your physician. Ask questions. If you can, have your x-rays done in the outpatient department of a medical school or major hospital or by a private board-certified radiologist.

What questions should I ask before I have x-rays?

You should ask the following questions:
- Are the x-rays clearly necessary for diagnosis?
- Are there any x-rays which I have had taken recently which might be used instead of taking new ones?
- What is the approximate dose of x-ray?
- What do you think you will find out from the x-rays?
- What dosage is the particular machine giving?
- When was the machine last inspected?
- What kind of shielding will be used during the procedure?

Is there really a difference between the machines used in one office and those in another?

Yes, there is definitely a difference. You should know that both the quality of the x-ray equipment and the quality of the technician or doctor doing the x-ray make a difference in whether or not you receive a low or high dose of radiation. The expertise of the operator also makes a difference in how good the x-ray will be. Another variable is in who reads the x-ray after it is taken.

What kind of training do x-ray technicians have to have?

There are some states which legally require that radiology technicians be trained and certified. The 1970 X-ray Exposure Study conducted by the Public Health Service shows that those x-rays supervised by radiologists in private offices involved less exposure than those supervised by non-radiologists in private offices. However, many states have been working with the FDA's Bureau of Radiological Health on radiation-control regulations and on training programs for personnel.

Are the machines inspected regularly?

There are presently no U.S. government inspection requirements. Although some states do have requirements,
in many states the equipment is not inspected every year.
Some machines, particularly those in doctors' offices, go
uninspected for long periods of time. There should be a
certificate posted near the machine. Look at it to see when
the last inspection was performed. If it was more than a few
years ago, go elsewhere.

When should x-rays be considered a necessity?

As noted earlier, x-rays are an important part of the diagnostic workup. When properly taken and read, they are one
of the doctor's most valuable tools. However, the benefits
of the x-ray must be weighed against the risks. A qualified
professional is a better judge of when x-rays are needed
than you are. You, however, need to know the right questions to ask so that you can assure yourself you are in the
hands of a skilled and competent practitioner.

What is the major risk of diagnostic x-rays?

The amount of radiation which x-rays deliver to your body
is the biggest risk. It is believed that the risks of x-ray dosage
are linear—that is, the more dosage a person receives during a lifetime, the greater his or her chance of developing
cancer or another abnormality.

Who can tell me what the approximate dosage should be for the various tests?

Your doctor should be able to give you approximate dosages
so that you can ask the technician where you are having
the test done what dosage his machine is giving. For example, a standard chest x-ray involves between 5 and 10
millirem (.005–.010 rem or rad); a mammogram should be
under 1 rad for both pictures of each breast.

Do the x-rays belong to me?

There is quite a bit of controversy over this issue. However,
you have a right to ask that the x-rays taken in one place
be sent to another doctor or hospital of your choice. Some

doctors and hospitals will give them to you directly; others will insist on mailing them to the other physician or hospital. It might be a good idea to explain that you are concerned about x-ray overexposure.

What is a fluoroscope?

This is a kind of x-ray in which a special machine (the fluoroscope) takes a continuous x-ray so that the doctor can see the movement of internal organs. A fluorescent screen, coated with a special substance, is mounted in front of an x-ray tube. The x-ray shadow is cast on the screen. The fluoroscopic image can be amplified and displayed on a television screen. Fluoroscopy can show the expansion of the lung or a barium liquid passing through a patient's esophagus to his stomach. Fluoroscopic techniques sometimes provide important information which cannot be obtained in any other way.

How much radiation exposure will I get from a fluoroscope?

Fluoroscopes take longer to perform and often expose you to more radiation than do the conventional x-ray exams recorded on film. There are new machines which give better images with less exposure, particularly those which amplify the light from the fluoroscopic screen and then provide a brighter image on a TV monitor, but the exposure is still higher than for a standard x-ray film. Make sure this procedure is done only by a board-certified radiologist and only when necessary.

Will the doctors use x-rays taken by someone else?

Some doctors will not use them because they are not aware they are available, they don't want to be bothered asking for them, they don't trust the manner in which they were taken, or the resulting film is not clear or detailed enough. There may be good reason for having x-rays retaken, such as if the first set is on poor-quality film. But you should make sure that your x-rays are being redone for good reasons and not just because a doctor or hospital does not want to share them. You should keep a record of your own x-ray history so that you can tell the doctor what has already been done, especially on high-dose film such as gallbladder or GI series. More and more doctors are accepting x-rays taken by others.

How is the dose of radiation measured?

You will hear the terms *rad* or *rem* used in describing the dose of radiation. *Rad* stands for *radiation absorbed dose.* A rem is equivalent to a rad. The terms apply to all types of radiation and take into account the energy actually imparted to the tissue. (Sometimes the terms *millirads* and *millirems* are used to describe the dosage.) The effects of diagnostic x-rays on the body depend in a complex way on a number of factors, such as the distribution of energies of x-ray photon in the beam, the total intensity or quality of radiation, the distance between the x-ray tube and the individual being x-rayed, the type and location of tissues and organs in the main beam, and the age and sex of the person being examined. The unit of exposure is the roentgen, named after Wilhelm Roentgen, who discovered x-rays in 1895. However, most radiologists now measure the absorbed dose, which is the amount of energy dumped by incident radiation into a gram of material. The dose absorbed by a gram of skin or muscle can be much less than that absorbed by a gram of bone placed in the same x-ray beam. This is because the heavy atoms of calcium in the bone absorb x-rays more easily than lighter elements abundant in tissue. X-rays pass through tissue more easily and don't leave as much energy behind.

What is skin dose?

This refers to the dose of radiation immediately on the surface of the skin. The outer layers of skin absorb x-rays readily; thus, particularly with older machines, the exposure inside a body will be less than the exposure at the skin. The absorbed dose in the outer layers of skin is often referred to as the skin dose, while x-ray energy deposited in a gram of bone, tissues, or an organ at a certain location inside the body is referred to as the depth dose at that location.

What x-rays give relatively high overall radiation doses?

Several examinations are of special concern because they involve relatively high overall radiation doses. They include examinations of the gastrointestinal system (upper and lower), thoracic spine (middle and dorsal), lumbosacral spine (lower), lumbar spine, cervical spine, gallbladder, kidney, ureter, bladder, skull, pelvis and hip or upper thigh, and fluoroscopic procedure.

What other things should I watch for when having x-rays taken?

A good operator will measure carefully the thickness of the part of your body which is to be exposed and consult a technique chart to set the tube current, voltage, and exposure time for each type of x-ray. If the operator hurries, there is more likelihood that a poor exposure will require additional x-rays. You must be careful not to move, since blurred images mean additional x-rays. The operator must also carefully align the beam, using the minimum beam-size possibilities.

When are lead shields used?

Shielding can help reduce the amount of scattered radiation absorbed, especially by reproductive organs. There are several kinds of shields such as lead aprons, lead-lined panels, scrotal cups, flexible lead-lined drape cloths, and shadow shields. If they are not offered to you, ask about them before being x-rayed. Newer machines have built-in shields to avoid scattering.

What kind of x-ray is a mammogram?

A mammogram is a soft-tissue x-ray of the breast. It is but one of several techniques used in diagnosis of breast cancer. The mammogram and the other techniques used in diagnosing breast cancer—xeroradiography, thermography, diaphonagraphy, graphic stress telethermometry—are discussed in Chapter 11.

What is endoscopy?

Endoscopy is the examination through optical instruments of the interior of the body. There are many different kinds of instruments designed to perform this examination on different parts of the body. Several new tools use fiberoptics for this procedure—tiny flexible fibers that carry a powerful light and a telescope which allows the doctor to peer inside the body. These instruments allow the diagnosis of various kinds of cancer without performing a major operation. Sometimes they are used in combination with other tests, such as x-rays, to confirm the diagnosis.

What are some of these endoscopic instruments called?

You can identify these instruments because they end in the suffix *scope*: cystoscope, hysteroscope, colposcope, laparoscope, peritoneoscope, bronchoscope, proctosigmoidoscope, esophagogastroduodenoscope, etc.

Why are these instruments important in diagnosing cancer?

For many years, these procedures have offered a fairly simple method of detecting malignancies, precancerous growths, and non-cancer-related diseases without the necessity for major exploratory surgery. This means you can return to work, be free from postoperative complications, and save money. The exact location of tumors can be determined and cytology can be done without a major operation. Since the introduction of fiberoptic equipment in the 1970s, new areas of the body can be examined without surgery.

What is a cystoscopy?

A cystoscopy exam allows the doctor to inspect the lining of the urinary bladder for the presence of diverticula, fistulas, stones, or tumors in the bladder. The bladder is first enlarged by filling it with air or water. A cystoscope—a thin, hollow tube with a light at the end of it—is inserted through the urethra. The doctor can then actually look at the walls of the bladder. Cystoscopic brushes can be passed along to the tract to obtain cells for microscopic examination. Small tumors can sometimes be removed through the hollow tube. This test is usually done if you have repeated urinary tract infections or if you have bleeding associated with urination.

When is a hysteroscope used?

A hysteroscope can determine the presence of fibroid and endometrial tumors; it can also be used to help locate lost IUDs or treat cases of infertility. The hysteroscope looks somewhat like a skin diver's spear gun, with an eyepiece and a trigger that controls a flexible tip that provides a full view inside the uterus. The instrument is inserted through the vagina and threaded through the cervix into the uterus to view the uterine cavity and entrance to the fallopian tubes.

What is a colposcope examination, and how is it done?

The colposcope is basically a microscope on a stand which gives a lighted, magnified view of the vulva, vagina, and cervix—an area which previously could not be seen without major surgery. It allows the doctor to look through a microscopic eyepiece into the area. No part of the instrument is inserted into the vagina. Further details about colposcopy are covered in Chapter 16.

Is the laparoscope used as a diagnostic tool?

Yes, the laparoscope is used to examine a woman's reproductive system for diagnosing disease as well as in performing a quick, relatively painless operation for sterilization. With the laparoscope, the doctor can inspect the uterus, the ovaries, the fallopian tubes, and even the appendix if the other organs are moved aside. He can sometimes use it to differentiate fibroid tumors from ovarian cancers and various other pelvic problems by looking inside the abdominal cavity. A small slit is made in the abdominal cavity near the navel. This procedure is usually done under general anesthesia in the hospital. Normally you can leave the hospital the same day. Sometimes the laparoscope is used for detecting liver lesions, either alone or in conjunction with an ultrasonic probe.

What is a peritoneoscope?

A peritoneoscope allows the doctor to decide whether or not to operate without making an incision in the abdomen; it is used instead of exploratory laparotomy in some cases. Liver metastases can be seen and biopsied with a peritoneoscope. It is used for people with lung, gastric, and pancreatic cancer, whose disease might have spread, and for people with lymphoma and with ovarian cancer. Depending on the location, either local or general anesthesia is used.

When is a bronchoscope used?

A bronchoscope is a slender, tubular instrument, that may be rigid or flexible, inserted into the patient's nose or mouth and threaded into the larger breathing passages. Its light at the far end allows the doctor to look directly into your bronchi. The doctor normally sprays anesthetic into the throat and bronchial tubes so that they are numb. Since it is inserted into only one bronchus at a time, you should have no trouble breathing normally during a bronchoscopy. The fiberoptic bronchoscope is a more flexible instrument which allows viewing of less accessible parts of the respiratory tract to locate early lesions.

What is a proctosigmoidoscope?

This is a lighted instrument that can be inserted to a maximum of 10 inches into the colon. It can be used for viewing the lower interior portion of the colon. Two-thirds of all cancers of the colon and rectum are accessible to detection by this means.

What is a colonoscope?

The colonoscope allows the doctor to examine the entire length of the colon. It is used to detect cancers which sometimes are not seen in x-ray studies. It is a highly flexible, four-directional instrument, no thicker than a finger, that can be maneuvered through the curves and around the bends of the colon. It gives off brilliant rays of light and gives the doctor an excellent view of any damage or abnormality in the tissue. The colonoscope permits tiny tissue samples, or biopsies, to be taken. Since the delicate walls of the colon can be penetrated by this instrument, a skilled physician is required to perform this test. Colonoscopy is often done in conjunction with a fluoroscope to help the doctor follow the course of the tube. It is usually performed under light anesthesia on an outpatient basis.

If the doctor sees polyps (cherrylike growths on the intestinal wall), he can sometimes remove them entirely, safely, and easily through working channels in the colonoscope which allow a variety of instruments to be inserted.

What are esophagoscopy, gastroscopy, and duodenoscopy?

These three procedures use flexible fiberoptic instruments to examine several parts of the gastrointestinal tract. A doctor can look at the esophagus (esophagoscopy), see problems in the stomach (gastroscopy) or in the pancreas (duodenoscopy). These instruments permit photography, biopsy, and collection of cytological materials. Several different models of instruments are available in varying lengths. They have working channels through which various tools can be inserted, and they have controls for air, water, and suction. Some anesthesia is used, especially in the area of the throat, to allow painless swallowing of the tube.

What kind of doctor should do these examinations?

Several of the new instruments require doctors who are qualified, trained specialists to perform the tests and to understand what is being seen by these tools. They can be dangerous in the hands of untrained practitioners. In most cases the average general practitioner has not had enough experience unless he has undergone special training. Make sure a trained proctologist, internist, or surgeon will be doing your tests.

What is involved in a barium enema with air-contrast examination?

This method uses a contrast medium to visualize the lower bowel. By carefully x-raying the colon, small and large lesions overlooked by other tests (such as palpation, proctosigmoidoscopy, or colonoscopy) may be seen. Sometimes if a barium-enema exam is negative, but suspicious signs and symptoms continue, the exam is repeated.

What is cytology?

Cytology is that branch of medicine which deals with the formation, structure, and function of cells. When it is mentioned in the area of diagnosis for cancer, it is sometimes called exfoliative cytology and refers to the technique of examining cells which have been normally shed or which are scraped from living tissue. The cells, which cannot be seen by the naked eye, are examined under the microscope, usually by a pathologist or a technician trained to know whether the cells look normal or not.

What kinds of tests are cytological exams?

There are several:
- Pap test to detect cervical cancer
- Vaginal pool aspiration or endometrial aspiration to detect uterine cancer
- Sputum tests to detect lung cancer
- Urine-sediment tests to detect cancer of the urinary tract, especially bladder
- Scrapings from the mouth to detect oral cancer
- Cell samples from the esophagus, stomach, pancreas, or duodenum
- Fluid tests from areas such as breasts, spinal cord, thyroid, prostate
- Bone-marrow tests

How are cytological exams performed?

A little fluid taken from the organ—either from cells which have been sloughed off, cells which have been scraped off, or body fluid which has been taken by needle—is spread on a glass slide. The fluid is stained with dyes and examined through a microscope. When cancer cells are present in the fluid, they can usually be spotted. The cytological exam of cells is based on the fact that cells on the surface of an organ are constantly being shed and falling off. In some places, these cells, both malignant and benign, can be scooped up in the normal fluid secretions. There are structural differences between the cancer cells and benign cells which can be seen under the microscope. The smear technique was first used in the Pap test. Today the new fiberoptic instruments make it possible to obtain smears from less accessible organs such as the stomach and the pancreas.

Can a final diagnosis of cancer be made with a smear test?

Most smear tests are used for screening to detect abnormal cells. Most doctors do not feel that the smear can be used to provide the final diagnosis of cancer. The smear consists only of individual scattered cells, sometimes clusters of them. A smear diagnosis gives strong evidence of the presence of cancer, but biopsy is still held to be essential for a final decision.

What are the advantages of the smear method?

There are several. Some smears, such as the kind used in the Pap test, can be done easily and cheaply for testing large groups for cancer. Some smears, like those for the Pap test and the lung sputum test, can detect the presence of cancer before any signs or symptoms appear. And in hard-to-reach areas such as the stomach, exfoliate cytology smears can provide evidence of the presence of cancer without the need for an operation.

Does the Pap test detect any cancers other than cervical?

The Pap test is approximately 97 percent successful in detecting cervical cancer; the cervix is the opening to the uterus and is where most cancers involving the uterus and female genitals begin. However, the Pap test will show only about 50 percent of cancers of the uterine lining (endometrium), and is of little or no value in detecting cancers of the ovary.

What are radioactive scans?

Radioactive or nuclear scans are tests in which the patient is given a weak radioactive substance—called a radioactive tracer—by injection into the bloodstream. The material is taken up by the body. A machine, which looks like an x-ray machine, moves over the area being tested and produces a series of pictures.

How can the doctor tell if cancer is present?

Deposits of cancer may show up as areas of either increased radioactivity or decreased radioactivity, depending upon the organ being studied, the type of radioactive substance used, and the kind of scan being done.

What kinds of substances are used in nuclear scans?

The kind of tracer used depends upon the part of the body which is being studied. Certain substances accumulate in certain body organs. An element like cobalt-60 allows doctors to track its progress as it makes its way through the digestive system by the radioactive trace elements it leaves behind. Radioactive iodine can be used for looking at the thyroid gland. Gallium is capable of showing rapidly dividing cells. New substances are constantly being tested and reviewed.

Where are radioactive scans done?

These tests must be done in special laboratories by doctors and technicians who are trained in handling radiotracers. Other conditions can, at times, look similar to cancer on the scans, so it takes a skilled practitioner to interpret them. Nuclear scans have been commonly used for detecting tumors since the early 1950s, and initially the tests were an offshoot of radiology. Now many hospitals have departments of nuclear medicine and it is a rapidly growing field in its own right. There is an American Board of Nuclear Medicine which certifies physicians in this field.

Who performs radioactive scans?

A skilled physician who has had special training after completing medical school—including several years of intensive postgraduate training to qualify as an expert in diagnosis with extensive technical knowledge of the machinery used, the chemistry of radioactive compounds, and nuclear physics and radiation safety—is responsible for nuclear scans. The American Board of Nuclear Medicine certifies doctors in this field. A nuclear medicine technologist assists the doctor, positions you, and operates the equipment during the examination. The technician has had special training and experience in nuclear medicine technology.

Are nuclear scans different from x-rays?

Yes, they are. X-rays involve passing radiation through your body from an external source (an x-ray tube) and recording the image on a film (radiograph) which the radiologist can examine. In a scan, the radioactive substance is introduced into your body, usually through an injection in your vein. The machine translates the substance into spots of light that expose the film, which is developed and called a scan. By observing how and where the radioactive compounds travel in your body, the doctor can detect changes in your body's processes.

What kinds of machines are used?

There are two main types. A "scanner" moves back and forth in straight lines, and as it moves it records images of the radiation given out. The other machine, called a "camera," records the radiation without the machine moving. It is larger than the scanner. The areas where the radioactivity is concentrated are seen as dots on the film. Places where there is high activity have more dots than those where there is low activity.

Is there any discomfort or danger to radioactive scans?

The scans involve little discomfort. The danger involved depends upon the part of the body. Some of the radiation given off by the tracer substance can be absorbed. However, the radioactive substance is weak, so the risks associated with nuclear scans are similar to those associated with diagnostic x-rays.

When are radioactive scans done?

It depends upon the kind of cancer suspected and the stage of the disease. Scans can be used to detect the primary source of cancer. They can also be used to estimate the progress of the treatment. Scans are also part of what is known as a metastatic workup—that is, checking the body for distant cancer. A metastatic workup is usually used before treatment is begun if there is a diagnosis of cancer or if a very high suspicion of cancer is present. Metastatic workups are part of the "clinical staging system" which determines the person's state of cancer at the time it is diagnosed.

What kinds of scans are done for a metastatic workup?

Again it depends upon the kind of cancer and knowledge of where that cancer is likely to spread. A metastatic workup can include bone scans, liver scans, and brain scans along with a battery of other tests.

How are bone scans done?

The liquid which has been "tagged" with the mildly radioactive substance is injected into a vein and carried by the bloodstream to the bones. Cancerous areas in the bone will usually pick up more of the radioactive material than normal bone, so these show up as "hot spots" on the films taken of the area. Most of the liquid injected into the body for the bone scan disappears within a few hours. The liquid is excreted from the body within 48 hours after the test is done.

Are bone scans difficult to interpret?

Yes, because injured bone, arthritis, infection, and certain other abnormal conditions may show up as hot spots on the bone scans.

Do bone scans show different things than routine x-rays?

Yes, bone scans can detect cancerous areas in some cases earlier than x-rays. They are more sensitive. Bone scans are also better than x-rays in following the disease; they can show progress or regression. Routine x-rays have some drawbacks. Approximately 50 percent of the bone tissues must be destroyed by cancer in a given area before it will show up on an x-ray. On the other hand, x-rays also have some advantages: they are quick, easily obtained, involve no discomfort and little risk, and are relatively accurate.

Do brain scans also show hot spots?

The picture that appears as a result of a scan depends on the person's individual situation, because each kind of lesion in each particular organ creates its own variation in the isotope's pattern. In a brain scan the picture is of the blood pools carrying the isotope around. The isotope accumulates within a lesion to form a hot spot. Regions that are only lightly represented on the scan of a normal brain usually show up much more darkly when they contain a lesion.

What are liver scans?

A substance is injected in a vein and circulates through the entire bloodstream. Because of the size of the particle injected, it is trapped by the normal cells in the liver and spleen (the major organs in the body which will trap particles of that particular size) accumulating enough of it to give an image. If there is a lesion, it is seen as a "cold spot" because the abnormal liver cells aren't performing their normal trapping function. Liver scans are used to evaluate liver size, shape, and position and to detect the presence of lesions in the liver. Liver scans are usually routinely recommended before major tumor operations in many sites.

When is a thyroid scan done?

A thyroid scan is done if a tumor is suspected after the doctor has examined the thyroid area with his hands. A small amount of radioactive material is swallowed or injected. A cold spot (showing decreased concentration of the radioisotope) makes the physician suspicious of cancer, although a great percentage of cold spots can also prove to be benign. A hot spot of great activity is usually a sign of a benign growth. A thyroid scan is used to determine the size, position, and function of the thyroid gland and to detect metastases of thyroid cancer. Sometimes two thyroid scan readings are taken—usually at 2 and 24 hours after administration of the radioactive material.

Would having a radioactive scan be a problem for a pregnant woman?

The radioactive material can be carried to your baby through your circulation system. The amount of radiation is small, but you and the doctor should discuss the problem and the alternatives together. Be sure you tell the doctor if you are pregnant or think you are pregnant.

What is a gallium scan?

A gallium scan is used to determine if the cancer has spread to more than one area of the body because it is capable of showing rapidly dividing cells. One of the main uses of this test is in detecting lymph-node involvement in lymphoma or other tumor masses.

Are lasers being used to diagnose cancer?

Yes. The carbon dioxide (CO_2) laser is being used to diagnose cancer of the vocal cord and colon, among others.

What is ultrasound?

It is one of the newer methods used to locate and measure solid tumors in the body. Ultrasound, or sonar, was used extensively during World War II for tracking submarines. Today it is used to clean teeth, age alcohol, and prospect for oil. It has been adapted for medical application and is a common technique for watching the heart in motion and for examining unborn babies.

How does ultrasound scanning work?

It works just like sonar. If a destroyer captain wants to locate a submarine, he sends bursts of sound through the water around him and waits for some of them to bounce off his target. By analyzing these echoes, he can tell where the submarine is and how large it is. An ultrasound technician, or sonographer, uses exactly the same principle.

How is ultrasound scanning done?

The technician presses a microphonelike probe across the patient's skin. This probe is called a transducer. The probe sends out sound waves at 1 million to 10 million cycles per second. When the probe picks up an echo, a dot registers on the screen (called an oscilloscope screen). The probe sends out sound waves 0.1 percent of the time it is on and listens 99.9 percent.

How can ultrasound tell a solid tumor from one that is not solid?

As the technician moves the probe across the skin surface, a composite picture emerges on the screen showing what's inside the body. A solid tumor looks solid on the screen because echoes are returning from all the particles inside it. But a cyst filled with fluid looks hollow, because fluid doesn't reflect ultrasound waves. The technician can make a permanent record of the picture with a special camera attached to the oscilloscope.

Can ultrasound tell the difference between a malignant tumor and a benign one?

No. Ultrasound can confirm that the mass is a tumor. It outlines it and shows the extent of it. But an ultrasound machine that by itself can distinguish a malignant tumor from a benign one has yet to be invented. A doctor, by looking at the shape and consistency shown by ultrasound and combining it with the clinical history of the patient, can say that a tumor is "highly suspicious" of being cancerous.

Is ultrasound like an x-ray?

No. Ultrasound has no radiation. It uses high-frequency sound waves to scan the body—sound waves that are far beyond the range of human hearing. The range of human hearing is about 20 to 20,000 cycles per second. The probe used in ultrasound scanning sends out sound waves at 1 million to 100 million cycles per second. The vibrations from these sound waves are reflected off body tissue and transformed into electrical signals that show up on a screen as a two-dimensional image.

Does the patient have to make any special preparation for an ultrasound scan?

No. You will be put on an examining table. Your skin in the area to be scanned will be covered with mineral oil in order to eliminate most of the air gaps that block sound transmission. You need no anesthesia and you will feel no pain. The ultrasound scan itself takes only a few minutes to perform, especially if it is being done on one small area of your body.

What are the advantages of ultrasound scanning?

With ultrasound, you have no radiation exposure. You need no incisions or injections. You do not have to swallow any substances. There is no discomfort. Ultrasound can be used many times on the same patient without side effects, as far as is known, even to pregnant women. Studies to date have revealed no known biological damage to humans from diagnostic exposure to ultrasound waves, although it is a form of energy being transmitted through tissues.

Is ultrasound new?

The procedure has been around for many years. In the past it was used mainly for obstetrical tests. Since 1970, there has been a dramatic change in its use in the United States. Now ultrasound is being used for the whole pelvis, and about two-thirds of the scans now being done are in the abdominal area. It is a field which is changing with new technology being introduced. However, there is a limited number of doctors who know how to use and interpret the tests accurately.

Is ultrasound being used in other areas besides diagnosis?

Yes. Ultrasound experts can measure a tumor's progress during therapy—whether it is getting smaller as a result of chemotherapy or radiation treatments. It can be used to tell the doctor whether or not the treatment is working. It is thought to be a good monitoring device because it can be used often, since there is no radiation involved. Ultrasound may be used to help the doctor more accurately aim radia-

tion during treatment. It is also used as a guide for operations. Sometimes it is used during an operation to help
determine the size, number and location of tumors.

What kinds of tumors are being diagnosed with ultrasound?

Ultrasound scanning has proved to be helpful in diagnosing
tumors of the stomach, pancreas, kidney, uterus, and ovaries. It has helped detect tumors of the eye and thyroid
gland. In the thyroid area, it acts as a complementary test,
mainly to estimate the size of the lesion. It is sometimes
used in breast cancer, especially to scan young, dense
breasts. It can actually differentiate between fluid or solid
tumors in about 98 percent of the cases.

How is ultrasound used in the gynecological area?

This is where the use of ultrasound began. It can be used
in the urinary area. In the ovarian area, it can detect whether
the tumor is cystic, partly cystic and partly solid, or all solid.

How is it used in liver and pancreas areas?

Ultrasound is useful in scanning the pancreas, especially
in thin patients. In the liver, ultrasound scans are often used
when a patient is jaundiced—since it can help to differentiate between normal consistency and pancreatitis. However, it cannot tell the difference between pancreatitis and
cancer of the pancreas. Small tumors of the pancreas can
be discovered by ultrasound.

Is ultrasound used in detecting breast cancer?

In some cases. It is useful in looking at the dense breasts
of younger patients. It cannot reveal calcifications and is
not useful in looking at breasts of older patients.

Is ultrasound useful in the chest area?

No, ultrasound has not been found to be useful in this area.

Is ultrasound used for detecting cancer of the kidney?

Ultrasound can be used for a more definitive diagnosis after
IVP (intravenous pyelogram) testing is done. It can help
differentiate between solid and cystic kidney masses.

Do ultrasonic scans give different information than standard x-rays?

Although ultrasonic scans can be used as a substitute for x-rays for certain kinds of examinations, they generally yield different types of information, so often both ultrasonic scans and x-rays are ordered. They are complementary tests. The boundaries between different types of soft tissue can be highlighted with ultrasonics, for example, and the characteristics of blood flow can be studied. However, for viewing structures such as bones, x-rays are presently preferable.

Can ultrasound be done on an outpatient basis?

Yes, it can. However, in many of the major centers which have the scanning equipment, inpatients take preference over the outpatients for use of the machine.

What is a CT scan?

"CT" stands for "computerized tomography." A newer way of looking inside the human body, it uses pencil-like x-ray beams to scan the section of the body being studied. It combines the speed of a computer with the sensitivity of the x-ray detectors. Sometimes you will hear the terms *tomographic scanner, ACTA scanner* ("ACTA" stands for "automatic computerized transverse axial scanner"), or *CAT* ("computerized axial tomography"). They all mean the same thing. In this book the term *CT scan* is used to refer to this procedure.

How does the CT scanner work?

The CT takes a three-dimensional look inside the body. The scanner has an arm which directs the beam through the body as it rotates around you. The x-rays pass through the body and are detected by an electronic device. About 160 scans are made in one position; then the detectors are rotated and the 160 scans are repeated.

What does the computer do?

As the beam moves around the body in the same plane, a minicomputer analyzes how much of the x-rays are absorbed as they pass through the various internal organs and structures. Up to eight slices 1 centimeter apart may be taken at any one time. Each target area in the slice has between 100 and 200 x-ray beams going through it. The approximately 100,000 bits of information are fed into a computer that performs a billion calculations to convert the data into an image. The image can be seen on a TV screen or in printed form.

How does the CT scan differ from the standard x-ray?

X-ray machines send a broad x-ray beam over a large area. CT scanners direct a pencil-point-thin line of electromagnetic energy through a narrow cross-section or slice of the body. Ordinary x-rays take a "flat" view, superimposing organs in the front of the body on organs in the back, giving a two-dimensional picture. CTs give a three-dimensional picture. CTs also give better pictures of soft tissues than do x-rays.

What is ECAT?

ECAT stands for "emission computerized axial tomograph." It is a cousin of the CT. Patients swallow radioactive material. The charged particles (positrons) given off from deep inside the body are recorded on the ECAT scanner, giving the doctor a picture taken from the inside of whatever organ is under study.

What is MRI?

MRI, which stands for "magnetic resonance imaging," is a new diagnostic device which produces pictures of the body's internal tissues that are similar to the computerized, cross-sectional x-rays made by CT scanners. The MRI method, which uses electromagnets instead of x-ray tubes, is safer than established techniques that depend on x-rays, injected contrast solutions, and radioactivity. Sharper pictures, with more distinction than CT scanners produce, are possible, especially for difficult areas such as the brain, liver, heart, and spinal cord. Brain scans, for example, are far more detailed than those from the best CT scanners. Without injecting anything into the body or exposing the body to radiation, the MRI pictures clearly show blood vessels and contours of brain tissue and distinguish between different types of soft tissues. MRI can show structure as well as function. It is capable of distinguishing normal from abnormal tissue—but at present cannot distinguish a benign tumor from a malignant one. Repeated scans can be done without risk of excessive radiation. Presently, the costly MRI machine is available on a limited basis at major medical centers.

Is it uncomfortable to have a CT scan?

There should be little discomfort. The total time needed to complete a series of scans making up a complete examination is about an hour. Sometimes contrast material is used. If it is needed, an intravenous needle is put in your vein and the solution passed through it.

Can I move during the CT scan?

No. It is very important that you not move during the examination. If you do, the examination may have to be repeated.

Do I need any special preparation?

Ordinarily not. If your head is being scanned, however, an elasticized stocking cap will be put over your scalp to assist the technician in positioning your head for the examination. Tape will also be used to ensure proper positioning. You will be asked to remove all jewelry, ornaments, dentures, and other similar objects in the head and neck area so that they will not interfere with the scanning examination. If the scan is of your chest, stomach, pelvic area, arms, or legs, you will be given a gown to wear.

Who will do the actual scan?

The technician will prepare you and position you for the examination, and will be operating the equipment. The diagnostic radiologist will view and interpret the scanning information. The report of the examination will be given to your doctor by the radiologist.

Has the CT scan taken the place of other tests?

The hospitals with CT scanners have reduced the number of pneumoencephalograms and angiograms significantly.

Both are conventional brain x-rays using contrast media, and both are high-risk procedures because of the injection of contrast medium. A CT scan is not considered a high-risk procedure.

How much radiation do you get from a CT scanner?

Some radiologists claim that the thin x-ray beams expose patients to less radiation than a conventional x-ray examination. They do not expose the patient to *more* radiation than the conventional x-ray. And the scan avoids the risks associated with the injections of contrast dyes needed in some of the conventional procedures.

How long does it take to do a CT scan?

It depends upon the question the doctor wants to have answered by the scan. A single scan takes anywhere from a few seconds to a couple of minutes, depending upon the type of scanner and the extent of the examination. A full body exam could take from 15 minutes to an hour, depending upon the questions to be answered. The CT scan can be done on an outpatient basis, with a minimum amount of discomfort.

What are CT scanners used for?

Originally, CT scanning was used only to see brain abnormalities. Today it is a tool which can be used for cancers such as those of the lung, bladder, prostate, liver, and pancreas. It is used to spot tumors, detect organ disorders and abnormal structures, follow blood vessels, spot blocked ducts, differentiate between normal and abnormal tissues, and see blood clots. It can detect small differences in the physical characteristics of tissues. It can tell the difference between white matter and gray matter and between blood and water. It can be used by radiologists in making out treatment plans because it can provide detailed information about the absorption of radiation by a particular tumor. Some scanners now take the scans in color, but these are not usually used for routine diagnosis, since the black-and-white image at this time gives more detail.

Types of Biopsies

Type	Procedure
Needle or aspiration biopsy	Fluid or tissue is removed by suction through a pointed needle.
Endoscopic biopsy	Fluid or tissue is obtained by using long instruments, usually with a needle or knife; the optical instrument allows the doctor to see into the body cavity.
Incisional biopsy	Part of the tumor is cut out to be looked at microscopically by the doctor.
Punch biopsy	Specimen is removed by means of a punch.
Total biopsy or excisional biopsy	The entire tumor is removed for examination under the microscope.

What is a biopsy?

A biopsy is the procedure in which a piece of tissue is obtained and examined under the microscope to determine whether cancer or other disease is present. This microscopic examination of the biopsy specimen is accepted by doctors in determining the nature of a tumor with complete accuracy. Therefore, whenever possible a doctor insists on obtaining a sample of every tumor that could be cancer before treatment is attempted. The biopsy provides the most reliable basis for a diagnosis of cancer.

Who determines if the biopsy cells are cancerous?

The biopsy is "read" by a pathologist—a physician who specializes in the study of normal and diseased body tissues.

What kind of training does a pathologist have?

In order to be certified by the American Board of Pathology, the person must be a licensed doctor of medicine or osteopathy and have four years of training in both clinical and anatomic pathology or three years of training in either specialty or eight years of practical experience under circumstances acceptable to the board. The doctor must also successfully complete the examinations administered by the board. The pathologist is a vital member of the health-care team, especially in the field of cancer.

Are all pathologists skilled in diagnosing cancer from slides?

As in all other specialties, the skill and the competence of pathologists vary. A decision regarding whether cancer is the disease in the tissue being examined depends on the interpretation the individual pathologist makes of the cellular structure of the biopsy. Frequently, tissue or slides are sent to experts of larger institutions for consultation, especially by pathologists practicing alone in small communities. If your diagnosis of cancer is based on the single pathological report of a single pathologist in a small community, be sure to ask that the slides or tissues be sent to other pathologists for confirmation. As important is the relationship between the patient's doctor and the pathologist. They need to be talking with each other and working together as a team.

How can the pathologist tell if cells are benign?

When a piece of tissue is taken from the body and examined microscopically, the normal cells have an orderly appearance. They possess the distinctive features of the organ from which they came. The cells from the thyroid gland, for example, are very different from those of the lymph nodes. Normal cells from different organs carry genetic "messages" that determine their structure and function.

What does the pathologist look for when he reads the biopsy?

The pathologist does many things. First he looks to see whether the specimen is malignant or benign. If it is malignant, he tries to identify the specific type of cancer cells present in the tumor and attempts to determine just how fast they reproduce themselves. With special stains and fixes, he can tell much from the tissue samples. He looks to see if the blood vessels or lymph channels have been invaded. With some kinds of tumors, he may test for hormone dependency. The pathologist gives the other doctors information which will allow them to determine the proper course of treatment.

How important is the pathologist in a cancer diagnosis?

The pathologist is the key to the entire diagnosis, since a diagnosis is nothing more or less than a carefully considered opinion. It is important first of all that there be adequate and properly prepared biopsy material, since no diagnosis is better than the evidence that it came from. Sometimes, it is found that the kind of specimen presented to the pathologist is inadequate for a true diagnosis to be made or the cellular structure is difficult to identify. Further, like everyone else, the pathologist is just one individual with the same burdens and problems we all have. He may be swamped with work and may not have the time to do an adequate job of preparation in, or reflection upon, the reports he makes. His relationship with the physician in charge of the patient may be poor. All these factors have a bearing on the kind of pathological study and report that is done on your biopsy—and underlines the need for a second pathological opinion. As was noted earlier, in large hospitals and medical centers where there is more than one pathologist, second opinions on biopsies are often routinely done.

What are the different kinds of biopsies?

There are three general techniques for getting the tissue for a biopsy: incisional, excisional, and needle.

What is an incisional biopsy?

In an incisional biopsy, a part of the tumor is cut out and looked at microscopically. This method is usually favored if the suspicious mass is a large one. The object is to get as large a sample as possible, cutting down on the chances of getting a false reading from a bit of tissue that is not representative of the whole.

What is an excisional biopsy?

In an excisional biopsy, the tumor is removed totally. This method is selected when the tissue has been identified as cancerous, when strong suspicion exists that part of it may

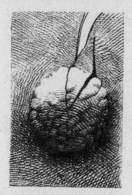
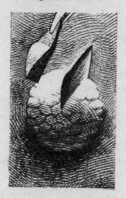
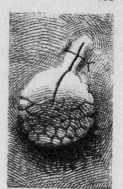

Incisional biopsy

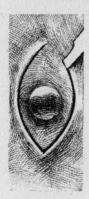
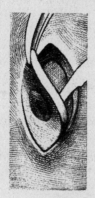
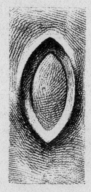
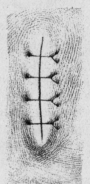

Excisional biopsy

be or become cancerous, or when the tumor is small. Many skin tumors, for example, are totally removed before the biopsy is performed.

What is a needle or aspiration biopsy?

In a needle biopsy, a needle is used to extract either fluid or tissue for a biopsy. In the United States, the usual needle biopsy is performed by inserting a fine needle into the lump to draw out fluid or tissue juice. A smear of this fluid is then examined for cancer cells. This method is also called an aspiration biopsy. In some places in the country, thin-needle aspiration is being used by urologists to take tissue samples to detect prostate cancer and by other physicians to detect breast cancer.

What is a wide-bore needle biopsy?

A wide bore needle is sometimes used to extract tissue for liver and bone marrow samples. This biopsy method is used extensively in the Scandinavian countries and in Great Britain. A tiny cutting instrument is inserted through the needle to obtain a tissue sample of the tumor and its immediate surroundings.

What are the advantages and disadvantages of the needle biopsy?

The advantages of the needle biopsy are that generally it can be performed in the doctor's office and requires only local anesthesia. It is a simpler and less expensive way to get the biopsy done. The big disadvantage, especially of the thin-needle biopsy, is that it is easy to get the needle in the wrong place and miss the tumor completely, especially if the growth is a small one. The wide-bore needle biopsy is more reliable.

How does the physician decide which kind of biopsy to perform?

There are no set rules. The size of the lesion, the location of it, and the suspected diagnosis affect the doctor's decision on the type of biopsy to perform.

I keep hearing the term *frozen section*. What kind of biopsy is that?

The frozen section can be done with either an excisional biopsy or an incisional biopsy. It refers to the procedure of preparing the tissue for the pathologist to read. There are two ways to prepare the tissue—via the frozen section, which is a quick procedure taking 15 to 20 minutes, or via a permanent section, which takes several days. The frozen section is a quick-reference method of determining whether or not cancer is present. The permanent section is a more accurate method.

When is a frozen-section biopsy used?

The frozen section is performed while the patient is in the operating room. It is used when a suspicious mass cannot

be reached to obtain tissue by means other than an operation. The patient is prepared for the major surgery; the
tissue is obtained, but the surgeon does not proceed with
the operation until the report is relayed to him from the
pathologist.

How is the frozen section done?

The surgeon sends the section of tissue he has cut to the
pathology laboratory. The tissue is cut and a "touch-prep"
slide is made by touching a slide against the tissue so it
makes an imprint. Solutions are added to another slice of
tissue (about 3/16 inch thick), which is put into a machine
(cryostat) for fast freezing. In about 3 minutes it is frozen
and cut into thin slices. The cut sections are placed on slides
and dipped in wood alcohol for about 10 seconds. These
slides and the touch-prep slide are stained. The frozen-
section slides are used to look quickly at the structure of
the tissue and the touch-prep slide is used to look at the
cellular structure. The two types of slides should agree.

How does the permanent section differ from the frozen section?

The permanent-section biopsy takes considerably longer
than a frozen-section biopsy. In this process, the tissue is
put through a time-consuming multistage procedure that is
highly complicated and that gives a high-quality slide. The
tissue is put through a series of solutions to take out the
water and fatty substances from it. It is then saturated with
warm liquid paraffin. When it has cooled and hardened, the
tissue in paraffin is sliced into thin slices. The slices are
placed on slides and stained so that the tissue can be studied
under the microscope. Proper staining, which brings out
cell formations and their nuclei, requires exact timing.

How is the permanent section done on an outpatient basis?

When the permanent section is being performed on an outpatient basis, the patient is told not to eat or drink after
midnight and checks into the hospital in the morning. The
patient receives a premedication injection for relaxation and
a small amount of local anesthetic in the area to be biopsied.
The lump or suspicious tissue is excised, and the wound

sutured closed. The patient returns home after a few hours and the pathologist returns a complete report within 3 or 4 days.

What are the disadvantages of the frozen section?

In the frozen technique, there can be some distortion of cells because of the freezing process, shrinking in alcohol, and the fact that the stain is a rapidly performed one. The technical appearance of the tissue may not be of the highest quality. The tissue can be wrinkled, torn, and fractured by the cutting processes of the frozen section. The pathologist must be able to understand which of the changes he sees are processing distortions and which changes are due to the actual abnormalities of the tissue.

Are there any advantages to a frozen section?

It depends upon the kind of cancer and the extent of it. If it is in an area where a permanent section *cannot* be done under local anesthetic, then the frozen biopsy eliminates a second operation. If general anesthesia must be administered to do the permanent section, then a frozen biopsy is called for because no anesthetic agent is perfect and each anesthetic entails a risk. In the area of breast cancer, however, since permanent sections can be done under local anesthetic and the risk of general anesthesia is not involved, it is usually to the patient's advantage to have a permanent section.

What are the advantages of a permanent section?

The advantages of this method are many. The tissue is first fixed in formaldehyde for from 3 to 12 hours. The fix is better, the tissue shrinkage is more uniform, and the whole process is slower and therefore reduces tearing of the tissue and distortion of its structure. The tissue cuts thinner in this manner. The method of fixation allows tissue to take up the stain better than the frozen section. The pathologist has the whole tissue block available for cutting samples at a later date. The definition and character of a single cell is much clearer and more precise than in a frozen section. The pathologist usually has better tissue to work with, and therefore you are assured of a more technically correct diagnosis.

Is a second opinion ever called for on a biopsy?

If the diagnosis is malignant, some surgeons send the slides to another pathologist, without including the conclusions of the first, for a second, uninfluenced decision. It is not possible to do this with a frozen section, only with a permanent section. You, as a patient, can request that the slides be sent to a consulting pathologist at another medical center for a second opinion.

Have there been advances in the kinds of microscopes being used by the pathologists?

The electron microscope sorts out tumor cells by exposing fine structures visible only at magnifications at least ten times as high as a light microscope provides. It gives information which the standard microscope cannot give and permits the pathologist to tell the difference between primary and metastatic tumors and often to identify where in the body the cancer began.

What is bone marrow aspiration? What is bone marrow biopsy?

These are two similar tests. A whole piece of the marrow is required for the biopsy. For both tests, the doctor, using novocaine, inserts a long, hollow needle through the skin and other tissues into the bone marrow—the soft, spongy center of the bone which produces blood cells. A small specimen of the marrow is then removed by suction. The specimen is examined under the microscope for the presence of cancer cells. For a bone marrow biopsy, the doctor pushes the needle in farther until there is a piece of whole marrow in it.

When will the doctor usually order a bone marrow study?

Usually bone marrow studies are ordered if some abnormality shows up in the complete blood count or peripheral smear. It is a routine test for suspicion of leukemia or to check if cancer has spread to the bone marrow. The presence of abnormal blood cells is frequently an early sign of tumor-cell invasion of the bone marrow.

What is a metastatic workup?

A metastatic workup is done to see if cancer has spread to other parts of the body. It usually consists of bone and liver scans; sometimes brain and lung scans are added.

Why would the doctor order a bone scan if my cancer is in the breast?

This is a relatively routine check, so don't let it frighten you. It is done because the bone is a common place for breast cancer to spread.

What does the doctor determine from the liver-scan test?

Although they are not truly diagnostic, these tests are valuable in alerting the doctor to the presence of liver involvement. The intravenous injection of radioactive material helps to accurately outline liver size, shape, and position and to detect the presence of abnormalities that alter the structure of the liver.

What specific tests does the doctor do to find out whether or not the cancer has metastasized?

For the most common sites to which cancer spreads, the general diagnostic techniques and treatment are as follows:

- *Lung*: This is the most common site for cancer of other organs to spread. X-rays, tomograms, bronchial brushings, scans, fiberoptic bronchoscopy, and biopsies are used in diagnosing lung metastases; chemotherapy and sometimes surgery are used for treatment.
- *Bone*: Metastases to the bone from cancers which start in other organs are more common than is primary bone cancer. Diagnosis is done by x-ray, bone scans, and gallium scans. Radiation, chemotherapy, and hormonal therapy are used for treatment.
- *Liver*: Metastases to the liver from cancers which begin in other organs are more common than is liver cancer itself. Ultrasound and liver scans are used to diagnose it. Radiation and chemotherapy can be used for treatment, depending upon the primary site of the cancer.
- *Brain*: Brain metastases are detected by physical ex-

amination and then usually confirmed by brain or CT scan. The treatment is usually radiotherapy or cortico-steroids.

Am I wise in not wanting to know the extent of my disease?

It is certainly your privilege to specifically tell your doctor not to inform you if your diagnosis is bad. However, knowledge of what is happening to you really is more valuable than not knowing.

Should I ask my doctor to explain my case to me?

If you are interested enough to be reading this book, you probably are interested enough in the progress of your own case to want to know the details. The fact is that the better you understand what is happening to you and what the alternatives are, the more likely you are to help in making the right decisions about your own care. The doctor has both a right and a duty to give the patient reasonable knowledge about his condition.

chapter 5

Treatment

Cancer can be treated in a number of different ways, depending upon the kind and the extent of the tumor. Among them are

- *Surgery:* removal of the tumor by cutting
- *Radiation:* the use of x-ray or radium
- *Chemotherapy:* the use of drugs and hormones
- *Immunotherapy:* the use of the body's immune system
- *New investigational treatments:* monoclonal antibodies, biological modifiers, and hyperthermia.

Questions to Ask Your Doctor About Treatment

- What treatments are available?
- What treatment do you recommend?
- Is this treatment necessary for me?
- Are there any other alternatives? What are they?
- Why do you think this treatment is preferable?
- What do you expect the results to be?
- How safe is the procedure?
- What are the side effects of the treatment and what can be done to relieve them?
- Can I be put on a program that doesn't interfere with my work schedule?

Types of Treatment

TREATMENT	DEFINITION	WHEN USED
Surgery	Removal of tumor by cutting	Most often used if tumor is small, if it is limited to a single area of the body, and if cancer has not spread to other parts of the body. It is the most frequently used method.
Radiation	Use of x-ray or radium	For those cancers extremely sensitive to radiation; used as cure attempt when cancer is localized; can be used to control growth; often combined with surgery (before or after); used to cure or palliate in 50–60 percent of all cancer cases.
Chemotherapy and hormone therapy	Use of drugs and hormones	Used after surgery or radiation as "adjuvant" or preventive treatment. Used when cancer is in body system rather than localized in one spot. Used to control growth and for palliation. Often combined with surgery and radiation.
Immunotherapy	Use of body's immune system	Stimulates or enhances body's own response.

- How will we determine how well the treatment is working?
- When can I call you to ask further questions?
- Can I leave a list with the nurse, or do you have hours when I can call and talk directly with you?
- Do I have a type of cancer which would be better treated at a specialized center?

Are there any general rules as to when the various treatments are used?

There are some general rules, but you must understand that the treatment will vary depending upon the kind of cancer, the extent of the disease, and how the person reacts to the treatment being given.

Are the kinds of treatment ever combined?

Yes. Often several types of treatments are given to the same patient in hopes of achieving better results than with one type of treatment alone.

How is my specific treatment determined?

Your doctor will consider many factors in determining the treatment for your cancer. Among them are
- What kind of cancer you have and its pattern of growth and spread
- Aggressiveness of the cancer
- Predictability of the spread of cancer
- The sensitivity of your cancer to specific drugs or other modes of therapy
- Morbidity and mortality of the treatment procedure
- Cure rate of the treatment procedure
- The areas of your body affected by your cancer
- Your physical state

Can I withdraw from a type of treatment once I have started the treatment?

This depends upon you and your doctor. Your doctor should explain in detail the pros and cons of your recommended treatment as well as alternative forms of therapy which might be available to you. Of course the final decision is yours, but you should understand you may be losing valuable time which can never be regained.

What are the newest types of treatments for cancer?

The newest treatments for cancer involve the harnessing of the body's own natural immunity. It is believed that cancer cells probably are present at some time in everyone, but that the immune system is usually able to stop the cells

before they have a chance to become cancers. The latest
cancer-fighting methods, now in clinical trials across the
country are known as biological response modifiers (often
referred to simply as biologicals). Many of these new treatments are still years away from being used for ordinary
treatment. Clinicians are just beginning to experiment with
ways of combining various biologicals with each other and
with standard treatments for more effective use. More information on these and other investigational treatments will
be found in Chapter 9.

**How can I, an ordinary cancer patient, take advantage of
the newest treatments?**

It depends upon what kind of cancer you have and the stage
of your cancer. Many of the newest treatments are available
only to patients with advanced cancer for whom all other
treatments have failed, since they are still considered experimental. A first step would be to discuss with your doctor
the treatment in which you are interested. You can ask him
or her to do a PDQ search. Many of the treatments are
available only at NCI-designated comprehensive cancer
centers or at the National Cancer Institute's Clinical Center.
Some are available in local communities through clinical
cooperative groups or through the community clinical oncology program. Chapter 23 gives information and lists of
key contacts for these four resources. For more information,
call the Cancer Information Service 1-800-4-CANCER.
Trained counselors can inform you of the kinds of treatments available and where they are being conducted. When
checking out any of these resources, it is essential that you
know the kind of cancer you have, the cell type, if possible,
and the stage of the cancer's progression.

**With so much new information about cancer and its treat-
ment, how does the ordinary doctor keep up with what's
going on?**

It is a serious problem, of concern to the National Cancer
Institute (NCI), which has created a computerized database
to tell doctors of the latest and best treatments for cancer
patients. Called PDQ, for Physician Data Query, it gives
information on the state-of-the-art treatment for each type

and stage of cancer, as well as information on more than 1,000 active treatment studies under way in this country. Also included is a directory of 10,000 doctors who devote a major portion of their practices to treating cancer and 2,000 institutions with organized programs for cancer. Patients can get information on the latest in cancer treatment by calling the NCI's Cancer Information Service, 1-800-4-CANCER.

How can the doctor measure the effectiveness of the various kinds of treatment on the tumor?

Different patients have different responses to treatment. The doctor uses physical exams, x-rays, scans, and various laboratory tests to measure each patient's tumor's response to therapy.

What if the treatment chosen for me does not work?

With the exception of a few cancers, there are many other treatment programs which can be used. One may result in controlling the disease even after another has failed to adequately control it.

Why are there so many different kinds of treatment?

Since no two cancers are truly alike and since people respond differently to treatments, patients with seemingly identical diseases may receive different treatments. Each type of cancer has its own way of growing and spreading. Therapy must be tailored to each individual cancer, to its size and location in the body, and to the physical condition of the patient.

What is meant by a curative form of treatment?

A curative treatment is one that is being used to cure the disease.

What is meant by adjuvant forms of treatment?

An adjuvant treatment is one that is being used in addition to a primary form of treatment.

What is meant by palliative treatment?

A palliative treatment is one that is intended to improve the condition of the patient. It may be to reduce pain, to eliminate the worst symptoms, to prevent complications, or to give a psychological uplift.

What is meant by treatment of choice?

The treatment of choice is usually the main kind of treatment for that stage of the illness. In many types of cancer, surgery is the treatment of choice, with radiation or chemotherapy used as adjuvant treatments.

What is the most frequently used treatment for cancer?

Surgery is still the most frequently used method of treating cancer, both alone and in conjunction with other methods of therapy, although chemotherapy and radiation are increasingly used today.

Why has there been a change away from using surgery alone for the treatment of some cancer?

There seems to be an increasing realization that cancer in many instances is a systemic disease—a disease of the body system rather than localized in one spot. Therefore, the use of surgery alone or radiation alone, two forms of treatment which are successful in treating tumors which are confined to one spot, are not adequate when the tumor has spread. In some kinds of cancers, although surgery might remove all visible signs of cancers, based on patients whose disease has recurred, it is thought that micrometastases (small colonies of cancer cells which cannot be detected by any known means) have escaped from the original tumor site and are looking for a home elsewhere in the body. Today there is much research being done using new approaches to assist in a systemic attack againt the disease.

Are the different kinds of treatment given one at a time or all together?

It depends upon many factors, including the tumor and the extent of the disease. Sometimes, they are given in sequence. Other times, two or more treatment modes are intermixed. Sometimes, radiation therapy is given first, after which surgery is used. For other kinds of tumors, surgery is the first kind of treatment used.

What is meant by "informed consent"?

Informed consent is a legal standard which defines how much a patient must know about the potential benefits and risks of therapy before being able to agree to undergo it knowledgeably with legal responsibility for the result. The question of informed consent is a very controversial and complex one, particularly if one is talking about surgery or other treatment procedures which carry some risks. Basically, you have the legal right to know everything you want to know about a treatment that is being proposed for you. In investigational treatment, you will be asked to sign a paper which explains the pros and cons of the treatments before they are performed. In most cancer treatment, however, it is up to you to ask about the major risks involved versus the benefits to be expected.

What is meant by the term *prognosis*?

Your prognosis is an estimate of what the outcome of your disease will be. The doctor bases his prognosis on your general physical condition plus his accumulated information about the disease and its treatment.

What is meant by the term *quality of survival*?

This term is often used when talking about cancer treatment. It means how good the life is that you will be leading after treatment. Some people feel that they would rather live a shorter period of time than undergo disfiguring operations or long periods of painful treatment. Influencing the quality of survival are such things as general health, the ability to function normally, pain, the patient's personal attitude, economic status, and physical condition. Each of these items needs to be examined as you assess the treatment for the illness.

chapter 6

Surgery

Surgery is used most often in cancer treatment for doing biopsies to remove the malignant tumor, to take out a growth that might become malignant, to relieve pain, or to remove a tumor that is the result of the spread of the disease. It is often the first step in a treatment plan when cancer is discovered. It is important to be certain that all the necessary diagnostic tests are performed before surgery is planned, to ensure that proper treatment is given. Choose your surgeon carefully. Remember that you're more likely to have a well-qualified surgeon if you choose one who is a fellow of the American College of Surgeons and is board-certified in his field. (Currently only about 55 percent of operations are performed by board-certified physicians.) It is important to ask questions before you agree to surgery so that you are fully informed about the reasons for treatment, the expected results, and the possible complications.

Questions to Ask Your Surgeon Before Operation

- Why do you want to do the surgery?
- Exactly what will you do? Please explain it to me in simple terms.
- What are the chances for cure with the surgery?
- What other kinds of treatment can you use instead of

General Types of Surgery

TYPE	DESCRIPTION	WHEN USED
Specific	Local removal of tumor	When tumor appears to be localized and there is hope of taking out all of cancerous tissue
Radical	Removal of tumor and adjacent tissues or organs affected by cancer cells as well as lymph glands	When surgeon believes this is necessary because of possibility of regional or local spread
Preventive	Removal of growth not presently malignant	If surgeon feels growth might become malignant if left untreated. Used for precancerous conditions such as polyps in colon and moles on skin.
Palliative	Treatment of complications incidental to the disease	To relieve pain; to try to stem spread of disease; to give patient several more years of useful life
Electrosurgery	Use of high-frequency current	For some cancers of skin, mouth, rectum
Chemosurgery	Use of chemotherapy drugs on tumor before or instead of surgery	Primarily for skin cancers and melanomas of eyelid
Cryosurgery	Destruction of tumors by freezing	Best for tumors easily seen or felt; usually head and neck and skin cancer
Laser Surgery	Use of laser beam	Being used as a surgical tool in treating cancer

doing the surgery? Are there any less extensive, less deforming, less painful operations than the one you are suggesting?
• What are the risks of having the surgery?
• What are the risks in the other kinds of treatment?
• What is the risk of death or serious disability?
• Do you feel the benefits outweigh the risks? Why?

- What are the consequences of postponing the surgery?
- What happens if I don't have the surgery?
- How much will the operation cost?
- How long will I be in the hospital?
- How long will the recovery period be?
- How disfiguring will the operation be?
- How disabling will the operation be? Temporarily? Permanently?
- Will I have drains, catheters, intravenous lines, transfusions?
- What are the possible aftereffects?
- How many times have you performed this operation?
- Whom do you recommend I see for a second opinion?
- Can the diagnostic tests be done on an outpatient basis?

Questions to Ask the Anesthesiologist

- What kind of medication will I be given before I go up to the operating room?
- Who will be administering the medication and anesthesia?
- How will they be given to me?
- Are you an anesthesiologist or an anesthetist?
- Will my allergies be a problem?
- What kind of anesthetic are you going to give me?
- What are the side effects?
- What are the risks?
- How long will the operation take?
- How long will it take before I regain consciousness?
- Will I go to a recovery room after the operation?
- What are the fees for your service?
- If you do not want to be fully unconscious during surgery, are elderly, or have lung problems, ask: Is general anesthesia absolutely necessary?

Questions to Ask When You Are in the Hospital

- What will be happening to me tomorrow?
- Why is this blood test/x-ray being taken?
- What will this test determine?

- What will this drug accomplish?
- What drugs have you prescribed for me to take and for what purpose?
- This pill/medicine is different from the one I have been taking. Will you please check to make sure it is prescribed for me?
- Do I have to stay in bed?
- Am I allowed to walk to the end of the hall?

Questions to Ask Your Doctor Before Leaving the Hospital

- How long will I have to take it easy after I leave the hospital?
- Will I be a bed patient at home? How long?
- Will I need help at home?
- Will I be able to take care of myself?
- When will I be able to engage in normal activities? (Ask specific questions based on your case: When can I drive a car? When can I play tennis? When can I resume sexual activities?)
- Will I have to have some special regimen?
- What symptoms, if any, should I report to you? (If you are under the care of several doctors, ask which doctor you should report to if you have questions or problems, and how you can reach the doctor at night.)
- What symptoms should I ignore?
- When can I safely go back to work?
- What medications should I continue to take?
- What exercises will I be permitted to do?

When does surgery offer the best chance of cure for cancer?

If surgery alone is being used, it offers the best chance for cure if the disease is still confined to one site and if the tumor can be fully removed by the surgeon's tools.

Do surgeons remove more than the cancer they can see?

Surgeons usually try to remove the visible cancer tissue plus some of the surrounding tissue, even if it seems normal. This is in case nearby tissue is hiding cancer cells that could later lead to the recurrence of the cancer.

Is surgery safer now than it was some years ago?

Cancer surgery, as well as surgery in general, is safer now than it was 20 or 30 years ago because of many advances in the areas of anesthesia, antibiotics to control infection, and transfusions to build up the patient's blood supply. All surgery has some risk to it. The complications of surgery are often related to the anesthesia. The problem is to weigh the benefits against the risks.

What is specific surgery?

That is when a tumor appears to be localized and there is hope of taking out all of the tissues which are cancerous.

What is radical surgery?

Radical surgery involves removal not only of the tumor but also of adjacent tissues or organs that may have been invaded by the cancer cells; in addition, lymph nodes in the vicinity of the tumor may be removed for staging the cancer to determine prognosis and treatment.

What is preventive surgery?

Preventive surgery is when a surgeon takes out growths which are not presently malignant but might become so if left untreated. These may be precancerous growths. They can be, for example, polyps in the colon, cysts in the breast, or moles on the skin.

What kinds of palliative surgery are performed on cancer patients?

Palliative surgery is sometimes necessary to treat complications incidental to cancer, such as abscesses which are a result of the tumor. The surgeon may sever nerves to relieve pain. Sometimes in patients with advanced breast cancer, for example, the surgeon may remove hormone-producing glands such as ovaries, adrenal glands, or pituitary glands.

What is electrosurgery?

Electrosurgery uses the cutting and coagulating effects of high-frequency current. This is applied by needle, blade, or disk electrodes. It is used as a treatment for some cancers of the skin, mouth, and rectum.

What is chemosurgery?

Chemosurgery is treatment with a chemotherapy drug before or instead of removing the tumor by surgery. The doctor coats the tumor with zinc chloride fixative paste; this paste destroys the upper layer of the tumor. The remaining tumor is then removed by surgery layer by layer until microscopic examination shows that all tumor cells have been eliminated. It is used primarily in the treatment of skin cancers and melanomas of the eyelid.

What is cryosurgery?

Cryosurgery destroys tumors by freezing them with liquid nitrogen. The liquid nitrogen is applied to the tumor through a probe. Instead of a scalpel, the cryosurgeon uses a hollow metal probe that contains liquid nitrogen which is circulating constantly at a temperature of about $-196°$ Celsius ($-320°$ Fahrenheit). The tip of the probe is inserted into the tumor or applied to its surface until the tumor has frozen solidly enough to kill the cancer cells. Sometimes liquid nitrogen is sprayed on the tumor surface to freeze the cancer cells.

Does cryosurgery take place in an operating room?

Yes. You are usually taken to an operating room, and local or general anesthesia is used just as it is in other surgery. When cryosurgery begins, the cold metal probe is applied to the tumor until it turns into a ball of ice. The temperature of the tissue around the outside of the tumor is measured by insertion of needle thermocouples—a kind of miniature thermometer. The surgeon takes regular readings from the thermocouples to determine just when the tumor has been cooled to the desired temperature.

Is the tissue then allowed to thaw?

When the tissue temperature drops below $-30°$ Celsius, the probe containing the circulating liquid nitrogen is taken out. The frozen tissue is then allowed to thaw slowly, because the process of thawing helps kill tumor tissue. Usually this process of freezing and thawing is repeated twice or three times at the same operation to make sure the tumor is destroyed. Within 4 to 5 days after the surgery, the treated area begins to slough off, as the body rids itself of the dead cells. This leaves a sore which eventually heals.

When is cryosurgery used?

Cryosurgery works best for tumors that are easily seen and felt. It is sometimes used to treat tumors of the head and neck and certain skin cancers.

Is the laser being used in surgery?

Lasers are being used in many different ways by surgeons. They have been found to be much less invasive than standard surgery, allowing surgeons to reduce the use of anesthesia, control bleeding to a degree never possible before, shorten operating times, and bring fast and effective treatment to previously inaccessible areas. They are being used to treat some early-stage cancers of the larynx as well as late stage cases of cancers of the lung and esophagus.

Are there any tests that will tell which patients will respond better to cancer surgery?

Experimental techniques are being used to analyze cancer cells to predict which patients will survive with simple surgery and which will have a poor prognosis unless additional treatment is given. For instance, the technique has worked in prostate cancer with 95 percent accuracy. Investigations are also being conducted on whether it is possible to determine which patients will do well with specific chemotherapy drugs before the drugs are given.

What should I know before agreeing to an operation?

Check the list at the beginning of the chapter of questions to ask the doctor before an operation is performed. The doctor should describe the operation in terms you can understand. He should be willing to answer your questions. You should ask what other types of treatment might be used instead of an operation. You should ask the kinds of risks involved in each of the treatments. You should talk with your doctor about getting a second opinion on the treatment.

Remember, once the operation has been performed, you cannot change that decision. Check your understanding of what the doctor has told you about your condition and the treatment of it before you leave the office; repeat to him what he has told you so you are sure you understand correctly.

What if the doctor won't take the time to explain what the surgery is all about?

If you think that his explanation is not satisfactory, you should tell him. If the doctor tries to pass it off—"Don't worry about it, I'll take care of you"—and won't answer your questions, you should seriously consider switching to another doctor, especially if you are the type of person who wants to share in the decision making. Before you agree to any operation you should know what is wrong with you and how the doctor arrived at his diagnosis. The surgeon should be able to tell you what benefits you might gain from surgery and what risks you will face. Be wary if the doctor is not willing to talk about these issues.

What if I think of questions after I've left the office?

This happens to almost everybody. The best thing is to have a list of questions you want to ask before you go into the surgeon's office. Bring paper and pencil with you so you can write down the answers. Bring another person in with you so that you have moral and mental support. If you have more questions when you get home, write them down and bring them to your next appointment. Or call the surgeon and arrange a time to discuss them with him.

Does it make any difference what day of the week I go into the hospital for surgery?

You usually do not have a choice, but normally go when there is an empty bed. But there are a few general rules that you should be aware of. It is better not to go into the hospital before a weekend or a holiday. It is best if your surgery is done during the week, rather than just before a weekend, when the hospital may not be as fully staffed. It is better to go into the hospital, if possible, at the beginning of a full work week.

Is it unusual to have drains, catheters, intravenous lines, and transfusions when you return to your room after an operation?

Doctors often forget how shocking it can be to a patient and his family to discover that a tube has been connected to his nose to drain his stomach, while another has been placed in his chest to drain air, that intravenous feedings are underway, and a catheter is in place to collect urine. Ask your doctor which of these procedures you should expect. Most of them are routine for many operations and if you are prepared for them, and have prepared your family, no one will be alarmed but will accept them for the routine procedures they are.

What kind of things should I know in order to make an "informed choice" about the surgery?

There are several things you should know if you want to make an informed decision. Among them are
- The likelihood of being cured, repaired, or made better by the operation
- The risk of death or serious disability from the operation or from its complications
- The benefit and the risks of *not* having the operation
- The alternative kinds of treatment which are available
- How disabling and disfiguring the operation is going to be

Are there some operations which are considered overdone?

In a study in which surgery done at a large medical-school-affiliated hospital was compared with that done at a smaller unaffiliated suburban hospital, results showed there were some operations performed much more often at the suburban hospital than at the medical-school-affiliated one. Among the overdone operations that had a relationship to cancer were D&C, hysterectomy, thyroidectomy, and radical mastectomy. In addition, overall, there were generally more operations performed at the suburban hospital than at the medical-school-affiliated hospital. Another study showed that these same operations were also performed more often in the United States as a whole than in either England or Wales.

What can a person do to make sure the operation being performed is necessary?

One of the best ways to make sure that your operation is necessary is to obtain the opinion of at least two surgeons before you agree to an operation. It is also best to choose someone other than a surgeon as your primary-care physician.

Is surgery dangerous?

Yes, all surgery has some risk to it. How much risk is involved depends upon many factors: the kind of operation being performed, the physical condition of the patient, the skill of the surgeon and his team performing the operation (especially the skill of the anesthesiologist), and the caliber of the hospital and its facilities. Again, however, the problem is to weigh the benefits against the risks. It is certainly a subject you should discuss with the surgeon before going ahead with the operation.

What determines whether the doctor will operate or whether another type of treatment will be used?

There are several items which the doctor considers before the decision to operate is made. Among them are the following:
- Is the person in good enough physical condition to survive the operation?
- Is the operation worth the risk in terms of choice of cure?
- What is the site and the cell type of the cancer?
- Is there any indication that the cancer may have spread outside the primary site?
- Is it technically feasible to remove the primary tumor and a reasonable margin of surrounding healthy tissue?
- Can similar results be obtained from a different kind of treatment?

What determines how radical the surgery will be?

Different kinds of cancer have different tendencies to spread. The surgeon must understand the history of the kind of cancer he is operating on, the growth rate, and how the tumor spreads. He takes into consideration whether or not the lymph nodes are involved and whether there is any indication that the cancer has spread to other parts of the body. The physical condition of the patient is also a determining factor. The surgeon will remove as much of the organ involved as is reasonable along with a generous margin of apparently normal adjacent tissues and often the neighboring lymph nodes.

What does the surgeon look for during the operation?

The surgeon gathers as much information as is possible about the cancer before the operation. But in most cases, all the questions cannot be answered before the doctor actually looks at and examines the diseased area.

How can the doctor determine if the tissue is malignant during an operation?

If the type of cancer and the degree of malignancy are not definitely known before the operation, the doctor cuts out a piece of the tumor and sends it to the pathologist for a frozen-section biopsy at the beginning of the operation. When the test results come back from the laboratory—it usually takes 15 to 20 minutes—the surgeon will then decide whether or not to continue with the operation to remove the tumor.

What if the doctor finds that the tumor has spread too far to remove it?

The doctor's decision in that case will depend upon the kind of operation being done, the condition of the patient, and the history of the disease. In lung surgery, for example, if the tumor has spread too far for the doctor to remove all of it, he may leave the lung alone and close the incision. Radiation or chemotherapy will then be used. In other kinds of cancer, the doctor may remove all he can of the tumor and then treat the patient with radiation or chemotherapy.

Are there some types of cancers which respond better to surgery?

The general rule is that the smaller the tumor, and the more differentiated or mature the tumor, the better the chance that the cancer will be cured by surgery.

What kind of evaluation should be done before the operation?

There are several things which should be done before any operation for cancer is performed. All the necessary testing should be done so that the diagnosis is as certain as it can be before the operation. More problems result from going ahead with an uncertain diagnosis than from the delay for more review and consultation. This does not mean, however, that you should shop around to try to find a doctor who will tell you that you do not have the disease. Also, the surgeon should consult with the other specialists who might be carrying on further treatment after the operation has been completed.

Is there a special kind of surgeon who works with cancer patients?

There are doctors known as oncologic surgeons who specialize in treating cancer patients, although oncologic surgery is not a board-certified specialty. These doctors specialize in performing surgery on patients with cancer. Before you have an operation, you should know whether or not your doctor has had special training in cancer treatment, and you should find out about his experience in treating your particular kind of cancer. There are no easy guidelines, but one or two cases of treatment of a particular kind of cancer a year does not qualify as extensive experience. Each cancer has its own special history of how it grows and where it spreads. The choice of a surgeon is a very critical part of cancer treatment. It is very important that the doctor know how your cancer might spread so that the proper operation can be done.

What is the American Board of Surgery?

The American Board of Surgery was established in 1937 by a group of prominent American surgeons, mostly college professors of surgery. Rigorous testing, written and oral, is administered to those who qualify with full training in approved surgical residencies. The board certification is a high point in the surgeon's career, proving to his fellow surgeons and to others that he has the judgment and ability to be a specialist in surgery. While it is true that some excellent surgeons are not board-certified, those who are not should be carefully checked before you allow them to operate on you. Although the board certification is not an absolute guarantee that the surgeon is a competent one, it is one of the criteria by which you can judge a surgeon.

What does F.A.C.S. mean?

The initials F.A.C.S. mean that the surgeon is a Fellow of the American College of Surgeons, a criterion to be used in evaluating the competence of the doctor. The American College of Surgeons, though it at present requires qualification for membership similar to that of the American Board of Surgery, does not demand rigorous testing before a candidate is admitted as a Fellow. Most first-class surgeons are members of the American College of Surgeons as well as being diplomates of the American Board of Surgery, and they operate in accredited hospitals. Either of these professional recognitions is indication that the surgeon is well trained and has proved to other surgeons that he is qualified in his area of specialization.

What kinds of qualifications does a doctor need to be a general surgeon?

To be certified as a surgeon by the American Board of Surgery, the person must be a licensed doctor of medicine, have had a minimum of 4 years of residency training in general surgery, and have successfully completed a written and an oral examination given by the board. Specialized surgeons must take additional years of training to be qualified.

Do all surgeons have to pass boards of the American Board of Surgery?

No. You should know that a doctor can be a surgeon without having passed the boards. It is worth checking to see what kind of qualifications the doctor has before you agree to let him operate on you.

What is a thoracic surgeon?

A thoracic surgeon is a highly specialized doctor. He operates on patients with problems in organs in the chest area. In the cancer field, this includes lungs and the esophagus. To be certified by the American Board of Thoracic Surgery, a doctor must have been certified by the American Board of Surgery, have had 2 additional years of training in thoracic surgery, and have successfully completed the written and oral examinations given by the board.

What are the qualifications of a plastic surgeon?

To be certified by the American Board of Plastic Surgery, the person must be a licensed doctor of medicine, have 3 years of training in general surgery or prior certification by any one of several surgical specialty boards, have had a minimum of 2 additional years of training in plastic surgery, and have successfully completed the written and oral exams given by the board.

What is a proctologist?

Doctors certified by the American Board of Colon and Rectal Surgery are often called proctologists. A proctologist is especially qualified to examine and perform operations of the colon and rectal area. To be certified by the board, a person must be a licensed doctor of medicine, have had 4 years of training in general surgery, and have had 1 year of training in colon and rectal surgery. The doctor could substitute 3 years of general surgical practice and 2 years of colon-rectal surgical training or certification by the American Board of Surgery if he plans to limit his practice to colon and rectal surgery and has demonstrated special competence in that field.

What is a neurosurgeon?

A neurosurgeon is concerned with the diagnosis and treatment of diseases of the nervous system (brain, spinal cord, and nerves) and its surrounding structures. To be certified by the American Board of Neurological Surgery, he must be a licensed doctor of medicine, have had 1 year of training in general surgery, 4 years of training in neurological surgery, and 2 years of independent practice of neurological surgery, and have successfully completed examinations given by the board.

What is the difference between a neurologist and a neurosurgeon?

The neurologist has many skills in common with the neurosurgeon but is not qualified to perform operations. Your internist will probably refer you to a neurologist if you have a problem of the nervous system. If you need an operation, the neurologist will send you to a neurosurgeon. The neurologist, certified by the American Board of Psychiatry and Neurology, must be a licensed doctor of medicine, have had 3 years of specialized training in neurology, have had 2 additional years of satisfactory experience in neurology, and have successfully completed the written and oral examinations. A neurological surgeon must be qualified as a surgeon, plus having completed 4 years in neurological surgery.

Is a gynecologist also a surgeon?

The gynecologist is trained to deal with problems related to the female genital system. He is also a surgeon with the skills necessary to correct diseases of the ovaries, fallopian tubes, uterus, and vagina. Many gynecologists also perform breast operations. Some gynecologists who specialize in cancer treatment are known as gynecologic oncologists. To be certified by the American Board of Obstetrics and Gynecology, the person must be a licensed doctor of medicine, have had 3 years of residency in obstetrics and gynecology, have successfully completed the written examination of the board, have had at least 12 months of independent practice, and have successfully completed an oral examination given by the board.

Does an ophthalmologist perform surgery?

The ophthalmologist treats the diseases of the eye and surrounding structures and has had extensive training and experience in the complex and delicate surgical treatment of eye diseases. To be certified by the American Board of Ophthalmology, the person must be a licensed doctor of medicine, have had 3 years of residency and basic science courses in ophthalmology, have had 1 year of independent practice or research, and have successfully completed the written and oral examinations given by the board.

What is an orthopedic surgeon?

The orthopedic surgeon is a specialist in the diagnosis and treatment of diseases of the bones, joints, tendons, and muscles. In the cancer area, he treats a great variety of bone tumors. To be certified by the American Board of Orthopedic Surgery, the person must be a licensed doctor of medicine, have had 4 years of general surgery, 2 years in the orthopedic area, and have successfully completed an examination given by the board. There are orthopedic surgeons in the larger medical centers who have special interest in cancer. If you have bone cancer, check to see if the specialist you are going to is treating a majority of cancer cases in his practice.

What kind of doctor is an otolaryngologist?

An otolaryngologist specializes in the diseases of the ear, nose, throat, and larynx. Sometimes this doctor is called an ENT specialist. He is qualified to examine and perform surgery on these organs. To be certified by the American Board of Otolaryngology, the person must be a licensed doctor of medicine, have had 1 year of residency in general surgery, have had 3 years of residency in otolaryngology, and have successfully completed oral and written examinations administered by the board. Again, some ENT specialists are primarily involved with cancer cases.

Does a urologist perform surgery?

The urologist is a specialist in the diseases which affect the kidneys, ureters, urethra, bladder, prostate gland, and male sex organs. He is an expert in both the diagnosis of the disease and in surgical treatment in the area. To be certified by the American Board of Urology the person must be a licensed doctor of medicine, have had 2 years of post-medical training, have had 3 additional years of training in urologic surgery and 18 months of independent practice, and have successfully completed the written and oral examination given by the board.

What are some suggestions for choosing a surgeon? How can I be sure I have a competent person?

You probably have as much influence over the choice of your surgeon as of your primary physician. Check out the surgeon's credentials and check out the hospital where he will operate to make sure you are getting "one of the best." (See Chapter 2.)

Remember these basic points:

- It is best to have a surgeon who is board-certified and a Fellow of the American College of Surgeons. Although this professional accreditation is just a guide, it tells you the doctor is well trained and has proved to other surgeons that he is qualified in his area of specialization.
- It is best to choose a doctor who has performed the operation many times. Although this does not prove he is competent, as a general rule the more experienced the surgeon, the more competent he is.
- It is best to be in a hospital which has an approved cancer program sponsored by the American College of Surgeons or is part of a comprehensive cancer center or is directly affiliated with a medical school. At the very least, the hospital should be accredited by the Joint Commission on Accreditation for Hospitals (JCAH) or the American Osteopathic Association.
- It is best to choose a surgeon who is willing to answer your questions and to give you the time and attention you feel you need. Check your understanding of what the doctor has told you about the operation by repeating it to him in your own words.
- It is best, if you wish, for you to know the risks of the surgery. Ask the doctor to tell you the risks based on your particular physical condition added to the statistical

evidence (both national and local) compiled over the years for the particular operation you will have. You should also ask what the risks are if you do *not* have the surgery.

- It is best to have a surgeon who knows and can work with your general practitioner or internist. Remember it is the surgeon who will most probably be in charge of your care while you are in the hospital.
- It is best to choose a surgeon who is part of a group or who is hospital-based, since this will probably offer you the best total care both before and after the surgery.
- If you are getting a second opinion, it is best to get it outside of the particular group practice where your primary physician is located, or where the first surgeon is located.
- It is best to get a second opinion before having the surgery done.

Are there different kinds of anesthesia used in operations?

Anesthesia primarily means the loss of feeling, particularly the senses of touch and pain. You will either have a general anesthesia or anesthesia applied to a specific part of your body. Among the terms you might hear are

- General anesthesia
- Regional anesthesia
- Topical anesthesia
- Inhalation anesthesia
- Intravenous anesthesia
- Spinal anesthesia
- Epidural anesthesia

Is general anesthesia dangerous?

Although anesthesia entails some risks, it is necessary for surgery. In most cases, general anesthesia must be given, so you will be asleep during the operation. In some cases, local or regional anesthesia can be used. In general, the surgery is less risky if local anesthesia is used. If you are aged or have a history of lung problems, you may want to ask your doctor and the anesthesiologist to explore whether general anesthesia is absolutely necessary.

When is general anesthesia used?

The doctors use this term when referring to any anesthesia which puts you to sleep so treatment can be done on any part of the body. The anesthesia may be light, such as for a superficial procedure upon the skin. You may be given a deep anesthesia so that operations upon the heart, lungs, or abdomen can be carried out. The anesthesiologist aims at producing a sleep of just enough depth to permit safe surgery.

What is regional anesthesia?

Needles can be put in various parts of the body and anesthesia such as novocaine can be injected to block or temporarily deaden those nerves supplying particular parts. That means that an arm, hand, neck, or side of the face alone, for example, can be anesthetized so that the operation can be performed. The advantage of regional anesthesia is that your heart, lungs, blood pressure, and general condition are not greatly affected because only specific nerves are blocked. This means many poor-risk patients can be operated on who could not withstand a spinal or general anesthesia.

What is topical anesthesia?

An anesthesia is sprayed or painted onto a mucous membrane surface (a lubricating layer lining an internal surface or an organ). Topical anesthesia is usually used for eye, nose, and throat procedures. Sometimes it is followed by injections of novocaine or similar local anesthetics. It is also commonly used when tubes are being put into the trachea (windpipe) or esophagus (food passage).

What is inhalation anesthesia?

This is a common type of general anesthesia. You inhale an anesthetic gas which is pleasant to breathe. The gas goes from the lungs into the bloodstream to the brain, where it induces anesthesia. Inhalation anesthesia is administered through a mask which is connected to a breathing bag and then to the anesthesia machine and gas tanks.

What is intravenous anesthesia?

This type of anesthesia is injected directly into your bloodstream through a vein. You will go to sleep almost at once. Sometimes an intravenous anesthesia is given to you before you get inhalation anesthesia. After the initial needle injection into the vein of the arm or foot, a solution containing the medication is allowed to drip into the bloodstream at a controlled rate of speed.

How is spinal anesthesia given?

A long, thin needle is put into the fluid surrounding your spinal cord and the drug is injected. This drug, actually a local anesthetic, blocks pain impulses in the spinal cord. You will have no feeling in your legs and pelvis. It is the kind of anesthesia often used during childbirth.

Are there different kinds of spinal anesthesia?

Spinal anesthesias are called by different names depending on where they are being injected. A high spinal anesthesia is used when organs in the mid- or upper stomach area are being operated on. A low spinal anesthesia is used when the rectum or genital organs in the lower area are the site of the operation. A saddle block is a form of spinal anesthesia used when the rectum or genital organs are being operated on. Spinal anesthesia completely anesthetizes that part of the body served by the nerves at the site of the injection into the spinal canal. Thus you can be awake and alert and your abdomen and lower extremities can be insensitive to pain.

What are epidural and caudal anesthesia?

These are similar to spinal anesthesia except that the drug is injected into the area outside the spinal canal rather than within it. It has some advantages, especially in protecting patients against the post-spinal headaches they sometimes get with spinal anesthesia. Its big disadvantage is that a skilled operator is needed to give it and it is not as complete an anesthetic as is the spinal.

What is meant by a nerve block?

Anesthesia can be given around the boundary of an area to make a nerve block. For example, lack of feeling around your hand can be caused by putting in a local anesthetic around the nerve in your elbow—the doctor has "blocked off" the sensory nerves some distance away from the actual site of the operation. It is a regional anesthetic.

Are different kinds of painkillers ever used in combination?

The anesthesiologist has many kinds of painkillers to choose from, such as sedatives, muscle relaxants, analgesics, narcotics, and gases. Sometimes one or two are used; at other times as many as six or more might be needed. Some are pills; others must be injected. Some can be given through a face mask or by putting a tube into the windpipe. The anesthesiologist combines various painkillers and uses one drug to reinforce another so that in total a lesser amount is needed. This keeps undesirable reactions to a minimum.

Will I be awake during spinal or local anesthesia?

You can be. Or if you wish, intravenous drugs can be given to you to put you to sleep during such anesthesia.

Who gives the anesthesia?

Anesthesia should be given either by an anesthesiologist or under the direction of an anesthesiologist. An anesthesiologist is a doctor specializing in anesthesia—the physician who can choose the most appropriate type of anesthesia to be used—and during surgery is responsible for maintaining all the body's vital functions.

What is an anesthetist?

Anesthetists are not physicians. Usually they are specially trained nurses who give anesthesia under the direction of a doctor. A hospital's department of anesthesiology, besides being responsible for the administration of anesthesia during surgery, usually sets the standards for the way in which the operating room and the recovery room are run.

Does the anesthesiologist work only in the operating room?

No, he works in the recovery room as well. It is the responsibility of the anesthesiologist to alleviate pain, relieve
anxieties before the operation, increase the safety in the
operating room, provide the best conditions for the surgeon
during the actual operation, and help ensure complete and
comfortable recovery afterward. Anesthesiologists have
made it possible to operate on patients who not long ago
would have been considered poor surgical risks because
they were too young, too old, or too feeble.

What will the anesthesiologist do during the operation?

He will be present during the operation and after it, monitoring your condition. He will watch your blood pressure,
pulse rate, temperature, and the electrocardiographic recording of the action of your heart. He can administer glucose, plasma, whole blood, and various other drugs as
needed.

What are the qualifications of a board-certified anesthe-siologist?

If the anesthesiologist is certified by the American Board
of Anesthesiology, he is a licensed doctor who has completed at least 2 years of specialized training in anesthesiology plus 1 year in other medical training, and has passed
qualifying tests. If he is listed as a Fellow of the American
College of Anesthesiologists, his proficiency has been certified by the college's board of governors after qualifying
tests.

Can I decide what kind of anesthesia I would like?

The decision on the kind of anesthesia to be used should
be made by your anesthesiologist and surgeon. However,
you can discuss any feelings and desires you have, and if
you do not want a particular kind of anesthesia, you should
discuss that with the doctors. If you wish to be asleep instead of awake during the surgery (even though you will
not experience any pain) you should talk to the doctor about
that.

How does the anesthesiologist decide what kind of anesthesia to use?

It depends upon the kind of operation, what the surgeon needs during the procedure, and the physical needs of the patient.

How long can a person stay under anesthesia?

It varies depending upon the kind of drugs used and the condition of the patient. Surgeons are not under the same pressure to hurry through operations as they once were, mainly because of advances in methods of anesthesia and better monitoring of patients during surgery.

Will I meet the anesthesiologist?

In many hospitals, the anesthesiologist comes to your room the evening before your surgery. He will try to ease any anxiety you feel, explain what will happen, and answer your questions. He will also ask you some questions, such as whether you have any allergies, whether you are sensitive to any drugs, and whether you have any illnesses other than the one for which you are being operated on. He might ask you whether you have ever had anesthesia before and whether you had ill effects from it. He will want to know about any past history of liver or kidney disease, since these organs eliminate certain anesthetic agents from the body. He needs to know what medications you are taking because anesthetics could cause dangerous reactions when combined with a number of other drugs, particularly tranquilizers, antidepressants, sedatives, and drugs used to lower blood pressure. The anesthesiologist will get some of this information from your medical history and other available medical records as well as by consulting with your surgeon.

Are there any special questions I should ask him if he comes to visit me before the operation?

You might want to know things such as the drugs he is planning to use, what discomfort, if any, you will have, when you will go to sleep, and when you will wake up consciously. If you have a special request—such as wanting to be asleep during a "minor" procedure that is ordinarily performed with a local anesthetic, or not wanting a spinal anesthetic—be sure to talk with him about it. The anesthesiologist will often do what you want if it is medically sound. Be sure you tell the anesthesiologist about all your allergies, whether they are drug-related or not.

How do I know that the doctor will not start the operation when I can still feel pain?

One of the jobs of the anesthesiologist is to make sure that you can feel no pain. He will conduct tests to make sure that before any surgery begins, you cannot feel the pain.

Will I have any medication the night before the operation?

It depends. The doctor might order tablets or injections the night before your surgery to make sure you have a good night's rest. If you are a heavy smoker or drinker, the doctor may tell you to stop for several days before the operation because tobacco and alcohol can cause complications with the anesthesia both during and after the operation.

Is anesthesia painful?

Not with today's procedures. Probably an hour or so before the operation, you will be given something to make you drowsy and relaxed. You may also be given medication to dry up mucous and salivary-gland secretions, which will help in the anesthesia. The anesthesia will be given in the operating room. Anesthesia, even types which were once painful, is now an almost painless procedure.

How will the anesthesia be injected into me?

After you reach surgery, the anesthesiologist will probably insert an intravenous (IV) needle into you so that any drugs which need to be used during the operation can easily be injected. If you are to be asleep during the operation, a drug will be injected and within seconds you will be sleeping. If a mask is to be used or an endotracheal tube is to be inserted, this will be done after you are asleep so you will not be aware of it. Sometimes you will be given a short-acting muscle relaxant to make it easier to pass a tube.

Will the IV needle be used for drugs other than the anesthetic?

It depends upon the operation. If you need additional drugs, these can easily be put in through the intravenous needle. The needle is joined to a length of flexible tubing attached to a bottle hanging over the operating table. The drops of whatever drug are needed, when released into the tube, will go immediately into the bloodstream.

What kinds of tests are done before the operation?

In cancer-related operations, many tests are performed to make as complete a diagnosis as possible. These tests are described in Chapter 4 and also in the chapters which discuss the particular kinds of cancer. There are some general tests which are performed for all operations. These include the following:

- Blood sample to test for hemoglobin (oxygen-carrying pigment of blood) to discover anemia; count of red and white blood cells; sometimes a routine test for syphilis
- Blood-type test if surgeon feels there is the slightest chance of need for blood transfusion
- Urine analysis for presence of sugar, blood, pus cells, crystals, and other materials

Is it important for me to know what blood type I am?

You should know your blood type, especially if it is a rare one. Ask your doctor and carry this information with you. If you do not know, blood types are quickly and easily determined in a laboratory by a simple slide or tube test.

What are the blood types?

Most people in the United States have either O Positive blood or A Positive blood. The frequency of the various blood types varies geographically and by racial or ethnic groups. In the United States whites are more likely than blacks to have type A blood, and blacks are more likely to have type B blood. Both races have about the same frequency of type O and type AB. This table shows the overall blood-type frequencies in the United States:

Blood Type	Rh Factor	Percent of the Population
O	Positive	39
A	Positive	35
B	Positive	9
O	Negative	6
A	Negative	5
AB	Positive	4
B	Negative	1.5
AB	Negative	0.5

Are there special procedures which are done the night before the operation?

Any of the following procedures may be done:

* *Shaving:* Since the skin and hair hide organisms which can cause infections, a wide area is usually shaved and cleansed before the operation. Usually a nurse or orderly will shave and clean with antiseptic an area larger than the proposed incision; skin preparation may start as much as 24 hours before the operation.
* *Enema:* Because there may be temporary interference with normal functioning of the intestines after some kinds of surgery and the bowels may not move for several days, an enema may be given the night before the operation to clear out the bowel.
* *Fasting:* You will usually not be allowed to eat or drink for about 12 hours before the operation so that it can be done on an empty stomach. You will probably be told to have a light evening meal and then nothing by mouth after midnight the night before surgery.
* *Sedatives:* Usually you will be given a sleeping pill so that you will have a good night's sleep before the operation. An hour or two before you go to the operating room an injection is usually given so that you will be in a calm, semiconscious state.
* *Stomach tubes:* If you are having an operation in the stomach area, a tube is usually inserted through the nose into the stomach so that the stomach and bowels will be empty and free of fluids and gas. Sometimes this is done the night before or in the morning. It is usually left in place throughout the operation.

- *Urinary catheter:* For some operations, especially those in the pelvic and bladder area, a catheter is inserted so that the bladder will be empty. This may be done in your room or in the operating room.
- *Blood transfusions:* Depending upon the operation and your own condition, you may receive a transfusion of blood before the operation. In many cases, blood is given before, during, and/or after the operation. Sometimes plasma is given instead of whole blood.

Are intravenous feedings usually a part of surgery?

The bottle of clear fluid is usually a part of both the pre-operative (before the operation) and postoperative (after the operation) procedures. Doctors have found that surgery is much safer when carried out on patients with normal blood chemistry. Various substances such as water, salt, sugar, protein, potassium, calcium, and vitamins can be given to the patient via the intravenous route, through the veins of the arms and legs, to substitute for the solid food which you cannot have until normal digestive processes are reestablished. (You will hear the term *IV*, which is the shorthand for *intravenous*.) It is not unusual for intravenous treatments to be continued for several days after a serious procedure has been performed.

What is meant by being "prepped" for an operation?

To ensure a perfectly sterile operation, several steps are taken. Usually a wide area around where the incision is to be made is shaved. The area is first washed with an antiseptic and all body hair is removed. The entire abdomen, genital area, and upper legs are often shaved for an abdominal procedure. For a brain operation, the head is shaved.

Why is a catheter needed for a surgical operation?

A catheter, a narrow tube which is inserted through the urethra to the bladder, is sometimes used during surgery to drain off urine. It is usually put in place before you are brought up to surgery. Thanks to modern materials, the flexibility of the catheter now permits it to be inserted with little or no discomfort.

What does the doctor mean when he says he'll write a "stat order"?

The medical profession uses the term *stat* fairly frequently and in several contexts. The word comes from the Latin *statim*, meaning "immediate" or "rush." A stat order is simply a request for fast service.

Who is usually in the operating room during the surgery?

Several people help with any operation, no matter how minor. The team, depending upon the extent of the operation, may be composed of:
* Surgeon
* One to three assistant surgeons, depending on the position, nature, complexity, or technical peculiarities (even some minor procedures require more than one pair of hands)
* Anesthesiologist or anesthetist
* Chief operating room nurse, who is the overall supervisor
* Nurse in charge of surgical supply
* Scrub or suture nurse, who handles instruments
* Circulating or chase nurse, who gets additional supplies and is responsible for the sponge counts (sponges are layered gauze pads used to blot blood so the surgeon can see)
* Additional persons, as needed, such as a cardiologist during a heart operation

How are stomach tubes inserted?

With the head tipped back, a thin tube is inserted in the nostril and pushed up and backward. You then swallow and the tube slides smoothly into the throat and to the stomach. Sometimes some kind of anesthetic is given when the tube is inserted. The tube is usually left in place throughout the operation and sometimes for a number of days after it to help suction off fluid and gas.

Does the length of time I spend in the operating room indicate the seriousness of the operation?

It depends upon the individual case. There are several situations which can make your time in the operating room longer but have no bearing on your own operation. For instance:

* The patient is sent for some time in advance of the actual operation.
* The anesthesiologist can make additional preparations that last 30 minutes or even an hour.
* The surgeon can take longer than he expected on the operation before yours, thus starting on your operation later than scheduled.
* You could spend more time than anticipated in the recovery room.

Your family and friends should never judge the length or seriousness of an operation by the amount of time you spend in the operating room.

Will I need to go into the recovery room after my operation?

Yes, it is the usual procedure so that you can be watched and checked by a medical team until you awaken. The recovery room has equipment for monitoring your heart action and respirators for assisting you to breathe if you need them. You can get intravenous fluids and blood in the recovery room. Normally the recovery room is run by a physician anesthesiologist so that you can be monitored when you wake up from the anesthesia. Respiration therapists will probably help you to cough and inflate your lungs as soon as you wake up. You may spend several hours or even days in the recovery room.

What if I have my operation late in the day—will I still go to the recovery room?

It depends upon the hospital. Some will take you to the intensive-care unit rather than the recovery room if you are on the afternoon surgical schedule, because in some hospitals the night-patient load in recovery rooms doesn't warrant maintaining a staff through the night.

How long will it take for the anesthesia to wear off after the operation?

Once the operation is finished, it can take anywhere from minutes to hours before you wake up. It depends upon the kind of anesthesia you are given and the dose. If you have had local, regional, or spinal anesthesia, it will usually wear off within 1 to 3 hours after the operation.

Will things seem hazy as I come out of the anesthesia?

Sometimes they do. Voices may seem to be coming from a long way off. You may not hear them distinctly. People may seem to be moving differently from the way you think they should. Vision, hearing, and sense of balance can all be affected by anesthesia, and it takes time for the effects to wear off.

Will I be able to get painkilling drugs after the operation if I need them?

You may experience some pain as you become fully conscious. There are many painkilling drugs which can be used with perfect safety. The doctor will be trying to balance your immediate comfort with your recovery. Some of the drugs tend to slow up vital functions. Since it is important after an operation that your vital functions get back to normal as quickly as possible, you may be asked to put up with some pain to speed your recovery. But if you are feeling a substantial degree of pain, be sure that your nurse and your doctor know about it. Try to keep your reports as factual as possible.

What are the general procedures that are followed after an operation?

It depends upon your doctor, the hospital, the operation performed, and your own physical condition. You will usually spend some time in the recovery room. Then, some of the following common procedures will probably be followed:

- *Bedrest:* You will most probably spend some time lying flat in bed. After your recovery from the anesthesia, you will be encouraged to change your position and move your legs often. This is to stimulate your circulation and make you breathe deeply so you will not get blood clots or pneumonia.
- *Getting out of bed:* Usually you will be made to get out of bed and walk a little the day after the operation with most major types of surgery, although sometimes it will

be a few days or even a week or longer. Again, it depends upon many factors. Getting out of bed as soon as possible speeds your recovery and minimizes complications of the operation.

* *Eating and drinking:* Unless you have had surgery of the stomach or intestinal tract, you usually will be given sips of water or tea within a few hours after your operation and will be allowed a bland diet the next day. Stomach and intestinal-tract patients usually don't eat or drink for anywhere from 48 to 72 hours.
* *Gas or urinary problems:* If you are having trouble with stomach gas, you will be encouraged to move about and walk as much as you are able. If the problem persists, a tube may be put through your nose and into your stomach for 24 hours. The doctor may also order pain medication. If you have trouble urinating, you can be given a medication to stimulate natural voiding. If the problem continues, you may have a catheter inserted to empty the bladder. The ability to urinate spontaneously returns usually within a week's time.
* *Pain:* If you have pain, your doctor may prescribe a pain medication. Many times pains involved with abdominal surgery are gas pains.
* *Other:* Depending on the operation and your condition, the doctor may order antibiotic drugs, intravenous fluids and medications, blood transfusions, and enemas.

Are there any common problems I can expect from my operation?

Side effects from operations vary widely, again depending upon the operation and your own condition. Many people never experience any serious problems. However, side effects can include any of the following:

* *Nausea and vomiting* due to the anesthetic, drugs, or the operation. The doctor may not allow you to eat or drink for 24 hours or may pass a tube into your stomach.
* *Gas pains* sometimes follow stomach operations. They usually disappear in a few days. Sometimes, for severe cases, a tube is inserted in the rectum or in the stomach. Usually by the third day, the bowel begins to function normally.

- *Soreness* in the wound area. Medication can be ordered.
- *Dizziness and weakness*, if they occur, usually disappear within a week or two without treatment.
- *Headaches* may occur when spinal anesthesia is used. The doctor may order a special medication plus lots of fluids. The headaches may last a week or two.
- *Tiredness.* Many people complain that they have little energy and feel like sleeping. It is important for you to nap when you feel tired and to limit visitors if you do not feel up to seeing people.

What is second-look surgery?

Though it sounds as if the doctor needs a second look because there was something wrong with the first, second-look surgery is an accepted procedure in a number of surgical circumstances, such as for recurrent disease, assessment of tumor in patients who have completed an initial course of treatment to determine the status of the tumor, to remove any residual tumor, or to determine what treatment should be instituted to give the patient a chance for cure. As with any surgical procedure, you should be certain to get a full explanation of the need for surgery before undergoing the procedure.

How can I be sure I am getting the right medication in the hospital?

If your doctor orders medicines for you on a regular basis, learn to recognize the ones he has prescribed, and if an unfamiliar capsule or liquid is offered to you, ask about it.

What will the nurses be checking me for during the first few days after my operation?

They will be checking your general color and appearance and your blood pressure, pulse, temperature, and rate of breathing. They will observe if your reflexes are getting back to normal and if you are swallowing properly. They'll come in to give you your medication and other things you may need. They will make you move in your bed, sit up, dangle your legs over the side of the bed, or walk—depending upon what your doctor has ordered for you. They will be checking for proper elimination of both urine and

stool. For the first few times after the operation, they will
help you get out of bed.

Why is deep breathing important?

It is important that you begin deep breathing early after an
operation to prevent pneumonia and other complications.
If your breathing is shallow, the air sacs around the edges
of your lungs don't fill out. You may be made to blow into
a special machine to help with your deep breathing.

What if I have soreness around my incision?

There is some soreness generally around an incision, but
if there is unusual soreness let your doctor or nurse know
at once.

When will the dressings be changed?

The time for changing dressings varies widely depending
upon the operation. Usually if the wound is clean without
a drain it is left alone until the doctor takes out the stitches.
Draining wounds or those which become infected might
need to be changed every day. If it is the kind which would
be painful, you may get a pain-relieving medication before
the dressing is changed.

When will the stitches be taken out?

They are usually taken out from the sixth to the tenth day,
depending on where the operation is. If it is in an area
where there is tension on it or if it is not healing firmly, the
stitches will be left in for a longer time. Sometimes metal
clips are used instead of sutures. These are usually taken
out on the fourth to sixth day.

The nurse does not seem to want to answer my questions. What should I do?

It depends upon the kinds of questions you are asking.
There are some questions which the nurse cannot answer.
But you should realize that the nurse in the hospital (and
in the doctor's and radiation therapist's offices) is one of
your best sources of information. If she can't answer the
questions herself, she might be able to get you the answers.
It is helpful to write down your questions so that when you

do see the doctor you can ask those that the nurse has not been able to answer for you.

What does surgery for cancer cost?

Surgery costs vary greatly from one area of the country to another, from one doctor to another, and from operation to operation. The one rule you should follow is to have a full and frank discussion of the costs of surgery before you go into the hospital. Extra charges may be made by the hospital for such items as x-rays, special drugs, medications and treatments, blood transfusions, anesthesia, the use of the operating room, the use of laboratory facilities, fees for consultations and/or second opinions while hospitalized, etc.

chapter 7

Radiation

Radiation therapy is the second most common treatment for cancer, following surgery. The National Cancer Institute estimates that more than half of all cancer patients receive radiation treatment sometime during the course of their illness.

Questions to Ask Your Doctor

- Exactly what type of radiation treatment will I be getting?
- Who will be responsible for my radiation treatment?
- If I have questions about my radiation treatment whom should I ask?
- Can I continue to work during these treatments?
- Is there a more convenient place where my treatments can be given?
- How long will it take for each treatment? For the whole series?
- What side effects can I expect?
- What should I do if these side effects occur?
- What side effects should I report to the doctor?
- How much will it cost?
- How much of a risk is involved?
- What is the alternative?
- What if I don't have this treatment at all?

Radiation Terminology

Type	Definition	Use	Other Terms
External beam	Machine delivers x-rays or gamma rays to tumor on or in patient's body. Machine usually some distance from patient's body. Neutron beam is a new experimental type of external-beam therapy.	Most frequently used kind of radiation	X-ray machine, linear accelerator, cobalt machine, superficial x-ray, orthovoltage machine, supervoltage equipment, megavoltage machine, cobalt 60 machine, betatrons, cobalt therapy
Internal radiation (radium implant)	Radioactive material such as radium placed directly into or on area to be treated. It is either sealed in a container and inserted into a body cavity or given orally or injected with a syringe.	Breast, vagina, bladder, mouth, tongue, prostate, thyroid	Radioactive cesium, radium needles, radium seeds, radioactive iodine, liquid radioactive gold, radioactive phosphorus, radium, iridium, interstitial implant, intracavitary implant, needle implant

Do I have a choice as to where I will have my radiation treatments?

Usually the doctor will advise you of where your radiation treatments will be given. It is a good idea for you to have a frank discussion with him about why he advises a specific radiotherapy department or a specific radiotherapist. You may want to explore whether it would be advantageous for you to use a large medical center versus a small hospital closer to home. You must weigh for yourself the advantages of convenience versus the technology and expertise a larger medical center usually has to offer. Radiology is a science, in which many recent advances have been made both in technology and in application, and the radiologist will be playing an important part in your treatment.

Is radiation therapy used alone?

Yes, it can be used alone. However, many treatments for cancer today include more than one form of therapy, and radiation is often used in combination with surgery or chemotherapy.

Is radiation therapy called by any other names?

You will hear it referred to by many other terms, including *radiotherapy, radiology, x-ray therapy, x-ray treatment, irradiation, radiation treatment, and cobalt treatment.*

What is radiation treatment?

Radiation treatment consists of using x-rays, at high levels— tens of thousands of times the amount used to produce a chest x-ray—to destroy the ability of cells to grow and divide. Both normal cells and diseased cells are affected, but most normal cells are able to recover quickly.

Is there more than one type of radiation treatment?

Radiation treatment is usually divided into two basic kinds: external-beam radiation and internal radiation.

What is external-beam radiation?

When external-beam radiation is used, a machine directs x-rays or gamma rays to a tumor on or in the patient's body. The machine is usually some distance from the patient.

What is internal radiation?

It is a procedure in which the physician places some radioactive material such as radium directly into or on the area to be treated. Sometimes, this is called a radium implant, brachytherapy, or interstitial or intracavitary radiation. Usually the radioactive materials are put into small metal tubes or needles which are then placed surgically within or near the cancerous tissue. The tubes or needles are usually removed after the required radiation dose has been given. Sometimes internal radiation is used alone; other times it is used in addition to external-beam radiation.

What are the categories of radiation treatment?

Again, as in surgery, there are three general categories: primary or curative treatment, palliative treatment for control of symptoms (not expected to cure), and treatment used as an adjuvant to other therapies.

What is curative radiation?

Curative radiation is so called when radiation is being used as the primary treatment to cure the cancer. It is the treatment of choice, for example, for some stages of Hodgkin's disease and of cervical, skin, and head and neck cancers.

When does the doctor choose radiation as a curative treatment rather than surgery?

The doctor usually chooses curative radiation instead of surgery when
- The tumor is the type that is especially susceptible to destruction by radiation.
- Radiation has as good a chance of success as surgery but will preserve function and appearance better than surgery will.
- The tumor is impossible to reach by surgery without destroying vital tissues, as in the case of some brain cancers.
- Radiation is clearly the treatment of choice in tumors of the lymph system such as in Hodgkin's disease and in some lymphomas.

What is palliative radiation?

Palliative radiation is a treatment that is not used to cure the patient but to treat other symptoms, such as to relieve pain or to shrink tumors.

How is palliative radiation used to relieve pain?

Sometimes radiation is used to relieve pain caused by tumors pressing on vital organs. By shrinking metastatic tumors, for example, radiation can relieve the pressure placed upon nearby structures, especially nerves. Radiation can also relieve headaches resulting from a metastatic tumor in the brain. In addition, it may also relieve other symptoms due to brain metastases, such as nausea, vomiting, and double vision. For some persons with bone metastases, if the bone where the tumor is growing is a weight-bearing bone (such as leg bone), radiotherapy may be used to avoid a fracture caused because part of the bone has been weakened or destroyed by the tumor growth.

How is radiation used to relieve tumors blocking other bodily functions?

It may be necessary to shrink a tumor that is blocking a passageway in the body, such as a large blood vessel, the breathing tube, the swallowing tube, or the intestines. Some tumors ulcerate and bleed. Radiotherapy can sometimes shrink these tumors and occasionally stop the bleeding.

When is radiation used as an adjuvant treatment?

Radiation is used as an adjuvant treatment when chemotherapy or surgery is the treatment of choice and radiation is being used in addition, with the hope of curing the patient or giving the patient a long disease-free survival. Radiation is used as a preventive measure in those cancers where research has shown that although they cannot be seen on the microscope, cancer cells may have already spread to other parts of the body. Sometimes, radiation is used after surgery if the operation was unable to take out all of the tumor or if the doctor feels that the tumor has spread to other parts of the body. It is also sometimes used before surgery to reduce the size of the tumor so it will be easier to remove. Or it can be used to treat the lymph-node area to which a cancer drains when it is possible to operate on the tumor itself but not on the draining nodes.

How does radiation treatment actually affect the cells?

X-ray treatments actually injure the cancer cells so they can no longer continue to divide or multiply. With each radiation treatment, more and more of the cancer cells die. The tumor shrinks because the dead cells are broken down, carried away by the bloodstream, and excreted by the body.

Isn't radiation only for people who have advanced cancer?

No. That is not true. Of those cancers treatable by surgery, radiation was originally used after the operation to get rid of any cancer cells the surgeons had left behind. At that time, it was difficult to treat the cancer cells without also destroying a great number of normal cells. Thanks to new technology, the use of radiation treatment has changed dramatically. The new machines give off rays which are capable of penetrating deeply into the body tissue. They give high doses of radiation to the tumor area with less injury to the surrounding tissue. Therefore, radiation today is used for primary treatment as well as in combination with other treatments for many stages of disease.

What is a cancer which is radiosensitive?

A radiosensitive cancer is susceptible to destruction by radiation.

What is a cancer which is radioresistant?

This means that the cancer, because of the type of cells from which it originates, is not usually destroyed by radiation that is within a dose range safe to surrounding tissues. Since some cancers are known to be radioresistant, radiation treatment is not used for them.

What is a tumor which is not amenable to radiation therapy?

This means that the cancer, either because of its location, size, or previous treatment, would not best be treated by radiation. Conventional radiotherapy would harm overlying vital organs, or the tumor may not be radiosensitive. Thus some other kind of treatment would be used.

What is localized radiation?

Localized radiation is radiation that is being used to treat one specific site. Sometimes radiation is given to a number of different sites or areas. Sometimes whole-body radiation is used, indicating that the radiation is delivered to the entire body.

Why isn't radiation treatment used for every cancer patient?

Each kind of tissue, each kind of cancer, and each patient has a different sensitivity to the effects of radiation. Some kinds of radiation treatment work better for some cancers than others. Different cancers spread and grow in different ways. The general theory in using radiation is that the radiation dose must be large enough to destroy the cancer cells but not so great as to seriously damage surrounding normal tissues. Sometimes the dose required to kill the cancer would also do permanent damage to the surrounding normal tissue. This is the major limitation in the use of x-rays and radium in the treatment of cancer.

After an operation, when is radiation therapy started?

If indicated, radiation therapy can be started as early as a few days after surgery, or when the wound has healed, usually by 6 weeks. Of course, this schedule varies depending upon the condition of the patient, the extent of the operation, the reason for the radiation treatments, and other factors.

Is radiation ever used both before and after an operation?

Sometimes, in special cases, radiation is done both before and after the operation. This is called the "sandwich" technique.

Is radiation therapy ever used during an operation?

This technique, called intraoperative radiation therapy, is being used at some cancer centers and major hospitals. The surgery is started, and the patient is given direct radiation therapy after the tumor is exposed or taken out. The operation is then completed. Intraoperative radiation therapy can deliver a higher dose of radiation to the tumor itself because surrounding organs sensitive to radiation, such as the skin, intestines, and liver, can be held aside or shielded. The exposed tumor can also be felt or seen directly, rather than viewed on a scan or x-ray. Intraoperative radiation therapy is being used on cancers for which the usual treatment is not possible or effective, such as in some cancers of the pancreas, colon-rectum, and cervix. There is more information about investigational treatments in Chapter 9.

Is hyperthermia ever used with radiation therapy?

Some centers are, on an experimental basis, employing hyperthermia—the use of heat on parts or all of the body—before radiation therapy. The theory being tested is whether heating the tumor before radiation is given will make the radiation more effective. Chemicals are also being tested which may make cancer cells more sensitive to heat. Experimental tests are also underway using iodine to make tumors more sensitive to radiation therapy.

Why does radiation work for some patients and not for others?

For many different reasons. Sometimes the tumor is too large for the radiation to have any real effect. Or it may be a tumor which for some reason is resisting the radiation. Or the cancer may have already spread too far for the radiation to be effective.

Is radiation therapy a new field?

Although radiation therapy is not a new field, research and improved technology especially in the past 15 years has made it a major treatment area for cancer. It is an area which is rapidly growing and changing. Also, since information about other kinds of cancer treatment is also new and expanding, new relationships are being found between the use of radiation treatment and the other treatments.

X-rays were discovered in 1895, and radium was discovered in 1898. Within a few years after that, scientists found that x-rays were capable of damaging body tissue. Subsequently researchers uncovered the curious fact that x-rays and radium did more damage to cancerous tissue than to normal, healthy tissue. The intricate details of the effects of these powerful radiations on living cells, especially cancer cells, are still being studied.

Is radiation more successful with some cancers than with others?

Yes, there are some cancers where radiation has been most successful. Hodgkin's disease and some lymphomas respond well to radiation, especially when the disease is diagnosed and treated in the early stages. Certain cancers of the head and neck and cancer of the uterine cervix have had good cure records with radiation. Early cancers of the bladder, prostate, and skin and certain brain and eye tumors, and some bone tumors (particularly if surgery is not done) respond well to radiation. For some cancers, radiation is better than surgery because, besides having a high potential for cure, it causes little or no loss of function in the irradiated part. Psychologically it is better for some patients, since their appearance is not changed as it might be with surgery.

What if a person is getting radiation to one area of the body but the cancer continues to spread in other areas? Does that mean that radiation is useless?

Whether the radiation is useless depends upon three factors: the kind of cancer the person has, the exact area being treated, and whether the treatment is given to cure the disease or to relieve other symptoms. Some kinds of cancer continue to grow for a short time during radiation, but then they shrink or sometimes disappear altogether. Sometimes the cancer will continue to grow outside the area being treated (known as the field of treatment) even while it is shrinking inside the field of treatment. Sometimes the radiation makes the person feel better or experience less pain even if the cancer continues to grow elsewhere. There are cases where a particular tumor in a particular person proves not to respond to the radiation treatment. Of course, this cannot be predicted before the treatment starts. In these instances, other forms of cancer therapy, such as drug treatment, are often considered.

What kinds of machines are used for radiation treatment?

Several types of machines with different characteristics are used for giving radiation externally, but usually either an x-ray machine or a cobalt machine is used.

What is the difference between an x-ray machine and a cobalt machine?

Both the x-ray machine (such as a linear accelerator) and the cobalt machine use high-energy beams to destroy the tumor tissue. Both are usually referred to as x-ray machines. However, the beams are produced by different energy sources. The linear accelerator produces electromagnetic waves; the machine must be turned on for it to change the electricity into high-energy beams. The cobalt machine uses a metal (cobalt) which has been made radioactive. This is also called a radioactive isotope. The rays are beamed to the body from a source. The radioactive material is enclosed in a shielded unit and the beams are emitted through a shutter. In other words, the cobalt machine is "turned on" all the time. When the cobalt is moved into position in front of a window in the machine, the radioactive beam can be used. How far the beams penetrate in both instances depends on the speed at which the electrons hit the target; methods have been developed to accelerate the speeds by means of electromagnetic boosts.

How is the amount of energy of x-rays measured?

It is measured in electron volts (eV). The low energies are measured in thousands of electron volts, called kilovolts (KeV). The high energies are measured in millions of electron volts, called megavolts (MeV).

What is meant by superficial x-ray or orthovoltage equipment?

This equipment gives out low-energy rays; usually any machine with energy less than 1 megavolt (1 million electron volts) is called an orthovoltage machine. This machine gives radiation to the surface of the skin; the dose which can be delivered to a tumor which lies at any depth beneath the skin is limited by the tolerance of the skin to radiation. This type of equipment has limited use today; usually it is used only for skin cancer.

What is meant by supervoltage or megavoltage equipment?

This term is usually used to describe any machine with energy greater than 1 million electron volts or 1 megavolt. These machines give the maximum dose beneath the skin rather than on it. Therefore much higher doses of radiation can be given to deep-lying tumors. Some examples of supervoltage machines are linear accelerators, cobalt 60 machines, and betatrons. Megavoltage radiation can direct a more precise, intense beam to a tiny target area in the body with less scattering of radiation to surrounding normal tissue and less skin damage.

What do people mean when they say they are getting cobalt treatments or radium treatments?

Many terms such as these are used imprecisely by the public. Actually cobalt is a radioactive material that is usually used in supervoltage machines as a source of radiation. Often people say they are getting "cobalt therapy" when they are really getting external-beam treatment with a supervoltage machine. Radium is a radioactive material which is placed inside the patient and then taken out after a specific period of time. Many times, however, people say they are getting "radium treatment" when they really are getting x-ray or radiation treatments with an external beam.

What is particle-beam radiotherapy?

This is a new, experimental kind of treatment. Sources of high-energy radiation in the form of neutrons, protons, and helium and heavy ions have been developed and are being evaluated in studies supported by the National Cancer Institute. This therapy uses high-LET (linear energy transfer) particle radiation and requires a cyclotron, linear accelerator, or synchrotron to produce the particle beam and a beam application system to direct the radiation to the tumor. Experimental treatment is being conducted in several centers in the United States and abroad.

Will my regular doctor be giving the radiation treatment?

No. This is a specialized field, requiring treatment from a doctor especially trained in therapeutic radiation. Your doctor will refer you to a specialist who can be called by several names: therapeutic radiologist, radiation therapist, radiotherapist, or radiation oncologist. We will be using the term *radiation therapist* when referring to the physician who specializes in treating the cancer patient with radiotherapy.

What does a radiation therapist do?

The radiation therapist will thoroughly examine you and all the pertinent information about your case to decide whether or not radiation treatment would be of benefit to you. If you are to have radiation treatment, the therapist will decide what treatment should be used and supervise its administration. The radiation therapist is well informed about the natural history of cancer and when radiation can be used in treatment. He carefully evaluates patients before treatment begins and at intervals during the course of the treatment to see whether the treatment is working. He knows how much radiation is enough to produce the best results while causing the least amount of damage to the normal organs near the tumor; he knows how much radiation is necessary for treating each kind of tumor as well as what radiation each normal organ can tolerate. He must be able to select the kind of radioactive energy best suited for the treatment of each case and to decide how to deliver it.

Is there a difference between a diagnostic radiologist and a radiation therapist?

Yes. The diagnostic radiologist is a specialist in interpreting x-rays. The radiation therapist is primarily a skilled clinical oncologist who is also an expert in the delivery of radiation therapy. The American Board of Radiology gives separate certification to these specialties.

Does the radiation therapist have special training?

To be certified by the American Board of Radiology, the person must have graduated from an approved medical school, have had 4 years of postgraduate training (3 in pathology, nuclear radiology, and therapeutic radiology), and have successfully completed the written and oral examinations given by the board. Thus this physician has had several years of additional specialized training in the treatment of human disease with radiation.

What other kinds of health professionals are on the radiation-therapy team?

It varies from place to place. But there are many other people on whom the radiation therapist depends to help and support him in his work. The *radiation physicist* has had extensive training in planning treatments designed to deliver the desired doses of radiation; the *dosimetrist* is especially trained in calculating the doses to plan the treatment; the *radiation-therapy technologist* is trained in a certified school of radiation-therapy technology and has had additional hospital training and experience; the *radiation-therapy nurse* has specialized knowledge in the care of cancer patients receiving radiation.

What does the radiation therapist need to know about me before treatment starts?

The radiation therapist needs to have a complete understanding of you and your medical problem in order to determine whether radiation treatments should be used and to plan the best method of delivering those treatments. You will probably be referred to the radiation therapist by your original doctor, who will have already discussed your particular problem with him. He will take a careful history, give you a physical examination, review all your previous records, such as x-ray films, pathology slides, and hospital records. You may also require additional special tests before your radiation treatment can be decided upon.

Will I have my first treatment at my first appointment with the radiation therapist?

In many cases you will not. The doctor must first get all the information he needs about your case. Then the treatment plan must be set up. Remember that the treatment plan is different for each patient, so it may take several visits to the radiation therapist before your treatment actually begins. Timing depends on the kind of cancer you have, the kind of treatments you have already had, the stage of your particular disease, your physical condition, and how complicated your treatment plan will be.

How is the dose of radiation decided on?

The dose varies with the size of the tumor, the extent of the tumor, the tumor type and grade, and its response to radiation therapy. Very complex calculations are needed to determine the dosage and timing of treatments. Sometimes a computer and three-dimension visualizing techniques are used to help determine the best method of delivering the amount of radiation that is needed. Often a contour of the part of the body to be treated is made to help in planning. This can be done with a ribbon of plastic, lead wire, or some other device.

Why is the radiation therapy sometimes given from different angles?

One way of giving the maximum amount of radiation to the tumor and the minimum amount to normal tissue is by aiming radiation beams at the tumor from two or more positions. The patient or the machine is rotated; the patient and machine are placed so that the beams meet each other where the tumor is located. The tumor thus gets a high enough dose of radiation to be destroyed but normal tissues escape with minimum radiation effects since the beams take different pathways to reach the tumor.

How does the doctor decide exactly where to apply the radiation?

Since the area to be treated must be located with extreme precision, many different devices can be used to pinpoint the location. You may have to have a number of x-ray films of the area taken either with a special x-ray unit (called a simulator) or with the treatment machine itself. Sometimes radioactive isotopes, ultrasound equipment, and other specialized diagnostic apparatus may be used to locate the exact area. Since many tumors are located deep inside the body, when their exact location in relation to the outside surface of your body is found, it is marked. This is called your "treatment port," the exact place on your body where the high-energy rays will be aimed. Finding your treatment port may take from half an hour to two hours.

Once the spot is found, how is it marked?

Generally, using your x-rays as a guide and with you lying or sitting on the treatment couch or chair, the radiation therapist marks the exact area to be treated on your skin with indelible ink. Sometimes purple ink is used, sometimes blue or red. Some therapists use magic markers. Sometimes a few small black india ink dots are used to permanently indicate the treatment area. It is important that the spots remain so that the beam can be aimed at the same spot each time. Sometimes bands or casts of plaster of paris or plastic are used to secure you in a particular position so that treatments can be delivered precisely and consistently each time you come in.

Will my normal cells be affected by radiation?

All cells are affected by the radiation, whether they are normal or malignant. The normal tissues have a greater capacity to recover from the damage induced by the radiation than do the cancer cells. The radiation therapist plans the treatment so that normal tissues are irradiated as little as possible. He also determines areas which are to be shielded and protected from the radiation.

Can I wear my own clothes while I am having a radiation treatment?

It depends upon where on the body the treatment is being given. You will probably have to undress, so wear clothing that is easy to get on and off. You might even want to bring your own robe. Some patients wear old underthings because sometimes the colored ink used to mark the spot comes off.

What safety devices are used to protect me from unnecessary radiation?

There are many safeguards used to protect you from unnecessary radiation to the parts of your body which do not need treatment. All the machines are shielded so that the significant radiation is only applied to a specific area. The treatment field is usually lit with a light that will outline the surface through which the radiation will pass; a series of safeguards in the machine limits the radiation to this lighted area of your body. Shields, usually lead blocks, are placed on special trays suspended from the machine to shield small areas of your body not needing treatment.

What parts of the body are covered by the shields?

This depends upon where the radiation is being given. Lead casts and blocks or plastic molds are custom-made based on your own anatomy and are used to protect the vital organs and to maintain the proper treatment position throughout the treatment course. For example, in giving radiation to the ovary, lead blocks would be made to shield your kidneys. The shields are usually arranged on a wire-mesh or transparent plastic tray held securely above your body; they are placed in position just before your treatment starts.

How are the molds made?

You are put in the position you will assume during treatment. The area to be radiated is outlined by the radiation therapist. The mold is made right on your body, using whatever material has been chosen. Small windows are cut into the mold to allow the beam to be directed to the precise area to be treated. The doctor can use the mold over and over again and will be sure that the beam is always directed to the correct area.

Do all patients need molds?

No, not all patients require molds.

Where do I go for my radiation treatment?

You will usually go to the outpatient clinic of a hospital to get your external radiation treatment. Sometimes you will begin the treatment while you are in the hospital and then continue it as an outpatient. The actual treatment time is usually a few minutes, though you will be in the treatment room for 15 to 30 minutes, and you will normally spend about an hour or more in the therapeutic radiology department of the hospital. Many patients bring a book or some handwork to help them pass the time if they have to wait. You are normally able to walk or drive to your appointment. Whether you can go alone or need someone to go with you will depend upon the treatment and the side effects you experience. It is always best to be accompanied by a relative or a friend for the first few treatments, until side effects, if any, are determined.

How many radiation treatments will I get?

The number of treatments depends upon the kind of tumor, the extent of the disease, the dose involved, and your physical condition. Radiation therapy is usually given 5 days a week for several weeks. For some kinds of cancers a few treatments are needed over a few weeks; for other kinds the treatments may last for months. Sometimes the radiation is given over the period of several days; sometimes there will be a treatment followed by several days or weeks with no treatments.

Why is the radiation given over a period of time instead of all at one time?

This is because the radiation must be strong enough to kill the tumor and still allow the normal tissues to heal. The radiation therapist determines the total radiation dose necessary and divides it into the number of single-treatment doses that will add up to the total dose by the time of the last treatment. In this way, although some of your normal cells will suffer radiation damage, they will recover between treatments. If the total dose were given all at once, many of the normal cells would be damaged beyond repair.

Why is it important to keep the appointments for radiation treatment?

Because the treatment program is very precisely planned. Sometimes a lapse of time which is not part of the treatment plan means that the course of treatment must be started all over again.

Will I be able to drive myself to the treatment?

It depends upon how often you are having your treatments. Some patients have been able to drive themselves. Discuss this with the doctor before you start the treatments.

How often will I have my treatments?

It depends upon your particular illness and the treatment schedule your doctor decides on. Most often the schedule is for five treatments a week—Monday through Friday—with the weekends saved as a rest period so that normal tissues can recover from the exposure to radiation. Sometimes radiation is given twice a week or three times a week. Treatments vary in duration from as short a time as a single day to 5 days to a number of weeks.

Will the treatment plan be changed during the course of treatment?

It could very well change. The plans for treatment depend on how you as an individual respond to the treatment as well as on other factors. Interruptions to allow for rest periods are common. The initial estimate of the time required to complete a series of treatments should not be taken as a rigid or fixed number of days.

Are any kinds of tests done when I go for my radiation treatments?

It depends upon your treatment plan. Usually tests such as blood counts are taken so that the doctor knows whether the radiation is doing damage to other structures. Sometimes x-rays and other tests are necessary to determine if the doctor should change the treatment plan.

How can the doctor tell whether or not the radiation therapy is working?

After you have had several treatment sessions, your radiation therapist will begin checking you regularly to find out how well the treatment is working. Your own reports of how you feel may be the best indication of the therapy's progress. You may not be aware of changes in your cancer, but you will be able to notice any decrease in pain, bleeding, or other discomforts you may have had.

For some cancers, the doctor can use regular x-rays to see whether the tumor is shrinking. Some tests will probably be done to be sure that the radiation is causing as little damage to normal cells as possible. For instance, you may have blood tests to check the level of white blood cells and platelets, which may be reduced during treatment.

What will actually happen to me when I have the radiation?

It depends upon what kind of radiation you are having and where on your body you are having the treatment. Usually you are put on a table, which is wheeled under the machine's lighted cylinder. Technicians will measure and focus the machine and put in place any shielding devices necessary. When you have been properly positioned on the treatment couch, the x-ray equipment has been adjusted, and the controls have been set, the technicians will ask you to lie very still and will leave the treatment room.

How can the technicians tell what is happening in the treatment room if they are not in there?

The technicians are in the next room, monitoring you on closed-circuit TV. An intercom system lets you talk with them at any time and allows them to hear everything you say. The TV system lets them watch you during the whole time of your treatment. You may feel very alone, but keep in mind that your treatment is being constantly checked and that you can talk with the radiation technologist through a speaker if you wish.

Will I feel anything when I am receiving radiation?

Most people experience no sensation while the treatment is being given. Sometimes a patient says that a feeling of warmth or a mild tingling sensation is felt. However, you will feel no pain or discomfort, and it will be unusual if you have any kind of sensation. If you feel ill or uncomfortable during the treatment, tell the technologist at once.

What should I do while the treatment is being given?

You should lie very still and try to relax. The treatment lasts only a few minutes.

How will I know when the treatment is finished?

Sometimes the machine will make clicking noises or a slight whirring sound when it is on. The machines are very large and may make noises something like a vacuum cleaner as they move around to aim at the cancer from different angles. Their size and motion may be frightening at first. If you are confused by anything happening in the treatment room, ask the technologist to explain it.

Why can't the technicians stay in the same room with me while I am having my radiation treatment?

Because the machine, although pinpointing the beam at a specific part of the body, does scatter some of the radiation. Although the amount of radiation outside the beam is tiny during any single treatment session, over months and years it could add up to a dangerous amount for the personnel. It is important for the personnel who are working with the radiation all day long not to be exposed to these scattered beams.

Does anyone monitor the amount of radiation hospital personnel are exposed to?

The Food and Drug Administration's Bureau of Radiological Health has the responsibility for monitoring radiation exposure. Maximum permissible doses have been set up for individuals who work with radiation. These are to protect anyone exposed to any radiation. Hospital personnel who work with patients who are getting radiation treatments must be carefully monitored with badges which measure the accumulated dose so that they will be able to tell when the maximum has been reached.

Is it safe for a pregnant woman to accompany me to my daily radiation treatments?

Basically, the levels in the radiation department should be acceptable for all people. However, some radiation therapists feel that pregnant women should not take any chances, since even small amounts of radiation may affect the fetus.

Does everyone have side effects from radiation?

The extent of the side effects in radiation, as in chemotherapy, varies. The health team involved with your treatment will discuss side effects with you and help you if you are having problems.

The side effects range from none to slight in some people to severe in a few instances, depending upon the intensity of the treatment, the location of the treatment, and the tolerance and condition of the patient. Some people go through their radiation treatments without suffering from side effects. Others do have serious problems with side effects. We have listed the side effects which have been experienced by people getting radiation treatment. It is important understand that no one experiences all of them, that the doctors and nurses can help you minimize some of them,

Side Effects of Radiation Treatment

POSSIBLE SIDE EFFECTS	THINGS YOU SHOULD KNOW
All sites	
Ink marks on skin where treatment is being given	Don't wash off the ink marks; they must stay on during the whole course of treatment, for they show the technicians where to aim.
	When taking a bath or shower, use lukewarm water only and pat skin dry. Do not wash treatment areas; let tepid water run over them. Gently sponge skin.
Dry or itchy skin; redness, tanning, sunburned look; skin may turn a shade darker than normal.	Ask nurse or technician to suggest lotion you can use.
	Don't wash area with soap or put on salves, deodorants, powders, perfumes, bandages, medications, cosmetics, suntan lotion, or other self-remedies during treatment or for 3 weeks after treatment unless specifically ordered by the doctor giving you radiation.
	Keep treated areas out of the sun. Be sure to prevent sunburn during treatment and after completion of treatment. You will always have to be careful about protecting the treated area from the sun. If treatment is to head and neck, wear wide-brimmed hat when outdoors.
	Do not apply hot or cold objects to the skin without doctor's permission. Do not use hot-water bottles, ice packs, hot-water compresses, electric heating pads, hot packs, or heating lights on treatment areas. Heat or cold may further shock your sensitive skin.
	Try not to rub, scrub, or scratch treatment area. Do not wear tight-fitting or irritating clothes over treated areas—no corsets, girdles, belts, or other articles of clothing that leave a mark on your skin. Do not shave the treatment area without asking the doctor or nurse. Use soft shirts and loose collars if radiation is in head or neck area.
	If skin blisters or cracks or becomes moist, be sure to tell the doctor. Remember these skin reactions are temporary and should disappear within a few weeks after treatment is stopped.

Side Effects of Radiation Treatment

POSSIBLE SIDE EFFECTS	THINGS YOU SHOULD KNOW
All sites (cont.)	
	After treatment, the use of a PABA sunscreen (number 15) or a sun-blocking product is recommended for the skin that has been irradiated to prevent further damage by the sun.
Hair loss	Depends upon the site of radiation; sometimes occurs where hair is present within the area being treated. Areas affected are scalp, beard, eyebrows, armpits, and pubic and body hair. Hair usually grows back after 3 months; might be a little thinner.
Extreme fatigue; a weak or tired feeling	This is a natural reaction to radiation therapy and one of the most common complaints. Get more rest. Sleep when you feel like it. Don't try to force yourself to do things if you feel tired. Limit your visitors. Take a daily nap. Rest for an hour or so a day.
Loss of appetite	See eating hints in Chapter 22.
Sluggish bowels	See hints in Chapter 22.
Head, neck, upper chest, mouth, throat	
Sore throat, red tongue, white spots in mouth, sore mouth, unable to wear dentures, lumplike feeling when swallowing, cough (rare)	Usually begins 2 to 3 weeks after treatment starts. Symptoms usually begin to decrease after fifth week of treatment and end 4 to 6 weeks after treatments stop. Make sure you report it to your doctor. See hints in Chapter 22.
Thick saliva	Usually occurs during third or fourth week of treatment. Rinse with club soda, which will refresh your mouth and can thin out the saliva. Check your local pharmacy for Xerolube (put two or three drops on your tongue and work it through your mouth). Use it as frequently as necessary.
Dry mouth	Usually occurs near end of treatment and lasts from several months to several years. See hints in Chapter 22.

Side Effects of Radiation Treatment

POSSIBLE SIDE EFFECTS	THINGS YOU SHOULD KNOW
Head, neck, upper chest, mouth, throat (cont.)	
Loss of taste or change in taste	Usually occurs during third or fourth week of treatment and returns to normal from 3 weeks to 3 months after treatment is completed; the x-rays may have destroyed some of the tiny taste buds on your tongue. Many patients prefer egg and dairy dishes instead of meat.
Problems with your teeth	If you have dentures, expect to remove them before each treatment. Have a complete dental examination before radiation therapy begins. Follow recommendations.
	Brush your teeth after every meal or snack with a soft toothbrush. Use fluoride toothpaste with no abrasives. Floss once or twice a day. Apply fluoride daily.
Earaches	Ear and throat are closely related—sometimes ears can be affected by treatment. If your ears bother you, tell the doctor. Sometimes ear drops will be ordered. Sometimes radiation to brain results in hardening of ear wax, which can impair hearing.
Drooping or swelling skin under chin	Fatty tissue under the chin sometimes shrinks after treatment, leaving loose skin which droops or swells.
	If you notice lumps or small knots on side of neck or in shoulder, tell the doctor.
Loss of hair	Whiskers, sideburns, and chest hair may disappear temporarily or permanently, depending on the dose and area treated. Do not use razor blades for shaving; you may shave with an electric shaver but not more than once a week. Radiation to brain area sometimes causes some hair loss. This is usually a temporary condition. Use a hairpiece or wig temporarily. See Chapter 8 for information on wigs.
Breast	
Dry, tender, moist, or itchy skin in armpit (axilla) or under breast	Can occur during third or fourth week of radiotherapy; if itchiness persists, ask the doctor for something to put on it.

Side Effects of Radiation Treatment

POSSIBLE SIDE EFFECTS	THINGS YOU SHOULD KNOW
Breast (continued)	
	If area is moist, be sure to talk with the doctor, who can give you something to put on it and have you expose it to the air several times a day.
	Sometimes a yellowish discharge appears 2 to 3 weeks after the treatment is completed. Make sure you contact the doctor, who can give you medication for it.
	Sometimes the side effects of radiation continue for 4 to 6 weeks, with skin reactions getting worse 2 to 3 weeks after radiation therapy. Do not be alarmed, but do discuss them with your doctor.
	If you have had a breast removed, it is best not to wear an artificial breast (prothesis) until a month or so after radiation treatment has ended.
Upper abdomen	
Nausea, vomiting, feeling of fullness	See Chapter 22 for hints on eating.
Lower abdomen	
Diarrhea	Usually occurs during third or fourth week of therapy. Varies from one to two soft stools a day to as many as ten watery stools a day. It is best to start diet with foods which are low in fiber early in treatment and not wait until you experience this side effect. See Chapter 22 for further information.
Feeling sick to stomach, cramps, rectal burning with bowel movement (rare), inflamed bladder (rare)	

and that your own attitude may play a role in determining how severe your side effects will be.

Are people usually very ill from radiation? Are they sick enough to stop treatment?

Not usually. The common belief that people get very ill from the radiation is not true, although most patients complain about extreme fatigue. Many patients are able to work, keep house, and enjoy some leisure activities while having radiation therapy. Very few people are unable to complete their entire treatments because of side effects. Sometimes the doctor will give you a rest from the treatments if a side effect is severe, or the doctor will decide to change the kind of treatment being given. It is very important that you tell the doctors, nurses, and technicians of the side effects you are experiencing.

Are there any specific problems I should report to my doctor or nurse?

Your doctor will advise you about what problems, if any, you need to watch for and how you should deal with them. As a rule, patients should contact the doctor or nurse if they have any cough, sweating, fever, or unusual pain over the course of their treatment. As soon as any of the side effects discussed in this chapter begin, you should tell the doctor, technician, or nurse immediately so they can help you to control the symptoms.

Are there some general dos and don'ts for patients receiving radiation treatment?

Yes, there are some general guidelines. Nearly all cancer patients having radiation therapy need to take a few extra measures to protect their overall good health and to help the treatment succeed. Later in this chapter there are comments on specific areas of radiation. But for patients receiving radiation to any part of the body, here are some general recommendations.

- Be sure to get plenty of rest. Sleep as often as you feel the need. Your body will use a lot of extra energy over the course of treatment.
- Good nutrition is important. Try to maintain a diet that will prevent weight loss.
- Do not remove the ink marks from your skin until your full course of treatment is completed. If the lines begin to fade, tell the technologist at your next visit. Do not try to draw over the faded lines at home unless they would otherwise be completely gone before your next visit. If you have to replace the marks, tell the technologist what you have done.
- Be extra kind to your skin in the treatment area. Do not wash or scrub. Use tepid (not hot) water, letting it run

over the area, and pat dry. Do not rub, scrub with a washcloth or a brush, or scratch the affected area.

- Tell the radiation therapist about any medicines you are taking before starting treatment. If you need to start taking medicines, even aspirin, let your doctor know before you start. Your doctor also needs to know if medications get changed during your treatment. If you are a diabetic and you eat less, your insulin dose may have to be changed.
- Do not apply any soaps, medications, powders, perfumes, cosmetics, suntan lotions, ointments, salves, bandages, tapes, or deodorants in treatment areas without checking with the doctor or nurse. Stay away from talcum powder; it contains an abrasive. Adhesive tape should not be used, because the skin is sensitive and may come off with the tape.
- Do not expose treatment areas to the sun during treatment or upon completion of treatment. You need to be careful about protecting the treated areas from the sun. If possible, cover treated skin with light clothing before going outside. Otherwise use a PABA sunscreen (protection factor 15) or a sun-blocking product.
- Do not wear tight or irritating clothing over the treated area (no corsets, girdles, belts, tight collars, or anything that leaves a mark on your skin). Use soft cotton clothing. Don't wear nylon clothing over the treatment areas; it is not porous and tends to keep the skin wet, causing tissue breakdown.
- Do not shave the treatment areas. If you must shave, use an electric razor but only after asking the doctor, nurse, or technician.
- Do, if your skin becomes dry, ask the nurse or technician to suggest a lotion for you to use. Don't use any soaps, creams, lotions, or powders without asking the nurse or technician. They may interfere with your treatment or contain materials which would irritate the skin.
- Do expect your skin to turn a shade darker than its normal color; this is usually a temporary condition.
- Do not apply anything—hot or cold—to your skin without asking your doctor. Don't use hot-water bottles, ice packs, hot-water compresses, electric heating pads, hot

packs, or heating lights on your treatment areas. Heat or cold may further irritate your already sensitive skin.

- Do expect there might be some hair loss, if hair is present within the area being treated. Areas that may be affected are the scalp, beard, eyebrows, armpits, and pubic and body hair. Usually hair grows back after 3 months, but it might be thinner. If you are having radiation in the head and neck area, you might wish to buy a hairpiece before your treatment begins. See Chapter 8 for information.
- Do, if you are having problems with nausea and vomiting, ask your doctor about anti-vomiting medicine and about how often you should be taking it. Read the information in Chapter 22 about solving eating problems.
- Do, if your throat or mouth is sore, tell your doctor. He can prescribe a mouthwash medication which, when swallowed or gargled, can numb the mouth so that you can eat normally.

Will I feel tired from the radiation?

Probably, but it depends upon the person, the dose, and the area of radiation. Most people find they tire easily. Some people complain of feeling tired a few hours after the treatment. Some who take daily treatments say they feel tired all of the time. If you feel tired, you should rest and take naps if you can. The feeling should start to wear off within a few weeks after the treatment ends. The following will help:

- Eat when you feel tired. Sometimes a small amount of food will give you the extra energy you need.
- Rest when you feel tired; some patients experience a tired feeling and need more rest during the course of treatments. Rest or sleep when you feel you need it. Don't feel that you must keep up your normal schedule of activities if you don't feel like it.
- Ask your family, friends, and neighbors to help with shopping, child-care, housework, or driving.

Will my skin get red or darker?

It depends upon the area of radiation and the condition and color of your skin. Usually about 3 weeks after your first treatment, you may find that your skin becomes red, or a shade darker than normal. You may get some irritation in the areas where you are being treated. Some people say their skin looks and feels sunburned. Be sure to tell the technician or doctor when you first note reddening of your skin.

What should I do if my skin gets irritated?

Some of this has already been covered in the list of dos and don'ts. However, the major points bear repeating. Try not to irritate the skin. Wear loose-fitting clothes. Don't scrub your skin in the area of treatment with a washcloth or a brush. Because the skin in that area is more sensitive, it needs more care in order to prevent irritation. Make sure you don't use soaps, creams, lotions, or powders on it without asking the nurse or technician. Don't apply anything hot or cold to it. Don't scratch or rub the skin in the radiation treatment area. Don't expose the area to the sun. If your skin looks as if it is going to blister or crack be sure you report it to the doctor immediately.

Can I get a skin burn from the radiation?

Some patients are afraid of skin burns from radiation. In the past, with the old-style x-ray machines, this was a serious problem. But with today's radiation equipment, the painful skin burns sometimes associated with radiation almost never occur. Sometimes the skin in the area being treated turns a light pink after a few days. Sometimes it looks tan. Sometimes it turns a bit rough and might even peel slightly. You may find that your skin is not as flexible or as movable as before.

Does the skin redness always come in the area being treated?

Sometimes not. For example, some people who have treatments in the chest area find they have a sunburn effect on their backs. This is because the machine's beam focuses its energy on a specific area just underneath the skin's surface, but as it goes on through the body, the beam spreads and leaves the body through a larger area in the back. As it goes out, it leaves the skin a bit red or darker in color.

Why can't I use lotions on my dry or itchy skin?

Many over-the-counter products for the skin, such as lotions or petroleum jelly, leave a coating that can interfere with your radiation therapy. Don't try any powders, creams, salves, or other home remedies while you're being treated or for several weeks afterward unless they are approved by your doctor.

Will the skin reactions go away after my treatment ends?

The majority of skin reactions should go away a few weeks after treatment is finished. In many cases, though, darkened skin areas will remain. Tell your doctor at once if your skin cracks, blisters, or becomes too moist.

What happens if my skin gets a wet feeling?

This is something which should be reported immediately to your doctor. It sometimes happens as the radiation treatment continues. It is called "weeping" of the skin because the upper layers have shed. It is not a burn. Usually the doctor will stop the treatments for a while, or will prescribe an antibiotic lotion or cream for you to put on the skin. He will usually also tell you to expose the area to air. You will probably be taught how to wash the area twice a day, by just letting warm water run over it, patting it dry, and applying the cream or lotion.

What is radiation pneumonitis?

Radiation pneumonitis is an inflammation of lung tissue resulting from radiation. It can be painful.

Will radiation therapy affect my emotions?

All people undergoing treatment for cancer are likely to feel some emotional upset. While radiation therapy may affect the emotions indirectly through tiredness or changes in hormone balance, the treatment itself is not a direct cause of mental distress. Some patients do report feeling depressed or nervous during their treatment. This may be because of the changes in daily routine, their fear about the cancer, or the fact that they can't do everything they could before. Such feelings are not at all unusual for a person with cancer. If you find yourself feeling unhappy or nervous while in treatment, try to remember that a positive outlook may be helpful. Researchers are studying the ways a patient's outlook could affect the body's functions. Some believe that using up your energies with unproductive emotions can only detract from the resources your body needs for health itself.

Does my diet have to change when I am having radiation treatments?

No, your diet does not have to change. However, it is important for you to eat well to speed tissue repair. You should try to maintain your normal weight through a well-balanced, nutritious diet and sufficient rest. Your appetite may be affected, but it is important that you eat properly. Good nutrition is essential also for several months after treatment. You should be careful to have both good nutrition and plenty of rest to help your body repair and replace the normal cells. Doctors have found that patients who eat well can better withstand both their cancer and the side effects of treatment. Try to keep emotional stress to a minimum. There is further information on ways to perk your appetite in Chapter 22.

Can I continue my usual activity during treatment?

Continue normal activities as much as possible and do whatever you feel you can without strain. Many people find they can continue to work during the treatment period. Others find they can continue some activity but less than the normal amount. Your daily activity will be determined by how you as a person feel and how much you think you can do. Your doctor may suggest you limit any activities, such as sports, which might irritate the area being treated.

Is there anything special I should do if I am getting radiation in the head and neck area?

Yes, there are several things you should know and some things you can do to minimize the changes in your system if you are getting radiation to the head and neck area (this includes radiation treatments in the area of the upper chest, mouth, throat, neck, and brain).

- Be sure you check with a dentist experienced in treating cancer patients before you begin radiation treatments.
- You may be sore in the area of the mouth and throat. You might notice that your tongue is red or that there are white spots in your mouth. You might have a hard time swallowing, feel a lump in your throat, or feel your food sticking in your throat due to irritation of the tissues in your throat and swallowing tube. You might not be able to wear your dentures. All of these are temporary side effects which usually begin 2 to 3 weeks after treatment starts and usually begin to decrease after the fifth week of treatment. They usually end some 4 to 6 weeks after the treatments finish. Of course you should report any of these side effects to your doctor.
- Smoking and drinking make your mouth and throat sorer. Don't use tobacco, alcoholic beverages, or hot, spicy, rough, or coarse foods like pepper, chili powder, nutmeg, vinegar, etc.; they can irritate your mouth.
- Avoid coarse foods such as raw vegetables, dry crackers, and nuts.
- Stay away from sugary snacks that promote tooth decay.
- If your mouth is irritated, frequent mouth care is needed, as often as every 1 to 4 hours depending on your need. Use a mouthwash made of 1 teaspoon of salt or 1 teaspoon of salt and 1 teaspoon of baking soda to 1 quart of warm water. A mixture of equal parts of glycerin and warm water is also effective. Do not use a commercial mouthwash without your doctor's permission. Do not use hot water; let it cool before using.
- Don't breathe in strong fumes such as paints and cleaning solutions.
- Brush your teeth with a soft toothbrush. Use dental floss to clean between the teeth.
- Use fluoride toothpaste with no abrasives. Apply fluoride daily.
- Don't shave with razor blades in the areas being treated. You may shave with an electric razor. You may find that whiskers, sideburns, eyebrows, head hair, hair in your armpits, or chest hair fall out temporarily, depending on the dose of radiation and the area being treated. Some men with much hair on their chests getting chest radia-

tion will find that the hair in the treated area falls out within a few weeks; it may grow back after about 3 months, sometimes a little thinner.

- Make sure if you are having radiation in the head area that you wear a wide-brimmed hat or scarf when you are out in the sunshine. Don't use any sunburn product on your skin during the course of your treatments.
- Don't use starched collars if you have radiation in the head and neck area; wear soft shirts and loose collars to prevent irritation to the treated area.
- You may have earaches, caused by hardening of the ear wax.
- You may have swelling or drooping of the skin under your chin. There may also be changes in your skin texture.
- See Chapter 22 for hints about eating during this period.

Why do I need to see a dentist before I begin radiation treatments to the head and neck area?

Dentists have become more aware of the effects of radiation on the teeth and now recommend that if you are having radiation in the area of the head and neck you should be taking special care of your teeth and mouth before, during, and after treatment. You should visit your dentist or a dentist who has had experience treating persons who have had head and neck radiation. Before your treatment starts, the dentist will probably take x-rays and examine your teeth. He will try to do any major work which he feels is necessary or will become necessary within the next year. He will explain the special care you should take to protect your teeth and mouth. Young people undergoing radiation treatment need to be closely watched, to ensure that the radiation does not lead to abnormal development of teeth that are still in the formative stages.

What is the special care I should be taking to protect my teeth and mouth?

The dentist will give you very detailed instructions. Most likely, you will be advised to

- Clean your teeth and gums several times a day, at least after meals and once more daily, with a soft brush.

- Use fluoride toothpaste that contains no abrasives.
- Floss between your teeth once or twice a day.
- Rinse your mouth well with a solution of salt and baking soda after you brush.
- Use a disclosing solution or tablet after brushing to reveal plaque you missed.
- Apply fluoride at least once a day to prevent tooth decay and decrease sensitivity. Your dentist will show you how this is done.
- Arrange follow-up visits more often than normal, both during and after treatment.

My mouth feels dry. Is there anything I can do for that?

Your glands may be producing less saliva than usual, making your mouth feel dry. It may be helpful to suck on ice chips and sip cool drinks often throughout the day. Sugar-free candy or gum may also help. Saliva protects your teeth against tooth decay. The dentist may prescribe a fluoride gel or fluoride mouth rinses. If the saliva flow is permanently reduced, you may need to continue preventive fluoride treatments after your radiation is completed. If you need it, ask your dentist about artificial saliva.

Will my eyes be covered during treatment?

Again, it depends upon where the treatment is being given. The lens and the cornea of your eyes are sensitive to radiation. Therefore, the therapist will block these areas if at all possible, if the treated area is close to your eyes.

Can I get eye cataracts from radiation treatment?

This depends upon the location of the treatment and the dose being given. You should be aware that patients can develop eye cataracts from radiation treatment.

Are there any special side effects for persons getting radiation therapy in the breast area?

Usually, patients receiving radiation treatment in the breast area do not have any serious side effects or problems. Sometimes, if radiation is given to the lymph nodes along the breastbone, the esophagus (the tube which connects your mouth to your stomach) may be affected and you might have some difficulty swallowing. Follow the suggestions given for side effects of head and neck radiation.

Some persons develop either dry, itchy skin or moist skin in the armpit area (axilla), or under their breasts. If this happens, tell the radiation therapist or nurse immediately so they can start treatment for it. In some cases, there may be a yellow discharge from the skin 2 or 3 weeks after the treatment has finished. You might also have soreness and swelling from fluid buildup in the treated area. If any of these occur, call the radiation therapist's office and discuss medication and treatment.

Many patients find it is better to wear a soft undershirt rathe. than a bra during the period when radiation therapy is being given to the breast area. It is important that nothing tight-fitting is worn to irritate the skin in the area of treatment.

Can I wear an artificial breast (prosthesis) during the time of my radiation treatment to the breast area?

If you have had a breast removed, it is best not to wear your prosthesis until a month or so after radiation treatment has ended.

Will my breast change in size?

One long-term side effect of radiation treatment to the breast is a change in size. Because women are so varied, it is not possible to predict the degree of change or whether the breast will become smaller or larger. But, like the skin darkening mentioned earlier, the change is usually slight and will not be noticeable when you are clothed.

I had a radium implant after my external treatment for breast cancer was completed, and now I have some side effects. Is that usual?

Some women receive a radium implant as a "boost" treatment after external radiation. Some find that the area feels tender or tight while the implant is in the breast. After the implant is removed, many women notice some of the same effects that occur with external treatment. Let your doctor know about any problems that continue.

Are there any particular side effects I can expect if I am getting radiation therapy in the stomach area?

While some people do not experience any side effects at all, most experience some nausea, vomiting, and/or diarrhea during their course of treatment. Others experience one or two of these side effects but not all three. Side effects are related to the size of the field and the dose being given.

What can be done about the nausea and vomiting?

Nausea and/or vomiting usually come on shortly after the treatment and last for a few hours. See Chapter 22 for information about eating during this period.

What can I do for diarrhea?

Many patients with treatments to the lower abdomen experience diarrhea, usually during the third or fourth week of treatment. It varies from one to two soft stools a day to as many as ten watery stools a day. Doctors feel it is best to start eating foods which are low in fiber early in the treatment and not to wait until you experience the diarrhea to begin your diet. There is further information on this subject in Chapter 22.

Can I become sterile from radiation treatment?

Whether or not you become sterile depends upon the location of the treatment and the dose of radiation being given. If your sex organs are in or very close to the field of radiation, the treatment can cause sterility in both men and women. If sterility is predicted, some males prefer to have their semen frozen and stored so that they may have children later on. In women patients, it is sometimes possible to block or move the ovaries before radiation to protect them from exposure. You should discuss the question of sterility with your doctor before radiation treatment begins.

Can external radiation therapy cause physical changes that will lead to sexual problems?

It all depends upon where the radiation beam is focused. Radiation therapy to male or female sexual organs, for example, may cause some problems. External-beam radiation to the prostate area can cause impotence as well as decreased sexual desire, though these effects are sometimes only temporary. In women, radiation to the pelvis may stop menstruation and cause menopausal symptoms as well as narrowing, dryness and thinning of the vagina, and itching. During treatment to the pelvis, many women are advised not to have intercourse. Others may find that intercourse is painful. Women will be most likely to resume having sex within a few weeks after treatment ends. To make it more comfortable, talk with your doctor about ointments, lubricants, and prescriptions that may help.

Ever since my radiation therapy, I've had a series of urinary-tract infections which make intercourse uncomfortable. Is this going to be a permanent condition?

About one-third of women who receive radiation therapy develop radiation cystitis—bladder irritation due to radiation. The urinary-tract tissues become very sensitive as a result of radiation treatment, and intercourse may cause the tissue surrounding the urethra to become swollen, inflamed, and susceptible to infection. Your gynecologist or urologist can prescribe treatment for irritation if it occurs. This condition usually clears up 4 to 6 months following treatment. You may find intercourse more comfortable if you lie on your side, with your partner placing his penis into the vagina from behind. Or your partner may lie on his side while you are on your back, buttocks against him and knees bent, up and over his side. Penetration in this position will not be quite as deep, as both partners have some control.

I am having radiation treatments and am afraid to have sex with my partner because I think I may be radioactive. Is there a danger?

If you are having external radiation therapy (in which a machine at some distance from your body beams high-energy rays to the cancer), you are not radioactive and will not be a danger to anyone around you. There is no reason not to have intercourse if it is comfortable for you.

If you are having internal radiation therapy (in which a small container of radioactive material is placed within the body close to the cancerous tissue), precautions are taken until the implants are removed or are no longer emitting radioactivity. You will be in the hospital during that time and will be given necessary instructions. The length of time depends upon the location and strength of the treatment. Be sure to discuss this with your doctor.

Are there long-term effects of radiation therapy to the pelvic area given to patients with cancer of the penis, testicle, or prostate? Can it affect sterility or sexual performance?

It is known that fertility is affected, since the body often stops producing sperm. Usually sperm production begins again within 6 months to a year after treatment, though radiation treatment close to sexual organs can cause permanent sterility. As insurance, it is advisable to discuss the possibility of sperm banking *before* your treatments if you are interested in having children. Your doctor can check sperm count to determine the quality of sperm and how much is being produced. There should be no specific sexual problems associated with radiation therapy in terms of erection or ejaculation capability.

How long can the side effects of the radiation last?

After your radiation therapy is finished, the side effects of the radiation can continue for the next 4 to 6 weeks. Some of the side effects, especially skin reactions, may get worse after your treatment stops. Do not be alarmed. Follow the instructions given to you, or call the radiation therapist's office if you need help during this period. (Since treatments are usually given in a hospital setting, nurses are available to answer your questions at any time.) You will usually be seen again by the radiation therapist some 4 to 6 weeks after the completion of the treatment. At that time, he can usually evaluate the effectiveness of the radiation treatments.

Is it possible for side effects to occur 6 months or a year after radiation treatment has ended?

Yes. Since radiation damages normal tissue as well as cancerous cells, late side effects in the radiated area are sometimes seen months or years after the treatment has ended.

Is there any special care I should take after my treatments are completed?

You should continue to bathe the skin in the treatment area in tepid water; wash gently, using a mild soap (talk to the nurse if you have questions about what kind to use). Do not rub or scrub. Ask the nurse or the technician to recommend a cream or ointment which you can use on the treated area after your therapy has been completed. Protect the treated area from the sun. Continue to wear soft clothing around the treated area. You can go back to other kinds of clothing after the skin has returned to its normal appearance. Gently wash off the marks. Do not scrub. The ink will wear off. Gradually return to your previous schedule of activity. If you notice any unusual sores in any of the treated areas, be sure to call the radiation therapist's office and discuss them.

What follow-up arrangements will be made after I have finished my course of treatment?

After the treatment is finished, a complete report is sent to the physician who referred you. You will usually be asked to return for checkup visits with the radiation therapist. It is important that you see both your primary doctor and the radiation therapist at the intervals they suggest.

Is radiation expensive?

Yes. It is costly because of the equipment used in the treatment and the number of persons needed to give the treatment. Most major health-insurance policies cover the cost of radiation therapy, both the charge from the hospital or clinic and the professional charge by the radiation therapist for the medical professional services. The exact cost varies depending on the type and number of treatments needed.

Is there any radioactivity left in me as a result of external radiation treatments?

No. There is no radioactivity left in you, and you are not made radioactive by external radiation treatment. The radioactivity of external radiation is confined to the treatment beam itself. Neither the normal tissues nor the malignant tissues become radioactive. When the treatment is completed, no radioactivity remains in the body.

Is it all right for me to be around people while I am having radiation treatments?

There is no need to avoid being with other people because of external radiation treatments. Your body will not contain any radioactive substance, so you are not a hazard to others—even in intimate contact.

Will my desire for physical intimacy change because of radiation treatment?

Your desire for physical intimacy may be lower, because radiation treatment can affect hormone levels and often causes some fatigue.

What are the different types of internal radiation?

There are two major kinds of internal radiation:

- Radioactive material which is sealed in a container and inserted into a body cavity at the site of the tumor. For example, a sealed tube containing radioactive cesium can be inserted into the vagina; radium needles are implanted in the tongue or breast; radium seeds can be used for prostate cancer.
- Radioactive material which is given orally or injected with a syringe; it mingles with body fluids and is transported to interior parts of the body. For example, radioactive iodine is swallowed and finds its way to the thyroid gland to attack a tumor there; liquid radioactive gold or phosphorus can be injected directly into the area of a tumor.

Why is internal radiation used?

The doctor is trying to put the radium or other radioactive material as close to the tumor as possible to control the growth. This also spares surrounding normal tissue. Because the radiation is concentrated in the tumor, it is possible to expose cancer cells to a higher dosage during a shorter period of time than would be possible with conventional radiation sources. For instance, it is known that radioactive iodine travels to the thyroid gland, and in some cases of thyroid cancer, the doctor can use it to destroy the gland and the cancer.

What kinds of radioactive materials are used as implants?

Some of the substances include radium, cesium, iridium, and others.

What kinds of devices are used in internal radiation?

Devices such as needles, seeds, wires, wax, molds, and capsules have been created to place the radiation source as close as possible to the cancer. For instance, needle implants, which the doctor can insert directly into the tumor, are often used for treating the mouth and tongue. Sometimes, hollow, flexible plastic tubes are put into the tumor and filled with a radioactive solution. Other times, the radioactive materials may be applied against the tumor in some kind of applicator.

What is an interstitial implant?

An interstitial implant is a procedure in which tiny bits of radioactive isotopes are temporarily implanted in and around malignant tissue in a solid organ such as the breast. Interstitial-implant treatment is usually left in from 3 to 5 days. It is sometimes used in some cancers of the tongue, lip, breast, and prostate.

How is an interstitial implant done?

Technically, the doctor places several hollow steel needles into the tumor and the area surrounding it. Thin plastic tubes are then threaded through the needles and anchored into place. The radioactive substance, usually in the form of tiny seeds embedded in a thin, stiff nylon ribbon, is inserted into the tubes. The outer layer of the seed is a steel sheathing which blocks dangerous ionizing beta rays (electrons) but allows the escape of the high-energy gamma rays that destroy the tumor. Sometimes the patient receives external radiation as well as an interstitial implant.

What is an intracavitary implant?

An intracavitary implant refers to the placing of radioactive material into a hollow space within the body. Intracavitary therapy is most commonly used in cancer of the uterus. The implants can either be put in permanently or are removed after a period of time. Sometimes the radioactive elements, such as radium, cobalt, and iridium, are used for removable implants; other times, radioactive elements such as radon, gold, and iridium are used for implants which are permanently left in the body. The removable implants are put into needles or plastic tubes which are fastened into the cancer.

What is a needle implant?

It is another term for an interstitial implant in a tumor using slender hollow needles in which a radioactive material is placed. Needle implants are used in the mouth and the tongue, for example.

How much radiation is given off by a needle implant?

This depends on the amount of radioactive material implanted and how long it is left in place. The decision is made by the radiation therapist when planning the treatment.

Are needle implants in the mouth and tongue painful?

There may be some pain associated with needle implants in the mouth and tongue. Pain medication is prescribed if needed.

How will the doctor implant the radiation into me?

It depends upon where the implant will be. Usually you will be hospitalized and put under general anesthesia. If you were having a radium implant into your uterus, for example, your doctor would, in the operating room, insert a hollow applicator inside your vaginal canal and carefully pack it into position with medicated gauze. In some hospitals, the radioactive material is placed into the applicator in the operating room; in others the radioactive material is put into the applicator after you have returned to your own room.

How long is the implant left in the body?

This depends upon the site and on the treatment schedule. The implant is usually left in from 1 to 6 days. During this time you are kept in an isolated room and visitors are limited as to the number and times they may visit you. Sometimes the implants are used along with other kinds of therapy such as x-ray treatments; this would influence how long the implant is left in.

Will I be giving off radiation while the implant is in place?

It depends upon the implant. Usually, if you have radium or other radioactive materials introduced into the diseased tissues, the radiation will pass through your body into the surrounding area. However, if the implant is in a sealed source (needle or hollow applicator), neither you nor any of your body excretions such as blood, urine, or stool become radioactive. Items you touch, such as bed linens, also do not become radioactive.

What happens once the implant is removed? Am I still giving off radiation?

No. Once the implant is removed there is no radiation to pass through your body, unless you have been administered a radioactive material by mouth or syringe. Then your body fluids do become radioactive, as do the bed linens.

Can the radioactive material which is put in the hollow applicator explode in my body?

No, you do not have to worry about that. The radioisotope is not explosive. The material will not explode.

Will I get regular hospital care when I have a radioactive implant?

Your hospital care will be a bit different than usual. The nurses and other hospital personnel are limited as to how long they can remain in your room and how close they can come to you and your bed. You might notice that they come into your room more often but for shorter periods of time. Your bed will probably be close to the window wall. The hospital personnel will probably not come close to the side of your bed, but will talk with you from the foot of the bed. They will probably be wearing film badges to measure the radiation. Naturally, the restrictions to the hospital personnel depend upon what part of your body the implant is in, the kind of radioactive materials used, and the dosage. Pregnant nurses will not be allowed to take care of you. Most times, you will be assigned to a single room. Although personal contact is limited because of the radiation implant, do not hesitate to call a nurse if you need her for any reason.

What about changing the bed and taking a bath?

Your sheets will probably not be changed routinely every day but only if they become dirty. The nurse will encourage you to take your own bed bath if you are well enough to do it yourself. If she must stay in your room for any length of time, she may use some kind of a lead shield for protection. If you have a vaginal applicator in place, the nurse will do as much as she can while standing at the head of the bed. When caring for a patient with seeds implanted in the head and neck area, the nurse will do as much of her work as possible while standing at the foot of the bed.

Will I be allowed to have visitors?

It depends. Usually visitors are restricted to persons over 18 years old, persons who are not pregnant, and persons who are not likely to become pregnant. Visitors are asked to keep a distance which allows for conversation but keeps them away from the bed. They will be allowed to stay only for a limited time to minimize their exposure to radiation.

How will the hospital personnel know I have a radioactive implant?

It depends upon what hospital you are in. A tag might be put on the front cover of your chart, at the foot of your bed, or on the door of your room—or in all three places. You will probably also be given a wristband which will say "radioactive precautions."

Will I be able to move around while the implant is inside me?

In most cases you must stay in bed while the applicator with the radioactive material is in place. (For breast interstitial implants, you may be allowed to be up and around in the room, but you will not be allowed to leave the room.) Depending upon the location of your tumor, part of your bed can be elevated. However, you must restrict your movements so that the radiation source will not become dislodged and harm sensitive, organs. You will not normally be allowed to turn from side to side or turn over onto your stomach. The nurse can put pillows under some parts of your body, depending upon where the radiation source is located, so that you can be tilted or propped up. You will usually be given exercises to do with the parts of your body that you can move.

Can I eat while the radiation implant is in my body?

Yes, you will usually be given a special diet with lots of fluids. The nurses will place the food where you can manage it without having to move your body. If your implant is in the vaginal area, you will be given pills to discourage bowel movements while the applicator is in the body. Sometimes you will be given sleeping pills or other medication to relax you. It is important that you not touch the implant while it is in your body. Although the container is sealed, touching it could cause radiation damage to your skin.

Do I have to go back into the operating room to have the implant removed?

Usually not. The implant is usually removed right in the room. Normally you are given some pain medication about half an hour before the doctor comes in to take out the applicator and the packing. You will then be allowed to get out of bed. Usually the nurse will help you move around until your strength comes back.

Will I have pain or feel sick while the implant is in?

Usually not. Some patients do experience a rise in temperature. Other patients complain of fleeting waves of burning sensations. If you feel hot or experience sweats, tell your doctor. Thyroid patients sometimes complain of a sore throat. Some patients are weak and tired from the anesthesia. Some patients find the applicator holding the implant to be slightly uncomfortable and lying flat for a period of time tiring. The doctor can order a sedative to relieve the discomfort. If you seem to have any side effects, be sure to tell the nurse.

Do I have to follow any special rules after my implant has been taken out and I go home?

You should avoid sunlight on the areas exposed to radiation. If you have dryness or itchiness, the doctor can give you a cream to relieve it. You should make sure you call the doctor if you have nausea, vomiting, diarrhea, frequent urination or bowel movements, a red vaginal bleeding or blood in the urine, a temperature above 100°, burning, or pain.

However, you should go back to your normal life. You can continue on your normal diet. You are no longer radioactive and are not a hazard to yourself or to anybody else. If you have had an implant in the gynecological area, you will be told not to take a tub bath, although shower baths or sponge baths are permitted. The doctor will also give you a list of other cautions; you may not douche, use tampons, or have intercourse for a time. You will be allowed to resume these activities gradually depending upon the condition of your vagina or cervix.

Will I feel tired?

Some people get tired easily and feel sleepy several times a day. If this happens, lie down and rest. It is better for you to do this than to get overtired. It is not unusual to take several naps the first few days.

Why is some radioactive material used in unsealed sources?

Some radioactive substances cannot penetrate casings, so they are used unsealed. The unsealed sources are usually liquids injected into the abdomen or the lung cavities. These liquids consist of particles that do not readily pass into blood and lymph; therefore they stay in one place. Another unsealed source is the iodine given by mouth to patients with thyroid cancer.

Are there any side effects from the liquids injected into the abdomen or the lung cavities?

Some patients may have nausea, vomiting, and diarrhea— similar side effects to those resulting from external radiation in the upper or lower abdomen. Also linens, dressings, and clothing can become contaminated if the unsealed source leaks. The patient's urine, feces, and vomit are not contaminated, since the liquids consist of particles that do not readily pass into blood and the lymph system.

Are there any special precautions if I am taking radioactive iodine therapy?

Yes. If you are taking iodine therapy, there may be a problem of contamination, since the body expels this substance through the kidneys, the salivary and sweat glands, and the stools. Therefore, the nurses will wear rubber gloves when handling bedclothes in case there is some urine on them; your bedpans will be thoroughly cleaned after each use and reserved for your use only; your urine will be stored in bottles placed in lead boxes. Even your tears and saliva will be radioactive.

How long will these special precautions have to be taken?

It depends upon the kind of radioactive material and the dose. The radioactivity of radioactive iodine decreases rapidly after a few days because of the decay in the activity of the substance and also because it is being excreted through the kidneys.

Will I be able to have visitors?

There will be restrictions as to how long and how close visitors can come, for anyone using unsealed-source radiation. Pregnant visitors will not be allowed.

What is a permanent implant?

This means that the radioctive material is left in permanently. Often radioactive materials are permanently implanted in the tongue or the palate or floor of the mouth. Permanent implants are also done in the prostate. The radioactivity of the material diminishes each day so that after a few days there is very little radiation coming from the patient's body.

Do special precautions have to be taken around persons with permanent implants?

It depends upon where the implant is and the dosage of the radiation. In some cases, the patients are hospitalized for the days when they have the greatest amount of radioactivity. The materials selected for permanent implant do not usually entail hazards to family members or others once the patient is ready to be discharged. If there is a need for special precautions, both the patient and the family are given full instructions.

Do radium implants in the prostate cause any aftereffects?

Radioactive implants into the prostate, though they require major abdominal surgery, usually result in fewer aftereffects than most other methods of treatment for prostate cancer. The quality of male erection generally is unaffected by the procedure. As with other forms of radioactive implants, there should be no fears of radiation aftereffects, since the life of the radiation implant diminishes quickly (usually before the patient leaves the hospital).

What are radioprotectors?

Radioprotectors are a group of chemical compounds that may be able to protect against short-term radiation damage. They appear to be able to keep normal cells from becoming cancer cells. Radioprotectors are presently being tested. If they are successful, they will allow radiation therapists to give higher doses of radiation than would normally be safe for the surrounding tissue. It is also believed that radioprotectors may eliminate the problem of second cancers sometimes induced by radiation treatment.

What is a radioactive bath?

This is an experimental technique where, during surgery, the abdominal cavity is rinsed with a radioactive solution to kill any cancer cells clinging to the lining.

chapter 8

Chemotherapy

Chemotherapy—which simply means the use of drugs or medications to treat disease—came into general use in the 1970s after clinical trials proved them to be effective in treating cancer. To many people, chemotherapy is frightening because of the fears of side effects that are sometimes caused by the use of the potent drugs needed to disrupt the cancer cells' ability to grow and multiply. The use of chemotherapy drugs has been greatly refined over the years, so that many of the earlier side effects have been modified. Chemotherapy may be given in several ways. Sometimes drugs are given in pill or capsule form and taken by mouth. Other times they may be injected into a muscle or given through a vein. How fast the cancer cells are destroyed may vary with the medication and the type of cancer. Because each drug acts on the cell in its own way, and at different times in the cell cycle, using them in combination can be more effective than using any one of them individually. Some are given on a weekly basis, others, monthly or daily, sometimes for periods of one or two years following the initial treatment. Because most anticancer drugs have the potential for dangerous side effects, they must be administered carefully by medical professionals experienced in their use. Chemotherapy has proven to be very effective in cancer treatment. It is estimated that more than 50,000 cancer patients are being cured each year with the use of anticancer drugs, either alone or combined with radiation therapy and/or surgery.

Questions to Ask About Chemotherapy

- Who will be giving me my chemotherapy treatments?
- What is the name of the drug/drugs I will be taking?
- What is/are the drug/drugs supposed to do?
- What are the possible undesirable side effects? What should I do if these side effects occur?
- Which side effects should I report to the doctor immediately?
- How will the drug be given to me? How often will the treatments be given?
- How long will each treatment take? How long will the whole series last?
- May I take other medication at the same time? May I drink alcohol?
- Is there any special nutritional advice I should follow?
- Are there any special precautions I should take while I am on chemotherapy?
- How much will it cost?
- How much of a risk is involved?
- What is the alternative? What if I don't have this treatment at all?

What is chemotherapy?

Chemo means "chemical," and *therapy* means "treatment"; thus chemotherapy is simply the treatment of cancer using chemicals (drugs).

What does chemotherapy do?

In simple terms, the chemicals destroy the cancer cells, either by interfering with their growth or by preventing them from reproducing. The various drugs work in different ways to interrupt the cell life cycle. Some affect the cell during one or more of its phases of growth and have no adverse effect on the cell during the other phases; others affect the cell throughout the whole cycle. The idea behind the use of chemotherapy is to slow down the multiplying of cancer cells or to destroy the cancer cells themselves.

Has chemotherapy as a treatment been used for a long time?

Although the use of chemicals to fight disease has been known for a long time, chemotherapy has been used against cancer only in recent years. Until the 1940s, attempts to find drugs that would selectively destroy cancer cells were not successful. The observation at Yale University that the potent World War I gas nitrogen mustard produced selective damage to the lymphatic system and bone marrow led to interest in the use of chemotherapy for cancer. The first successful use of chemotherapy was at Yale in the mid-1940s. During the 1960s and 1970s the uses and successes of chemotherapy expanded rapidly.

When is chemotherapy used?

Chemotherapy is used for many different reasons:
- It can cure some kinds of cancer.
- It can be used to achieve long-term remissions in some kinds of cancer.
- It can be used to reduce a large tumor, making it small enough to remove by surgery.
- It can be used after surgery to kill the cells which may have been left or are in another part of the body.
- It can be used to shrink tumors which cannot be surgically removed.
- It can be used to make radiation treatment more effective.
- It can prevent or relieve pain or control unpleasant symptoms.

Is chemotherapy usually used alone as a treatment?

Like other treatments for cancer, chemotherapy is sometimes used alone. Most of the time chemotherapy is used in combination with another kind of treatment—radiation therapy or surgery.

What does chemotherapy do that is different from the other kinds of treatments?

The chemotherapeutic drugs enter the bloodstream either directly by intravenous injection or indirectly by absorption through the stomach tissues. Therefore, the drugs are transported wherever tumor cells may be growing. This is different from surgery and radiotherapy, which concentrate on a specific part or region of the body for treatment. Chemotherapy is used when there is the possibility that cancer cells may be deposited in a different place from the primary tumor or may be circulating throughout the body via the bloodstream.

Can chemotherapy ever cure cancer?

According to the National Cancer Institute, the drugs can produce cures in about 15 percent of clinical cancer. In many of the remaining cases, they often temporarily stop the growth, or relieve pain and allow the patient to live a longer, more comfortable life. In some cancers, in some patients, chemotherapy can cause the tumors to disappear. In other cases, chemotherapy makes the tumor shrink. When this doesn't happen, the drugs may at least stop the tumor from growing or make it grow more slowly. There are a few cases, however, in which chemotherapy has no effect on the growth of the tumor.

Isn't chemotherapy used only as a last resort for advanced cancer cases?

During the early years, when chemotherapy was an investigative treatment, it was used primarily on patients after other treatments were no longer working. Today, many doctors are using chemotherapy to prevent the spread of cancer for persons with minimal disease. When the drug is used early, the main idea is to remove the micrometastases which are not yet seen under the microscope, but are believed to be present, especially in some stages of breast cancer.

What are the different types of chemotherapy?

Chemotherapy drugs are classified by their structure and function. They fall mainly into the following five classifications:
- *Alkylating agents* are known for their chemical action, which interferes with cell division. They are called non-cell-cycle-specific agents because they attack all cells in a tumor whether the cells are resting or dividing. They work by stopping or slowing down cell growth.

- *Antimetabolites* are drugs which interfere with the cells' ability to replicate. These drugs are designed to starve cancer cells by interfering with vital life processes. They fool the cell by introducing the wrong building elements or blocking synthesis of the right ones.
- *Natural products* include plant alkaloids and antibiotics. Plant alkaloids stop cell division at one of its phases. Antibiotics are made from molds like penicillin but are stronger and do not act in the same way as regular antibiotics. Rather, they interfere with cell division and damage more cancer cells than normal cells.
- *Hormones* are naturally occurring substances in the body that stimulate or turn off the growth or activity of specific cells or organs. In cancer treatment, the environment is changed either by adding or removing the hormones, thus antagonizing the growth-stimulating hormones that promote growth of cancer cells in certain tissues.
- *Miscellaneous agents* which don't fit into any of the other categories.

Who prescribes chemotherapy?

Chemotherapy should be prescribed by a doctor who has had special training in the use of drugs and drug combinations for the treatment of cancer. This may be a medical oncologist (chemotherapist), who is a specialist in internal medicine with special training in the overall care of the cancer patient, or a hematologist, who is a physician who specializes in blood diseases. Most chemotherapy drugs are too risky to be prescribed by general physicians without special training.

Do nurses play a role in actually administering the chemotherapeutic drugs?

Absolutely. There are specially trained chemotherapy nurses in many parts of the country, both in doctors' offices and in hospitals (outpatient clinics and inpatient facilities), who actually give the majority of chemotherapeutic drugs under the supervision of a physician. These nurses are well trained in the administration of the drugs and know what side effects to look for.

Why is it important to have specially trained personnel dealing with chemotherapeutic drugs?

Chemotherapy, and especially combination chemotherapy (in which more than one drug is used), may be a highly toxic form of cancer treatment. Patients who are not closely monitored could die from the side effects, because the drugs are very potent. In addition, it is a field of medicine that is new and changing quickly. New forms of therapy may not always reach the doctors who are not specializing in this field. If you are living in a community that does not have a specialist to administer the drugs, you should make sure your doctor seeks a consultation with a cancer center, a medical school, or a large medical center for guidance from experts who know the latest drugs in use, the administration technique, how to adjust doses, and what the side effects are on the normal cells.

Where are the drugs given?

Chemotherapy can be given either in a doctor's office or in a hospital—the latter either in an outpatient clinic or as a patient in the hospital. Most times oral drugs can be taken at home. Many times the first doses of the drugs are given in the hospital so that a trained health-care team can give them and closely monitor your reactions to them. This is usually only a 1- or 2-day stay, with the remaining drugs given in the doctor's office or outpatient clinic. In other cases, the drugs are given in the doctor's office or outpatient clinic from the beginning. Occasionally, you may have to stay in the hospital when drugs have to be given intravenously for a long period of time.

How does the doctor decide on what kind of drug to use?

The doctor must look at your general condition, the type of tumor you have, and the extent of its growth. He evaluates the responses of chemotherapy in similar patients and selects that kind of chemotherapy which is most likely to damage or kill the tumor. However, not enough is known yet about the effects of the anticancer drugs on various kinds of cancers and individual differences among patients to make this an exact science. Thus the medical oncologist cannot always specifically predict how the drug will affect the tumor of any given patient, although he can usually predict the amount of toxicity of the drug. It has been said that using chemotherapy is like trying to kill crabgrass without killing the whole lawn.

What is meant by combination chemotherapy?

That is when more than one drug is being used for treatment. Most often two to five drugs are used in combination. These combinations are often used in an attempt to kill cells in different phases of their reproductive cycle and to delay or prevent resistance of the tumor to the drugs from occurring.

Does each patient get the same dose of the drug?

No. The doses are based on many things, including body size. Some of the dosages are calculated in milligrams of drug per kilogram of body weight. Others are calculated in milligrams of drug per square meter of body surface area. More and more drugs are being based on surface area because the surface area changes less during the course of the treatment and thus allows a more constant amount of the drug to be given during therapy. When more than one drug is used in a combination treatment plan, the dose for each drug is usually lower than when it is used alone. What the doctor is trying to do for each person is to give him the "maximum tolerated dose"—that is, the amount of the drug which will give the greatest anticancer effect with the least amount of damage to normal cells.

Are there any new developments in chemotherapy drugs and how they are administered?

The following techniques and developments are currently under early investigation:

- Attaching a drug to monoclonal antibodies that will find and kill cancer cells, leaving normal cells alone
- Using implanted, refillable pumps to deliver anticancer drugs directly to organs
- Isolating cancer cells from a patient's tumor in the laboratory and testing different drugs against those cells

before chemotherapy is begun on the patient. It is hoped that this will allow doctors to match drugs more closely with an individual's disease.

* Finding new drugs which have fewer or less-drastic side effects than the present drugs
* Using biological drugs—that is, those made by the body itself—which may be less toxic than conventional chemotherapy.

There is more information about new developments in cancer treatment in Chapter 9.

Why is it that some of the drugs are given by intravenous injection while others are given in pill form?

It is because chemotherapy drugs differ in many ways, and this affects the form in which they are given. Some drugs are not absorbed when given by mouth and have to be given by injection.

How is chemotherapy given?

Chemotherapy can be given
* *Orally*, by mouth, in pill, capsule, or liquid form (PO)
* *Intravenously*, either injected into a vein as a shot (IV push) or as a fluid drip (IV or IV drip)
* *Intramuscularly*, by injecting it into a muscle in the arm, buttocks, or thigh (IM)
* *Subcutaneously*, with an injection beneath the skin (SQ)
* *Intra-arterially*, by injecting it into an artery (IA)
* *Intrathecally*, by injecting it directly into the spinal fluid (IT)
* *Intracavitarily*, by injecting it into the pleural space (lung) or into abdomen (for fluid accumulation)

How is the method of administration decided?

Some drugs can be given only in one or two ways. Adriamycin, for example, can be given only intravenously or intra-arterially. If the drug can be given in different ways, the decision will hinge on the necessary dose, preferences of the doctor and the patient, what kind of cancer it is, and so on.

Can drugs be given directly into the bloodstream without putting the needle into your vein each time?

There are several different ways this can be done, especially for people who need to have drugs or other fluids injected often into the bloodstream. The doctors may insert an indwelling catheter, implant a drug delivery system or use a pump to give the drugs.

How does the indwelling catheter work?

The doctors insert one end of a catheter—a thin silicone rubber tube—into a larger vein or artery deeper inside the neck, chest or abdomen. The other end comes out through a small incision in the skin. Drugs or fluids are injected or infused through the end of the catheter and then go directly into the bloodstream. This device can be left in place for days, weeks or even months.

How is a drug delivery system inplanted?

The system is placed completely under the skin, usually on the chest. It consists of two parts—a portal, a small stainless steel chamber, and a catheter, a thin flexible rubber tube. One end of the catheter is placed in a vein or artery inside the body and the other end is firmly attached to the portal with a special lock. The operation takes from 30 minutes to an hour. Both parts of the system are placed completely under the skin. There is no permanent opening. Drugs and fluids can be put directly into the bloodstream through a simple injection through the skin.

Can pumps be implanted to give chemotherapy drugs?

Physicians at a number of hospitals are using infusion therapy as a treatment. This method, known as intra-arterial infusion, uses either an external or internal pump to give the drugs. It delivers high concentrations of the drug to a specific target—unlike the intravenous (IV) infusion, which distributes the drug throughout the entire body. An external pump can be used, but it restricts the person's activities.

How does the internal pump work?

The size of a hockey puck, the internal pump is like a balloon that is sensitive to pressures within its own walls. The pump is implanted in the body. The drug can be delivered at an even rate over time. Since the pump is inside the patient's body, the patient can carry on normal activities. When the drug supply is used up, it is refilled by injecting more drug through the skin into the pump. The pump is being used for liver, head and neck, and brain tumors.

Does it hurt to get a chemotherapy drug?

It depends upon where and how it is being given. If you are taking it in pill, capsule, or liquid form or applying it as an ointment, it is no different from taking any other medicine in the same form. If you are getting a drug which is injected into the muscle, it is like getting a vaccination or penicillin shot. You usually feel a pinprick. If you are taking a drug which needs to be injected in the vein, the process takes longer than the muscle injection but does not usually involve pain. It is similar to having blood drawn for a blood test. A needle is put into the vein under the skin and the drug is pushed in or drips into the body from an intravenous setup. The time of the whole procedure varies from 2 minutes to 1 or 2 hours. Some people having certain drugs injected say they feel a temporary burning sensation in the area of injection. Others feel warmth throughout the body. Some patients say the needle insertion hurts. With a few drugs, extreme care must be taken when they are administered intravenously.

What determines how the chemotherapeutic drug will be given to me?

It depends upon the kind of drug being used, the kind of cancer you have, the extent of the disease, and the location of the cancer. For example, some drugs are given by IV (injection into the vein) because they reach the bloodstream better and thus reach the cancer cells better this way. IV is a way of making sure that the correct amounts of the drugs are carried to all parts of the body where the cancer may be growing. Some drugs are made only in a form which can be given in one manner.

Does one particular drug ever stop being effective in a particular patient?

Yes, sometimes the drugs lose their effectiveness against the particular cancer. Scientists believe that in some cases the cancer cells are multiplying more quickly than the drug can kill them. Other times the doctors have to reduce the doses or stop giving the drugs entirely because they are producing side effects on the patients. Sometimes the cancer cells have undergone change and are now able to survive and even grow rapidly in the presence of the once-destructive drug. When this happens the cells are called "drug-resistant."

How do cells become drug-resistant?

Cancer cells often find ways to avoid a drug's effect and "turn off" its anticancer activity. If that happens, doctors usually try to overwhelm the resistant cancer cells by introducing new drugs or combinations of drugs. Unfortunately, for some reason, cancer cells are often able to resist these new agents as well, even drugs they haven't encountered before or drugs that have different structures and mechanisms of action. Researchers have found that some cancer cells, through genetic changes, "learn" to produce large amounts of an enzyme that overrides a drug's usefulness and allows the cancer to grow again. In other cancers, the cell membrane changes in a way that allows it to block the entry of the drug into the cell or reduce the time the active drug remains in the cell. Some cancer cells show increased amounts of a certain protein on the cell membrane which may influence the way a drug enters or leaves the cancer cells.

What kind of research is being done on drug resistance?

Many studies are being conducted in this field. Researchers have found ways to overcome drug resistance in cells grown in the laboratory. Several of these approaches are now being used on patients in clinical trials. These include different ways of administering drugs, such as alternating treatment with different combinations or injecting the drug directly into a region like the abdomen in order to increase the local concentration of drug delivered to a cancer site.

What is meant by regional perfusion?

That is when the drugs circulate in a closed circuit through the bloodstream of the cancer-affected region. A tourniquet prevents the drug from reaching and damaging sensitive organs beyond the cancerous area. The drug is injected through an artery to the cancerous area, is withdrawn from a vein by special tubes, and then recirculated through artery and vein by means of a pump oxygenator. Regional perfusion allows large doses of drugs to be directed to one spot in the body. It is especially suited to treating certain tumors in the arms and legs.

For how long and how often will I be getting chemotherapy treatments?

The length of time and how often you will be having treatments depend upon the kind of cancer you have, the drugs being used, how long it takes your body to respond to the drugs, and how well you tolerate them. Treatment schedules vary widely. Chemotherapy may be given daily, weekly, or monthly. Some drugs are given every 4 to 6 weeks, with other drugs given weekly in between. There are also drugs that may be given every day for a short time or drugs that may be taken orally once or twice a day over a long period of time. When used as a preventive measure (adjuvant therapy), chemotherapy may continue for 1 or 2 years, depending on where the primary tumor is located. Some people have to stay on chemotherapy off and on for the rest of their lives.

How does the doctor measure whether or not the drug is working?

The nurse and doctor will use several methods for measuring the effectiveness of the drugs: physical examination, laboratory tests, scans, x-rays, blood counts, and blood chemistry tests. All patients on chemotherapy will have certain laboratory tests on a regular basis. Blood counts, for instance, will be used by the doctor to help adjust the doses of drugs. Other chemical tests will monitor your blood sugar and kidney and liver function. Scans and x-rays allow the health team to determine if the treatment is working. Team members will also be checking your weight, eating patterns, side effects, amount of pain you have, energy level, and how you are feeling in general.

Will I be able to continue working while I am having chemotherapy treatments?

Most people find that they are able to work and perform the physical activities to which they are accustomed, such as swimming, golf, tennis, etc. Often working people can be put on a program that doesn't interfere with work schedules, such as receiving the drugs just before the weekend or late in the day. Some patients, however, do feel tired when they are on drugs.

Does it make any difference what time of day the drugs are given?

It depends upon the drugs. Some drugs must be taken or given at a specific time in order to be sure that certain levels of the drugs are in your blood at all times. This is a subject that you need to discuss with the health team that is caring for you. It is important to follow your doctor's instructions very carefully. In addition, there is some research under way indicating that time of day—circadian rhythms—may influence side effects of the treatment.

I am taking my chemotherapy at home. What if I forget to take it?

You should set up a schedule so that you will not forget. Take the drugs at mealtime or at certain times during the day so it will be easier for you to remember. If you forget at any time, make sure you tell the doctor as soon as possible.

Will I be able to drink wine and cocktails while I am on chemotherapy?

Usually you can drink in moderation. That means not more than one or two cocktails daily or wine with your dinner. Double-check with your doctor first. In some circumstances it may be absolutely essential that you have no alcohol. If your platelet count falls, for example, or if you develop any bleeding, your doctor may advise you to stop drinking alcoholic beverages. Alcohol may interfere with your liver function and destroy vitamins. Chemotherapy may have to be stopped if this occurs.

Can I take other pills or drugs during treatment?

A few things may interfere with or in some way affect your chemotherapy, so to be safe you should tell your doctor the dose, frequency, and use of any medicine—pills or liquid, prescription, nonprescription, or over-the-counter—that you are taking. It would be most helpful if you bring your prescription medicines with you when you visit the doctor. If you begin taking new medicines while on chemotherapy, be sure to tell the doctor.

Some of the drugs which can interfere with your chemotherapy include antibiotics, anticoagulants, blood medicines, anticonvulsant (anti-seizure) pills, aspirin, barbiturates (such as Seconal and Nembutal), blood-pressure pills, cough medicines (including Robitussin), Darvon, diabetic pills, hormone pills (including birth-control pills), sleeping pills, tranquilizers (nerve pills), and water pills.

Will I be able to have dental work done while on treatment?

Generally you will. Again it depends upon your illness and the drugs you will be taking. Regular teeth cleaning and cavity repairs are not usually a problem. However, be sure to tell your dentist that you are on chemotherapy drugs. If the dentist is going to perform oral surgery, take out a tooth, or give you an injection, tell your doctor so that blood counts can be taken a few days before the dental work is going to be done. If the counts are normal, your dentist can do minor surgery as he would if you were not receiving the drugs.

Do all chemotherapy drugs produce some side effects?

The extent of the side effects (you will sometimes hear the word *toxicity* used when referring to side effects) varies greatly from patient to patient and from drug combination to drug combination. The side effects range from slight in some people to severe in a few instances. Some drugs have more noticeable side effects than others. Some people go through their entire chemotherapy treatment without suffering from side effects. Others do have serious problems. We have listed the side effects as known for each drug. It is important to remember that no one experiences all of them. Remember too that the doctors and nurses can help you minimize some of them. Your own attitude plays a large role many times in determining how severe your side effects will be. Some believe that patients who have a relaxed attitude toward chemotherapy may experience milder side effects.

Why does a patient get side effects from the chemotherapy?

The drugs that kill the cancer cells may also harm the normal cells, especially those cells that are growing fast or are not fully developed. The mouth, stomach, and intestines, the hair follicles (roots), and the bone marrow are areas of the body which normally have fast-growing cells and are thus affected by the chemotherapy. To allow the normal tissues to repair themselves, drugs are generally given in cycles to provide drug-free intervals. The drugs work against cancer over the long term because the normal cells repair themselves faster than the malignant ones.

Are the side effects of all the drugs the same?

No. Each drug has its own potential side effects. When drugs are combined, the side effects can change. You should talk with your doctor about what the side effects are for the kind of treatment you are getting.

What can be done to minimize the side effects?

It depends upon the drug, the dosage being given, the tumor being treated, the stage of the disease, and the severity of the side effect. Sometimes, as in the case of some cancer where there are several different kinds of drugs which can be used, as soon as a sign or a symptom is noticed, the drug is discontinued and another given in its place. In other cases, the dose may be decreased to just below the symptom level. Or the doctor may prescribe medicines to lessen the side effects if he feels they will not interfere with the chemotherapy drugs. There are several suggestions in this chapter (and in Chapter 22) of ways to deal with side effects.

How long do the side effects last?

Most of the problems last a few hours to a few days. For example, most nausea and vomiting will usually disappear in a few hours. At the other end of the scale of side effects is hair loss, which may not abate until the chemotherapy treatments are finished.

Do the side effects mean that the drugs are working?

There does not seem to be any relationship between the side effects and what is happening to the tumor. Neither the appearance of side effects nor the absence of them seems to have any relation to the effectiveness of the drug. A patient may have no side effects and yet the drug may be making the tumor shrink greatly. Another patient's tumor may also be shrinking greatly but that patient can be experiencing considerable side effects. It depends upon the individual's tolerance to the drugs being given and the responsiveness of the cancer cells to them.

Are there any serious side effects for which I should call my doctor immediately?

You should promptly report the following symptoms to your doctor:
- Fever over 100°
- Any kind of bleeding or bruising
- Development of any rash or allergic reaction such as swelling of eyelids, hands, or feet
- Shaking chills
- Marked pain or soreness at the chemotherapy injection site
- Any pain of unusual intensity or distribution, including headaches
- Shortness of breath or inability to catch your breath
- Severe diarrhea
- Bloody urine

Any new, unexpected symptoms, especially severe ones, that arise during chemotherapy should be promptly reported to the doctor.

Major Chemotherapy Drugs: Their Uses and Most Common Side Effects

DRUG	KIND OF CANCER COMMONLY USED FOR	HOW GIVEN	COMMON SIDE EFFECTS	OCCASIONAL OR RARE SIDE EFFECTS
Alkylating Agents*				
Busulfan (Myleran)	Chronic myelogenous leukemia	Oral	Nausea and vomiting, diarrhea	Bone marrow depression, skin darkening, hair loss, breast enlargement, impotence, sterility, chronic lung problems, eye problems
Chlorambucil (Leukeran)	Chronic lymphocytic-leukemia, lymphomas, breast, ovarian, testicular, choriocarcinoma	Oral	—	Bone marrow depression
Cisplatin (Cis-diamminedi-chloroplatinum, CDDP, platinum, Platinol)	Testicular, ovarian, head and neck, lymphomas, sarcomas, bladder, lung, esophagus, cervical, prostate, myeloma, melanoma, osteogenic sarcoma	Intravenous	Severe nausea and vomiting	Bone marrow depression, kidney damage, hearing problems, eye problems

Drug	Cancer	Route	Common Side Effects	Other Side Effects
Cyclophosphamide (Cytoxan, Endoxan, Neosar)	Lymphomas, leukemia, breast, ovarian, myeloma, lung, neuroblastoma, retinoblastoma, Ewing's sarcoma, mycosis fungoides, testicular, rabdomyosarcoma, endometrium	Intravenous, oral	Nausea and vomiting	Bone marrow depression, hair loss, bloody urine (can be prevented by drinking lots of fluid), sterility (may be temporary), chronic lung problems, skin darkening, nasal stuffiness, second cancers (bladder, acute leukemia), eye problems
Dacarbazine (DTIC-Dome, imidazole, carboxmide)	Melanoma, Hodgkin's disease, sarcoma	Intravenous	Nausea and vomiting, burning pain where needle put in (if drug leaks out during IV)	Bone marrow depression, flu-like symptoms, metallic taste, sensitivity to sun, liver damage, flushing of face, skin rashes
Estramustine phosphate (Estracyt, Emcyt)	Prostate	Oral	Nausea and vomiting	Diarrhea, feminization, bone marrow depression, heart problems, skin rashes
Mechlorethamine (HN2, Mustargen, nitrogen mustard)	Lymphomas, lung, mycosis fungoides	Intravenous (For mycosis fungoides, intravenous, local instillation, and topical)	Severe nausea and vomiting, irritation of veins, burning pain where needle put in (if drug leaks out during IV)	Bone marrow depression, hair loss, skin rashes, menstrual irregularities, fever

*Can cause gonadal dysfunction (sterility) and long-term use can lead to a slight increase in leukemia.

Major Chemotherapy Drugs: Their Uses and Most Common Side Effects (continued)

DRUG	KIND OF CANCER COMMONLY USED FOR	HOW GIVEN	COMMON SIDE EFFECTS	OCCASIONAL OR RARE SIDE EFFECTS
Melphalan (phenylalanine mustard, Alkeran, l-pam, l-sarcolysin)	Breast, ovary, myeloma	Oral	Mild nausea	Bone marrow depression, especially platelets, second malignancies, lung problems, menstrual irregularities, hair loss, mouth sores
Thiotepa (triethylene thiophosphoramide)	Breast, ovary, bladder, Hodgkin's disease	Intravenous, intramuscular, subcutaneous, topically into bladder, intrathecal	Nausea and vomiting, bone marrow depression	Headaches, fever, allergic reaction, dizziness, local pain
Antimetabolites Cytarabine (ara-C, cytosine arabinoside, Cytosar-U, arabinosyl cytosine)	Acute leukemia, lymphomas, head and neck	Intravenous, intrathecal, subcutaneous	Nausea and vomiting, diarrhea, anemia	Bone marrow depression, mouth sores, liver damage, ulcers, dizziness, headache, lung problems, tiredness, bone pain, fever, rash

Drug	Uses	Administration		Side effects
Floxuridine (FUDR, 5-FUdR, 5-fluoro-2'-deoxyuridine)	Head and neck, liver	Intra-arterial	Loss of appetite	Nausea and vomiting, mouth sores, hair loss, bone marrow depression, skin rashes, itching, diarrhea, abdominal pain and cramps, ulcers, liver damage, catheter problems
5-Fluorouracil (5-FU, Adrucil, fluorouracil)	Stomach, colon, pancreas, liver, ovary, breast, bladder, prostate (basal-cell skin cancer—used as a cream)	IV push or drip, infusion into liver, oral less dependable	Nausea and vomiting, diarrhea, bone marrow depression	Mouth sores, bone marrow depression, skin darkening (sensitive to sun), hair loss, skin rash, poor muscle coordination, nail loss or brittle nails, increase of tears, euphoria
Hydroxyurea (Hydrea)	Chronic myelogenous leukemia, acute leukemia, head and neck, melanoma, ovarian, colon	Oral	Mild nausea and vomiting	Bone marrow depression, skin rashes, mouth sores, diarrhea, hair loss, hepatitis, itching
6-Mercaptopurine (Purinethol, 6-MP)	Acute leukemia, chronic myelogenous leukemia	Oral (IV experimental)	Occasional nausea and vomiting	Bone marrow depression, liver damage, mouth sores, skin rash, diarrhea, fever

Major Chemotherapy Drugs: Their Uses and Most Common Side Effects (continued)

DRUG	KIND OF CANCER COMMONLY USED FOR	HOW GIVEN	COMMON SIDE EFFECTS	OCCASIONAL OR RARE SIDE EFFECTS
Methotrexate (amethopterin, Mexate, Folex)	Choriocarcinoma, acute leukemia, lymphomas, sarcomas, head and neck, breast, colon, lung, testicular, mycosis fungoides	Intravenous, oral, intramuscular, subcutaneous, intra-arterial, intrathecal	Nausea, diarrhea, mouth sores, bone marrow depression	Gastrointestinal problems, liver damage, kidney problems, cough, fever, hair thinning, headache, mental impairment, anemia, flank pain, eye problems
6-Thioguanine (thioguanine, Tabloid)	Acute nonlymphocytic and chronic myelocytic leukemias	Oral	Occasional nausea and vomiting	Bone marrow depression, jaundice, appetite loss, diarrhea, mouth sores, skin rashes, possible liver damage
Natural Products (Plant Alkaloids and Antibiotics)				
Bleomycin (Blenoxane)	Squamous-cell cancer of head and neck, penis, vulva, cervix, skin, anus, lymphomas, soft tissue sarcomas, testicular, esophagus, melanoma, lung	Intravenous, intramuscular, subcutaneous, regional arterial infusion	Nausea and vomiting, fever, chills	Skin rash, darkening, discoloration, peeling or tenderness, chronic lung problems, mouth sores, hair loss, headache, swelling and pain in joints, unusual taste sensation, loss of appetite

Drug	Cancer treated	Route		
Dactinomycin (actinomycin D, Cosmegen)	Testicular, melanoma, choriocarcinoma, Wilms' tumor, neuroblastoma, rhabdomyosarcoma, Ewing's sarcoma, retinoblastoma, Kaposi's sarcoma	Intravenous	Nausea and vomiting, swelling of vein, hair loss	Mouth sores, bone marrow depression, skin rash, acne, second malignancies, loss of appetite, diarrhea, fever, fatigue
Daunorubicin (rubidomycin, daunomycin, Cerubidine)	Acute leukemia	Intravenous	Nausea and vomiting, fever, red urine, hair loss, burning pain where needle put in (if drug leaks out during IV)	Bone marrow depression, heart problems, mouth sores, liver problems
Doxorubicin (Adriamycin)	Breast, bladder, thyroid, lung, ovary, acute leukemia, sarcomas, neuroblastoma, lymphomas, Ewing's sarcoma	Intravenous	Nausea and vomiting, red urine, burning pain where needle put in (if drug leaks out during IV), hair loss, bone marrow depression	Mouth sores, liver damage, heart problems (dose related), skin darkening (nails, creases), can reactivate skin reactions from past radiation, kidney problems, fever, chills, eye problems
Mithramycin (Mithracin)	Testicular, Paget's disease of bone	Intravenous	Severe nausea and vomiting, diarrhea, burning pain where needle put in (if drug leaks out during IV)	Bleeding, bone marrow depression, liver and/or kidney damage, mouth sores, fever, headaches, depression, drowsiness, facial flushing

221

Major Chemotherapy Drugs: Their Uses and Most Common Side Effects (continued)

Drug	Kind of Cancer Commonly Used For	How Given	Common Side Effects	Occasional or Rare Side Effects
Mitomycin (Mutamycin)	Gastric, breast, lung, cervix, bladder	Intravenous	Nausea and vomiting, burning pain where needle put in (if drug leaks out during IV), fever	Bone marrow depression, kidney problems, hair loss, fatigue, tiredness, lung problems, diarrhea, fever, mouth sores, blurred vision
Vinblastine (Velban)	Lymphomas, testicular, head and neck, breast, kidney, Kaposi's sarcoma	Intravenous	Bone marrow depression, burning pain where needle put in (if drug leaks out during IV)	Nausea and vomiting, hair loss, mouth sores, loss of reflexes, severe constipation, skin rashes, mental depression, headache, diarrhea
Vincristine (Oncovin)	Lymphomas, breast, acute leukemias, Wilms' tumor, brain, testicular, cervix, neuroblastoma, rhabdomyosarcoma	Intravenous	Burning pain where needle put in (if drug leaks out during IV), hair loss	Pain in arms, legs, jaw, or stomach, numbness or tingling in hands or feet, bone marrow depression, severe constipation, metallic taste, hoarseness, mental depression

Hormones

Adrenocorticoids Cortisone, hydrocortisone, prednisolone, prednisone, methylprednisolone, methylprednisone, triamcinolone, paramethasone, fluprednisole, dexamethasone, betamethasone, fludrocortisone	Lymphomas, leukemias, breast, myeloma	Oral	Gastrointestinal upset, weight gain, fluid retention	Ulcers, increased susceptibility to infection, paper-thin skin, increased appetite, sleeplessness, agitation, skin rash, increased blood sugar and blood pressure, increased bruising

223

Major Chemotherapy Drugs: Their Uses and Most Common Side Effects (continued)

Drug	Kind of Cancer Commonly Used For	How Given	Common Side Effects	Occasional or Rare Side Effects
Androgens: Testosterone propionate (Neohombreol, Oreton), fluoxymesterone (Halotestin, Ora-Testryl), nandrolone phenpropionate (Durabolin), testolactone (Teslac), nandrolone decanoate (Deca-Durabolin), calusterone (Methosarb), dromostanolone propionate (Drolban, Masteril, Macleron, Permastril)	Breast, kidney	Oral	Nausea and vomiting, increase in facial and body hair, deepening of voice, prominent muscles and veins, increased libido	Fluid retention, jaundice, liver damage, personality changes

Estrogens: Diethylstilbestrol, diethylstilbestrol diphosphate (Stilphostrol, Stilbestrol diphosphate), chlorotrianisene (Tace), ethinyl estradiol (Estinyl), conjugated equine estrogen (Premarin)	Prostate, breast (post-menopausal)	Oral	Nausea and vomiting, bleeding, fluid retention, elevated blood calcium	Breast tenderness or engorgement, fluid retention, voice change, decreased libido, increased thirst, drowsiness, constipation, excessive urination, incontinence, heart problems
Progesterones: Medroxprogesterone acetate (Provera, Depo-Provera), hydroxyprogesterone caproate (Delalutin), megestrol acetate (Megace, Pallace)	Endometrial, breast, prostate, kidney	Oral, intramuscular	—	Nausea, fluid retention, liver problems, skin rashes, abscesses
Miscellaneous Aminoglutethimide (Cytadren, elipten)	Breast, prostate, adrenal	Oral	—	Lethargy, dizziness, skin rashes, facial fullness, bone marrow depression, fever, loss of appetite, nausea, vomiting

Major Chemotherapy Drugs: Their Uses and Most Common Side Effects (continued)

DRUG	KIND OF CANCER COMMONLY USED FOR	HOW GIVEN	COMMON SIDE EFFECTS	OCCASIONAL OR RARE SIDE EFFECTS
Carmustine (BCNU, BiCNU)	Brain tumors, lymphomas, multiple myeloma, lung	Intravenous	Nausea and vomiting, swelling and burning of vein	Delayed blood-count depression, lung problems, facial flushing, liver problems, dizziness, eye problems
L-asparaginase (Elspar)	Aute lymphoblastic leukemia, lymphoma	Intravenous, intramuscular	Nausea and vomiting, fever, allergic response, abdominal pain, diabetes, chills, fever	Liver damage, pancreatitis, drowsiness, weight loss, mental depression, clotting problems, seizures, lack of consciousness, flu-like symptoms
Lomustine (CCNU, CeeNU)	Brain tumors, lymphomas, kidney, lung, melanoma	Oral	Nausea and vomiting	Delayed blood-count depression, mouth sores, hair loss, liver problems, kidney problems, eye problems
Mitotane (O,p'-DDD Lysodren, 1-dichloro-2-[0-chlorophenyl]-2-[P-chlorophenyl]-ethane)	Adrenocortical carcinoma	Oral	Nausea and vomiting	Diarrhea, mental depression, tremors, visual disturbances, skin rash, lethargy, drowsiness, headache, hypertension, fever, general aching

Megestrol (Megace, Pallace)	Endometrial, breast, prostate, kidney	Oral	Changes in menstrual cycles and amount, vaginal bleeding	Nausea and vomiting, stomach cramps, weight gain, skin rash, headaches, hair loss, fluid retention
Procarbazine (Matulane)	Lymphomas, lung, brain	Oral	Nausea and vomiting, mental depression, confusion	Second malignancies, diarrhea, bone marrow depression, mouth sores, skin rashes, eye problems (See text for restrictions in diet.)
Streptozocin (streptozotocin, Zanosar)	Malignant insulinomas, carcinoid, Hodgkin's disease, liver, colon, pancreas	Intravenous	Kidney damage, nausea and vomiting, local pain, liver problems, second malignancies	Diarrhea, mild anemia, bone marrow depression, hypoglycemia, diabetes, liver problems
Tamoxifen (Nolvadex)	Breast, prostate	Oral	Nausea	Bone marrow depression, vaginal bleeding and discharge, menstrual irregularities, hot flashes, bone and tumor pain, visual changes, skin rashes, dizziness, hair loss, depression, light-headedness, headache

227

Major Chemotherapy Drugs: Their Uses and Most Common Side Effects (continued)

DRUG	KIND OF CANCER COMMONLY USED FOR	HOW GIVEN	COMMON SIDE EFFECTS	OCCASIONAL OR RARE SIDE EFFECTS
Investigational*				
Amsacrine (M-AMSA, 4'-[9-acridinylamino]-methansulfon-m-anisidide acridinyl anisidide)	Leukemia, lymphomas, colon, melanoma, breast, T-cell, lymphoma	Intravenous	Nausea and vomiting, bone marrow depression, burning pain where needle put in (if drug leaks out during IV)	Liver problems, mouth sores, seizures, heart problems
5-Azacytidine	Acute granulocytic leukemia, melanoma, gastrointestinal	Intravenous	Nausea and vomiting, diarrhea, fever	Blood-count depression, liver damage, lethargy, skin rash, mouth sores
Chlorozoto-cin (DCNU, CZT)	Colon, kidney, pancreas, ovarian, Hodgkin's disease, stomach, melanoma, breast, lung	Intravenous	Bone marrow depression	Nausea and vomiting, kidney problems, lung problems
Dianhydrogalactitol (DAG, galactitol)	Brain, ovary, cervix, lung	Intravenous	Bone marrow depression, burning pain where needle put in (if drug leaks out during IV)	Nausea and vomiting, mouth sores, skin rash

Drug	Used for	Administration	Side effects	Additional side effects
Carboplatin (cyclobutane dicarboxylate platinum, CBCDA, JM-8)	Lung, ovary, head and neck	Intravenous	Mild nausea and vomiting, bone marrow depression, anemia	
Dibromodulcitol (Mitolactol, elobromol)	Melanoma, chronic myelogenous leukemia, breast, head and neck, lymphoma, sarcoma, brain, lung, gastric, kidney, colon, ovary, uterus	Oral	Bone marrow depression	Nausea and vomiting, loss of appetite, diarrhea, shortness of breath, skin darkening, itching, hair loss, difficulty in urination, allergies
Dichloromethotrexate (DCM)	Colon, lung, liver breast, ovary	Intravenous, intramuscular, intra-arterial infusion	Hepatitis, jaundice, kidney problems, mouth sores, nausea and vomiting, abdominal pain, diarrhea, bone marrow depression	Hair loss, anemia, appetite loss, skin rash, lung problems
Etoposide (VP-16-213, Vepesid, epipodophyllotoxin)	Lymphomas, acute nonlymphocytic leukemia, small-cell lung, testicular, bladder, prostate, hepatoma, rhabdomyosarcoma, uterine	Intravenous, oral	Nausea and vomiting	Bone marrow depression, hair loss, lung problems, fever, chills, loss of appetite

All side-effects information is preliminary; additional or more severe adverse effects may be reported.

Major Chemotherapy Drugs: Their Uses and Most Common Side Effects (continued)

Drug	Kind of Cancer Commonly Used For	How Given	Common Side Effects	Occasional or Rare Side Effects
Hexamethyl-melamine (HMX, altretamine)	Lung, ovary, breast, lymphoma, cervix, head and neck	Oral	Nausea and vomiting	Bone marrow depression, mental depression and confusion, hallucinations, diarrhea, abdominal cramps, cystitis, impaired sense of touch, hair loss
Ifosfamide (Ifex, ifx, isophosphamide)	Non-Hodgkin's lymphoma, sarcoma, lung, ovarian, pancreas, testicular, melanoma, acute and lymphocytic leukemia	Intravenous	Urinary-tract problems, nausea and vomiting, hair loss	Bone marrow depression, confusion and drowsiness, liver damge, burning pain where needle put in (if drug leaks out during IV), nasal stuffiness, sterility, mouth sores, darkening of skin, lung and heart problems, anemia, nail ridging
Interferon (IFN)** and biological response modifiers	Lymphoma, myeloma, vocal cord, kidney, melanoma, breast, colon, rectal, lung	Intravenous, intramuscular, subcutaneous	Fever and chills	Bone marrow depression, fatigue, chills, flu-like symptoms, headache, loss of appetite, weight loss, hair loss, nausea and vomiting

Drug	Cancer types	Route	Side effects	
Methyl-gag (Methylglyoxal-bis-guanyl-hydrazone, MGBG, mitoguazone, methyl-G)	Melanoma, esophagus, lung, leukemia, lymphoma, myeloma, head and neck	Intravenous, intramuscular	Flushing, numbness —usually in facial areas but could involve entire body, nausea, mouth sores	Bone marrow depression, vomiting, bloody diarrhea, tiredness, fatigue, skin rash
Mitoxantrone (Novantrone, DHAD)	Leukemia, lymphoma, breast	Intravenous	Bone marrow depression, mild nausea and vomiting, mouth sores, green urine	Hair loss, heart problems, blue streaking in or around the vein, liver problems
Razoxane (ICRF-159, razoxin)	Lymphomas, acute leukemias, lung, gastrointestinal, osteogenic sarcoma, head and neck, breast	Oral	Mild nausea and vomiting, hair loss	Bone marrow depression, diarrhea, skin rash, flu-like symptoms, mouth sores, headaches
Semustine (methyl-CCNU)	Melanoma, gastrointestinal, lymphoma, brain tumor	Oral	Nausea and vomiting, second malignancies, kidney problems, delayed bone marrow depression	Lowered blood count
Tegafur (florafur, 5-fluoro-1-tetrahydro-2-furyl-uracil)	Breast, colon-rectal, stomach, esophagus, genitourinary tract	Intravenous, oral	Nausea and vomiting, flushing, dizziness and apprehension with rapid administration	Mouth sores, loss of muscle co-ordination, diarrhea, lethargy, confusion, dizziness

**Interferon (Intron, Roferon) has been approved by the FDA for use in treating hairy cell leukemia.

Major Chemotherapy Drugs: Their Uses and Most Common Side Effects (continued)

DRUG	KIND OF CANCER COMMONLY USED FOR	HOW GIVEN	COMMON SIDE EFFECTS	OCCASIONAL OR RARE SIDE EFFECTS
Teniposide (VM-26,4'-demethyl-epipodophyllotoxin-B-D-thenylidene glucoside)	Lymphoma, brain, bladder, lung, ovary, leukemia, breast, kidney, melanoma	Intravenous	Bone marrow depression	Nausea and vomiting, hair loss, fever, liver problems, loss of reflexes
Triazinate (TZT, Baker's antifol, ethanesulfonic acid)	Brain, kidney, stomach, breast, colon, lung	Intravenous	Nausea and vomiting, bone marrow depression, skin darkening, skin rashes, mouth sores, diarrhea	Visual disturbances (blurring, double vision, headaches, crossing of eyes)
Vindesine (Eldisine, desacetyl, vinblastine amide sulfate)	Lymphomas, lung, leukemias, colon, breast, testicular, melanoma	Intravenous	Bone marrow depression, burning pain where needle put in (if drug leaks out during IV), loss of reflexes, hair loss	Nausea and vomiting, jaw pain, constipation, loss of taste, fatigue, tiredness, skin rash, mouth sores, loss of appetite, diarrhea
Zinostatin (neocarzinostatin)	Acute leukemia, bladder, gastric, pancreas, melanoma	Intravenous, intramuscular, subcutaneous	Bone marrow depression, burning pain where needle put in (if drug leaks out during IV)	Nausea and vomiting, diarrhea, loss of appetite, fever, liver problems, skin rash, chills, headache, mouth sores, fatigue, lung problems

What can be done to help control my nausea and vomiting?

Drugs called antiemetic agents are used to help lessen nausea and vomiting. They are usually given before the chemotherapy treatment begins. Nausea and vomiting vary from person to person and also depend upon the chemotherapy agent being given. Among the drugs that may be prescribed to help combat nausea and vomiting are Compazine, Thorazine, Phenergan, Torecan, Trilafon, Inapsine, Haldol, Decadron, and Metoclopramide. Most are given orally, intramuscularly, or rectally. Some suggestions regarding food and nausea and vomiting are given in Chapter 22.

Can I take drugs at different times of the day to help control nausea and vomiting?

It depends upon the drug. Some must be taken or given at specific times or else they will not be effective. However, most nausea and vomiting seem to occur 2 to 4 hours after the treatment and last less than 24 hours. For some drugs, and some people, getting the drug early in the morning (along with antinausea medicine), then taking the antinausea medicine again 4 hours later and eating a light meal, allows them to eat a large meal at dinnertime, free of symptoms. Others say that taking their treatment late in the day along with antinausea medicine and a sleeping pill seems to work. These people say they can sleep through the night and feel only slightly nauseous in the morning. Talk with your doctor or nurse to see if there is any way to experiment with the times you take your antinausea medicine, depending upon the drugs you are being given.

Do nausea and vomiting usually occur at specific times?

Generally there seem to be three different kinds of nausea and vomiting experienced by cancer patients on chemotherapy:

- Nausea and vomiting which start a few hours after treatment and last a short time (this is the most common)
- Violent nausea and vomiting which is of 12 to 24 hours' duration
- A feeling of nausea which seems to be always with you (with this symptom you must force yourself to eat)

Is it true that marijuana can reduce nausea and vomiting?

The active chemical compound of marijuana, called THC—tetrahydrocannabinol—has been reported by researchers to be helpful in controlling nausea and vomiting in some cancer patients. The researchers feel that the drugs used in chemotherapy often cause the patient to feel nauseous by triggering a response in the brain rather than a response in the stomach. Marijuana, they theorize, acts on the brain to block or at least suppress the response. Over the past 10 years, the National Cancer Institute has tested THC on 20,000 patients.

Is the THC tablet available to cancer patients?

Yes, it is now available in prescription form under the trade name Marinol (dronabinol) and is manufactured by Unimed, Inc.

Does the THC tablet have any side effects?

Since THC is a mood-altering drug, some cancer patients on chemotherapy reported problems in tolerating the mood-altering effects, even when THC was helpful in curbing nausea and vomiting. Particularly in some older patients, problems were severe enough to require hospitalization for psychiatric care. Side effects of THC include anxiety, hallucinations, disorientation and dizziness. Many doctors feel that other drugs available are effective for nausea and vomiting without exposure to mood-altering problems. THC is probably most useful for those patients who have had a history of pot smoking and are accustomed to the drug's mood-altering effects.

Has hypnosis been used to curb nausea and vomiting?

Some people are plagued with nausea and vomiting before the chemotherapy treatment begins. For some, just a glimpse of the highway leading to the hospital or the smell of the clinic will trigger an attack. Several centers are using mind-control techniques to help ease the anxiety that brings on this anticipatory nausea. Among the mind-control techniques under study are relaxation, biofeedback, and self-hypnosis, which patients can do before leaving home. Some centers are using classical music and pictures of pleasant scenes to help patients. Most are having some success with mind-control techniques in giving their patients relief from the anxiety that can trigger attacks of anticipatory nausea and vomiting.

Sometimes the nausea takes away my appetite. Other times, even when I am not nauseated, I don't feel like eating. Is there something I can do?

It is important for you to eat well—especially a diet high in protein—during your treatment period. Your appetite may be poor, but you need to make sure you are eating a balanced high-protein diet in order to maintain your strength, to prevent body tissues from breaking down, and to rebuild the normal tissues that have been affected by the drugs. See Chapter 22 for additional information.

Will I lose my hair?

Many people find hair loss the most upsetting side effect of chemotherapy. The rapidly growing cells that make up the hair roots (follicles) are sensitive to chemotherapeutic drugs. Not all drugs cause hair loss, however. There are several important things to remember. The hair loss is temporary. Body hair generally returns once the chemotherapy drug is stopped. Occasionally, the hair will begin to regrow while you are still being treated with the chemotherapy drug. Complete baldness occurs generally within two to three cycles of the drug. When your hair begins to regrow it will be thick and soft and sometimes even better than before.

If I am bald to begin with, will I grow hair when chemotherapy stops?

No. If you are already bald before starting your chemotherapy treatments, there will be no new hair growth.

Will I lose my hair in places other than on my head?

The hair follicles of the beard, eyebrows, mustache, eyelashes, armpits, legs, and pubic area are all rapidly growing cells and are sensitive to some of the drugs used in chemotherapy. Sometimes the loss is partial, but many times there is a complete loss of scalp and body hair.

What should I do to prepare for the hair loss?

You should buy a hairpiece, a wig, or a toupee before you start the treatment. Eyebrow pencil and false eyelashes may be needed. Some people find that horn-rimmed glasses or other glasses that are fitted with rims coming just in front of the eyebrows can conceal this hair loss. Turbans, hats, or scarves can be used instead of a wig, but most patients feel more comfortable if they have made the effort to buy a wig before their hair starts to fall out. Wigs are tax-deductible medical expenses and may be covered by some medical insurance policies. Some hospitals and some American Cancer Society units have wig banks where you can get them free.

If you have long hair, cut it short before it begins to thin. If you buy a hairpiece, use it as the hair begins to thin out. Some black patients find they can delay hair loss by braiding their hair instead of vigorously combing it.

What is a cold cap and how does it help to prevent hair loss?

Researchers are investigating ways to prevent hair loss through the use of scalp hypothermia—the cooling of the scalp with a cold cap. The cap is usually put on the head about 10 minutes before the drug is given and is left on during the treatment and for 30 to 50 minutes afterward. The cold cap causes a narrowing of the blood vessels of the scalp, lessening the amount of drug that reaches the hair follicles. The cap does not prevent hair loss in all patients. The best protection seems to be obtained in those receiving low drug doses.

Can the cold cap be used for all cancer patients?

The National Cancer Institute researchers caution that cold caps should not be used in patients with cancers that might spread to the scalp, such as leukemia, lymphoma, and mycosis fungoides. The use of a cold cap in treating these cancers could prevent the skull and scalp area from receiving necessary treatment. Additional studies of scalp hypothermia are being done. You should discuss the pros and cons of cold caps with your doctor.

Are there any side effects to using the cold cap?

Some patients have complained of headaches, a sensation of cold, and a feeling that the cap was heavy.

When hair falls out from radiation or chemotherapy treatments, does it fall out gradually or all at once?

Though hair loss differs from patient to patient, and from drug to drug, don't be surprised if your hair falls out in huge hunks, and your head becomes sensitive. Your scalp may also become flaky and irritated. A mild dandruff shampoo or some olive oil rubbed into the scalp may help.

Do you have any general hints about buying wigs and hairpieces?

Yes, we have a few hints.

- Buy the wig before you start losing your hair. This is very important. It is really best to get the wig before you start having the chemotherapy treatments if at all possible.
- Buy the wig yourself. Bring a friend with you if you like, but don't send someone else to do it for you. It is essential that the wig or hairpiece fits you well, looks nice on you, and pleases you.
- The less-expensive wigs tend to look synthetic. If this is the kind you are buying, dust it with a little baby powder to take away the shiny look.
- Get your first wig the same color as your hair. You can start wearing it while you lose your hair.
- Many people find it useful to buy more than one wig. Having a second wig is especially helpful if you tend to perspire.
- Buy a good synthetic, rather than a real-hair wig, because it washes better, is less expensive to maintain, is cooler, and is cheaper than the real-hair wigs.

Is there any kind of wig that is better if I am only going to have partial hair loss?

If your doctor expects you to have only partial hair loss, it is better to get a capless wig.

Will it be hard to hold the wig on my head if I have complete hair loss?

It may be. It is generally recommended that you use beautician's tape folded upon itself to hold the wig in place. Tape it to the crown and the temple areas of the wig. There is a company that makes wig retainer pads, which can be attached to any wig by a simple basting stitch. The pads cushion the scalp by conforming to the natural contour of the head. (International Foam Products, Inc., 711 Commercial Ave., Carlstadt, NJ 07072. 201-935-9065.)

You should also have the wig styled to fit your face. Styling is usually included in the cost of the wig, but if it isn't, you can have it done at a beauty parlor. If you are expecting complete hair loss, make sure that the inside of the wig is smooth.

Can I wear a headband underneath my wig?

Yes, if you prefer. People who wear headbands under their wigs usually like cotton scarfs instead of silk or synthetic scarfs. Cotton is cooler and helps keep the wig from sliding.

Are there any special scarfs or turbans made for women with hair loss?

There are several manufacturers of special scarfs and turbans. One style, called Hide & Chic, is a combination scarf and hat of light cotton and polyester that has body and shape to disguise the lack of hair beneath. There is also a child's version. (Marebar, Inc., P.O. Box 547, Marlton, NJ 08053.) The Sweetie Cap is a comfortable, inexpensive cover-up complete with bangs, which can be used as a cool, featherweight alternative to a wig. (Lan Care, Inc., 2747 17th Ave. Ct., Moline, IL 61254–9990.) A lightly padded headband, called Scarf Shapers, gives height and shape to scarfs. It is made of soft poly-cotton and padded with batting; it fastens at the back with velcro and is washable. (Scarf Shapers, 42 Winthro Drive, Riverside, CT 06878.)

How often should I wash a wig if I am wearing it every day?

People who wear wigs all the time usually wash them every week. Wigs tend to trap dust, and then they become hotter to wear. You should use shampoo to wash your wigs. Deodorant soaps will leave a coating on them.

Are there specific things I can do while losing my hair?

You can wear a soft fabric nightcap to catch the hair. If you use a nightcap, make sure it is a soft one, not a stiff netting type. Check the elastic on it so it will be comfortable for your head size.

What about when my hair starts growing in again?

As your hair starts growing in, shampoo it often. You might also want to go back to a hairpiece rather than wearing your full wig while your hair is growing back.

Will coloring my hair or having a permanent while I am having chemotherapy make my hair fall out?

It does not seem so. There has been some limited research done on this subject, and the women who colored their hair or had permanents during chemotherapy did not seem to have any more or any less hair loss than those who did not.

What can cause my urine to change color while I am on chemotherapy?

Some drugs can temporarily change the color of your urine. Some may turn it red, orange, or bright yellow. This is a temporary side effect and is not due to blood in your urine. The doctor can tell you if your drug can cause this side effect.

What can I do for bloody urine?

It depends upon what is causing it. If it is due to infection, the doctor will need to provide medication. However, if it is a side effect of your drug, you can do some things yourself to help. You can avoid it by drinking about 2 quarts of non-alcoholic beverages every day, if you are on a drug such as cyclophosphamide where this can be a problem. The bloody urine (or cystitis) caused by drugs is due to irritation of the lining of the bladder. This gives you discomfort or bleeding when urinating. Usually the doctor will tell you that if you are taking the particular drug at home daily, you should take it early in the morning. If you are taking it twice a day, take one dose in the morning and one in the early afternoon so that you will have plenty of time to drink a lot of fluids and flush your bladder well before bedtime. Otherwise the urine and drug will be sitting in your bladder for several hours. If you see blood in your urine or have a burning sensation and the urge to urinate often, increase your fluid intake and call your doctor's office.

What can I do about the sore spots inside my mouth?

Good mouth care such as brushing your teeth several times a day and frequent use of a mouthwash can help lessen the soreness. Even if you do not now have mouth sores, it is a good idea to take extra care of the mouth as a preventive measure when taking these drugs. Salt, baking soda, glycerine, or peroxide mixed with water can be used several times a day as a rinse. Commercial mouthwash usually irritates the sores. A soft-bristle brush or swab can be used to clean your mouth if your regular toothbrush is too stiff. You should also floss every day as part of your oral health program. Topical anesthetics, such as those used for teething children, may be soothing. You might ask your doctor to prescribe a topical anesthetic to use before meals. If your mouth is sore, try to plan your menus around bland, nourishing foods that are heated only to a medium temperature. There are additional hints in Chapter 22.

Will chemotherapy affect my teeth?

Certain chemotherapy drugs cause a reduction in saliva in your mouth. Saliva protects your teeth against tooth decay. The dentist might prescribe the daily use of a fluoride gel in a small tray that fits over your teeth. Fluoride mouthrinses may also be recommended. It is important to be under the care of a dentist who has experience in treating people undergoing chemotherapy.

Will I get tired?

It depends upon you—your physical condition and how your body reacts to the drugs. Some people do complain about becoming tired easily. Some people find they can continue their normal daily activities. Do whatever you feel like doing at your own pace. Understand that increased cellular activity is taking place as cancer cells are being destroyed. If you find you are getting tired, plan rest periods during the day. Don't get overtired. The fatigue will gradually decrease as your therapy progresses. Don't get discouraged or alarmed if you find that you are getting tired; it is a normal reaction and it does not mean that you are getting worse. Patients say they continue to have a fatigued feeling for a period of time even after the treatments have stopped. The feeling gradually goes away.

What is meant by temporary damage to the bone marrow?

Many types of chemotherapy, while stopping the growth of tumor cells, also stop the growth of cells in the bone marrow. The bone marrow is where your body manufactures

- *White blood cells* (leukocytes), which help fight fungal and bacterial infections. They capture, destroy, and remove germs from your body.
- *Red blood cells*, which help carry oxygen to the various parts of your body. They also bring back waste products such as carbon monoxide.
- *Platelets*, which help blood to clot where there is a cut. They act as a tiny plug that stops the flow of blood.

Why are these cells particularly sensitive to chemotherapy?

Since bone marrow cells duplicate rapidly in order to maintain normal blood counts, these cells are particularly sensitive to chemotherapy. Bone marrow is responsible for producing most of the blood cells, and thus you may experience a drop in some of your blood counts while on chemotherapy.

What does the doctor mean when he says he is going to take a complete blood count?

When the doctor takes a complete blood count (CBC) he will test some or all of the following:

- *White blood count,* which gives the number of white blood cells per cubic millimeter
- *Differential count,* which refers to the distribution of the various types of white cells in the blood, usually expressed in a percentage
- *Platelet count,* which gives the number or quantity of platelets per cubic millimeter in the blood
- *Hemoglobin,* which gives the amount of oxygen-carrying protein present in a known volume of blood, expressed in grams per centigram
- *Hematocrit,* which is the percentage that red cells occupy of the whole blood volume
- *Retic or reticulocyte count,* which is the percentage of young (non-nucleated) red cells present in the blood

What is meant by the term *bone marrow depression?*

It refers to the decreased ability or the inability of the bone marrow to manufacture the platelets, red blood cells, and/ or white blood cells normally produced there.

What is a drop in the blood count called?

It depends upon which cells it affects. A drop in the white blood cell count is called leukopenia. A drop in the red blood cell count is called anemia. A drop in the platelets is called thrombocytopenia. If all of them drop, it is called pancytopenia.

When does the doctor check my blood count?

Your doctor generally will be checking your blood count before he gives you any chemotherapy. If your counts are slightly low, he may hold up giving you your next dose of chemotherapy or wait and check your counts in a few days. This is not a bad sign; it simply means the effects of the drugs are still in your system.

What if my blood count falls very low?

If your blood count falls very low, you will be carefully followed and in some cases you may be admitted to the hospital for observation and for transfusion of blood cells, either white blood cells, red blood cells, or platelets.

Is there anything special the doctor will tell me to do if my platelet count is low?

Too few platelets will affect the clotting of your blood. This means that your blood will clot more slowly than usual so that bleeding may be prolonged following a cut or injury. If you should cut yourself, apply pressure over the cut for at least 5 to 10 minutes. If the cut is on an arm or leg, elevate it to slow the bleeding. It is best to avoid situations which might result in an injury—such as contact sports or heavy work. Be especially careful when using knives or razors. Avoid noseblowing or forceful sneezing. For shaving, an electric razor is safer than a straight razor.

A lack of platelets may also cause small red dots called petechiae on your skin. These spots are not harmful, but you should tell your doctor about them. You may also notice that you bleed easily from your nose or gums. Applying pressure or using ice or cold water will usually stop bleeding. If it lasts more than 15 to 20 minutes, call your doctor.

You will be given injections only if absolutely necessary. Your chemotherapy drugs might be suspended until your bone marrow recovers. Your doctor will probably suggest that you avoid sun, alcohol, and aspirin and any other medication unless approved by him. If severe bleeding develops, platelet transfusion may be necessary.

How does a shortage of red blood cells affect me?

A lack of red blood cells makes it difficult for your body to get enough oxygen to do its work. This may cause you to have the symptoms of anemia: tiredness, dizziness, pale skin color, and a tendency to feel cold.

What should I do if I have symptoms of anemia?

Even though you may have some of the symptoms of anemia you can still be fairly active. You'll need to have a balance of rest and activity in your day. Don't get overly tired. Set aside rest periods during the day. Allow yourself 7 to 9 hours of sleep a night. If anemia gets too severe, your doctor may transfuse you with packed red blood cells to correct your condition and decrease your symptoms.

What kind of problems will I have if my white blood count is too low?

A low white blood count makes it difficult for your body to fight infection. Even the common cold can be a problem.

If your white blood count is low you should take the following precautions:

- Try to stay away from crowds and people who have colds and flu; this is particularly important the first 10 days after receiving your drugs, because your white blood count will automatically drop before it goes back up.
- Keep cuts and scratches clean with an antiseptic such as alcohol and keep the area clean with soap and water until the sore heals.
- Inspect your body for signs of infection in your nose, on your lips, in your eyes, or in the rectal area. If an infection should develop, tell the doctor about it right away.
- If you contract a cold or flu, ask your doctor for advice. Do not take any medicine that has not been prescribed by the doctor, including aspirin, cough medicine, vitamins, antibiotics, painkillers, or any other type of medicine.

When I have a low blood count, are there any special symptoms I should watch for?

You should be alert to the following symptoms and report them to your doctor at once:

- *Signs of infection*: fever, sore throat, cough, sputum (phlegm), cold symptoms, chills or sweating, burning on urination and/or increased frequency of urination and/ or voiding small amounts, wounds that do not heal or that become red and swollen, boils and pimples that do not clear, vaginal discharge or itching
- *Signs of bleeding*: oozing gums, nosebleeds, bruising (especially without known injury), cloudy, pink or red urine, black or bloody stools, vaginal bleeding, long menstrual periods or too heavy or too frequent menstrual flow
- *Signs of anemia*: extreme weakness or fatigue

When I have a low white blood cell count, are there any special symptoms I should look for?

You should be alert to the following symptoms and report them to your doctor's office at once:

- An area of redness, swelling, or increased warmth on a part of the body
- Increased bruising and bleeding from your mouth or rectum; blood in urine or sputum; black bowel movement
- Extreme weakness or fatigue; a rise in temperature, runny nose or cough; chills or diarrhea

Are special isolation rooms used for patients with lowered blood count?

Special isolation rooms are in hospitals and are sometimes used for people who need to be protected from infection. Although still regarded as experimental, special germ-free rooms are used for patients while they receive massive doses of cancer drugs.

What is a laminar-air-flow unit?

This is an enclosure in which the patient is surrounded with a steady stream of sterile bacteria-free air, giving him sterile air to breathe and at the same time protecting him from contamination from the environment and from the attendants. All persons who enter wear a sterile gown, cap, mask, gloves, and shoe cover. Sometimes patient isolation systems are called life islands, with the hospital bed enclosed in a plastic canopy.

What is leukapheresis service?

This is another way of controlling infection in cancer patients. Patients who are treated intensively with drugs which produce a dangerously low white cell count can be given white cell transfusions. Doctors remove white blood cells from healthy donors for transfusions into patients who need them. In some study projects, the white cells are being given regularly to patients who have not yet developed an infection, as a preventive treatment.

What are some of the nerve and muscle effects one can get from chemotherapy?

They include numbness and tingling in the hands and feet. Some patients describe the feeling as similar to having one's hand "fall asleep." Some people experience a clumsiness in movement. Sometimes there are weakness and lethargy in moving the muscle. In rare cases, some people have problems with keeping their balance. They are temporary effects of the medicine on nerve cells.

Will having sexual relations hurt my partner who is undergoing chemotherapy?

There is no reason for sexual relations to hurt an individual receiving chemotherapy, though touch perception—the way touching feels—can be altered as a result of the changes in body chemistry. Of course, much depends upon where the cancer is and what stage it is in. Do not hesitate to talk with your partner as well as the doctor or nurse about sexual intimacy.

My partner's emotions seem to swing from depression to real "highs" since he's been on chemotherapy. Is this normal?

Though emotional problems such as those you describe are not unusual, it is important for the doctor to be aware of these reactions. Mood swings, including periods of depression followed by spurts of activity, have been observed in patients on chemotherapy. These emotions may be part of how your partner feels about the disease. Being tolerant, understanding that chemotherapy is a cause of unusual stress and realizing that as time passes, these side effects usually subside, will help you deal with his moods. For the patient who has been on chemotherapy for some time, the treatment can wear down mental and physical reserves. Therefore, the love and understanding of family and friends as well as of the health-care staff, are necessary for emotional stability. If the quality of the patient's life is being seriously changed by medication-related depression, the doctor may wish to adjust the medication schedule.

I'm worried because my menstrual cycle is all mixed up since I started on chemotherapy. Is such disruption usual?

Some drugs may change your menstrual cycle. Periods may come earlier or later than is usual for you and may last longer than normal. Sometimes women's periods stop temporarily, and sometimes they stop altogether in conjunction with menopausal symptoms such as hot flashes.

Is it all right for me to become pregnant while I'm on chemotherapy?

Your doctor will explain that you should not become pregnant while you are on chemotherapy. Prevention is important, because even if your period stops, it is possible for you to conceive. The effects of chemotherapy on unborn children are unknown, and it is important to prevent pregnancy during chemotherapy treatment. Once treatment is completed, menstrual periods may return and conception and normal pregnancy may be possible. If you are of child-bearing age, it is important to discuss the subject of birth control and childbearing thoroughly with your doctor.

I never had a vaginal infection until I started my chemotherapy treatments. The infection I've developed makes my vagina very itchy. Is it dangerous to continue having sexual relations?

Rubbing of the area during intercourse can be irritating and painful, and some doctors counsel patients to avoid intercourse for at least a few days. Since chemotherapy can lower the body's ability to fight infection, some women get vaginal yeast or bacterial infections which produce intense itching or burning sensations on the vulva or just inside the vagina. In some cases, the male partner also reacts, developing itching, burning, or redness of the penis after intercourse. It's a good idea to have your doctor check any vaginal infection symptoms so the problem can be diagnosed and the proper treatment prescribed. To help lessen irritation and prevent infection, it is suggested that you wear cotton underpants rather than those made of a synthetic fabric and panty hose with ventilated crotch and avoid shorts or slacks that are restricting.

What are the effects of chemotherapy on the male sex organs?

Often, men who are undergoing chemotherapy have a reduced sperm count, sometimes resulting in sterility. This, of course, does not mean that erection or intercourse is affected. Production of sperm may return to normal when chemotherapy is completed, although in some cases men have become permanently sterile. Since the effect of chemotherapy on the sperm and unborn child is not really fully known, it is advisable to use contraceptive precaution during this period.

The doctor said I might become sterile as a result of chemotherapy. Can I store sperm for future use?

For men desiring children, freezing or storing sperm for future use, *prior* to chemotherapy treatments, may be an option. This alternative should be discussed with the medical staff before treatment. Unfortunately, the technique is not always successful, since the quality of sperm may be such that conception may not occur. Production of sperm may return when chemotherapy treatments are stopped, although it is possible that sperm counts, and the effectiveness of the sperm, may be permanently reduced by some drugs.

My doctor told me that my chemotherapy treatments may have changed my sperm genetically. Is this possible?

There is some indication that some genetic changes in sperm may occur as a result of chemotherapy. Ask your doctor to recommend a urologist or genetic counselor who can evaluate the quality of your sperm and give you information on any possible effects on your ability to father a healthy child.

I notice I have black-and-blue bruises all over me since I've been on chemotherapy. Is there a reason for that?

Low blood-platelet counts are a side effect of many chemotherapy drugs. Low platelet counts may cause bruises or may cause you to bruise more easily. Strenuous sexual activity, when you are so susceptible to bruising, can result in black-and-blue marks on sensitive parts of the body. It is advisable to use a lubricant during intercourse to avoid injury to vaginal tissues while platelet counts are low.

Since I've been on chemotherapy, sex is uncomfortable because my vagina seems to be very dry. What lubricants can help?

Chemotherapy may cause the vagina to become dry. A water-based lubricant such as KY Jelly or Lubrifax can help. Vaseline is *not* recommended, because it is greasy, rather than water based, and can increase chance of infection. Saliva, your own or your partner's, can be applied by mouth or by fingertip to enhance lubrication and sexual excitement. You should also have your physician check your estrogen level, which provides information on how well your ovaries are functioning and whether the dryness is due to a physical change in your vagina.

What will the doctor recommend if I am retaining fluids?

He will probably tell you to avoid salty foods and to cut down the amount of salt you are using in your foods.

Can I expect side effects from hormone therapy?

Men taking estrogens sometimes get enlarged breasts and/or decreased sexual desires. Women taking androgens may find that their voices deepen, hair growth increases, and sexual desire increases. Women who are menopausal may have bleeding. You should discuss any of these symptoms with your doctor or nurse. These changes usually disappear when you stop taking the drugs.

Are skin rashes common during chemotherapy?

This side effect is sometimes seen. A drug may cause a slight rash around the injection site. It usually disappears within 30 to 90 minutes. Localized or generalized rashes are usually red and sometimes very itchy.

I have dry skin. Is that a result of the chemotherapy?

Dry skin can be a side effect of chemotherapy. Sometimes the cells of the skin become sensitive to the drugs. You may notice changes in skin color. The change may be in one small area or may cover a large area of your body. Both color changes and dry skin are temporary effects. Your skin should return to normal once you are off the medication.

What kind of personality changes might a cancer patient on chemotherapy expect?

Again, this is not a very common side effect. It is difficult to differentiate personality changes due to disease from those due to drugs. However, sometimes the person will experience changes in emotions, such as depression or confusion, because of the drugs. There are many things in life which affect your moods, but it is important that you and your family recognize that some drugs may cause these side effects so that you will be prepared for unusual feelings and keep them in proper perspective.

What flu-like symptoms do some patients experience?

Some of the drugs may cause a flu-like reaction after they are given. Many people experience fever and chills, aching bones, and a general tired feeling. Like other side effects, these should be reported to your doctor.

Is the metallic taste in my mouth a common side effect?

No, but it can happen to people on some of the drugs. Patients often try washing out their mouths frequently to try to mask the taste. Some also suck on citrus fruits or sugar-free hard candies as a remedy.

What can I do for heartburn or pain in the upper stomach?

This side effect can usually be relieved by taking half a glass of milk or 1 or 2 tablespoons of an antacid preparation; if it is severe and unrelieved, contact your doctor's office.

Is it unusual for dark circles to form on my fingernails?

Some drugs cause darkening of the fingernails. This is a harmless side effect and will usually disappear when the drug is stopped.

Do veins ever get darker when a patient is on chemotherapy?

Sometimes the drugs will irritate the veins and some discoloration may develop along the pathway of the vein.

Sometimes it looks as if someone has marked it with a dark-brown felt-tipped pen. The darker your skin, the darker the vein becomes. Exposure to the sun makes the vein even darker. Don't be alarmed; veins are not damaged, and the coloring fades within a few weeks.

Do patients sometimes suffer from irritation where the drug is being injected?

This may happen. If it is a rash it normally disappears in 30 to 90 minutes. However, tissue burns from leakage of medications at the site of the injection should be reported to the person giving the drug immediately. Cold compresses such as ice and pain medication may be used to help alleviate discomfort.

What kinds of eye problems can patients on chemotherapy experience?

Eye problems for patients on chemotherapy are relatively rare. They can include blurring of vision, tearing, double vision, headaches, crossing of eyes and formation of cataracts. Most of the problems are temporary, disappearing when the patient stops taking the drug. Sometimes the loss of eyebrows and eyelashes, which can be a part of hair loss caused by chemotherapy, can cause irritation and excessive tearing of eyes.

Are there any foods which cannot be eaten while taking procarbazine?

Procarbazine (Matulane), a drug sometimes given to patients with Hodgkin's disease, lung, and brain cancers, can sometimes cause reactions in some people in combination with certain foods and drinks. This is because of a complicated interaction of the drug with foods containing tyramine. Typical reactions include headache, flushed face, fast heartbeat, and a rise in blood pressure. Among the foods which can cause these reactions are ripe cheeses (especially cheddar), spicy sausages (salami, pepperoni), Chianti wine, chicken livers, pickled herring, alcohol, and foods that are aged or overripe. Reaction to these foods, however, is rare. You may continue to eat foods from this group if you wish, but start in small amounts to be sure that they still agree with you. You are most likely to get a reaction during the second week you are taking procarbazine and the week following when you stop taking it.

Does everybody have to follow these restrictions regarding procarbazine (Matulane)?

It depends. Patients on MOPP protocol are usually told by their doctors and nurses to follow the instructions. There is a wide variation with some people having no reactions at all and others having severe reactions. People with lung and brain cancers who are taking procarbazine are also usually already having difficulties in eating anything at all. They should be encouraged to eat foods they wish. You should talk with your health care team about these problems.

My veins are difficult to find. Is there anything I can do?

Many people who receive chemotherapy develop problems with their veins. You can help by squeezing a tennis ball or other piece of equipment which develops hand strength. Do the exercise 50 to 100 times three or four times a day. You can do the exercise while you read, watch TV, or even while you are waiting in the clinic.

Do any of the chemotherapy drugs cause a gain in weight?

Some of the drugs, such as prednisone or dexamethasone, do increase your appetite and cause weight gain in some patients. Sometimes your blood pressure also gets higher. If this happens, the doctor will probably tell you to not add salt to your food and to avoid salty snacks such as pretzels. It has also been noted that many women with breast cancer tend to gain weight while on chemotherapy regardless of what drug they are taking.

Will I experience constipation if I am on chemotherapy?

It depends upon the drugs you are being treated with. Most of the pain medications are likely to make you constipated. For some drugs, such as vincristine, constipation can be an early symptom of a more serious problem. Try to prevent constipation before it occurs by drinking lots of water (at least eight glasses a day) and fruit juices. Eat fruits and vegetables if your diet allows. A glass of prune juice or a few tablespoons of bran in the morning may help you. Keep active with hobbies and light exercise such as walking. You can try a stool softener such as Metamucil, which you can buy at a drugstore without a prescription. If you do become constipated, discuss it with your nurse and doctor. They may tell you to take a regular laxative or prescribe something for you. It is important to discuss the side effects with the health team taking care of you so they will know if there is anything unusual happening. There are additional hints for dealing with this problem in Chapter 22.

Will I experience diarrhea?

The patients who get diarrhea are usually those taking antibiotics and antimetabolites. You should try a diet low in roughage, high in constipating food like cheese and boiled milk. Diarrhea can easily cause you to lose fluid and become dehydrated. It is important that you drink plenty of fluid every day. If you have tenderness in the anal area, use a substance such as a medical ointment. If it does not stop in 1 or 2 days or if you have more than two or three loose stools a day, be sure to talk with your doctor. You should not take any medicine for diarrhea without your doctor's permission. There are additional hints for dealing with this problem in Chapter 22.

What can I do about sensitivity to the sun?

You should be careful when going outside, even if you are walking outdoors. Wear a hat, and use sunblock lotion. Be careful when you are at the beach. Be sure to wear sunblock lotion that contains para-amino benzoic acid (PABA).

What is meant by the term *Leucovorin rescue?*

This is an experimental technique which is used to spare normal cells from the toxic side effects of high doses of methotrexate. Methotrexate has been used in low doses for many years to treat cancer. It is now being tested in high doses for the treatment of several diseases, including head and neck cancer, leukemia, and osteogenic sarcoma. Large amounts of methotrexate are given for a prescribed period of time, followed by the administration of another drug, citrovorum factor (Leucovorin), at a predetermined time.

The Leucovorin rescues or protects the patient from the life-threatening effects of high doses of the methotrexate.

Are cancer patients on chemotherapy at a higher risk for getting shingles?

Cancer patients, especially those with lymphomas, are more susceptible to shingles. Other patients receiving chemotherapy drugs which suppress the immune system are also at a higher risk. Shingles (or herpes zoster) is a painful viral infection of certain sensory nerves that causes a skin rash along the course of the affected nerve.

Can I be vaccinated or take flu shots when I am on chemotherapy?

Vaccination can be dangerous for patients with lymphomas. It is important that you check with your doctor before taking any type of immunization shots.

Is there a risk of developing a second cancer as a result of drug treatment?

Some researchers have reported an increased risk of acute nonlymphocytic leukemia among patients who had been treated for ovarian cancer and Hodgkin's disease and in research with laboratory animals. Alkylating agents and the drug procarbazine are the agents involved.

Does the risk of developing a second cancer as a result of chemotherapy mean that I should not be taking chemotherapy?

Reports of such potential risks do not suggest that chemotherapy drugs should be avoided. Rather, you and your doctor need to discuss the potential risks of chemotherapy against the potential gains. Chemotherapy has cured many people and has enabled others to live for longer than they could have expected to without it, since the drugs are used to delay, and possibly prevent, a recurrence of the cancer.

What does the doctor mean when he says a breast or prostate cancer is "hormone-dependent"?

He means that the cancer is depending on the hormones in your system to make it grow. How this mechanism works is not clearly understood. But it is known that about 40 percent of the breast cancers and over half the prostate cancers fall into the "hormone-dependent" category. In the case of hormone-dependent prostate cancers, sometimes the testicles are removed to take away the hormones which are supporting the growth and the female hormone estrogen is given to change the environment. In the case of breast cancer, particularly in younger women, the ovaries may be removed to change the environment. In three out of ten cases, the tumor will actually be reduced in size and occasionally will disappear. Tests (called estrogen receptor tests) have been devised to determine whether or not a tumor is hormone-dependent.

Why are female hormones used to treat prostate cancer and male hormones used to treat breast cancer?

Scientists are uncertain as to the exact mechanism by which hormones influence the growth of cells. Some cancers of the breast, prostate, and uterus occur in tissues which are influenced by hormones; sometimes they appear at a time of life when hormonal activity in the body has changed, such as after menopause. Cancer that starts in tissues such as the breast in women and the prostate gland in men depends for its growth on the presence of the hormones to which these tissues normally respond. Scientists feel that treatment with hormones may affect these cancers through changing the normal environment. Thus androgens (male hormones) are sometimes used to treat women with breast cancer. Older women who have passed menopause sometimes respond to treatment with doses of estrogens (female hormones). Female hormones help to suppress the growth of cancer of the prostate. Other hormones used are corticosteroids such as cortisone and prednisone for certain types of leukemia and lymphomas. Doctors also sometimes remove glands which secrete hormones (such as the ovaries or testicles) to help slow down malignant growth.

How many different kinds of chemotherapy drugs are now in use?

Over fifty different chemotherapy drugs have been developed that are useful in the treatment of some kinds of cancer. Some of them are still in the experimental or investigational stages.

Who discovers these new drugs?

The National Cancer Institute sponsors an international co-operative chemotherapy program, involving many research laboratories of the federal government, the universities and medical schools, and the pharmaceutical industry. This program encourages scientists of all kinds to search for drugs to cure cancer. Chemotherapy is one of the most heavily studied areas in cancer treatment. Scientists are creating new chemical compounds, studying plant specimens, and extracting antibiotics from natural fermentation products and soil samples. At the same time, many of the world's top chemists are searching for ways to improve the activity of known drugs.

How many new materials are tested each year?

According to the National Cancer Institute, each year about 50,000 materials are tested, including chemicals, antibiotics, natural products, and newly synthesized compounds related to known drugs. Of almost equal importance is the testing of new doses and schedules which alter the anti-tumor activities of some of the older drugs.

How are the new materials tested?

The first series of tests for new materials are performed on animals. They are tested against particular kinds of cancer in rats and mice that have been shown to predict anti-tumor activity in man. If the drug appears to work in the small rodents, it is then tested in larger animals such as monkeys and dogs to see what kind of side effects it produces and to make sure that the drug kills cancer cells without damaging normal tissues excessively. If the drug passes these tests, it is then put through a series of tests on human patients.

How are the drugs tested in patients?

After a new cancer drug comes out of the laboratory testing, there are several years of careful, step-by-step "clinical trials" before it can be approved for general use. Before a new drug may be used in clinical studies with cancer patients, the Food and Drug Administration (FDA) must license the compound as an Investigational New Drug. The National Cancer Institute coordinates these clinical trials, using investigators who participate on a voluntary, cooperative basis. These scientists determine the suitability of candidate drugs for evaluation in the treatment of one or more malignant diseases. Only one out of every 5,000 drugs originally screened is considered promising and safe enough to be studied in patients.

What are the phases of drug evaluation?

- *Preclinical*: This is the phase in which drugs are tested in rodents, and if they pass those tests are then tested in large animals.
- *Phase I*: This phase involves patients with advanced disease who have exhausted other forms of treatment. The first trials are usually begun at one-tenth the dose that produced side effects in the most sensitive animal species. The drug is usually used on patients with a wide range of cancers. During this phase the dose is gradually increased in subsequent patients until the dose that produces tolerable side effects is reached. Effects on the tumor are also evaluated. The data collected in this part of the study indicate the side effects which can be expected in humans. The drug can be used only if the person gives informed consent and can stay nearby to be closely monitored during the first few treatments.
- *Phase II*: The anti-tumor activity of the drug is determined in several specific cancers during this phase. Tumor masses are measured and x-ray studies are done so that the effectiveness of the drug can be evaluated before the decision is made to continue the trials. Again, the tests are performed on patients with advanced disease for whom no effective treatment is available. During this phase, the types of tumors which respond to the drug and how often they respond are closely measured to determine the effects of various dosages and how frequently they must be given to produce good results.

- *Phase III*: If the drug is found to be effective in the Phase II trial, this phase establishes whether the drug is more useful and/or has fewer side effects than other drugs already being used. The drug is tested on patients on a large scale, comparing it with the best standard therapy (drugs currently being used) to determine which is better.

The doctors say they are going to use a "Phase II" experimental drug. Should the word *experimental* scare me?

The words *experimental* and *investigational* are used when the new anti-cancer drugs are in the research stages. They are understandably alarming words unless you understand the stringent guidelines which govern drug development. The experimental drugs are only available through persons working under the auspices of the National Cancer Institute, using U.S. Food and Drug Administration regulations governing the use of experimental drugs. If your physician is using a Phase II drug, it has already been screened in the preclinical and Phase I evaluation.

How do I know whether or not my doctor is using an experimental or investigational drug?

You will know because you must sign a consent form. The person giving the investigational drug must clearly explain to the patient both the potential value and the possible risk. This procedure allows the patient to weigh the advantages against any additional problems it might create. A patient may receive an investigational drug only if he qualifies under very specific criteria. Before any of the investigational drugs are administered, the doctor must have a diagnosis (from a biopsy), x-rays to determine the extent of the disease, and studies to determine the patient's blood picture.

Who is allowed to give investigational drugs?

The federal regulations allow only qualified oncologists (cancer specialists) to prescribe investigational cancer drugs. This is to ensure that the patient will receive every possible benefit with a minimum of risk.

Does the doctor giving the investigational drug have to follow any rules and regulations?

Yes. All drug investigations have written guidelines, called protocols, which spell out the overall plan, the criteria for selecting patients, and requirements for monitoring patients, and they give general directions to the investigators. The three distinct phases of drug evaluation on patients are carefully controlled experiments which reveal dosages, side effects, and anti-tumor activity.

During a Phase III drug evaluation, does the doctor or the patient know which patients are getting the experimental drugs and which are getting the drugs already considered standard therapy?

It depends on several factors. The drug evaluation may be done in what is called a randomized trial. In some, neither the doctors nor the patients know whether the drug which is being given is the new experimental drug or the standard therapy. These are called "double-blind" studies. In others, the persons giving the drugs and sometimes the patients know whether they are getting the new drug or the standard therapy.

How am I, as a patient, protected in these investigation trials supported by the National Cancer Institute?

All patients participating in the National Cancer Institute-supported research programs are protected by Department of Health, Education and Welfare regulations (45 CRF, Part 46) pertaining to studies with human subjects. The institutions in which the research is carried out must have review committees of medical scientists who decide whether the importance of the knowledge to be gained outweighs the risks to the patients who participate. In addition, the patients must give their informed consent to participate. The major elements of informed consent as noted in the regulations include the following:

- A fair explanation of the procedures to be followed and their purposes, including identification of any procedures that are experimental

- A description of the discomforts and risks reasonably to be expected
- A description of the benefits reasonably to be expected
- A disclosure of any appropriate alternative procedures that might be advantageous for the patient
- An offer to answer any inquiries concerning the procedure
- A disclosure that the person is free to withdraw his consent and to discontinue participation in the project or activity at any time without prejudice to the subject

Do the hospitals using the investigational drugs have any say in what drugs are being used?

All investigational drugs used in accredited hospitals must be approved by a committee (usually called the human investigations committee or the human experimentation committee) which usually includes administrators, pharmacists, and physicians. They study all available information on a drug to decide whether or not it is appropriate for use with patients in their institution.

I hear the word *protocol*—what does that mean?

Protocol is the term used to describe your treatment program. It means a predetermined treatment plan for groups of patients with similar medical problems. It is usually used when referring to treatment with experimental drugs.

What does the term *randomization* mean?

Randomization is part of being on a clinical trial. Some protocols have several treatment groups or "arms." People are assigned to an arm on an unbiased basis. This is called randomization and is considered the best way to remove bias on the part of the doctors and to clearly establish if one treatment is better than another. These studies are not done unless there is a question as to whether one treatment is better than another.

How expensive is chemotherapy?

The cost associated with chemotherapy varies depending upon the drugs being used, how often they are given, and even where they are being given. The cost of the visit to the doctor, the tests involved, and the charge to administer the drug must be added to the cost of the drug itself.

Will my insurance cover chemotherapy?

It depends. Some major medical policies cover chemotherapy. It is important that you discuss the costs with your doctor and clarify your coverage with your insurance company.

chapter 9

Investigational Treatments

New cancer treatments—be they immunotherapy, hyperthermia, biological response modifiers, or new chemotherapy drugs—start in the basic research laboratories with studies in test tubes and on animals. Careful trials are conducted. Then, if the experimental or investigational treatments show promise of being better than standard ones, they are tested in patient studies, called clinical trials. Important information about a new treatment is obtained from clinical trials: whether it is safe and effective, its risks, and how well it may or may not work. Many new treatments are currently being investigated at cancer centers and clinical centers around the country. You may hear or read about them and consider learning more about how they can be applied in your own treatment. The Cancer Information Service 1-800-4-CANCER toll-free number can give you information on where these treatments are being carried out.

Questions You Should Ask Before Agreeing to Investigational or Experimental Treatment

- What is the purpose of the study?
- What does the treatment involve? What kinds of tests will be needed?

- What will happen in my case if I don't have this treatment?
- What will happen in my case if I do have it?
- Are there standard treatments for my case? If so, how does this study compare with them?
- What are the risks involved? What are the side effects from this treatment compared with the standard treatment? Could I be harmed by the research?
- How will my daily life be affected? Will the treatment make me sicker?
- How long will the study last?
- Will I have to be hospitalized? If so, how often and for how long?
- What are the benefits of the new treatment?
- What are my alternatives?
- How much will the treatment cost?
- Is there any long-term follow-up care as part of the study?
- Do I need to sign an informed consent form?
- Can I stop treatment at any time?

What kinds of treatments are considered investigational?

There are investigational treatments of all kinds. Some involve trying new chemotherapy drugs or new combinations of chemotherapy drugs. Others add one treatment to another, such as giving radiation while operating on a patient. The use of heat to treat tumors, called hyperthermia, is another investigational treatment. Much of the current research is in the field of immunology or biological response modifiers.

What is immunology?

Immunology is the study of the body's defense system, which is called the immune system. The body uses this mechanism to protect itself against infection and disease.

Is immunotherapy new?

Although the idea that the immune system might hold the secret to the cure of cancer dates back to the 1800s, its use in treating the disease is still in its infancy. Immunotherapy is a relatively new and experimental form of treatment with varying results. All forms of immunotherapy are considered investigational at this time, and clinical trials to evaluate these treatment methods are currently under way at a number of medical centers around the country.

What is immunotherapy?

Immunotherapy is a method of managing cancer by making use of the body's own immune system. In immunotherapy the patient is given either a vaccine or a stimulating material which may boost the patient's ability to make antibodies or to mobilize lymphocytes and other cells capable of killing the cancer cells. In other words, immunotherapy is an attempt to strengthen the immune system of the patient to fight off the disease. It is important to understand that as a treatment, immunotherapy is in an investigational stage and is being used only in major medical centers around the country.

Why does the immune system let cancer cells grow?

Researchers have found that cancer cells often have a way of hiding from the immune system. They may add a chemical disguise that prevents the system from knowing they are foreign bodies. Scientists also speculate that the body's immune system can destroy only a certain number of cancer cells; they theorize that by the time its defense is mounted, too many cancer cells may have formed. New research is showing that changing one part of the immune system may make it react, leading to changes in another part. Other research indicates that stimulating one part of the immune system may lead the body to make substances that may weaken the immune responses and even lead to tumor growth.

How does the immune system work?

The immune system is a complex natural watchdog. If a person gets a cut, for instance, as bacteria invade the system and infection starts, the body is warned by its immune system. It mobilizes cells to survey the invading agents and then to form specific neutralizing proteins (called antibodies) as well as specific cells able to engulf, destroy, or neutralize. Another example of the work of the immune system is in diseases such as measles or smallpox. It has been known since early times that people who recovered from such diseases were nearly always safe (immune) from getting the disease if ever exposed a second time. This protective mechanism is the immune system.

How does the immune system recognize invading foreign bodies?

White blood cells—some of which are lymphocytes—are constantly circulating through the blood and lymph system. These lymphocytes recognize cells that are different and foreign, such as bacteria and viruses. When the lymphocytes recognize the foreign cells, they multiply and attack and kill them. The lymphocytes essentially are a surveillance system—they watch over the body cells and try to get rid of those which do not belong in it.

Does the immune system recognize cancer cells?

One of the most important recent advances in immunology is the demonstration that the lymphocytes recognize tumor cells in much the same way they recognize bacteria and viruses. It seems, however, that in some persons the immune system may not work perfectly and fails to recognize cancer cells or to respond appropriately to them, allowing them to grow. Some scientists feel that the changes in the surface of cancer cells are not as foreign to the body as viruses or bacteria, since cancer cells are closely related to normal body cells. Many scientists feel that cancer cells occur in our bodies more often than we realize, and that most of us repel these early cancers without ever being aware of it.

What is meant by "spontaneous tumor regression"?

When tumors in untreated patients get smaller for no apparent reason or disappear completely, it is called spontaneous tumor regression. In some rare cases when a tumor disappears spontaneously it may remain undetectable for long periods. It is more usual, however, for the tumor to shrink temporarily, for the patient to get better, and then for the tumor to grow back again. Scientists feel that it seems logical to assume that the immune system is responsible for these regressions. However, it is possible that the supply of nutrients to the tumor or other factors play a role in this phenomenon. The phenomenon of spontaneous tumor regression has stimulated much research into possible immune mechanisms.

What kinds of cells are in the immune system?

The immune system has many components, some of them discovered so recently that they are still being categorized. Most functions of the immune system are performed by cells called lymphocytes, which fall into two categories: B lymphocyte cells make special molecules called antibodies, which then attack invading cells; T lymphocyte cells kill invading cells and sometimes tumor cells directly. Scientists estimate that the body contains more than 1 million lymphocytes and that about 1 percent of that total are replaced daily. Other cells—killer cells, natural killer cells, suppressor cells, and macrophages—are also involved in the body's immune defense.

What are biological response modifiers?

Biological response modifiers are substances used to trigger the body's own defenses against cancer. Scientists have discovered hundreds of biological (manufactured by the body) and chemical substances that boost, direct, or restore many of the normal immune defenses of the body. Many of these substances occur naturally in the body, while others are made in the laboratory.

What is the difference between immunotherapy and treatment with biological response modifiers?

Treatment with biological response modifiers includes the traditional immunotherapy but also encompasses the use of highly purified biologic substances with anticancer activity.

What are the various kinds of biological response modifiers?

Biological response modifiers—the entire field of immune system research—are usually classified into several categories:
  • Antigens, such as monoclonal antibodies and vaccines
  • Interferons

- Thymosins
- Lymphokines and cytokines (such as interleukin and tumor necrosis factor)
- Immunomodulating agents, such as BCG and lavamisole
- Effector cells, such as macrophages and natural killer cells
- Miscellaneous approaches, such as bone marrow transplantation

A major National Cancer Institute program is presently testing the efficiency of several of these promising substances.

How do scientists think biological response modifiers will be used to fight cancer?

A number of potential uses for biological response modifiers are being explored, including the following:

- Helping normal cells to control cancer cells by boosting the immune system or by eliminating or suppressing the bodily response that permits cancer growth
- Making cancer cells more sensitive to being destroyed by the patient's immune system or stimulating cancer cells to grow and to mature into less harmful cells
- Blocking the processes that change a normal or precancerous cell into a cancerous one
- Enhancing the body's ability to repair normal cells damaged by other forms of treatment such as chemotherapy or radiation
- Using biological response modifiers as direct agents on some parts of the immune system

What are monoclonal antibodies?

Research into biological response modifiers has led to the discovery of monoclonal antibodies, invisible bits of protein manufactured by animal and human cells, which can also be grown in the test tube. Each type of antibody—and there are hundreds of them—has the incredible ability to recognize and latch onto a specific target. The target can be any living matter, down to and including a single biological molecule. Monoclonal antibodies are powerful new tools for cancer treatment, and monoclonal antibody technology is a giant step toward developing treatments that attack specific cancer cells.

How are monoclonal antibodies used to kill cancer cells?

There are several studies under way to research use of monoclonal antibodies in different areas of cancer treatment. They include

- Injecting antibodies into a patient's bloodstream and letting them work on their own, searching out and destroying cancer cells
- Adding a protein (called a complement) to monoclonal antibodies before they are injected to strengthen their ability to destroy cancer cells
- Attaching chemotherapy drugs to monoclonal antibodies before they are injected. When an antibody finds a cancer cell, the chemotherapy agent is released, destroying the cancer cell—but leaving the normal tissue surrounding it
- Attaching radioactive isotopes to the antibodies so that the isotopes can deliver radiation directly to cancer cells

Monoclonal antibodies have been tested with limited success on patients with colon, bone, breast, skin, and lymph cancer and leukemia. Most of the research is in early stages. In Boston, a combination of monoclonals is being used, in addition to standard treatment, to treat leukemia patients, mostly children. Drugs and radiation are used to eliminate the visible leukemia cells. Bone marrow is removed, treated with monoclonal antibodies to destroy remaining cancer cells, and then returned to the body. In Baltimore, radioactive iodine has been chemically bonded to monoclonal antibodies to treat patients with liver cancer. There are trials in progress to test the use of monoclonals in treating B-cell chronic lymphocytic leukemia, cutaneous T-cell lymphoma, melanoma, and advanced lymphoma.

How is interleukin being used in treating cancer patients?

Scientists at the National Cancer Institute and at selected other centers have been working with experimental animals for several years to identify normal cells in the immune system that can kill cancer cells. In 1980, a natural body substance, known as interleukin-2, was used to treat white blood cells to generate immune system cells that reacted against cancer cells. These cells were named lymphokine-

activated killer (LAK) cells. There is now a genetically en-
gineered form of interleukin-2, called RIL-2, which has been
used in the most recent animal and human studies.

Researchers used RIL-2 to treat white blood cells from
normal mice and then injected the resulting LAK cells into
mice with lung and liver metastases, giving them repeated
injections to enhance the effect of the LAK cells. This treatment reduced the size and number of lung and liver metastases in the mice. Scientists have begun to treat cancer
patients with advanced disease with RIL-2. White blood
cells are removed from the patients, treated with RIL-2 to
convert them into LAK cells, and then injected back into
the patients' blood. At the same time, the patients also receive RIL-2 intravenously. Other varieties of interleukin,
interleukin-1 and interleukin-3, are being tested. Besides
the National Cancer Institute, other centers which are conducting NCI-sponsored trials using interleukin-2 are the
New England Medical Center, Boston; Montefiore Medical
Center, Bronx, New York; Loyola University Medical Center, Maywood, Illinois; University of Texas Health Science
Center, San Antonio, Texas; Cancer Research Institute of
the Medical Center at the University of California, San
Francisco, and City of Hope National Medical Center,
Duarte, California.

What are the interleukin-2 TIL studies?

This is a new immunotherapy approach also developed at
the National Cancer Institute. The treatment is with new
cells, called tumor-infiltrating lymphocytes (TIL), powerful
anti-cancer cells in the body which scientists say appear to
be 100 times more potent than the LAK cells. The tests
have only been done in mice. Trials will be conducted with
a small number of patients to see whether what works in
mice will also work in humans.

How does tumor necrosis factor work?

Tumor necrosis factor (TNF) occurs naturally in very small
amounts in humans and other animals and has an ability to
destroy tumors. Laboratory tests on animals show that animals with cancer have lost the ability to produce tumor
necrosis factor in their own bodies. Research conducted in

Japan found that TNF could be produced artificially from a human gene by genetic engineering techniques, and can selectively destroy malignant cells in many different forms of cancer when applied in the laboratory to cancer cells. It is hoped that tumor necrosis factor will combat a long-standing problem in cancer treatment. Heavy doses of chemotherapy and radiation can make some patients more susceptible to a second cancer while curing the first. It is hoped that tumor necrosis factor will bolster the patient's immunity to other cancers, allowing patients to withstand greater doses of chemotherapy and radiation. Normal cells are virtually unaffected by TNF. TNF is currently in clinical trials at the National Cancer Institute and at a few selected other facilities nationwide.

Is research being done on ways to turn cancer cells back into normal cells?

Yes. Differentiation research, as it is called, is being conducted in several areas of the country. In laboratory experiments, scientists have successfully used chemical agents to halt the continuous reproduction of cancer cells. The cells do not become normal; that is, they do not perform the activities of regular cells. However, they are no longer young cancerous cells, and eventually they die as a normal cell would. Researchers have also found that some of the agents used to make the cells "mature" can increase the efficiency of anticancer drugs and radiation, and may be useful in treating advanced disease. This promising research is in very early stages, with Phase I trials under way in the United States and Europe.

What new methods are being used in chemotherapy treatment?

Some new methods are being tried; others are being researched. Among them are

- Using combinations of drugs, each of which attacks the cancer in one of a number of ways but has a different toxic effect on normal cells. This kind of treatment, first used successfully for leukemia and Hodgkin's disease, is now being used in many kinds of cancer.
- Using more intensive drug treatments for a shorter pe-

riod of time, making sure that patients get full doses of
drugs as quickly as possible
- Using chemotherapy before surgery or radiation treatments to shrink tumors. Some previously inoperable
  cancers can now be removed or destroyed. Other cancers
  need less-radical surgery or less-extensive radiation
  treatment than would have been needed without the
  preliminary chemotherapy. Head and neck cancer and
  osteogenic sarcoma are two cancers that have responded
  well to this treatment.
- Linking chemo drugs to monoclonal antibodies that are
  able to find their way to specific cells, delivering drugs
  directly to the tumors, sparing healthy tissues. This technique is still in early testing stages.
- Giving drugs directly to a limited area of the body, such
  as the liver, to destroy cancer cells with little damage to
  normal tissues. Pumps are used to deliver the drugs continuously to the area of the tumor. There are portable
  infusion pumps as well as pumps that can be implanted
  in the body. Sometimes a catheter will be implanted for
  delivering the drug into the tumor area.

Among the plans for future chemotherapy research are
- Finding new drugs that can overcome the resistance
  often developed by cancer cells to chemotherapy agents.
  Doctors have learned to alternate treatments by using
  different drug combinations and are seeking new and
  different ways to overcome the cancer cells' resistance.
- Learning more about how cancer metastasizes, determining why cells that leave the original site have a different chemistry than other cells, and devising drugs to
  counter them. This research is in its very early stages.
- Developing a laboratory test with computer measure-
  ments to determine how effective a specific chemotherapy drug will be on a particular patient, thus allowing
  a doctor to immediately decide on the best drug for that
  person.
- Discovering drugs which cause cancer cells to behave
  in more normal fashion—allowing them to mature so
  that they do not divide and multiply

New drugs, combined with new ways of using old drugs,
make the research in the field of chemotherapy very prom-

ising. The future holds hope for the development of drugs that attack cancer cells without damaging normal ones.

Does interferon, once promoted as a major cancer cure, still have a place in cancer therapy?

Research on interferon is continuing and is proving to be an important part of cancer treatment—although not the magic cure that was once envisioned. Interferon is a protein molecule made by the body's immune system in minute amounts. The molecule somehow helps the body to combat certain diseases, including those caused by some viruses and possibly including cancer. It is normally produced by cells. Researchers originally believed there was only one interferon. They have found, however, that there are many different interferon genes, each with a specific job, each different, but all working together in ways that scientists have yet to sort out. They have now divided interferons into three classes: alpha, beta, and gamma. They are further divided according to the cell types from which the interferon comes: leukocytes (white blood cells), lymphoblasts (precursors of immune cells), and fibroblasts (connective tissue cells). In addition, two different types of interferons are available: those produced naturally by the body and those produced synthetically by taking interferon genes, inserting them into bacteria, and raising a large quantity of the substance.

How effective has interferon been in treating cancer?

In animal trials, interferon has been most effective when it has been given at the same time or shortly after an animal has been inoculated with a tumor. Large tumors have not responded well to interferon. It is thought that interferon may not directly kill cancer cells, as do the conventional drugs, but may slow their rate of growth and division so that they become sluggish and die. It also seems to be a better anticancer agent when combined with a chemotherapy drug. Phase II trials (where the anti-tumor activity of the drug is determined in several specific cancers) have shown at least a 50 percent decrease in tumor size in occasional patients with breast cancer, melanoma, and a few miscellaneous solid tumors. Response rates in patients with kidney cell cancer appear to be higher. More than half of the lymphoma patients tested have responded to alpha interferon, and very high response rates (over 50 percent) have been seen in hairy-cell leukemia and chronic granulocytic leukemia. There are dozens of investigational trials under way using different kinds of interferon for various cancers.

What is thymosin, and is research into its use in cancer continuing?

Research on thymosin is being conducted at several centers in the United States and Europe. Thymosin is the name given to a family of hormones naturally produced by the thymus. The parent hormone of interferon, thymosin was first isolated from the thymus gland in 1965. Two forms of thymosin are being tested: thymosin fraction V, which is an extract from calf thymus tissue, and Alpha 1, which is synthetically produced. Patients with small-cell lung cancer, head and neck cancer, and renal cancer are participating in these early trials. Other thymosin preparations—such as thymopietin, thymic extract, and *facteur thymique serique* are under investigation in other parts of the world. One of the trials is using thymosin combined with radiation therapy. Thymosin is also being used with patients who are at risk for AIDS as well as for patients with AIDS, as a preventive to help ward off opportunistic infections.

What kinds of research are being conducted with lymphokines and cytokines?

Lymphokines and cytokines are proteins secreted by cells in small amounts to help regulate a variety of cell processes. Lymphokines and cytokines provide one of the means by which cells involved in the immune process "communicate" with each other and direct the overall process. The list of lymphokines and cytokines is long, and their potential seems great. Among the research projects under way are some involving interleukin, T-cell replacing factor, transforming growth factor, macrophage activation factor, and tumor necrosis factor.

What does intraoperative radiation therapy do?

Intraoperative radiation therapy gives a direct single dose of radiation to the tumor and potential areas of spread nearby at the time surgery is being done. The radiation therapist can see the tumor directly, rather than relying on x-rays and other means of pinpointing the cancer. In some centers, high-dose intraoperative radiation is used alone. In others, conventional external radiation is used, with the intraoperative radiation given as a boost at the time of the operation.

How is intraoperative radiation done?

The procedure requires a great amount of planning and cooperation between the surgeon and the radiation therapist. The surgeon performs the operation but does not close the incision. In most hospitals, the patient is then taken from the operating room to the radiation therapy area, where the radiation therapy is given. The surgeon then completes the operation.

Is intraoperative radiation new?

The concept of radiating the tumor during surgery is not new. It dates back to the early 1900s, but at that time x-ray dosages were too low to be effective. Over the past 15 years, the Japanese have been the most active in using intraoperative radiation. Several centers in the United States have recently begun investigational trials using intraoperative radiation therapy, with some promising preliminary results.

For what kinds of cancer is intraoperative radiation therapy being used?

Intraoperative radiation is used mainly in treating stomach, pelvic, and rectal cancer. Investigational trials are being conducted for gastric, pancreatic, colon-rectal, and cervical cancers and for soft-tissue sarcomas. Most of the trials are being carried out at the National Cancer Institute, Howard University, Massachusetts General Hospital, the Mayo Clinic, and the New England Deaconess Hospital.

What is particle-beam radiation therapy?

Particle-beam radiation therapy uses neutrons, protons, helium ions, negative pi-masons (pions), and heavy ions. It is in the early research stage. All types of particle beams are produced with physics equipment and are highly experimental. Systems designed especially for neutron therapy have recently been put into operation. Opportunities to treat patients with charged-particle beam radiation therapy have been few because of the physical limitation of the equipment and because the technology for sophisticated planning of treatments has only recently become available. Neutron-beam systems are the least expensive and most extensively studied. The other particle beams are still highly experimental and far more costly to produce than neutron beams.

Can my doctor refer me for particle-beam radiation therapy?

Yes. The many studies being conducted, mainly through the Radiation Therapy Oncology Group (RTOG), include research on cancers of the brain, uterus, head and neck, gastrointestinal (GI) tract, lung, and urinary tract, as well as ocular cancer and melanoma. A listing of the institutions accepting patients for research studies is in Chapter 23.

How does neutron-beam treatment differ from the usual x-ray radiation treatment?

Neutron beams work differently than x-rays. Neutrons are uncharged bits of nuclear matter. In neutron-beam radiotherapy, these neutrons travel at nearly the speed of light. When directed into the body, the neutrons collide with atomic nuclei, breaking some apart to produce a number of charged particles that in turn cause very dense damage in the area of collision. Neutron-beam radiation causes much denser damage than x-ray radiation.

What are the advantages of neutron-beam therapy over the usual x-ray treatment?

It is believed that neutron-beam therapy will offer several advantages in treatment:

- Neutrons are less dependent than x-rays on the presence of oxygen for their cell-killing ability. This fact may be important in the treatment of large tumors, many of which contain oxygen-deficient (hypoxic) areas.
- Neutron beams seem to be effective at killing cells regardless of the stage of the cell cycle.
- Cancer cells are less able to repair the denser damage done by neutron beams, so fewer cells recover.
- A lower physical dose of neutron beams kills the same number of cells as a higher dose of x-ray beams.

Where in the United States are there cyclotron neutron-therapy facilities?

The National Cancer Institute has funded development of cyclotron neutron-therapy facilities at the M.D. Anderson Hospital and Tumor Institute in Houston, at the University of California at Los Angeles (including the VA Hospital, the Jonsson Comprehensive Cancer Center, and the UCLA School of Medicine), and at the University of Washington in Seattle. In addition, the National Cancer Institute is supporting clinical research with a deuterium-tritium (D-T) generator made specifically to treat cancer patients at the Fox Chase Cancer Center in Philadelphia.

There are also facilities at the Cleveland Clinic Foundation Lewis Research Center (NASA) and at the Fermi National Accelerator Laboratory in Batavia, Illinois, both for neutron therapy. There is a physics cyclotron for proton therapy at Harvard University, and physics machines for helium and heavy-ion therapy at the University of California's Lawrence Berkeley Laboratory in Berkeley.

What are protons, and where are they being studied?

Protons are positively charged particles found in the nucleus of every atom. When accelerated to high speeds, a beam of protons can be accurately focused and delivered to tumors. Protons and other electrically charged particles also cause great damage as they slow down in tissue, resulting in what is called a "Bragg peak": a distinct maximum of radiation dose and consequent damage caused by these particles just before they stop. The Bragg peak can be made to coincide with the tumor, allowing a large dose of radiation to be delivered to the tumor region, with relatively little damage to the normal tissue beyond it. Cancer treatment experiments with proton beams are being carried out at the physics cyclotron at Harvard.

What are alpha particles, and where are they being studied?

An alpha particle consists of two protons and two neutrons—a helium atom stripped of its electrons. Removing the electrons from larger atoms, such as carbon and oxygen, results in what are called heavy ions. Alpha particles and heavy ions are positively charged, have a much greater biological effect in the Bragg peak area than protons, and are very expensive to produce. They are being studied for cancer treatment in physics facilities at the Lawrence Berkeley Laboratory in Berkeley, California.

What are hypoxic cells?

Hypoxic cells are cells that do not require much oxygen. The most commonly used forms of treatment work best on cancer cells that contain a lot of oxygen, because the oxygen molecules block the damaged DNA molecules from quickly coming together and repairing the damage. But most cancers, as they grow larger, develop areas that are deficient in oxygen, since the development of blood vessels to the tumorous tissues does not generally keep pace with the growth of the tumor itself. Some of the newer forms of treatment, such as radiation sensitizers and particle-beam radiation, are aimed at oxygen-deficient cells.

What are radiosensitizers and radioprotectors?

The development of radiation sensitizers and protectors may create a promising new method in cancer treatment. Most treatments now used are not able to kill off all the cancer cells, either because some cells are resistant or become resistant to the therapy, or because doses of the treatment that are high enough to kill all cancer cells will do too much harm to normal tissue. Radiation sensitizers are chemicals that replace the oxygen in a tumor's hypoxic cells (cells that contain little oxygen), thereby making them more sensitive to the treatment. Radioprotectors are agents that protect normal tissue against radiation, allowing higher doses to be given to kill the cancer cells.

Radiosensitizers are referred to as hypoxic cell sensitizers, thio-depleting agents (BSO and DEM), PDL repair inhibitors, and pyrimidine analogs. Terms referring to radioprotectors include sulfhydryl compounds with long chemical names and abbreviations such as MEA, WR-2529, WR-2923, and WR-638.

Are radiosensitizers and radioprotectors being tested on patients?

Yes, they are being used in early investigational trials. The treatments show promise in tumors of the brain, sarcomas of soft tissue, and bone cancer. Scientists feel that in the future, extensive combinations of radiation, chemotherapy sensitizers, and radioprotectors may create significant improvements in the treatment of cancer.

What is radioimmunoglobulin therapy?

Radioimmunoglobulin therapy is a method of delivering radiation directly to cancer tumors, via the bloodstream, using radioisotopes piggybacked to cancer antibodies. It allows continuous radiation to the tumor for days and even weeks, rather than short bursts of conventional radiation. Radioimmunoglobulin therapy, an investigational treatment, is being used in liver cancer. Proteins produced by the patient's tumor are taken out, purified, and then injected into rabbits, which in turn manufacture antibodies against the protein. These antibodies are then "tagged" with radioiodine and injected into the patient. The radiolabeled antibodies bind to the tumor, and then the radioiodine proceeds to destroy much or all of it.

Is the laser being used for cancer treatment?

In the past few years, lasers have been used increasingly in cancer treatment. A laser beam produces a narrow shaft of hot, concentrated light. When focused with lenses or mirrors into very small spots with high power concentrations, a laser beam can cut and vaporize living tissue with remarkable speed and precision. A doctor is able to zero in on a lesion without damaging the surrounding cells. The beam is set at high intensity to minimize charring and any threat to surrounding cells.

Are there different kinds of lasers?

Yes. Three different kinds of lasers are used in surgery. Their names come from the type of energy used to produce the light: carbon dioxide (CO_2), argon ion (Ar), or neodymium-yttrium aluminum garnet (Nd-YAG). The CO_2 and the Nd-YAG lasers are used in cancer treatment.

What does the carbon dioxide (CO_2) laser do?

The carbon dioxide laser bombards the tumor with continuous high-powered waves that not only kill the cancer cells, but literally vaporize them. The carbon dioxide laser is well absorbed by water. Thus, because body tissue is 70 to 90 percent water, the laser beam superheats the cell water to 100° C, vaporizing it. The vapor comes out as steam, which is removed with a suction device. The laser seals the nerves as well as most blood vessels, accomplishing its results without blood being shed.

How is the Nd-YAG laser used?

The YAG laser, so named because it employs a crystal made of yttrium, aluminum, and garnet, has the deepest penetration into tissue of any of the lasers. It can be used with fiberoptics. The laser is inserted into a patient's body through an endoscope, a slender, flexible tube with a fiberoptic core through which the insides of the area to be treated can be seen. Television and still-photography cameras can be connected to the scope to record what is found. Doctors can thread thin wires or tiny instruments down the endoscope to snip off tiny pieces of tissue, remove polyps or stones, and halt bleeding. A second fiberoptic tube the size of pencil lead can be fed through the endoscope, and the laser beam is then directed through the tube. The heat of the laser beam is used to cut or cauterize tissue. The depth of the cut and size of the burn can be controlled by adjusting the beam's power.

For what kinds of cancer are laser treatments used?

The CO_2 laser is being used in treating cancers of the vocal cord, oral cavity, bronchus, cervix, vagina, vulva, rectum, and brain. The YAG laser is being used in treating cancers of the stomach, colon, esophagus, rectum, bladder, and penis.

What is photodynamic therapy?

Photodynamic therapy—also called phototherapy, photo-chemotherapy, and photoradiation therapy—is the use of light-absorbing chemicals in treating cancer. In most cases, oxygen is required in addition to a photosensitizer and light. Some scientists consider photodynamic therapy a form of laser treatment.

How does photodynamic therapy work?

A chemical, called hematoporphyrin derivative or dihe-matoporphyrin ether, jumps to an "excited" and destructive chemical state when it is exposed to light. It then transfers its energy to the oxygen found in tissues, causing the oxygen molecules to become highly energetic. While it is in this state, which lasts about 1/1,000,000 of a second, oxygen is toxic to the cells around it. To allow deeper penetration of light into the tumor, some scientists are using fiber optic techniques in which light, reflected many times over, can be "curved" through a thin quartz fiber and inserted into the tumor.

What are the advantages of photodynamic therapy in cancer treatment?

One of the major advantages of photodynamic therapy is that it can be used following other treatments such as sur-gery, chemotherapy, and radiation therapy, thus adding one more possible treatment to those already available. Al-though it can be used on relatively large tumors (4 to 5 centimeters), photodynamic therapy appears to be espe-cially useful to people with early disease or early recur-rence. It has been used to relieve obstructions in the bronchial area, and it may also be an alternative to surgery for people who are not able to withstand an operation. Pres-ently, it is an investigational treatment.

How many patients have been treated with photodynamic therapy?

Since 1976, about 2,000 patients worldwide have been treated with photodynamic therapy. Most of the patients, who had advanced disease that was recurrent or unresponsive to other treatments, responded to the photodynamic therapy. There is some research under way using photodynamic therapy in conjunction with hyperthermia. Photodynamic therapy has been effective in treatment of tumors of the skin, lung, esophagus, bladder, and head and neck as well as in gynecologic tumors. It shows promise in many other areas as well.

Is it true that chemotherapy and radiation interfere with or damage the body's own immune system?

It is true that radiation and chemotherapy can suppress the immune system. It is also true that some cancer patients seem to start out with an immune system which is not fully normal. It is thought that gaps in the body's immune system may allow emergence of cancers and that, at some time in the future, we will find ways to strengthen the body's own defenses so that drugs and radiation will no longer be needed. At present, when treatment must be given for established cancers, it is felt that the least immunosuppression occurs with the off-again, on-again therapy now being used, permitting immune defenses to recover and thus protect the body's other functions.

What is hyperthermia?

Hyperthermia is the use of heat to kill cancer cells. The treatment is still investigational. Scientists are trying to determine whether the technique may prove valuable, particularly in combination with other methods of treatment such as surgery, radiation, and chemotherapy.

Why do scientists think that hyperthermia may work?

The idea of using heat for the treatment of cancer has been around for a long time. Some say it goes back to 600 B.C. Cancer cells do not tolerate slightly higher temperatures as well as do normal cells, so researchers have been investigating methods of applying heat to tumors with the least amount of damage to surrounding tissue. Some researchers feel that the heat stimulates the immune system and thereby enhances the anticancer activities of other treatments such as radiation therapy and chemotherapy.

Is there more than one kind of heat treatment?

Yes. There are several ways to bring heat into a tumor. It can be directly transferred by using water or hot wax. Electromagnetic radiation with microwaves, infrared rays, or radiowaves are sometimes used. An entire limb may be heated. Or a small antenna may be implanted directly into a tumor. The whole body may be treated by using a thermal suit or by placing the person within a series of hot-water blankets. Blood may be removed from the body, heated, and then returned to the body.

How is the heat concentrated in the tumor?

Tumors tend to have poor blood flow, and heat tends to concentrate in areas with poor blood flow. The normal tissue around the tumor has good blood flow and so is able to resist the heat.

Is hyperthermia safe?

There may be some discomfort in the area of the hyperthermia. The greatest risk is thermal burn, which can occur either in deep tissue or tissue nearer the top of the skin, depending on the kind of treatment. Whole-body hyperthermia may have severe complications. The temperature of the treatment, how long it lasts, how the heat is distributed, and the experience of the physicians doing the treatment are all important aspects. It is a treatment which should only be done by experienced, qualified professionals.

Is hyperthermia being used with other treatments?

Yes. Hyperthermia may be used to shrink a tumor before surgery. It may also be used in combination with radiation therapy and chemotherapy. Researchers believe that hyperthermia helps other treatments to work better.

Is hyperthermia being done in many hospitals?

There are approximately sixty medical centers in the country using hyperthermia in some form for treating cancers of the breast, head and neck, brain, lung, bladder, bone, and abdomen and gynecologic tumors. Research is continuing at a rapid pace.

Where is hyperthermia being tested?

Hyperthermia is being tested in several medical centers in the country and at the National Cancer Institute. Most patients being treated are those for whom all other standard treatments have been tried. Call the Cancer Information Service 1-800-4-CANCER to find out if there is a center near you using hyperthermia on an investigational basis. Several of the studies are being performed by doctors who are members of the Radiation Therapy Oncology Group, one of the Clinical Cooperative Groups that assist the National Cancer Institute in evaluating new approaches to cancer treatment.

What is BCG?

BCG, or Bacillus Calmette Guerin, is a vaccine that has long been used to immunize patients against tuberculosis. In recent years, cancer researchers working with BCG found that it could stimulate resistance against transplanted tumors in animals. Researchers also found that BCG could bring about shrinking of early-stage transplanted tumors in 50 to 75 percent of the animals.

Is BCG being studied as a treatment for cancer?

Yes, it is. The National Cancer Institute is sponsoring clinical studies of BCG in many leading universities and medical centers. Studies have shown that putting BCG directly in the bladder can be effective for treating bladder cancer that has recurred. BCG, mixed with a patient's own cancer cells which have been treated with radiation, also seems to be useful in treating advanced colon cancer. A large investigational trial of the effectiveness of BCG in cancer treatment is presently under way.

Is there new research in bone marrow transplants?

There has been a great deal of progress in bone marrow transplants. Transplants are discussed in Chapter 14.

What results have been found from research on patients' attitudes toward cancer and their chances of cure?

Considerable research is focused on whether mental attitudes have any influence on cancer treatments and cures. Researchers are looking at issues such as how hopeful a patient is, what kind of support the patient is receiving from people around him, and the patient's view of his own health and life status. One study undertaken at the University of Pennsylvania has reported that a positive mental attitude, good social contacts, and a happy life did *not* help patients with *advanced* high-risk cancers live longer or prevent the cancer from recurring. The study did not address the possibility that psychosocial factors or events might influence either the cause of disease or the outcome of patients who have cancer at an earlier stage. Many additional studies are planned to investigate the role of psychosocial attitudes and social influences on cancer.

What is AIDS?

AIDS—Acquired Immune Deficiency Syndrome—is a disease in which the body's ability to defend itself against disease is reduced as a result of a dramatic decrease in the type of white blood cells called T-helper cells. The decrease in T-helper cells disrupts the ratio of them to another kind of white blood cell, the T-suppressor cells, whose job it is to suppress antibodies. The normal ratio is two T-helpers to one T-suppressor. People with AIDS have just the opposite: two T-suppressors to one T-helper. Bacteria, viruses, and other microorganisms that ordinarily do no harm can simply run free in the system, with the body unable to fight them.

Is AIDS cancer?

No. AIDS is not cancer in the usual sense. AIDS includes a lowered resistance to certain infections and a wasting away. Some patients with advanced disease also have cancer, usually a tumor called Kaposi's sarcoma, and some lymphomas. Some AIDS patients suffer from severe neurological problems affecting speech, movement, and memory—similar to Alzheimer's disease.

Is the drug AZT being used to treat patients with AIDS?

AZT (azidothymidine) is an experimental anti-AIDS drug which has been cleared for wider use because initial tests show that it can prolong the survival of some patients with the disease. Although the drug shows promise, it is not a cure for AIDS. To be eligible for treatment with AZT, the AIDS patient must meet certain medical criteria, must not be in another drug test program and must have the recommendation of a doctor who is an expert on AIDS and is licensed to practice in the United States. The patient must have pneumocystis carinii pneumonia, a form of pneumonia common to AIDS patients. The drug is manufactured by Burroughs Wellcome Company which is offering it free of charge for the tests. The drug causes side effects, including nausea, mild headaches and a temporary reduction in the body's ability to generate new blood cells.

Are other drugs being tested to use in treating AIDS?

There are many other agents being studied for testing against AIDS. Among them are 2'3' dideoxycytidine, ribavirin, interferon, interleukin-2, and combinations of these and other agents.

What is Kaposi's sarcoma?

In people who do not have AIDS, Kaposi's sarcoma is a disease which affects mostly older men of Jewish and Mediterannean backgrounds. It is an uncommon cancer. Patients develop purple to red-brown lumps, spots, or patches on the skin, usually on the legs, without other symptoms. Kaposi's sarcoma in these people develops slowly, and usually the person dies *with* it, not *because* of it. The disease is confined to the skin.

How does Kaposi's sarcoma differ in AIDS patients?

In AIDS patients, Kaposi's sarcoma tends to be aggressive and may produce significant deterioration in the organ af-

fected. The tumors develop most commonly on the skin
surfaces anywhere on the body, such as inside the mouth,
gastrointestinal tract, lymph nodes, and lungs. In some cases,
however, involvement inside the body produces no symptoms. About 30 percent of AIDS patients develop Kaposi's
sarcoma.

What is the treatment for Kaposi's sarcoma?

For the patient who does not have AIDS, Kaposi's sarcoma
is usually treated with radiation therapy with surgery or
chemotherapy sometimes used. For the patient with AIDS,
radiation therapy is used for either localized or widespread
disease. Investigational treatments include chemotherapy
and various biological response modifers, including interferons.

I have heard that vitamin C is a good treatment for cancer. Are there any studies to back up the use of this vitamin?

Nobel laureate Linus Pauling and Dr. Ewan Cameron are
the champions of the use of vitamin C for treating cancer.
According to Dr. Cameron, cancer cells produce an enzyme,
hyaluronidase, that can destroy substances that make normal cells whole. He feels that if it were possible to reduce
the production of this enzyme or strengthen the "cement"
of the cell—the collagen—then cancer cells could not grow.
Linus Pauling feels that vitamin C provides reinforcement
and strength to the collagen. They tested their theory in
Scotland, giving 100 patients vitamin C every day and
matching them to historical control patients—by searching
records and finding similar patients treated at the same
hospital over 10 years. Two studies at the Mayo Clinic attempted to reproduce the Pauling/Cameron work but did
not find that vitamin C was of any benefit to cancer patients.
Dr. Pauling continues to dispute the manner in which the
Mayo trials were conducted. In the meantime, vitamin C
is among the vitamins being studied both in the laboratory
and in clinical trials sponsored by the National Cancer Institute, mainly in the prevention of colorectal cancer.

Is the National Cancer Institute doing research on using vitamins or diet to treat cancer?

Most of the research being conducted by the National Cancer Institute on the subject of diet and cancer is in the area of prevention. (The National Cancer Institute and the American Cancer Society have issued dietary guidelines to help prevent cancer. You can get these guidelines plus booklets to help you follow them by calling 1-800-4-CANCER.) For patients undergoing treatment, the highest priority is a diet adequate in calories, protein and vitamins (see chapter 22). After completing treatment, you may wish to modify your diet in order to lower fat and raise fiber levels. The National Cancer Institute is currently conducting research to see if a diet lower in fat will prevent recurrence of breast cancer.

What is a clinical trial?

In cancer research, a clinical trial is a study conducted with cancer patients, usually to evaluate a new treatment. Each study is designed to answer scientific questions and to find new and better ways to help cancer patients.

Before a new treatment is tried with patients, it is carefully studied in the laboratory. The laboratory identifies the new methods most likely to succeed and, as much as possible, indicates how to use them safely and effectively. However, since no laboratory research can predict exactly how a new treatment will work on patients, clinical trials must be conducted before any new treatment can be approved for general use.

What are the standards under which investigations of experimental treatments are usually done?

The standards under which investigations of experimental treatments are performed are the same type of scientific standards which are required to judge any claim. They include the following:

- The drug or therapy used should be tried and analyzed on experimental animals. These experiments must be able to be repeated by other impartial investigating groups or researchers with the same results under the same circumstances.

- The results of the treatment given should be compared with the natural course of the disease and with the usual treatment to be sure the new treatment is better or as good but with fewer side effects.
- The effects of the treatment should be studied on a large number of people who have a biopsy of proven cancer so that the nature and consistency of the results can be recorded.
- Other previous treatments and/or other treatment methods being used at the same time should be noted and analyzed in determining the effectiveness of the treatment.
- There should be clinical evidence—including seeing and examining treated patients, reviewing microscopic slides of biopsy, x-rays, and other *objective* evidence— which is open for complete examination. (*Objective* means free from or independent of personal feelings and opinions.)

How are these standards usually applied to an investigational or experimental treatment before it is put into widespread use?

Drugs used in clinical chemotherapy trials are a good example of the rigorous testing that is required. The drugs, created in the laboratory, are first tested on rats and mice. If a specific drug works on tumors of these small animals, it is then tested on larger animals such as monkeys and dogs to see what kind of side effects the drug produces and to make sure that the drug kills cancer cells without damaging normal tissues excessively. If the drug passes these tests (and only 1 out of 5,000 drugs tested does), the FDA approves it as an investigational drug and allows it to be put through a series of tests on humans.

How is human drug testing done?

Human testing is done in three phases. The first two involve people with advanced disease who have exhausted other forms of treatment. All patients must have had a biopsy to prove that they actually have cancer, with appropriate tests to determine the extent of it. The first phase (Phase I) tests the amount of the drug which the patient can tolerate, and side effects are studied. The drugs are then tested for their anti-tumor activity—that is, for the types of tumors which respond to the drug and how often the tumors respond. These are all closely measured to determine the effects of various doses and how often they must be given to produce good results (Phase II). The drugs are then tested on patients on a large scale to see whether or not the drug is more useful or has fewer side effects than other drugs or treatments already being used. This phase (Phase III) is designed to compare the new treatment with the standard treatment and the normal course of the disease to see which treatment is more effective.

Who regulates the use of new drugs or substances for treating cancer?

The Food and Drug Administration (FDA) is the agency which regulates the introduction and clinical testing of the new drugs. The National Cancer Institute or drug companies may be involved in conducting the tests, but neither the American Cancer Society nor the National Cancer Institute is a regulatory agency. The regulations governing the introduction and clinical testing of new drugs have been established and are administered by the FDA. These regulations require that certain standards of safety and effectiveness be met and that a carefully planned clinical study be undertaken.

Aren't American scientific standards very strict? Is it easier to get drugs approved in Europe?

Yes, U.S. standards are very strict. It is easier to get new drugs approved in Europe. The original U.S. Food, Drug, and Cosmetic Act of 1938 was amended in 1962, after the problems caused by the drug thalidomide became evident. (Thousands of pregnant women around the world who took the drug produced deformed babies.) The amendment requires a demonstration of the effectiveness of the drug as well as of the safety of the drug before it can be licensed for use in the United States. This means that there is a lag between when drugs are used in the United States compared with many other countries of the world. The new drugs in the United States must go through animal tests before they can be used on humans, and it takes 5 to 10 years to do all the necessary testing before new drugs are considered safe and effective for use in this country.

Why are clinical trials important?

New cancer treatment must prove to be safe and effective in scientific studies with a certain number of patients before they can be made widely available. Through clinical trials, researchers learn which approaches are better than others. Many of what are now standard treatments were first shown to be effective in clinical trials.

How are clinical trials conducted?

Every clinical trial is designed to answer a set of research questions. Each study enrolls patients with certain types and stages of cancer and certain health conditions. A study that involves two or more treatments can give reliable answers only if all the patients fit approximately the same clinical profile so that they can be compared with each other. Patients become part of a network of clinical trials carried out around the country. This network enables doctors and researchers from many specialties involving cancer treatment and care to pool their ideas and experience to design and monitor clinical studies.

How can I find out what clinical trials are available for my type of cancer?

There are many ways. Talk with your doctor. Get a second opinion if you wish. Your doctor can check with a new computer information system called PDQ (Physician Data Query), supported by the National Cancer Institute. PDQ can give your doctor the latest information on clinical trials being offered around the country for each type and stage of cancer. Your doctor can check PDQ from a library or personal computer. Calling the Cancer Information Service's toll-free number (1-800-4-CANCER) enables you to get information about the treatments available for different kinds of cancer, including investigational trials being conducted all over the country, using information from PDQ.

Can I leave a trial study at any time?

Just as you can decide whether or not you want to join the study, you may leave a clinical study at any time. Your rights as an individual do not change because you are a patient in a clinical trial. You may choose to take part or not, and you can always change your mind later, even after you enter a trial. If you decide to leave, it will not be held against you. Don't be afraid that you will receive no further care. You can freely discuss other possible treatments and care with your doctor and nurses.

How can I learn if a trial is sound and well run?

You need to know the following facts in making up your mind:
- The purpose of the study
- Who has reviewed and approved it
- Who is sponsoring it
- How the study data and patient safety are being checked
- Where information from the study will go

Who needs to approve clinical studies?

The ethical and legal codes that govern medical practice apply to clinical trials. In addition, most clinical research is federally regulated or funded with built-in safeguards to protect patients, including regular review of the study plan and progress by researchers at other institutions. Most clinical research must be approved by an institutional review board located at the institution where the study is to take place. These review boards are designed to protect patients and are made up of scientists, doctors, clergy, and other people from the community. The job of the review board is to see that the study is well designed, with safeguards for patients, and that the risks are reasonable in relation to the potential benefits.

Are there private companies that develop treatments for individual cancer patients?

Yes. This is a fairly new approach to cancer treatment which custom-tailors the newest types of treatments for individual cancer patients. The most credible group of this type is

Biotherapeutics, Inc., formed by two former senior investigators at the National Cancer Institute. For a fee, a patient can have his or her cancer researched and treatment tailor made. The costs are high, ranging from $1,500 for basic testing of tumor tissue to $35,000 for treatments with individualized monoclonal antibodies. The private company believes it has more flexibility than does the government. It takes patients for new experimental therapy for which there are long waiting lists in government-sponsored trials. To be eligible, patients must meet strict criteria. Biotherapeutics, Inc. is run by Dr. Robert K. Oldham and Dr. William H. West, Riverside Drive, Franklin, Tennessee, 37064; (615) 794-4797.

chapter 10

Unproven Methods of Cancer Treatment

Cancer patients are frequently lured by the promise of a cure to try unproven methods of treatment using products that are claimed to be natural and without harmful side effects. The cures most commonly offered include diets, devices, and drugs. Many promoters of unproven methods claim there is a conspiracy to keep cures from the American people or that the cancer establishment is hiding a cure because it does not want to lose the business it gets from cancer patients. Some years ago, a great deal of controversy swirled around the use of laetrile, a product made from apricot pits.

Many patients and their families are swayed into trying new so-called "sure-cure" methods that can actually delay or interfere with treatments of proven benefit. Some can cause dangerous reactions. It is important to be an informed consumer in assessing any cures reported in the popular press. Ask the hard questions about the treatment being offered, and do your own research into what it promises. Patients and families need to use common sense and good judgment in assessing unproven treatment methods.

Cancer, as all the scientific advances recently explored have shown, is a very complex disease that involves the very basis of human life. Friends who care about you may impose tremendous burdens upon you by urging you to try unproven cures they've heard about. Anticipating the possibility of receiving unsolicited advice is the first step in dealing with it. Knowledge of the various unproven cures outlined in this chapter will be helpful to you. Although hundreds of unproven methods have been reported in the press, ranging from asparagus oil to unsulfured raisins, we will limit discussion to those most popular at the present time.

Questions You Should Ask Yourself Before Using Unproven Methods

- Why do I want to use this kind of treatment?
- What do I think the treatment will accomplish?
- What evidence is there that the treatment will work?
- Has the treatment been written up in a scientific journal? Why not?
- Does it sound too good to be true?
- Am I jeopardizing my chances by using this type of treatment?
- Have I discussed the treatment with my doctor?
- Will the doctor continue to care for me if he knows about my plans?
- Is there some way my doctor and I can come to a compromise?
- Can I continue my regular treatments and try the unproven treatment at the same time?
- Is there some kind of investigational or experimental treatment that would give the same or better results?
- Is there some approved, alternative treatment I could try instead of my regular treatments?
- What costs will be associated with the unproven treatment?

What is the difference between investigational or experimental treatment and unproven methods?

Investigational or experimental treatments are done under specific standards set up by the scientific community. The treatments have some basis for being tested in humans— that is, they work against some tumors in animals. The term *unproven method* is used to describe cancer treatment in which either the substance or the treatment method has not been shown *scientifically* to be effective against cancer.

What are some of the most common unproven methods?

There are at least fifty different unproven treatments. One of the best known is laetrile, which has been used by an estimated 50,000 to 75,000 Americans. There are many others, including a large variety of food cures, serums, and herbs. The American Cancer Society has published a booklet entitled *Unproven Methods of Cancer Management* which provides information on both the most prevalent and most promoted unproven treatments.

Are there some treatments that were once known as unproven methods which have become standard treatments?

There are some treatment methods—the use of heat (hyperthermia), for example—which on and off for hundreds of years have been thought to have some effect on cancer cells. However, scientific evidence was scanty and inconclusive. New methods of producing and directing heat—such as using spacesuit underwear, radio frequencies, microwaves, and ultrasound—have brought the subject back into the forefront. However, the role of hyperthermia in the treatment of cancer is not fully established. It is still considered an investigational method.

Are the scientific standards used for investigational or experimental drugs also used in testing unproven methods?

No. Usually those who promote unproven methods lead patients and their families to believe that the method can produce a cure—without the scientific evidence to back it up. There are several shortcomings common to most unproven methods:
- Usually the amount of experimental evidence is very small.
- Sometimes the treatment has shown little or no effect on animals, but the persons giving the treatment feel that it will work on people.
- Often there is no biopsy evidence available, or if it is available, it is found that the whole tumor had been

removed by surgery or destroyed by radiation or chemotherapy before the unproven method was started.

- Current, reputable scientific journals are not used for
reporting scientific information. Instead of publishing
findings in reputable journals or presenting them at
meetings of their medical peers, those using unproven
methods may take the publicity route and report findings
to laymen who are in no position to evaluate statements
critically and scientifically.

- Claims of persecution by organized medicine and science are often made. Investigation usually shows that
papers are not published because the reports do not offer
scientifically objective evidence of effective results.
There are over 400 high-quality medical journals and
over 2,600 health-science journals where new medical
developments are regularly communicated. There are
also thousands of regularly scheduled meetings of doctors and scientists at which to present well-documented
scientific evidence.

- Records of unproven treatments are often scanty, inadequate, or nonexistent. Often no biopsy has been done
to confirm the cancer. As a result, many of the claimed
cures may not have been cancers in the first place.

- Often proven treatment is used along with the unproven
method. If the patient reacts favorably, the improvement
is credited to the unproven therapy.

- Many of the cures are claimed by doctors with unrec-
ognized degrees such as N.D. (Doctor of Naturopathy),
Ph.N. (Philosopher of Naturopathy), DA BB-A (Diplomate of American Board of Bio-Analysts), and Ms.D.
(Doctor of Metaphysics). In addition, unproven methods
may be used without any explanation and without your
signing a consent form.

Is the subject of unproven methods new?

No. Unproven remedies for the treatment of cancer are as
old as the disease itself. In 1748, the House of Burgesses
of the General Assembly of Virginia, of which George Washington was a member, passed a resolution appointing a committee to make a trial of Mary Johnson's "receipt of curing
cancer," consisting of garden sorrel, celandine, persimmon

bark, and spring water, and to report on its effect. In 1754, the committee, after hearing the testimony of many witnesses who had taken the remedy report that they had been cured of cancer, put the report into the minutes of the House of Burgesses and voted Mrs. Johnson a reward of 100 pounds.

What is the macrobiotic diet?

The macrobiotic diet, also known as the Zen macrobiotic diet, consists mainly of cereal products such as rice. Individuals following the diet must not eat any sugar, meat, or animal products and must restrict their intake of fluids. There are many variations of the macrobiotic diet. The principle of all of the diets is to recommend that liquids, usually in the form of miso or tamari broths, be used only sparingly. Meats (including poultry), dairy products, tropical or semitropical fruits and juices, sugar, honey, or anything artificial are to be avoided. The most restrictive of these diets, not usually followed today, uses only cereals, usually in the form of brown rice. Those who recommend the diet for cancer patients believe that cancer is a toxic blood condition which has developed because of poor habits.

Was Dr. Sattilaro cured by the macrobiotic diet?

In the fall of 1976, Dr. Anthony Sattilaro, president of Philadelphia's Methodist Hospital, was diagnosed for prostate cancer, with many metastases. He was treated with surgery and hormone therapy. Because he felt he was not responding after 6 weeks of this standard treatment, Dr. Sattilaro placed himself on the macrobiotic diet while continuing with hormone therapy. He remained on the hormone therapy for 1 year while on the diet. The diet consisted of 50 percent cooked whole grains such as brown rice, wheat barley, and millet; 25 percent locally grown vegetables; 15 percent beans and other vegetables; and small quantities of fish, soup, condiments, fruits, seeds, and nuts. His articles credit his cancer cure to the macrobiotic diet.

Has the National Cancer Institute evaluated Dr. Sattilaro's claims?

In the opinion of the doctors at the National Cancer Institute, about 70 or 80 percent of patients with prostate cancer have a favorable response to treatment with the type of surgery and hormone therapy that Dr. Sattilaro received. In many patients, the response to hormone therapy may not be evident until more than 6 weeks of treatment have been given. Therefore, the doctors at the Cancer Institute feel that Dr. Sattilaro's improvement was due to the surgery and hormone treatment he received. His case history, they believe, does not contain any evidence to show that the macrobiotic diet was the sole cause of his improvement. In addition, the doctors note that in cancer of the prostate, the response to hormone therapy may continue for many years, so that the length of response noted in Dr. Sattilaro's case may be the result of the hormone treatment rather than the macrobiotic diet.

Can the macrobiotic diet be harmful to cancer patients?

The macrobiotic diet lacks nutritional elements needed even by healthy people. It is low in many vitamins and minerals. Since milk products are excluded, getting enough calcium can be a problem. For cancer patients there can be additional difficulties. Many are already experiencing weight loss and lack of appetite. It is common for cancer patients to feel full both during and after eating. Persons on the macrobiotic diet need to eat large amounts of food, mostly bulky foods, to obtain the number of calories required by the diet. The diet does not allow vitamin and mineral supplements.

Isn't Dr. Lawrence Burton curing cancer at his clinic in the Bahamas?

Lawrence Burton, Ph.D., is a zoologist who claims that his treatment—known as immuno-augmentative therapy or IAT—is effective against cancer. He has a clinic in the Bahamas. In newspaper interviews, Dr. Burton has described great success in treating patients with a serum created from a combination of agents of human blood. His treatment materials have not been licensed for sale in the United States by the Food and Drug Administration. Although Dr. Burton has described his success in treating cancer patients in newspaper, magazine, and television interviews, he has never formally reported in the scientific literature details of his treatment methods or results of studies he has conducted at the clinic. Since the research results have not been published, other scientists have not been able to evaluate his claims.

Has the National Cancer Institute evaluated Dr. Burton's therapy?

Representatives of the National Cancer Institute visited Dr. Burton's clinic and reviewed patient records. The information provided in these records was not sufficient to determine how effective the treatment is. In addition, the composition of the treatment materials was not disclosed, so there was no evidence on which to determine the value of the treatment. The National Cancer Institute has offered to screen Dr. Burton's materials to evaluate them for anti-tumor qualities and to test them for purity and side effects. Dr. Burton has not supplied material for testing or identified the treatment for the National Cancer Institute. Five American patients who had been to the Burton clinic in the Bahamas gave the National Cancer Institute sealed IAT specimens. The analysis of these specimens showed that they were dilutions of blood proteins with no biological activity, that they were contaminated with bacteria, and that four of them were positive for hepatitis. One of the patients developed hepatitis. These findings were confirmed by the Center for Disease Control, which also reported that sixteen individuals developed abscesses at injection sites after receiving IAT. In early 1986, according to a report in the Journal of the American Medical Association, the Bahamian clinic was closed by the government because it was dispensing AIDS-contaminated products. The report noted the drugs consisted primarily of a protein found in egg whites. The clinic has again reopened.

What is the Livingston-Wheeler Clinic?

This clinic, run by Dr. Virginia Wheeler Livingston and her husband, Dr. Owen Livingston, in San Diego, California, claims that a microbe (which is referred to by the clinic as *progenitor cryptocides*) in the same family as tuberculosis and leprosy, is the cause of cancer. The clinic uses inoculations with a vaccine made by an undisclosed method to strengthen the immune system. The Livingstons believe that the bacteria is transmitted through eating fowl, and the clinic advocates eliminating chicken and eggs from the diet. No scientific data of any kind have been made available to the medical community.

What is laetrile?

Laetrile is a product made from apricot pits which contains a chemical called amygdalin. Amygdalin occurs in the seeds of many plants—it is abundant in the kernels of peaches, apricots, bitter almond, and apple seeds. Promoters of laetrile claim that it is a harmless and effective treatment for cancer, and some patients who have taken it say that it has helped them. However, no clear-cut scientific evidence supports these claims. The National Cancer Institute has tested laetrile in laboratory animals but has not found convincing evidence that it is effective against animal cancers. Because of widespread public use and interest in this subject, the National Cancer Institute conducted a clinical study of laetrile with cancer patients. The conclusion of the researchers who participated in the trial was that laetrile was ineffective as a treatment for cancer and did not substantially improve symptoms of the disease in the patients studied. A detailed report of the study was published in the *New England Journal of Medicine* in January 1982 (Volume 306, No. 4).

How is hydrazine sulfate used in cancer treatment?

Hydrazine sulfate has been proposed for two purposes: as a cancer treatment and as an aid to patients who suffer from loss of appetite and weight. The National Cancer Institute has evaluated it as a cancer treatment but has found insufficient evidence to justify testing the drug in clinical trials. NCI has also studied the work of researchers who have conducted limited clinical trials but has again found that hydrazine sulfate does not have enough anti-tumor activity to warrant further study. Two researchers, Dr. Joseph Gold of the United States and Dr. M. L. Gershanovich of the Soviet Union, have reported that hydrazine sulfate helps patients with weight loss and loss of appetite. NCI has reviewed their studies and found they can draw no firm conclusions from them. Preliminary results from several investigators in this country suggest that hydrazine sulfate may improve the way the cancer patient's body uses sugar, but the studies do not yet show whether or not hydrazine sulfate will improve appetite or reverse weight loss. Therefore, hydrazine sulfate cannot be recommended for general use.

What is the Janker Clinic?

The Janker Clinic is a private hospital located in Bonn, West Germany, that was founded in 1936 as a radiation hospital. National Cancer Institute physicians have visited the Janker Clinic on two separate occasions and the clinic's treatment methods have been formally reviewed by the NCI's Division of Cancer Treatment. NCI scientists found the data provided by the Janker Clinic inconclusive. In addition, the NCI has said it was aware of no publications in the scientific literature to substantiate claims made for the effectiveness of the Janker Clinic treatment methods.

Who is the medical director of the Janker Clinic?

Dr. Wolfgang Scheef, the medical director of the hospital, is chiefly responsible for developing treatment methods for the Janker Clinic.

How can I go about getting information about the Janker Clinic?

You may contact the German Cancer Research Center (Deutsches Krebsforschungszentrum), Postfach 101949, Im Neuenheimer Feld 280, 69 Heidelberg, Federal Republic of Germany (Tel. 01149-6221-4841). Information may also be provided by the German Cancer Society, Karl/Weichert/ Elle 9, 3000 Hanover 61, Federal Republic of Germany (Tel. 01149-511-523-2923).

What are antineoplastons?

Antineoplastons are substances derived from peptides present in human urine. Dr. Stanislaw Burzynski, a physician in Texas, advocates these substances as a treatment for cancer. The National Cancer Institute notes that the information required to support the claim for the effectiveness has not been made available, suggesting that the studies necessary in developing a new anticancer agent have not been done. At the request of Canada's Bureau of Human Prescription Drugs, Health and Welfare, the National Cancer Institute evaluated two antineoplastons used by Dr. Burzynski (A2 and A5) and found no activity that would warrant further investigation.

What is the Greek cancer cure?

Dr. Hariton Alivizatos of Athens, Greece, has developed a cancer diagnostic and treatment method. He claims to have invented a blood test to detect cancer and a nontoxic cancer cure, which he administers as a vaccine at his clinic in Greece. The National Cancer Institute notes that none of Dr. Alivizatos's claims have been substantiated and that although the treatment appears to be immunological in nature, it has not been scientifically confirmed. To date, Dr. Alivizatos has not published reports of his work in the scientific literature and no follow-up information is available on the patients treated at his clinic.

chapter 11

Breast Cancer

Breast cancer has received a great deal of publicity in recent years, and most women are familiar with the importance of regular breast self-examination as a routine good health habit. Because early detection of a developing cancer is an important factor in its treatment and cure, any suspicions of a change in the breasts should be followed up with a visit to the doctor. Eight out of ten lumps prove to be noncancerous. But for those who have a lump which is cancerous, early treatment is important and essential. New techniques developed in recent years have made breast reconstruction possible, and breast reconstruction has become an important part of treatment and rehabilitation.

Women Most Likely to Get Breast Cancer

Major risks:
- Women age 50 or over
- Women whose mother or sister have had breast cancer, particularly if it was pre-menopausal
- Women who have already had cancer in one breast

Other risks:
- Women with precancerous breast disease
- Women with breast cysts proven by aspiration or surgery

- Women who have not had any children
- Women who had their first child after age 30
- Women who began menstruating at 12 or younger
- Women who have experienced menopause after 55
- Women who are obese

Symptoms of Breast Cancer

- Lump or thickening of the breast
- Discharge from the nipple
- Dimpling or puckering of the skin
- Retraction of the nipple
- Scaly skin around the nipple
- Other changes in skin color or texture, such as "orange peel" skin
- Swelling, redness, or feeling of heat in breast
- Lump under arm

To Find Breast Lumps As Early As Possible

Procedure	Explanation
Check breasts each month.	If you do this each month, 3 to 5 days after the end of your period or on the same day each month if you are post-menopausal, you'll recognize a change as soon as it occurs. Over 70 percent of breast lumps are found by the woman herself; about 80 percent of them are benign.
Make certain gynecologist, internist, or family physician checks breasts at least once a year if you are over 40 or every three years between ages 20 to 40.	This double-checks your examination and gives you the opportunity to make certain you are examining yourself properly.
Look for changes in appearance of breast and call doctor immediately if any of these are present:	Cause for concern is any change from what is normal for you—and you are the one who can detect the changes fastest.

To Find Breast Lumps As Early As Possible (continued)

PROCEDURE	EXPLANATION
Any change in size or shape of the breast.	You are asked to do this by watching your breasts in a mirror as you raise your arms to determine if any area reacts differently from the comparable area in the opposite breast. This is usually found to be the result of fibrocystic changes — but it can signal the presence of cancer, and only the doctor can determine this.
Unusual pain or an area of unusual tenderness should be reported to the doctor if it persists after your menstrual period.	Pain is not usually one of the signs of breast cancer, but it is a common sign of a developing cyst and should be checked by the doctor even if there is no evidence of a lump.
Dimpling, puckering, or retraction of nipple or flaking of nipple skin should be called to the doctor's attention.	This may indicate the development of a cancer of the ducts beneath the nipple or of the nipple itself.
Nipple discharge is another cancer sign that should be immediately reported to the doctor.	Any noticeable nipple discharge should be checked. Any bloody discharge must be checked immediately, because it indicates that there is some trouble in the nipple duct.
Have a baseline mammogram at 35, annual or biannual mammograms from ages 40–49 and annual mammograms after 50 or if you fall into a high-risk group.	This will give the doctor something to check back on at a later date to determine if there has been a change, or to discover cancer at a very early stage.

If You Find You Have a Lump in Your Breast

STEP	EXPLANATION
Call the doctor for an appointment today.	This gives you the chance to tell the nurse that you have found a lump and that you want an immediate appointment. Delaying can prove to be a fatal decision.

If You Find You Have a Lump in Your Breast
(continued)

STEP	EXPLANATION
Remind yourself that 8 out of 10 times the lump will turn out *not* to be cancer.	Don't naively assume, however, that since you feel well and the lump hasn't changed, you can afford to wait to see the doctor.
If the doctor suggests he will watch the lump over a few months' time, discuss having a mammogram or a biopsy. Also think about asking for a second opinion.	Many physicians feel that having a baseline mammogram is important at this time because it gives him something to compare with at a later date. Also, it jolts the doctor into action, rather than passively deciding to wait and see.

Questions to Ask Your Doctor If You Have a Lump in Your Breast

- What does the lump feel like? What do you think it is?
- Should I have a mammogram? What does the mammogram show?
- What kind of biopsy do you do? Can it be done on an outpatient basis? Why not?

If he recommends a mammogram:

- Do you know how many rads I will be exposed to with the techniques being used by the radiologist you are sending me to?

Questions You Must Ask Yourself

- How important are my breasts to me?
- Am I willing to have a limited operation and later have a second operation if it is found that the cancer has spread? Can I live with that fear?
- Do I want to have breast reconstruction? (If you do, it is best if the doctor knows before he operates.)

Steps to Take if Doctor Suggests Biopsy

STEP	EXPLANATION
Arrange to have someone—husband, mother, sister, friend—come with you into the doctor's office.	Having a trusted person with you helps in getting answers to the questions you want to ask. It also helps to write down the questions before you go and the answers while you are there.
Ask the doctor if he believes in the two-step procedure—doing the biopsy separate from the operation.	This gives you several options which you will not have if the doctor proceeds with the biopsy and is given the okay to continue with removing the breast if he feels this is necessary.
Explain that you want the pathologist to have the full three or four days needed for a detailed study of the tumor and its spread.	Time is essential to the pathologist in determining the nature of the tumor.
Ask if you will be premedicated and semi-awake during biopsy and if it can be done on an outpatient basis.	This eliminates the hazard of going under anesthesia twice and leaves several options open to you.
Explain that you want to get a second opinion.	A second opinion at this point will help to establish a fuller view of what is involved and help you determine how you want to proceed.
Make sure you have a mammogram before you have a biopsy.	After the biopsy, scar tissue will form inside the breast where the tissue was removed. A mammogram should be made before the biopsy so that any future changes can be compared with the original.
Make sure you have confidence in the doctor who will be doing your surgery. Find out how many breast operations he has done in the past month.	You are best off with a surgeon who specializes in breast disease—preferably a surgical oncologist. At least you should get a second opinion from such a doctor.

Steps to Take if the Biopsy Shows Malignancy

STEP	EXPLANATION
Ask the doctor his opinion about doing lesser surgery and using radiation instead of removing the breast if the malignant lump is small and has not spread to other organs.	Many cases have been treated in this manner with success. This is still controversial with some physicians, but it should definitely be an option for discussion.
Ask the doctor what kind of operation he will be doing—a lumpectomy, segmental or partial mastectomy, or a simple, modified radical, or radical mastectomy.	New evidence is showing that there is no difference in survival statistics between women who had the most radical surgery (removal of breast and underlying and adjacent tissues, including pectoral muscles) and the modified radical (which does not remove the muscles of chest and fatty tissue under the arm). It is very important to discuss the operation with your doctor before surgery.
Ask the doctor about having an estrogen and progesterone receptor test on the tissue.	If you have breast cancer that has spread, this test can help determine future treatment and should be done before chemotherapy starts.
Ask the doctor about breast reconstruction.	Though most surgeons feel that reconstruction cannot be done at the same time as initial surgery, it is wise to let the surgeon know if you are interested in reconstruction before he operates so that the original surgery is planned with the future reconstruction in mind. Talk to him about seeing a plastic surgeon before the operation.

Tests for Breast Cancer

TEST	EXPLANATION
Physical exam	Includes clinical history; physical; routine blood, urine, and heart exams; close examinations of breasts.
Mammography	Gives the doctor visualization of breast, showing natural contrast provided by fat content of breast. Sometimes possible to differentiate benign tumor from malignant. Allows doctor to see if additional tumors are present. Make sure it is done with a dedicated machine, giving under one rad per breast and read by a radiologist who reads mammograms every day.

Tests for Breast Cancer (continued)

TEST	EXPLANATION
Thermography	Not as accurate in detecting preclinical cancers as mammogram, but is preferred by some doctors because it does not use radiation. May prove helpful in predicting cancer development. Should not be used alone as diagnostic tool.
Needle aspiration	Insertion of fine needle into lump to draw out fluid or tissue.
Surgical biopsy	Removal of sample (whole lump if small) of suspicious breast tissue to be examined for cancer cells. Minor surgical procedure, but only positive way of identifying malignant tumor. Can be done on an outpatient basis.

If Biopsy Shows Lump to Be Cancerous

Scans, bone and liver	Painless, routine outpatient diagnostic procedures similar to x-rays. Used to determine whether cancer has spread to bones and liver. Also known as metastatic workup.
Gallium scan	Sometimes used to determine if cancer has spread to more than one area of body. Capable of showing rapidly dividing cells.
Ultrasound scan	Sometimes used especially for young, dense breasts. Sometimes used as a follow-up for patients who have had lumpectomy and radiation therapy.
X-rays	May sometimes be part of workup.
CT scan	May sometimes be used.

Questions to Ask Your Doctor Before Agreeing to a Breast Operation

- How big is the lump?
- Where is it?
- What specific kind of breast cancer do I have?
- Do we have the opinion of more than one pathologist on that?
- Have you talked directly with the pathologist about my report? What did he say?
- Can you feel any lymph nodes?

- How fast does this type of breast cancer grow?
- Is there any evidence of metastases?
- What kind of operation do you plan to do?
- How often do you perform mastectomies? lumpectomies?
- Are there any alternative kinds of treatment for my case?
- Will you explain what the scar will look like?
- Will you do the operation with the thought that I am interested in having breast reconstruction?

What kind of doctor should I see if I have symptoms of breast cancer?

If you have a lump or other symptom of breast cancer, you should first see the doctor who normally takes care of you—your internist, family practitioner, gynecologist, or general practitioner. He will order whatever tests are necessary to determine whether or not your symptom is actually cancer. The doctors who specialize in treating breast cancer are usually surgical oncologists. Reconstructive breast surgery is the specialty of plastic and reconstructive surgeons. Since several options exist for treatment, make sure you get second opinions and read this chapter so that you can decide what options you wish to follow.

Is the National Cancer Institute supporting any studies on breast cancer?

Yes, the National Cancer Institute's clinical cooperative groups are presently supporting many studies on breast cancer. (See Chapter 23.)

What is the function of the breast?

The breast is a very complicated organ. It has tens of thousands of tiny cells able to secrete milk on order, preparing itself throughout pregnancy to supply the infant's nutrition, receding when no longer necessary, prepared to start all over again when called upon by another pregnancy. Each month, during menstruation, changes occur in the breasts. The growth, maturation, and function of the breast are the result of a sequential stimulation by several separate hormones—secreted from the ovary, anterior pituitary gland, adrenal cortex, and thyroid.

How are most breast cancers found?

Most breast cancers—over 70 percent—are found by the women themselves, either during monthly self-examinations or by accident when showering or looking in the mirror.

Are most breast lumps cancerous?

No, they are not. With all the information on breast cancer that has been written in the past few years, it is important for you to know that chances that a lump in your breast is *not* cancer are really excellent. In fact, eight out of ten lumps are found to be benign. However, it is important for you to know that lumps found in post-menopausal women are more apt to be cancerous than those found in women who are still menstruating. Ninety-three percent of women never develop cancer of the breast. Those are really very good odds. Further, the cure rate is 85 percent if the cancer is detected early.

Do men ever have breast cancer?

Yes. However, less than 1 percent of all breast cancers occur in males. When they do occur, it is usually at middle age or older. Almost all breast cancers in men are carcinomas, with the most common kind being infiltrating ductal carcinoma. Men can also develop Paget's disease and inflammatory carcinoma.

What are the symptoms of male breast cancer?

A painless lump, usually discovered by the man himself, is by far the most common first symptom. Nipple discharge, nipple retraction, and a lump under the arm are also symptoms commonly seen in male breast cancer. Diagnosis is the same as for women, using mammography, physical exam, medical history, and biopsy.

What are the treatments for male breast cancer?

The treatments are similar to those used for women: surgery, radiation, and chemotherapy, depending upon the stage of disease. Hormonal therapy, used for advanced disease, is even more effective in men than in women.

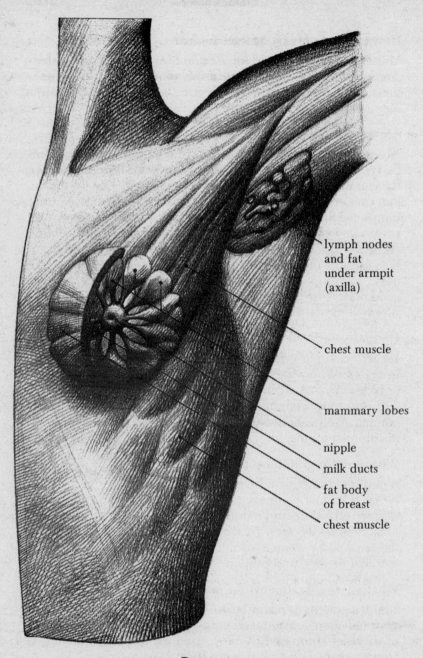

lymph nodes
and fat
under armpit
(axilla)

chest muscle

mammary lobes

nipple

milk ducts

fat body
of breast

chest muscle

Breast

What is meant by *fibrocystic changes*?

At one time, doctors believed that fibrocystic disease—also referred to as lumpy breasts, cystic disease or chronic cystic mastitis—meant that these women were at a higher risk for developing cancer. Doctors now find that 70 percent of the women with fibrocystic changes who have a biopsy have no increased risk of developing cancer. Of the remaining, only those with a specific kind of cell, called ductal or lobular atypical hyperplasia, are in a moderately increased risk group—about 4 percent of those biopsied. The term fibrocystic disease is no longer being used. Rather, the condition is called fibrocystic changes or fibrocystic condition.

Can doctors tell the difference between cystic lumps and cancerous lumps?

It depends upon many factors. Cysts are usually movable, spherical in shape, and relatively soft, unlike many malignant tumors. They are caused by a buildup of fibrous tissues which is related to the changes that normally take place in the breast during each menstrual cycle. These changes may be exaggerated if the menstrual cycle becomes irregular, particularly if there is a long time between periods. The lumpiness may disappear slowly after menopause. Fibrocystic lumps seem to appear and disappear with the menstrual cycle, while most cancerous lumps are stable. Many women have breasts with cysts of many sizes, giving the breast a "cobblestone" feel. Women with cystic breasts should be examined frequently, and doctors often recommend that cysts that do not change in size be biopsied and/or surgically removed. If the cyst disappears after aspiration with a syringe and needle, this is a good sign it is benign.

What are micro-calcifications?

Micro-calcifications are minute flecks of calcium which can be seen on the mammogram. The diagnostic radiologist looks for clustering of these micro-calcifications which might signal the presence of cancer. Larger calcifications, in contrast, are most often associated with benign conditions.

Is breast cancer inherited?

It seems that heredity may account for some familial patterns of breast cancer, although shared dietary, social, and other environmental factors probably play a role. Women whose mothers or sisters had breast cancer before menopause are more likely to develop the disease than women with no family history of the disease. Those whose aunts or grandmothers had breast cancer before menopause are also at a higher risk. Women who fall into any of these higher-risk categories should be followed closely by a physician who specializes in breast disease.

Do women with inverted nipples have a greater chance of developing breast cancer?

No, not if this is your normal condition. Inverted nipples are subject to infection if not kept clean and dry, but there does not seem to be a relationship between inverted nipples and breast cancer. However, if your nipple is normally erect and retracts—or if you see dimpling or puckering in your breast—you should see the doctor so he can check this symptom.

Is discharge from the nipples of the breast a cause for alarm?

It is wise to call any discharge from the nipples to the attention of your doctor. If the discharge is bloody or has a green or brown color, this probably means that a small quantity of blood or other substance is being discharged and is reason for the doctor to look at it to determine the cause. Some young women may have a slight clear or yellowish nipple discharge at the time of menstruation; this is not unusual and should not cause alarm but should be mentioned to the doctor. Most discharges occur prior to menopause when other changes are taking place in the body and should be seen by the doctor to determine if there is a problem. Some of the fluid can be put on a slide and analyzed to see what is causing the discharge.

Why does the doctor try to see if the tumor will "move"?

Most cancerous tumors tend to invade breast tissue and cause the breast to form scar tissue in and around the cancer.

This causes the lump to become "fixed." Benign tumors such as fluid cysts or solid fibrous growths tend to be more movable because they neither invade the surrounding breast tissue nor cause the breast to deposit scar tissue around them. However, in some cases, movable tumors have been found to be cancerous, and this is the reason why a surgical biopsy is necessary to determine the nature of most lumps.

Can blows or injuries to the breasts cause breast cancer?

No. But such injuries often draw attention to a lump in the breast even though the lump is not a result of the injury.

Does diet play a role in breast cancer?

Research findings, especially of large population groups, indicate that diet may be a possible factor in breast cancer. In areas of the world where breast cancer is common, diets are high in fat and animal protein. Americans, for instance, consume three times as much fat and more animal protein than the Japanese, and have proportionately more breast cancer. When Japanese women move to the United States, their rate of breast cancer begins to rise and continues in each generation until the rate approaches that of American women. In addition, post-menopausal women who are overweight have an increased risk of developing breast cancer. There are presently underway research projects which are studying whether reducing the amount of fat eaten by women at high risk for breast cancer will affect the number of breast cancer cases.

Does the birth control pill increase my risk of getting breast cancer?

Researchers, in a study published in the *New England Journal of Medicine* in August 1986, concluded that overall, oral contraceptive use does not increase the risk of breast cancer. Among the findings:
- The risk of breast cancer was the same for women who had never taken the pill as for those who had, regardless of the length of time users had taken it, be it less than 12 months or more than 15 years.
- The brand and formula of the birth control pill had no relationship to the risk of breast cancer.

- The age at which a woman began using the pill or whether she had been pregnant or had a child before starting the pill did not matter.
- Women with a history of benign breast disease or a family history of breast cancer were not at increased risk.

The study did not answer questions about the effects of birth control pills on developing breast tissue when they are taken by adolescents. And because the pill has been available only since 1960, the study did not show what happens after many decades of use.

Is there any connection between breast feeding and breast cancer?

For many years, it was thought that nursing helped to immunize women against breast cancer. Later studies seemed to indicate that women who nursed were more prone to cancer. Today, most scientists feel it is neither protective nor a risk.

Does cancer occur more often in any one part of the breast?

Yes. About half of all breast cancers develop in the upper outer portion of the breast, the part of the breast closest to the underarm. The second most common site is the area surrounding the nipple, where about 18 percent of breast cancers are found.

I try to examine my breasts, but I'm not really sure what I'm looking for. What do I need to know?

The first thing you should know is that it is important to do the breast exam not just to look for problems but mainly to get to know your own breast tissue so that you will recognize a change when you feel it. The exam should be done once a month. If you are menstruating, probably the best time to do it is within the week following your period. If you are no longer menstruating or have had a hysterectomy, you need to pick a day of the month that you will always use. Some women pick their birthdate. Some feel that the first day, the last day, or the fifteenth day of the month is the easiest to remember.

When you have an appointment with your doctor, you should ask him to teach you breast self-examination after he has examined your breasts. Then you will know what

your breast feels like when it is normal and he can answer
any questions you have about what you are feeling. You can
also get an illustrated pamphlet on breast self-examination
by calling the American Cancer Society office near you or
the Cancer Information Service.

Just how should I examine my breasts?

Your breast self-examination should be done in three steps.
First, look in the mirror with your arms down at your side.
Make sure you have a good light that is not casting any
shadows and a big enough mirror. Look at the shape of your
nipples, and notice the contour of your breasts. The nipples
are usually more or less equal and pointing outward. The
contour of both breasts is usually sloping downward. Although the shape and size of each breast may be different,
the contour is usually the same. Now look at the same features with your arms over your head. Then rest the palms
of your hands on your hips and press down firmly to flex

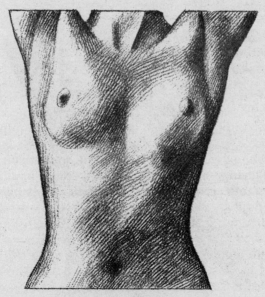

arms over head

Breast self-examination

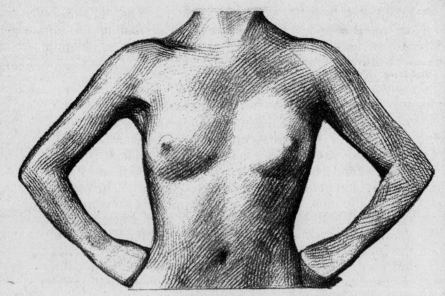

arms on hips

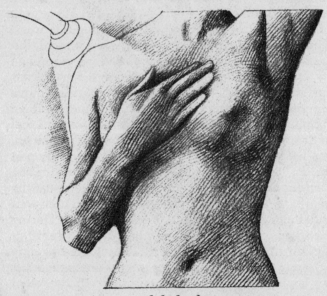

while body is wet

Breast self-examination

your chest muscles. In all these views you are looking for any changes—a swelling; any puckering, scaling, or dimpling of skin; nipples which have retracted; a change in contour. If you regularly inspect what is normal, you will have confidence in your examination and your ability to see something not normal.

What is the second step?

The second step is to examine yourself when you are wet—either during a shower or a bath—with soap on your breast. Some of the lumps most difficult to find can be picked up most easily in a soapy breast. Your hands will easily glide over your wet, soapy skin. With your fingers flat, move gently over every part of each breast. Use your right hand to examine the left breast and your left hand for your right breast. Raise the opposite arm while you examine the entire breast. You are looking for any lump, hard knot, or thickening. Pay special attention to the area between the breast and armpit, including the armpit itself.

What is the third step of the breast self-examination?

Next you lie down. To examine your right breast, put a pillow or folded towel under your right shoulder. Place your right arm behind your head. This will distribute the breast tissue more evenly on your chest. With your left hand, fingers flat, press gently in small circular motions around an imaginary clock face. Begin at the outermost top of your breast (imagine that is 12 o'clock on the clock), then move around the breast (to 1 o'clock, 2 o'clock, etc., until you get back to 12). At the lower curve of your breast, you will feel a ridge of firm tissue. That is normal. Then move in an inch, toward the nipple, and keep circling to examine every part of your breast, including the nipple. This will require you to make at least three more circles. Now slowly repeat the same process on your left breast with a pillow under your left shoulder and your left hand behind your head. During this process you are again looking for lumps, hard knots, or thickening. Finally, squeeze the nipple of each breast gently between your thumb and your index finger. You are making sure there is no discharge. If there is any discharge, clear or bloody, you should immediately report it to your doctor.

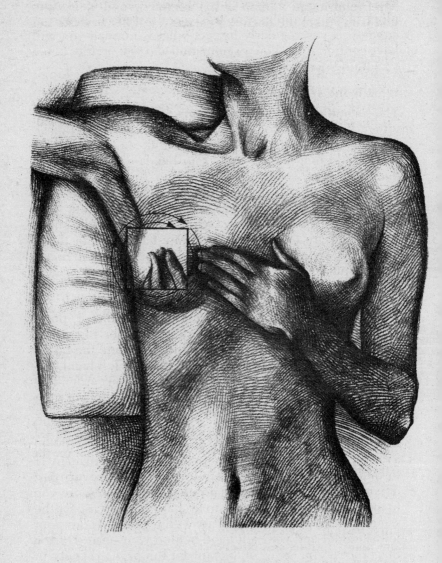

Breast self-examination (lying down)

My friend found a lump in her breast several weeks ago and won't go to the doctor. What can I tell her to make her go?

There are several things you can try:

- First of all, tell her that about 80 percent of the lumps which are found prove to be non-cancerous. Her chances are eight out of ten that it will prove to be nothing. For her own peace of mind, she should have a doctor evaluate the lump.
- Second, if the lump does prove to be cancerous, her chances of the cancer being arrested are much higher if it is found at an early stage than if she lets it continue to grow.
- Suggest that you or a family member make the appointment for her. It is sometimes hard for people to take the first step, to pick up the phone and call the doctor, to admit that something might be wrong.
- Offer to accompany her to the doctor's office or talk to a family member about going with her. If she is frightened, it could be very helpful for her to have someone go along with her to share the experience.

What happens after either the doctor or I find a breast lump?

There are numerous ways your case can proceed. This is an important decision point. You must prepare yourself to make a decision about how you want to proceed if, after the examination, the doctor suggests there is a possibility that the lump may be cancer. You need to decide, for example, whether you wish to have a second opinion on the kind of treatment you will have.

Is a second opinion important in breast cancer?

In our view, a second opinion is always important. It is more important in treating breast cancer simply because there are many options and differences of opinion in this area. A second opinion can help you think through your choices.

What will the doctor do if he has any doubts about my lump?

If the doctor has any doubts, he will suggest further studies. These may include a mammogram, aspiration of the lump with a needle and syringe to see if it is a cyst, or an excisional biopsy. These tests are used to make sure that the lump is *not* cancerous or to determine treatment if it should be cancerous. *Remind yourself again* that eight times out of ten it usually turns out that the lump is *not* malignant.

I am still confused. Tell me again what the steps are that would lead up to the operation for breast cancer.

Let us take it from the time when you find a lump or something unusual about your breast and go to the doctor. He will probably proceed as follows:

- He will look at what you have found and examine both breasts for lumpy areas.
- If he has any doubts, he may advise further studies, such as mammography, aspiration of the lump with needle and syringe to see if it is a cyst, a needle biopsy, or an excisional biopsy (taking out the whole lump for examination).
- If the biopsy shows that the lump is cancerous, the doctor will order a bone scan, x-ray of the chest, blood studies, and other tests to determine whether or not the cancer has already spread to distant parts of the body such as the bone, lungs, and liver.

What is a mammogram?

A mammogram is a soft-tissue x-ray of the breast. It shows breast masses and helps to identify those which may be malignant. Mammograms can show tiny concentrations of calcification or perhaps other abnormalities that may indicate a tumor in the breast. Tumors can often be observed by this x-ray technique before they can be discovered by physical examination.

Can a mammogram tell whether or not cancer is present?

Mammograms are diagnostic tools. They may indicate to a trained doctor whether cancer is present or not. They are used by surgeons to locate the site of the tumor and to check if there are additional tumors in the breast. However, they should never be used alone. They should be used in addition to a careful breast examination by a doctor who regularly treats breast cancer. In order to make a definitive diagnosis of breast cancer, a biopsy must be done of those suspicious areas seen on the mammogram.

What is a Xeroradiograph?

A Xeroradiograph is a mammogram which basically uses the Xerox techniques. It processes the x-ray image on Xerox paper. A selenium-coated metal surface is substituted for x-ray film, and after being exposed to x-rays, it is dusted with calcium carbonate powder. This produces an etching-like image. The Xeroradiograph is blue and white. The mammogram is black and white. Sometimes this test is called Xeromammography.

Who performs mammography?

Radiological technologists who are specially trained in mammography normally conduct the tests and process the mammograms. The mammograms are then given to a radiologist, who studies them, interprets them, and reports the findings to your own physician. It is very important that you go to a qualified radiologist who reads many mammograms, for as with other diagnostic tools, the results are only as good as the skill of the person who conducts and interprets the tests.

What is digital mammography?

Digital mammography uses sensitive detectors rather than film or a Xerox-type device to measure x-rays passed through the breast. It is a new, developing technique which should increase the amount of information while reducing the radiation received.

Can mistakes be made in reading a mammogram?

As with any diagnostic tool, errors can be made in mammography or Xeroradiography. For instance, the position of the breast on the plate can distort results. The doctor reading the mammogram can make a mistake. This is why both the technicians involved in taking the films and the radiologist who reads them must be extremely qualified. Interpreting the films requires skilled and trained persons who read mammograms daily and can see the subtle differences.

Why is it a good idea to have a mammogram before having the breast lump removed?

A mammogram of the breast before surgery can serve several purposes:

- It can be used as a record for the doctor to use in future comparisons.
- It can tell if there are additional lumps in the areas of the breast which cannot be felt.
- Used in conjunction with other findings, it can sometimes help to determine if the lump is benign or cancerous.
- It will guide the surgeon during the operation.

What does the doctor look for in the mammogram to help him determine if the lump might be cancerous?

The doctor knows that benign tumors tend to show sharp edges in x-rays and are frequently surrounded by a halo of fat and seem to be homogeneous in density. Malignant tumors usually look as though they have tentaclelike tissue reaching into the surrounding areas. Fine, sandlike calcium deposits can be seen, and the skin in the area is often distorted. Even with his expert eyes, however, the doctor needs other guidelines besides the x-ray to help him make a positive diagnosis.

What dose of radiation does a woman get when she has a mammogram done?

The dose of radiation for mammograms should be less than 1 rad per breast, with two views of each breast on a machine dedicated to mammography. You should ask when your physician makes the appointment for your mammogram or you should call the radiologist yourself before you have the examination to be certain that the machine being used is used only for mammograms. If the dose is more than 1 rad per examination, try to find another facility with lower-dose equipment. Many "dedicated" machines today give considerably less than 1 rad per two-view examination.

What does the mammogram tell the doctor that he can't learn in some other way?

If the doctor finds a suspicious lump, the mammogram may give the doctor some indication as to whether or not the lump is cancerous. He will also see whether or not there are other lumps which might be cancerous in the breast and which cannot be felt by manual examination. This information is important to the doctor if he is to perform an operation on the breast. If the woman has large breasts or fibrocystic disease, mammography is especially useful.

Can the doctor tell definitely from a mammogram whether or not cancer is present?

A negative mammogram *does not* guarantee there is no cancer in the breast. A mammogram can identify certain lumps as benign. However, the mammogram is only one phase in the total picture. In most cases, surgical biopsy is necessary to finally determine whether or not a suspicious lump is cancer.

I have heard so much controversy over mammography that I don't know whether or not to have a mammogram.

The controversy on the question of mammography has been over the use of it for *routine* screening, to detect breast cancer. The concern over mammography grew from the risks involved in radiation. When mammography was first introduced, some of the techniques exposed women to 10 rads of radiation or more per exposure. (A rad is a unit of radiation that measures the amount of energy absorbed from radiation at a given point.) If mammography was given regularly as a routine exam over a 10- or 20-year period, there was fear that this exposure could be hazardous. However, newer techniques have been developed which have lowered the doses in some cases to a third of a rad or less for each exposure.

Because of the controversy, the American Cancer Society has issued guidelines on screening exams to detect breast cancer. According to these guidelines, you should:

- Do breast self-examination monthly starting at age 20
- Have a physical examination of the breast by a physician at 3-year intervals between the ages of 20 and 40, and annually thereafter
- Have a baseline mammogram between the ages of 35 and 40, followed by annual or biennial mammograms from 40 to 49 and annual mammograms from 50 on.

The National Cancer Institute, American College of Radiology, and American College of Obstetricians and Gynecologists have also issued similar guidelines. Some physicians recommend annual mammograms should continue at least until the age of 75.

So is mammography safe enough that if I have a lump in my breast and my doctor tells me to get a mammogram I should go ahead with it?

Yes, definitely. There is no question about the use of mammography in making a diagnosis when symptoms are present. In this instance, the true risk would be in not having the mammogram done.

What are the benefits of a mammogram?

According to the National Cancer Institute, at the ACS/NCI screening centers, mammography has helped detect 45 percent of breast cancers that were missed by the doctor when he examined the breast manually. For earlier cancers, called minimal tumors, which cannot be felt and are only detectable through mammography, cure rates of up to 95 percent are being reported.

I am still worried about getting too much radiation. What should I ask before I get a mammogram?

When making your appointment for mammography, be sure to ask whether the facility is using a dedicated machine, how many mammograms are taken there (a radiologist needs to be reading mammograms every day to be able to detect subtle changes), and how many rads you will be exposed to. A breast examination should require no more than 1 rad per breast when proper equipment and techniques are used.

What preparations are necessary before having my mammography?

There are no special diets or other procedures. However, on the day of the examination you may be asked not to use any deodorant, perfume, powders, ointment, or preparations of any sort in the underarm area or on your breasts, since these can obscure the results of the Xeroradiographic mammograms. Also, it is more convenient to wear a skirt or slacks with a blouse or sweater, since it is necessary to undress to the waist for the examination.

What happens when I go for the mammography examination?

You will be asked to remove all clothing above the waist. Then you will sit, stand or lie in various positions to obtain the best pictures of your breasts. Both breasts will usually be x-rayed, since it is important to compare images of each breast. The technologist sometimes uses a cone-shaped device, a sponge, large balloon, or a similar object to help position your breast for a better picture. You may feel some pressure when the machine flattens your breast. The entire procedure usually takes about half an hour. After the radiologist studies the results, he reports his findings to the physician.

How accurate is a mammogram or Xerogram?

It is accurate, but not as accurate as a biopsy—nothing is. The test is also not as reliable in young women because the density of the tissue makes it more difficult to forecast a malignancy accurately. The test is also not as accurate on women with very small or very large breasts. However, it can be an important part of the whole picture as far as a diagnosis of breast cancer is concerned. Radiologists feel that it has about an 85 percent accuracy rate. Furthermore, it should be in your records for future reference if you have any history of lumps.

How much will a mammogram cost?

A mammogram usually costs between $100 and $250. Routine screening mammograms may or may not be covered by your medical insurance, depending upon your policy.

Is ultrasound used for diagnosing breast cancer?

Sometimes. Ultrasound is a painless way to detect abnormalities in the breast by projecting high-frequency sound waves into the breast. The pattern of echoes from these sound waves is converted by computer into a visual image of the interior of the breast. It is most useful in telling the difference between solid masses and cysts, especially in younger women whose breasts are very dense. It does not, however, show microcalcifications or identify very small cancers, so it is not as good as mammography for screening. Ultrasound is being used in some medical centers to follow high risk patients who have had lumpectomy and radiation therapy treatments.

Is CT scanning used in detecting breast cancer?

A CT scan, which takes a series of pictures shot from different angles, is synthesized by a computer to produce a detailed picture of a section of tissue. So far, CT scans have been useful in detecting cancer in small dense breasts which are difficult to examine by mammography. However because CT scans require a relatively high x-ray exposure, the injections of a chemical into the body and the use of complicated and expensive equipment, it is not suitable for routine screening and diagnostic studies.

Is MRI a screening method for breast cancer?

MRI, or magnetic resonance imaging, uses a combination of magnetic fields and radiowaves to detect abnormal tissue. Preliminary studies indicate that MRI can successfully image breast cancers—at least large, palpable ones. MRI can not at this time distinguish between breast cancer and benign tumors.

Are monoclonal antibodies being used in diagnosing breast cancer?

Monoclonal antibodies are presently being tested for use in diagnosing breast cancer. No trials of monoclonal antibodies for breast cancer treatment are under way at present.

Is thermography used in diagnosing breast cancer?

Sometimes. Thermography, also referred to as contact thermography and graphic stress telethermometry, is a technique for measuring heat given off by various parts of the breast. A cancer gives off more heat than normal tissue because of its fast metabolic rate and abnormally rich blood supply. Thermography is safe because it does not use any radiation; it simply measures heat radiated by the breast.

How is thermography done?

You take off your clothes and sit in a cool room for about 10 minutes to allow your skin temperature to cool. For contact thermography, the breasts are held against or wrapped with material containing liquid crystals which change color with changes in temperature. For telethermometry, the heat is measured by an infrared sensor. In all cases, the heat emissions are then recorded by a camera.

Is thermography as good as mammography?

Thermography is best at showing large cancers in women with symptoms. It is not as accurate as mammography, especially in finding very small cancers deep within the breast. It may prove helpful in predicting cancer development. Work to improve the technique as well as trials to determine its effectiveness are under way. At present, it should not be used alone as a diagnostic tool.

What is transillumination?

Transillumination, or diaphanography, is used by some doctors to further their knowledge of the nature of a lump. With the help of a powerful light beam, they interpret the contours of the lump. It is used mainly in addition to other clinical devices available to give the doctor further insight into the kind of lump being examined and can help distinguish a cyst from a solid tumor. Quite simply, in a darkened room, the doctor beams a powerful light through the breast area being examined. Different types of tissues transmit and scatter light in different ways, and these differences can be more clearly seen with an infrared-sensitive television camera and display. Current studies show that transillumination does not identify the very small cancers routinely detected by mammography. The technique remains experimental.

What is a needle aspiration?

Sometimes, when the character of the lump and the mammogram suggest that the lump is a cyst, the doctor will withdraw fluid from the lump with a needle and syringe (aspirate). The fluid which is taken out is examined by the pathologist for possible cancer cells. If the lump is solid, the doctor may be able to get a sample of cells to be analyzed in the laboratory.

Are both mammograms and needle aspirations done on the same breast?

Sometimes both are performed. However, if the needle aspiration is performed before the mammogram, there is usually a 2-week wait between the two procedures, since blood collects inside the breast around the site where the needle aspiration is performed and can complicate the reading of the mammogram.

What is needle localization?

On a mammogram, a doctor can see a small area of change in the breast tissue or can see a change which is deep inside the breast—neither of which can be felt manually. Taking a piece of tissue from the area in question is the only way to know if the problem is cancer. Because the doctor cannot feel the location of the area which is to be removed for biopsy, a way of pinpointing and marking the area before the biopsy is needed. This procedure is called needle localization.

How is needle localization done?

Using your mammogram, the radiologist finds the area of change in the breast and marks with a pen the skin lying directly above it. A thin, hollow needle that contains a wire is put into your breast at that spot. A new mammogram is taken to check that the needle is in the correct spot. If it is not, the needle is partly taken out of the breast and put back into the right spot. Another mammogram will be taken to check the needle position. When it shows that the needle is in the exact spot, the needle is removed, leaving the wire to mark the spot.

How big is the wire?

The wire is about the size of a strand of hair, with a tiny hook at the tip holding it in place in the breast. During the biopsy, this wire guides the surgeon, who will cut along the wire and follow it inside your breast to the suspicious area which cannot be seen with the naked eye. The surgeon will remove the area along with the marker wire.

Is needle localization painful?

Not usually. Before placing the needle, the doctor numbs the skin with a painkiller. The skin of the breast is sensitive to pain, but the tissue inside the breast is not. Most women say the insertion of the needle is painless. You may feel a slight tugging or twinge if the needle needs to be moved into a different position.

What is a needle biopsy?

If the lump is solid—that is, if it does not have any fluid in it—the doctor may do a wide-bore needle biopsy. This needle is larger than the one used for needle aspiration. It has a sharp point which cuts a piece of the lump as it passes through the tumor. This tissue needs to be analyzed by a specialized pathologist.

What is a surgical or excisional biopsy?

Usually those terms refer to taking out the whole lump for examination. This will leave you with a scar, but it can be done in a way that disturbs the shape of your breast as little as possible. There is a fuller explanation of biopsies in Chapter 4.

What kind of doctor will perform the biopsy?

Physicians who specialize in treating breast cancer are usually called surgical oncologists. Talk to your family doctor about whom he would recommend.

Will I have to go to the hospital for the breast biopsy?

Breast biopsies can be done either on an outpatient basis or in the hospital. If performed on an inpatient basis, they can be done either as a separate operation or as part of a mastectomy. If the biopsy is done as a separate operation, it is known as a two-step procedure.

What is meant by a two-step procedure?

A two-step procedure means that the biopsy will be done separately, usually at the outpatient clinic in the hospital or even in a doctor's office. If cancer is found, the treatment takes place several days to a week later.

What is the alternative to a two-step procedure?

The alternative to the two-step procedure is to have both the biopsy and the mastectomy operation done at the same time. You go to the operating room and are put under general anesthesia as if the mastectomy were definitely going to be performed. The surgeon takes a biopsy and immediately sends it to the pathologist, who will determine whether or not it is cancerous from a test called a frozen section. If the biopsy shows that the lump is cancerous, the mastectomy will be performed immediately. Under this one-step procedure, a woman who signs the permission slip for surgery does not know whether she will wake up with or without her breast.

What are some good reasons for wanting a two-step procedure?

There are several.

- First of all, eight out of ten women will prove to have benign lumps. If you have a one-step procedure you may be subjected needlessly to the danger of general anesthetic.

- The one-step procedure uses a frozen-section biopsy, which does not tell the doctor as much as the regular biopsy. The two-step uses both a frozen and a permanent section to analyze the tissue.
- Unless all the tests (such as bone or liver scans) are done before the biopsy, the doctor has no way of knowing how widespread the disease is. Doing this whole range of tests on every woman who needs a biopsy is unnecessary, since 80 percent of the women biopsied will be found not to have cancer. A two-step procedure allows additional time to determine the extent of disease.
- You can get a second opinion and discuss different forms of treatment.
- You have time to prepare yourself emotionally.
- You will have time to make arrangements at work and at home for your recovery period.

Why should the bone and liver scans be done before operating?

These tests will help to tell the doctor the extent of the disease. Most doctors feel that doing a mastectomy on a woman who already has disease which has spread beyond her breast is performing needless surgery. Some statistics show that the removal of the breast and all the lymph nodes in these cases does not affect the cure rate. A woman who has positive bone and liver scans cannot be cured by surgery. Therefore, some doctors feel she need not be subjected to the trauma of a mastectomy when this may not provide a positive cure for her disease. The two-step method of determining the nature of a breast tumor seems like a sensible approach. However, there are some physicians who prefer the one-step procedure. There are also some women who feel that they would like to make the decision quickly and get the surgery over with as promptly as possible.

What is the difference between a frozen section and a regular biopsy?

The main difference is in how much the pathologist can tell about the nature and the type of cancer. A full discussion of the two kinds of biopsies is in Chapter 4.

What if the doctor insists on a one-step procedure and I want a two-step procedure?

Our advice would be unequivocal: Find another doctor, fast.

Do most doctors recommend a two-step procedure—that is, a time lapse between the biopsy and the removal of the breast?

Many doctors today subscribe to the belief that a two-step procedure is a useful alternative.

Won't all this time delay mean that the cancer has more chance to spread?

No. Studies have shown that a short delay between biopsy and treatment will not affect the spread of disease or reduce the chances for successful treatment. An interval of 2 days to a week between the two procedures is not a problem. Many medical professionals now agree that this time delay is perfectly acceptable and in most cases is a wise way to proceed. The advantages of getting all of the necessary information about the extent of the cancer far outweigh the advantages of performing a quick, disfiguring operation.

I feel I need some time to think, but everybody keeps pushing me to have the biopsy and the operation done right away. What should I do?

It is important to have the time to think and to look at the alternatives. You may want to talk it over with your husband and children, your sisters, your mother, or your friends. You may want to get a second opinion. It is all right to take a few extra days to make the right decision. It is better to take the time to study than to make a hasty choice. On the other hand, some people want to have it done and over with. If you are that kind of person, go ahead as long as you feel comfortable with your choice.

If I knew I could have a breast reconstruction, maybe the decision wouldn't be so hard to make. Is this something I can decide at this time?

Yes. This is something you should discuss with your doctor. You should ask your surgeon for a consultation with a plastic surgeon before the mastectomy if possible, even though the full extent of the reconstruction can't be determined until after the incision has healed. In some cases, the plastic surgeon can be in the operating room at the time of the mastectomy. Some women feel that the prospect of reconstruction makes a great deal of difference in their attitude toward the mastectomy. There is additional information on breast reconstruction at the end of this chapter.

What is meant by lymph-node involvement?

The doctors check to see whether or not the cancer which started in the breast has spread to the lymph nodes under the arm. This can be done during the biopsy stage. Treatment for breast cancer which has spread to the lymph nodes is different from treatment for localized breast cancer which has not yet begun to spread.

Can the doctor check whether there is any involvement with the lymph nodes if the biopsy is done as part of a two-step procedure?

Yes, he can.

What happens when a biopsy is done on an outpatient basis?

The patient is prepared for surgery and premedicated with a relaxant. A dose of local anesthetic is injected into the skin, the incision is made, and the lump is removed. There should be no pain. The sutures are carefully made, a pressure bandage is used to cover the incision, and the patient is taken back to her room and allowed to relax until the medication has worn off. Usually the operation is performed in the morning and the patient is ready to leave the hospital in the afternoon. The stitches are usually removed within 3 or 4 days, at which time the doctor will give the patient the result of the pathologist's report.

Is there any pain with a biopsy?

It is common to have some pain in the area of the operation, but the following suggestions can help to ease it:
- Take pain medicine as directed by the doctor or nurse.
- Wear a supportive bra 24 hours a day.

- For a few days, don't make lifting and pulling motions with your arm on the side of the biopsy.
- Try to stay warm, as cold temperatures will cause your nipple to contract, which may result in pulling on the stitches.

Will my breast look different after the biopsy?

Yes, it will, but within a few months it will look better. You will probably have a bruised area around the biopsy; it will fade in about 2 weeks. You may notice a flat spot where the biopsy was done. It will take about 6 weeks for this to fill in and for your breast size and shape to be almost as they were before. Your nipple may be pulled to one side. It should go back to nearly normal in a couple of months. You may also feel some numbness in the area of the biopsy and in the nipple for a couple of months.

Will my scar be red and swollen?

Probably you will see a slight redness and swelling along the incision or find a small amount of pink draining from the scar area. These symptoms are normal. If there is a lot of redness and swelling or pus around the area or if you have heavy bleeding, call the doctor right away. Your scar will be red for a while but will soon fade in color.

What if when I ask for a separate procedure for the biopsy, the doctor says that I will be doubling my risk of undergoing general anesthesia twice?

Your doctor, if he uses this argument, has overlooked the fact that a general anesthetic is not usually needed for a biopsy. In most cases, a biopsy can be performed under local anesthesia, with the patient fully conscious or, if she prefers, semiconscious. Most biopsies are now performed on an outpatient basis.

What happens next if the pathological report shows that the tumor is cancerous?

Eight out of ten times, the lump will prove to be benign, but if the report shows the tumor to be cancerous, the next step will be for you to have a metastatic examination or workup. The workup may involve bone and sometimes liver scans to see if the cancer has spread. In addition, a chest x-ray, blood studies, and mammogram—all of which have probably already been done—will be part of the decision-making process before the treatment is decided upon.

I am about to go into the hospital for a biopsy for a lump in my breast. I am very depressed. Is it normal for me to feel this way?

It is not unusual for women who are about to have a breast biopsy, and possibly face having breast cancer, to be very distressed. Studies show that women, particularly those who have had a friend or relative with cancer and are now facing that possibility themselves, tend to be depressed. On the other hand, there are some women who are optimistic in this situation, either feeling that the lump will be benign or that their doctor will be able to take care of it. It is important, if you can, to discuss how you feel with someone. Some people find it easy to talk with their husbands or their mothers, sisters, or close friends. Others feel more at ease talking with someone who is not close to them—such as one of the members of the hospital team. If you are in the hospital and feel you need this kind of discussion, ask for a cancer nurse, a doctor, social-service worker, or the chaplain. There is also a toll free cancer information service (1-800-4-CANCER) where trained volunteers can help answer your questions and discuss alternative kinds of treatment with you.

Understanding the Doctor's Terms

TERMINOLOGY	WHAT IT MEANS	REMARKS
Excisional biopsy	Removal of tumor only	Usually this operation can be performed under local anesthesia. If the lump proves to be benign—as in 8 out of 10 cases—no further steps are necessary. If the diagnosis is cancer, after the biopsy specimen is carefully studied, the type of treatment will depend on decisions you and your doctors must make.
Incisional biopsy	Removal of part of tumor	

Understanding the Doctor's Terms (continued)

TERMINOLOGY	WHAT IT MEANS	REMARKS
Lumpectomy tylectomy local excision	Removal of breast lump followed by radiation therapy. Underarm lymph nodes usually removed.	Lumpectomy removes only the breast lump and is followed by radiation therapy. Most surgeons also remove and test some of the underarm lymph nodes for possible spread of cancer. *Advantage:* The breast is not removed. *Disadvantages:* Small-breasted women with large lumps may have a significant change in breast shape. Scar tissue from the treatment may make it more difficult to examine the breast later. If underarm lymph nodes are not removed, cancer spread may be undetected.
Segmental or partial mastectomy, quadrantectomy, wedge resection, hemimastectomy	Removal of part of breast, some underarm lymph nodes, followed by radiation therapy	Any of these terms may be used to describe operations in which part of the breast is removed. Usually the tumor plus a wedge of normal tissue surrounding it, including some skin and the lining of the chest muscle below the tumor, are removed. Surgery is followed by radiation therapy. Many surgeons also remove some or all of the underarm lymph nodes to check for possible spread of cancer. *Advantages:* If the woman is large-breasted, most of the breast is preserved. There is little possibility of loss of muscle strength or arm swelling. *Disadvantages:* If woman has small or medium-sized breasts, this operation will noticeably change the breast's shape. Cancer in the underarm lymph nodes may be undetected unless nodes are removed for examination.

Understanding the Doctor's Terms (continued)

TERMINOLOGY	WHAT IT MEANS	REMARKS
Simple mastectomy, total mastectomy, complete mastectomy	Removal of the breast. Chest muscles left intact. A few lymph nodes closest to breast may be removed. May be followed by radiation therapy.	Not a simple operation at all. The entire breast is removed. *Advantages:* The chest muscles are not removed, and arm strength is not diminished. Most underarm lymph nodes remain, so the risk of arm swelling is greatly reduced. Breast reconstruction is easier. *Disadvantages:* The breast is removed. If lymph nodes are not looked at and cancer has spread to them, it may remain undiscovered.
Modified radical mastectomy, total mastectomy with axillary dissection	Amputation of breast, lymph nodes in armpit, and lining over chest muscles. Variations: partial removal of lymph nodes in the armpit, partial removal of muscles of chest, complete removal of chest muscles, or a combination of these.	This operation is the most common treatment of early-stage breast cancer. *Advantages:* It leaves a better appearance than the radical mastectomy, because the chest muscle and muscle strength of the arm are retained. Swelling is less likely, and when it does occur, it is milder than the swelling that can occur after a radical mastectomy. Survival rates are the same as for the radical mastectomy when the cancer is treated in its early stages. Breast reconstruction is easier and can be planned before surgery. *Disadvantages:* The breast is removed. In some cases there may be arm swelling because of the removal of the lymph nodes.
Radical mastectomy (sometimes called the Halsted mastectomy)	Amputation of the breast, the fat under the skin surrounding the breast, the muscles on front of chest that support the breasts, and all the fat and lymph nodes that are contained in the armpit.	This operation was the standard treatment for breast cancer for more than 70 years and is still used today for a few women. *Disadvantages:* It removes the entire breast and chest muscles and leaves a long scar and a hollow chest area. It may cause swelling of the arm, some loss of muscle power in the arm, restricted shoulder motion, and some numbness and discomfort. Breast reconstruction is also more difficult.

Understanding the Doctor's Terms (continued)

TERMINOLOGY	WHAT IT MEANS	REMARKS
Extended radical mastectomy	Radical plus removal of internal mammary nodes and possibly thoracic nerve.	Insist on complete discussion of operation, disfigurement, and alternative treatments.
Supraradical mastectomy	Radical neck dissection or at least removal of supraclavicular areas in continuity with breast and armpit lymph nodes.	Same as above.

The General Stages of Breast Cancer

STAGE	OTHER CLASSIFICATIONS	EXPLANATION
In situ	Tis, N0, M0	Noninvasive cancer that has not spread below membrane and glands of breast
Stage I	T1, N0, M0	Confined to the breast; no wider than 2 centimeters
Stage II	T2, N0, M0 T0-T2, N1, M0	Tumor is between 2 and 5 centimeters or smaller, but has spread to underarm lymph nodes
Stage IIIA	T0–T2, N2, M0 T3, N0-N2, M0	Tumor is larger than 5 centimeters or involves chest wall or skin but can be surgically treated

The General Stages of Breast Cancer (continued)

STAGE	OTHER CLASSIFICATIONS	EXPLANATION
Stage IIIB	any T, N3, M0 T4, any N, M0	Tumor, regardless of size, has lymph nodes that are fixed to one another or involves lymph nodes above or below the collarbone or tissues near breast. Inflammatory breast cancer is either IIIB or IV depending on whether metastases are present
Stage IV	Any T, any N, M1	Cancer believed to have spread to other parts of the body

How does the doctor classify the stages of breast cancer when it is found?

Staging will usually include three sets of letters and numbers. The first two in the classification column grade the tumor size, the second two indicate the nodal involvement, and the third pair relate to whether or not the tumor has metastasized. The general categories of staging and more information on how it is done and what it means can be found in Chapter 3.

What size tumors are indicated by the "T" classifications?

T0 means there is no evidence of primary tumor. T1 refers to a tumor that is 2 centimeters or less in its greatest dimension. T2 refers to a tumor which is more than 2 centimeters but not more than 5 centimeters. T3 means that the tumor is more than 5 centimeters. A T4 designation indicates a tumor of any size with direct extension to the chest wall or skin.

Tumor Sizes

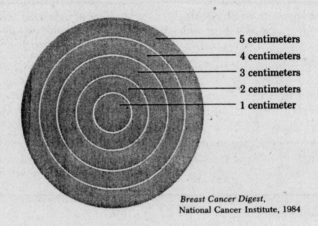

Breast Cancer Digest,
National Cancer Institute, 1984

Is there more than one kind of breast cancer?

Cancer of the breast is not a single disease. There are at least fifteen distinct varieties. The doctor and the patient need to know which variety they are dealing with before making the decision as to how to proceed. Among the types of breast cancer are intraductal, inflammatory, medulluary, papillary, tubular, lobular and Paget's disease.

What is inflammatory breast cancer?

This is a rare type of breast cancer which often spreads rapidly to other parts of the body. In inflammatory breast cancer, the breast looks like it is inflamed. Ridges may appear on the skin, or the breast skin may thicken, displaying the pitted appearance known as *peau d'orange*, or orange peel. Inflammatory breast cancer does not cause a fever or other signs of infection. The breast's redness and warmth develop as the result of cancer cells blocking the lymph vessels in the skin of the breast. Most inflammatory breast cancers are treated as Stage IIIB or IV.

What is the difference between a lumpectomy and a segmental mastectomy?

A lumpectomy removes only the breast lump with a small margin of surrounding tissue. A segmental or partial mastectomy removes the lump plus a wedge of normal tissue. The lumpectomy leaves only a small scar—generally 2 inches or less—with minimal puckering or distortion of the breast. The segmental mastectomy leaves a much larger scar. A separate incision is made for both procedures at the armpit to remove some lymph nodes. Both operations are followed by radiation therapy. Women with relatively large tumors and small breasts are probably not able to have a lumpectomy or segmental mastectomy, since taking out the tumor and some normal tissue would remove most of her breast tissue.

Is there any difference in the effectiveness of these two operations?

No, there seem to be no differences. The National Cancer Institute is conducting clinical trials for both treatments. Results have been reported from the study of segmental mastectomy that was begun in 1976 and involved 1,843 patients with Stage I and Stage II breast cancers 4 centimeters or less in size. The 10-year results of that study show that the segmental mastectomy, with removal of underarm lymph nodes to determine if cancer had spread there and followed by 5,000 rads of radiation therapy given to the breast 5 days a week for 5 weeks, is as effective as total mastectomy (removal of the whole breast). Those women who had cancer cells in their underarm lymph nodes were treated with chemotherapy. The second National Cancer Institute clinical trial, begun in 1979, compares mastectomy with an option of breast reconstruction with lumpectomy. Women who receive lumpectomy have a much smaller scar than those who have segmental mastectomy. The early results of this study also show that the less-disfiguring surgery followed by radiation is as effective as removal of the entire breast for many women with early-stage breast cancer. Since these are early results of the second study, the findings will continue to be followed.

Is cancer more likely to spread in a woman who has had lesser surgery for her breast cancer?

The results of the clinical trials presently being conducted will hopefully answer this question. It was once thought that more extensive surgery meant there was less chance of the cancer recurring in the breast and of it spreading to other parts of the body. It was believed that tumors spread in an orderly fashion, from the tumor to the lymph nodes and then to other parts of the body. Breast cancer does not seem to follow this pattern. Many scientists today believe that breast cancer is a systemic disease and that the different breast operations do not affect the spread of it to another part of the body. When it comes to surviving breast cancer, women who had segmental mastectomies and radiation therapy have so far fared as well as those who had their breast removed.

Are there some women who should not have the lesser surgery?

Yes. There are several groups. Among them are those with small breasts, those who have a lump fixed to the skin or underlying muscle, those with more than one cancerous lump or area in the breast, and those who are too sick to undergo the radiation therapy following the operation.

Can cancer recur in the breast after lesser surgery?

Yes. But if and when that happens, a woman can still have a mastectomy.

Is it necessary to take out the lymph nodes as part of lesser surgery?

It is important, because taking out some or all of the underarm lymph nodes allows the doctor to tell whether or not the cancer has spread beyond the breast area. If cancer cells are found in a lymph node, the node is said to be "positive" for cancer. A node is "negative" if there is no evidence that cancer cells have spread to it. If the lymph nodes are positive, chemotherapy treatments will probably be given.

What happens during lymph-node surgery?

It will depend upon your doctor and your hospital, but the general procedure is as follows. Lymph-node surgery can take from one hour to several hours, depending upon the number of lymph nodes taken out. When you awaken from surgery, your underarm area will be bandaged, and a tube may have been placed at the site of surgery to drain any fluid that may accumulate. You may feel some discomfort: tingling, numbness, or pain in your chest, shoulder area, or upper arm. The numbness under your arm will go away gradually, but you may not have total feeling back for a long time. You will be in the hospital 7 to 10 days for a lymph-node dissection; the stay is 2 to 4 days if only a sampling of nodes is taken. Before you leave, the tube that drains fluid from your incision will be taken out. Your stitches will be taken out in 1 to 3 weeks at the doctor's office or clinic. Additional general information about what to expect when you have an operation can be found in Chapter 6.

What should I do to take care of my scar from the lymph-node surgery?

Before you leave the hospital, ask the doctor or nurse for instructions on taking care of your incision. When you have permission to bathe or shower, do so gently and pat, don't rub, the area of your incision. To keep your skin soft and to promote healing, you may want to massage your incision gently with vitamin E cream or cocoa butter. As time goes by, the redness, bruising, or swelling will disappear. But you should watch for any signs of infection such as inflammation, tenderness, or drainage. If you develop any of these signs or a fever, call your doctor. Although each woman recovers from surgery at her own rate, most women are ready for the next part of their treatment, radiation therapy, about 1 to 2 weeks after their lymph-node surgery.

Will I need to do arm exercises after lymph-node surgery?

At first you will have to be careful not to move your arm too much. But by the second or third day, you may be ready to begin exercises to ease the tension in your arm and shoulder. If you have lymph-node sampling rather than dissection, you will probably recover your arm motion more quickly, because the operation is not as extensive. The nurse, doctor, or physical therapist will show you what exercises to do. You will probably begin with these simple movements and be given others to do at home:

- Lie in bed with your arm at your side. Raise your arm straight up and back, trying to touch the headboard.
- Raise your shoulders. Rotate them forward, down, and back in a circular motion to loosen your chest, shoulder, and upper back muscles.
- Lying in bed, clasp your hands behind your head and push your elbows into the mattress.
- With your elbow bent and your arm at a 90 degree angle to your body, rotate your shoulder forward until the forearm is down, then up.
- With your arm raised, clench and unclench your fist.
- Breathe deeply.
- Rotate your chin to the left and right. Cock your head sideways.

Does radiation therapy have to follow the lesser surgery?

Yes. In the National Cancer Institute study, women given radiation treatment after their segmental mastectomies had much lower rates of the cancer recurring in the breast.

What is involved with the radiation therapy following lesser surgery?

High-energy x-rays are aimed at the breast and sometimes at nearby areas that still contain some lymph nodes, such as under the arm (if only a sample of lymph nodes was taken during surgery), above the collarbone, and along the breastbone. The goal is to destroy any cancer cells that may still remain in the breast or surrounding areas. The high-energy x-rays are delivered by a linear accelerator or cobalt machine. Usually treatments are given 5 days a week for about 5 weeks. A single treatment takes about 20 to 25 minutes. Only a few minutes of this time are for the treatment; most of the time is spent putting you in the proper position. Most people continue with work or their regular activities during the treatment period.

About 1 to 2 weeks after the treatment has been completed, most women receive a concentrated "booster" dose of radiation to the area where the breast lump was located. The dose is given either externally, using an electron beam, or internally with an implant of radioactive material. The electron-beam booster is delivered by a type of linear accelerator machine and requires daily visits for 5 to 10 days. You may notice an increase in skin redness at the site of the treatment. This is normal. The implant procedure requires a short hospital stay of 2 to 3 days. Thin plastic tubes are threaded through the breast tissue where the original lump was removed; the tubes are then filled with radioactive seeds. The implant will remain in the breast for 2 to 3 days. Read Chapter 7 for information on radiation treatment.

Does it cost more to have a lumpectomy than a mastectomy?

Lumpectomy is a more expensive treatment. Although you stay in the hospital less with a lumectomy, you must pay doctor bills to both a surgeon and a radiotherapist, along with the extra cost of radiation therapy.

I want to have lesser surgery, but my doctor does not want me to. What shall I do?

First, you need to find out why your doctor does not want you to have it, because there are times when mastectomies are the best treatment. Second, you need to get another opinion at a medical center where doctors are experienced in doing lesser surgery, node samplings, and radiotherapy. Call the nearest large medical center and ask for a radiation therapist or a surgical oncologist. Call the 1-800-4-CANCER line and ask for the name of a major medical center near you or of physicians who specialize in breast surgery.

What is the difference between a radical mastectomy and modified radical mastectomy?

In the radical mastectomy (also known as the Halsted mastectomy) the doctor removes the breast tissue, the lymph nodes under the armpit, and the muscle under the breast.

The modified radical, which most surgeons are now using, removes the breast tissue and the lymph nodes, but

Treatment Choices for Breast Cancer

STAGE	POSSIBLE TREATMENTS
In situ	Removal of lump, and lymph-node dissection, with radiation in selected cases. Mastectomy in selected cases.
Stage I	Diagnostic biopsy as separate procedure with lymph node dissection.
	Limited surgery—lumpectomy, or segmental resection with lymph-node dissection—plus radiation. Provides results equivalent to more extensive surgery. May be considered experimental by some physicians.
	Modified radical mastectomy. Radical mastectomy in highly selected cases.
	Investigational: Surgery or limited surgery plus radiation, plus chemotherapy or hormone therapy.
Stage II	Diagnostic biopsy as separate procedure with lymph node dissection.
	Limited surgery—lumpectomy or segmental resection with lymph-node dissection—plus radiation and/or hormonal therapy. Provides results equivalent to more extensive surgery. Considered experimental by some physicians.
	Modified radical mastectomy. Radical mastectomy in selected circumstances only. Adjuvant combination chemotherapy, following treatment for local disease, for premenopausal women with lymph node involvement. Tomoxifen for post-menopausal women with lymph node involvement and positive estrogen receptors. Investigational: new types of chemotherapy and hormone therapy.
Stage IIIA	Modified radical mastectomy or radical mastectomy plus radiation and chemotherapy, with or without hormones.
	Surgery and/or radiation followed by hormone therapy.
	Investigational: Combination chemotherapy with or without hormonal treatment.
Stage IIIB and inflammatory breast cancer	Biopsy for diagnosis, receptor assay followed by radiation and chemotherapy or hormonal treatment.
	Mastectomy if necessary.

Treatment Choices for Breast Cancer

STAGE	POSSIBLE TREATMENTS
	Investigational: Combination chemotherapy followed by surgery and/or radiation therapy. Newly developed chemotherapy drugs or biologicals.
Stage IV and inflammatory breast cancer	Biopsy for diagnosis, receptor assay followed by radiation or mastectomy. Hormone therapy may be first treatment depending on extent of disease and receptor status. Combination chemotherapy.
	Investigational: Hormone treatment; combination chemotherapy with or without hormone treatment. Newly developed chemotherapy drugs or biologicals.
Recurrent	Hormone therapy, type depending on extent of disease and receptor levels. Surgery and/or radiation. Combination chemotherapy. All depend on extent of disease, response to other treatments and receptor status.
	Investigational: combination chemotherapy with or without hormone treatment. Investigational hormonal treatments. Newly developed chemotherapy agents and biologicals.

the muscle is left intact. The advantage of the modified radical is that it is cosmetically more attractive and does not handicap the motion of the arm. Studies indicate that the survival rate for the two operations is the same.

Is the choice of what surgical procedure I will have up to me or up to the doctor?

Of course your doctor is responsible for the surgery. But he cannot perform any operation unless you give your signed consent to have it done. You should have your doctor give you his complete explanation of what he recommends as his best judgment and ask him all the questions that concern you about the operation. Do not sign anything until you are certain you understand what you are signing. It is your right to refuse to sign the hospital form that gives blanket permission for a radical mastectomy. It is your right to refuse to sign the form that allows the hospital to do the biopsy and the mastectomy as a one-stage procedure. It is your right to modify the form in your own handwriting to indicate you are giving permission only for a biopsy.

What will happen to a cancerous breast lump if it is not removed?

That is not a feasible alternative. Since cases differ, results differ. But the cancer will, in almost every case, continue to grow and spread, either in the breast area or to other parts of the body. Uncontrolled cancer of the breast is not a pretty or painless choice. In general, the life expectancy of women with untreated breast cancer is about 2½ years.

What can I expect to happen immediately before mastectomy surgery?

As for most surgical procedures, the area will be shaved and your breast washed with germ-killing soap. The nurse will administer a sedative that should relax you completely and put you into a drowsy, semiconscious state. An IV (intravenous) needle will be placed in a vein in your forearm or hand on the side opposite the side to be operated on, and the needle will be taped to your skin. The IV will be used for intravenous feedings, to administer anesthesia, and to administer blood if needed. Depending on the procedure, the surgery will take between 2 and 4 hours. You will stay in the hospital from 7 to 10 days. Additional general information about what to expect when you have an operation is given in Chapter 6.

Will there be a drain in the area where I had surgery?

Yes. Your breast area will be bandaged, and a tube will be placed at the surgical site to drain away any fluid that may accumulate. Before you leave the hospital, the tube will be removed. Some of your stitches may also be taken out before you leave. The remaining stitches will be removed within 1 to 3 weeks at the doctor's office or clinic.

Is it unusual for my chest and arm to feel numb after a mastectomy?

No, it is not unusual. This is a normal reaction. The entire operated side will feel this way for quite some time after the operation, sometimes for months, although the time var-

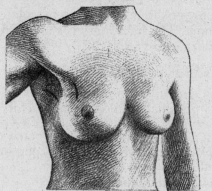

lumpectomy with axillary node dissection

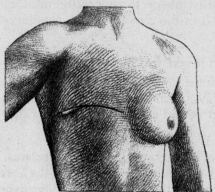

simple mastectomy

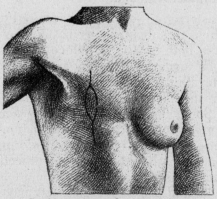

radical mastectomy with skin graft
Examples of breast operation scars

ies from person to person. In a few persons, some numbness may be permanent. The numbness is the result of nerves injured or cut during surgery.

What does a mastectomy scar look like?

The appearance depends upon the extent of the operation and the doctor's personal method. Some doctors use a vertical cut, others a horizontal one. If you have a preference, you should discuss this with your doctor before the operation so your wishes can be considered and discussed.

How dangerous is a mastectomy?

Not dangerous at all as far as the surgery involved is concerned. Mortality rates referring to the mastectomy operation itself put it in the almost-no-risk category. It is a very safe operation.

How long will it take for the incision to heal?

The incision for a lumpectomy will usually heal within a week or 10 days. Wounds of more-radical operations are usually healed within a month to 6 weeks after the operation.

I am thinking of having a preventive mastectomy. My mother and aunt died of breast cancer before they were 40. My breasts are lumpy, and the doctor has done several biopsies with a diagnosis of precancerous condition. Would I be wise to have both breasts removed?

Preventive mastectomy—sometimes referred to by physicians as prophylactic subcutaneous mastectomy—is the removal of one or both breasts to reduce the risk of cancer. It is sometimes suggested to women considered to be at high risk of developing breast cancer. There is some controversy about the advisability of this operation for high-risk women. Some doctors recommend instead that the women perform monthly breast examination and have checkups every 3 months. If you are considering a preventive mastectomy, you should discuss the procedure, reconstructive surgery, possible complications, and follow-up care with your doctor and plastic surgeon. You may want to get a second opinion as well as requesting some information from a genetics counseling clinic affiliated with a university medical school. Furthermore, you may wish to talk with someone who has had a preventive mastectomy before you make this decision. It is a question that only the individual involved can answer. Part of the decision must be based on how worried you are about getting cancer and how important your breasts are to you. You need to carefully study the pros and cons before you make this decision.

Questions You Will Want to Ask Your Doctor Following a Mastectomy

- What arm exercises can I do?
- When can I start to shower again?
- What restrictions do you put on my affected arm?
- When will I be able to drive?
- Will you arrange for a Reach to Recovery volunteer to see me?
- When will the stitches be removed?
- Are there any restrictions on sexual activity?
- What kind of therapy is prescribed?
- Why is it being prescribed?
- What will it do?
- Can I lift things?
- When can I start doing my household chores?
- When can I start active sports again?
- When can I get a permanent prosthesis?
- When can I have reconstructive surgery?
- Will I have to have any additional treatment such as radiation or chemotherapy?
- Why? Does that mean that the cancer has spread?
- How long will I have to have those treatments?

How shall I care for my incision?

Wash with soap and water gently and pat, don't rub, the area of your incision. You may take a shower within 2 to 3 days after the stitches are removed. If the stitches are not removed before you go home, they will probably be covered with a gauze pad to protect them from irritation. Your doctor will tell you when they are ready to be removed. Do not use any medications—salves, creams, or lotions—on your incision unless told to do so by your doctor. Watch for any signs of infection—redness, swelling, pus discharge, tenderness, or fever—and report them to your doctor as soon as possible.

One last word. Before you are discharged from the hospital, please force yourself to look at your incision carefully (even if you may not want to). This will help you to be alert to any changes that may occur. Ask the nurse for assistance and for guidance in evaluating it. It will appear swollen and red. This is normal. The swelling will go away, the color will return to normal, and the stitches will heal. But for your own sake, please don't avoid looking at the incision.

What is the role of Reach to Recovery?

This is a volunteer program sponsored by the American Cancer Society. It is based on the idea that women who have been through breast surgery and have experienced the pain, anxiety, and convalescence are able to help others through the initial period following the mastectomy. The program is set up so that only the surgeon or doctor, with the patient's permission, can arrange to have the volunteer visit the patient in the hospital. In some areas of the country, the patient can request a visit from a Reach to Recovery volunteer after she leaves the hospital.

Some doctors still do not know about Reach to Recovery or misunderstand its goals and methods, feeling that somehow it will interfere with the doctor–patient relationship. So, if you are interested, be sure to ask your doctor specifically if he will arrange for a Reach to Recovery volunteer to see you. Her visit offers help during the emotional, tense period of postoperative adjustment and allows you to talk frankly and honestly about a mutual problem. In addition to lending an understanding ear, the Reach to Recovery volunteer brings an invaluable kit with a realistically written manual of information and exercise materials as well as a temporary breast form and bra. She will demonstrate some of the basic exercises needed to facilitate recovery, and since she is a mastectomy patient herself, she is available to answer questions and give moral support.

Why is everyone so anxious to make me move my arm?

There are good reasons for this. First of all, it will help prevent swelling of the arm and help the drainage of the wound. Changing the position of the arm will limit shoulder pain and help you to gradually build your affected arm back up to its fullest capacity as quickly as possible. Moving your arm is very important because it helps prevent the forming of adhesions which will later limit how much you can move it. Frequent exercising is necessary to relieve stiffness and a heavy feeling. Your doctor will tell you when you can safely begin to exercise. The amount and the extent of surgery will determine the problems you will have with your arm.

Are there any suggestions for activities I should be doing with my arm after the operation?

The American Cancer Society's Reach to Recovery program makes the following suggestions:

- Use your elbow and hand as much as you can for normal activities.
- For the first few days after the operation, practice deep breathing often. Lying on your back, breathe in deeply, expanding your lower chest as much as possible. Then let the air out and relax. Concentrate on relaxing while letting the air out. Do this three or four times, breathing in deeply and relaxing.
- Check with the doctor about exercises you can do at various times after surgery.
- You should get full motion and strength back in your arm about 2 to 3 months after your mastectomy. If you are having difficulty regaining shoulder motion, ask your doctor for help or for a referral to a physical or occupational therapist.
- You will have normal shoulder motion when you can reach across the top of your head and touch the opposite ear without feeling a stretch in your armpit. Your upper arm should be right next to your ear. Do not put your arm behind your head so you can grab your ear more easily. Keep your head straight up. Another test for

shoulder motion is to raise your arms as high as possible about your head with the upper arm touching your ears.

- You can begin exercises for shoulder motion when your doctor gives permission. It is usually all right to stretch your shoulder until you feel a mild pull. Any stretching should be done slowly and smoothly. The way to get your motion back is to work gradually, doing a little more each day.

- The stiffness and tightness felt in the tissues of the chest and armpit after surgery or radiation therapy will come and go for a while. Continue to work to improve your motion at least three times a day until that feeling of tightness is no longer a problem.

- Start on activities that are helpful in your regular routine—for example, reach into cabinets, wash and brush your hair, put your arms behind your neck, fasten your bra.

What kind of arm exercises should I do?

Your doctor will tell you when you can begin exercising and will probably give you his own list of exercises. A nurse or physical therapist will be happy to review them with you. Start exercising gradually and work up to doing each exercise five times a day, working up to a maximum of twenty times per day per exercise. Here are some of the suggested exercises:

- Squeeze a ball, a rolled-up bandage, or a crumpled sheet of paper. Lying in bed, lift your arm straight up and alternately squeeze and relax the ball. If it is uncomfortable to hold your arm straight up, support the arm using several pillows.

- Stand erect, feet apart, with toes 6 to 12 inches from and facing a wall. Bend elbows and place palms against the wall at shoulder level. Work both hands up the wall parallel to each other until the incision pulls or pain occurs. Mark the spot so that you can check your progress. Work hands down to shoulder level. Move your feet and body closer to the wall if it is more comfortable. Rest and repeat.

- Stand erect, feet apart. Place the hand on the unoperated

side on your hip for balance. Bend the elbow of the arm on the operated side, placing the back of the hand on the small of your back. Gradually work the hand up your back until your fingers reach the opposite shoulder blade. Slowly lower your arm. Rest and repeat.

Information given to you by the Reach to Recovery volunteer will also include exercises for you to do.

Some people have swollen arms after a mastectomy. What causes that?

The lymphatic system which normally drains fluid from your arm is disrupted with mastectomy surgery. Your arm may be more likely to swell or to become red, warm, or unusually hard if you develop an infection. Therefore, it is important for you to take special care to avoid injury, infection, and swelling of the arm. You must always be careful what you do with the arm on the side where the mastectomy is performed, since the swelling can occur even several years after the operation.

When can I start using deodorant again?

It depends upon where the incision is made. You should wait until all the stitches are removed and the incision heals before using a deodorant.

What kinds of things should I watch for in order to protect the arm on the side where my mastectomy was performed?

- Do not allow blood samples to be drawn from or blood pressure to be taken on the affected arm.
- Avoid injections and vaccinations on the affected arm.
- Do not wear tight jewelry or elasticized or tight sleeves on that side.
- Keep that side covered when you are out in the sun. Avoid insect bites by using protective insect repellent.
- Wash cuts promptly, treat them with antibacterial medication, and cover them with sterile dressing. Check often for redness, soreness, or other signs of infection.
- Avoid burns while cooking.
- Pamper your arm by carrying your purse or packages on the other side.

- Wear a thimble when sewing to avoid pinpricks.
- Wear gloves or mitts when gardening and working with sharp objects or hot objects. Use a mitt when taking hot dishes out of the oven. Use rubber gloves when washing with harsh detergents.
- Use an electric razor to avoid cutting this area. Underarm shaving may be a problem for a while because of the lack of mobility or numbness, so take great care.
- Never pick or cut cuticles or hangnails. Apply lanolin hand cream to hand and arm several times a day.
- If you do notice pain, swelling, or redness on your scar or arm, with or without fever being present, call your doctor. In the meantime, put your arm over your head and pump your fist.
- Though you should be cautious, it is also important to use your arm normally. Don't favor it or keep it dependent.

What can I do if I have a swollen arm?

The swollen arm (edema) is due to the disruption of the lymph channels. It is very important that you do the exercises described (or similar ones which your nurse, physical therapist, or doctor has ordered) and follow the suggestions for arm care so that the swelling is prevented. If swelling does occur, elevating the arm may help to reduce it. You can use a pillow, trying to keep your hand higher than the elbow and the elbow higher than the shoulder. You should maintain this position for at least 30 minutes and repeat the exercise several times each day. When you are lying down, keep your arm elevated on a pillow. Isometric exercises (such as making a fist and tightening your arm muscles for 3 seconds, then relaxing them) several times a day help to increase circulation of fluid from the arm. An elastic cuff that inflates and deflates, applying pressure, can be helpful. In addition, sometimes salt-free diets are used. Some doctors will perform surgery if the swelling continues over a long period of time.

What is a lymphadema sleeve?

It is a sleevelike apparatus into which you place your affected arm. It forces the fluids back into the lymph system and reduces the swelling. Although using it once or twice a day helps to control the swelling, it will not cure the problem. The doctor will tell you how long to leave your arm in the sleeve and the correct pressure setting. Usually the unit is used at a physical therapy department at a hospital, although some units are about the size of a train case and can be used at home. The doctor can write a prescription for one, and some insurance companies will cover its cost.

Will all the pain, numbness, and tingling sensations eventually disappear?

Yes, they should. However, some women continue to have symptoms for many months after the operation has healed. Some patients say they have pain radiating from under the arm to the waist when they touch under the armpit. As with other operations, the symptoms are affected by the weather. If you have unusual sensations, discuss them with your doctor. Some people feel pain in the breast that was removed. Doctors are not sure why this phantom pain occurs, but it does exist. It is not imaginary.

Will I get full muscle strength back in my arm?

That depends upon the operation which has been performed. In some radical mastectomies, you may be limited in the strength of certain motions and feel some permanent muscle weakness.

Will I have trouble sleeping?

Some women do have trouble sleeping on the side of the operation. Others say that they cannot wear their prosthesis to bed because the elastic in the bra is too tight (you can get a "sleeping brassiere" which is much softer and more comfortable to wear). Some women described the feeling as like being in a cast, saying it is difficult to sleep because it is hard to find a comfortable position. Others talk about the difficulty of lying flat on their backs because of the pulling sensation. Yet others experience very little difficulty with this problem.

When can I expect all the stiffness, heaviness, and tautness to be gone?

As with most surgery, you shouldn't expect it all to be gone in a month. You may have to exercise many more weeks before the stiffness eases up, and you may, as with other surgery, feel some recurrent stiffness and pulling. If by 6 weeks after you have had the operation, when you are fully healed with all the stitches out, you don't have the full range of motion, you should tell your doctor or nurse. They may order additional exercises.

When can I go back to doing my regular work?

Again, this depends upon the extent of your operation and your own personal condition. You should discuss this with your doctor before you go home from the hospital. Most doctors recommend early resumption of work, including household chores and office duties.

Can I continue with sports such as bowling, golf, tennis, skiing, and swimming?

You can certainly go back to them, but you should check with your doctor as to when you can take up active sports again. Swimming is very good exercise for breast patients, and there are many styles of bathing suits which you can use.

Are there some medical reasons why I should wear a prosthesis?

Yes, there are medical reasons why you should wear a form to replace the missing breast. The weight of the remaining breast, particularly for women with medium-to-large breasts, can cause shoulder, neck, and back pain. You may find that your posture will change, with the affected shoulder rising, if you do not have a prosthesis. The larger the remaining breast, the more vital the need, not only for appearance but also for weight. For your own well-being, emotional comfort, and self-confidence, you should plan to buy a prosthesis. In many cases, a well-fitted prosthetic device means the difference between prompt, cheerful, total recovery and long-term personal distress. You will need some device to make your clothing fit well.

Can I wear the prosthesis all the time?

Yes. Many patients wear it all the time, around the clock. Some patients start by wearing it a few hours a day and gradually increasing the number of hours of wear. Wearing the form to bed at night may help prevent a stiff neck and shoulder problems. Waterbeds have also been recommended by some, since they provide support and conform to the body.

Where do I go to buy a prosthesis?

There are several places: corset shops, surgical supply houses, foundation departments of some large department stores, and some special outlets. Some American Cancer Society offices offer a variety of forms that a woman can examine (but are not for sale) in a noncommercial setting. The Reach to Recovery volunteer or the American Cancer Society office can give you material describing the various forms and a list of suggested outlets available. Most of the outlets have fitters who can help you. The large mail-order houses also have prostheses available.

When should I go to get a breast prosthesis?

Most doctors will tell you to wait until the scar is fully healed before you get fitted for a breast prosthesis. Most patients can begin using a full prosthesis a month or 6 weeks after surgery. However, soft forms can be worn from the very beginning. For instance, at the very beginning you can use simple clean padding in your brassiere. The Reach to Recovery volunteer who visits you may provide you with a temporary Dacron-filled prosthesis to wear while the wound is healing and the area is tender and swollen. Some patients tell us they use items such as cotton balls, lamb's wool, handkerchiefs, sanitary napkins, or padded bras during the period between their operation and being fitted for a prosthesis. You should check with your doctor before wearing the permanent prosthesis.

How can I be sure I find the right prosthesis?

First of all, you should not shop for the prosthesis by your-self. It is much better if an involved person, such as your sister, mother, husband, or a good friend, goes along with you. Second, you should make sure you try on several different kinds and models so that you can be sure the one you finally buy is what you really want. There are more than a dozen different breast forms on the market. You should try on several to compare the way they feel and look. The breast form should feel comfortable, have a natural contour and consistency, and should remain in place when you stretch, bend, or reach. Make sure you shop around and try on different types and different brands. It is important to pay close attention to how the prosthesis feels and how it fits—the form should match your other breast from the side, the bottom, and the front. Remember you will be wearing it every day for a long time to come.

Can I make my own prosthesis?

Some people do make their own prostheses. Some of the material put out by the American Cancer Society has instructions for making your own breast forms and night bras. Some small-breasted women or women who have had both breasts removed find that they can use homemade forms. However, in many cases, the homemade forms are too light-weight and tend to ride up. Again, you must be careful because you might end up with aches in your shoulders, backaches, and posture change if you wear a prosthesis which is not of the proper weight for you.

What is a special mastectomy bra?

It is a bra with a built-in pocket to hold the form in place. It also has extra material under the arm and above the breast. The form is placed in the pocket of the bra, which holds it in place. You can bend, stretch, or stoop without jarring it out of place. Some patients have complained that the special mastectomy bras do not fit properly. Many patients have altered their own bras with pockets, and still others have had seamstresses make pockets for their bras. In some stores, fitters will sew pockets into your bras to hold the prosthesis.

What should I wear when I shop for the prosthesis?

You should bring along some figure-revealing clothes to see how natural the form will look—a sweater or one of your more revealing dresses. If you want to use your own bras, make sure you bring them along so they can be altered if needed.

What is meant by a cover on the form?

Some of the forms, both lightweight and heavy ones, have nylon or cloth covers. The covers are made of washable, fast-drying materials. The cover allows the forms to be pinned directly into regular brassieres for occasional use instead of in the specially made pocket. Some women prefer to wear the covers on the forms at all times. They like the way they feel. The tricot covers, especially, are easy to wash out every night and dry so that they can be worn the next day.

I have a depression under my arm left from the surgery. Is there any way to fill that?

There are "back" pads which can be worn under the form or along the side. These are sold with most prostheses and can fill in the depressions left by the surgery.

What are the different kinds of prostheses available?

There are several different kinds of breast forms made by several companies. Generally they fall into these classifications:

- *Silicone gel-filled:* Form usually made of silicone skin. Very soft and flexible with the look, feel, and weight of the natural breast. Worn with regular bra. Adjusts to body temperature. Filled with silicone glycerine or gel, fluid, or sponge. Some can leak if fingernail or pin pricks it. OK for swimming. Most expensive. ($75–$300)
- *Liquid- or air-filled:* Form usually a plastic shell or a soft plastic form. Soft form has natural feel, look, and weight. Usually comes with covers. Depending on make,

can either be worn with regular or specially made bra. Air-filled has pocket that can be inflated to vary shape or size. Liquid-filled can leak if pricked. OK for swimming. ($60–$100)

- *Foam rubber:* Lightweight (molded foam or foam chips) but weights can be added. Spongy feeling. May get stiff and yellow with wear. Good for leisure wear, swimming (needs waterproof cover). Especially useful with lounging bra for postoperative period. Some people like them for general wear. ($10–$50)
- *Polyester:* Lightweight and long-wearing. Soft pads with tricot filling. Good for sleepwear and postoperative wear. ($10–$25)

Ask the American Cancer Society or the Reach to Recovery volunteer for a complete up-to-date list of prostheses manufactured in the United States.

Can I get a breast form with a nipple?

Some forms are made with nipples. Others can be worn with nipples that are sold separately and can be easily attached.

Can I get a form in a dark skin color?

Some forms are made in both light and dark skin colors.

Are there any cosmetics to cover the scars I have after surgery? I find that the ordinary kinds just don't seem to work.

There is a special brand of cosmetics, Covermark, which is designed to blend into one's individual skin color. The cosmetics are waterproof and when carefully applied are particularly useful for swimming. Available from Lydia O'Leary, (One Anderson Ave., Moonachie, NJ 07074) and in many drug and department stores.

The tight elastic bothers me in my bra, but I like the way this particular one fits. Can I do anything about that?

Notion stores and girdle and corset shops sell bra extenders which can be used to make a bra more comfortable. They also sell shoulder-strap pads which some women use to relieve discomfort on the shoulder-strap area.

Can I have a prosthesis custom-made?

There are a few manufacturers who custom-make prostheses. The American Cancer Society can give you an up-to-date listing.

What does a prosthesis look like?

Usually it is flesh-colored. The prostheses are sized to match the remaining breast both in its shape and its weight. Normally, they are teardrop-shaped. The flat side goes against the wall of the chest and the tail end goes toward the armpit. One manufacturer makes a reversible one which can be used on either side.

Does a prosthesis feel cold against the chest?

Most of them feel a little cold when they are first put on. But after they have been worn for a few minutes, they warm to body temperature and feel like a normal breast to the touch.

Will my insurance cover a prosthesis?

It depends on your insurance plan. Some health insurance (and Medicare) covers part or all of the cost of the first prosthesis. The doctor should write the prescription for the form. Breast forms and mastectomy bras may also be tax-deductible when medically prescribed. In most cases, only the first prosthesis is covered. A replacement form is not covered. Be sure to read your insurance policy, because some say you must buy the form within a specific period of time and buy a certain type. Keep all your receipts. Most prostheses are covered by warranty.

During the summertime, I perspire under the prosthesis. Can I do anything about that?

You can buy a sheepskin pad, which you wear facing the body, behind the form, to absorb perspiration. Some patients sometimes use facial tissue under the form during the summer.

Is anyone making special bathing suits for women with mastectomies?

Many of the major bathing-suit companies make special bathing suits for mastectomy patients. You can usually get them through the same source where you got your prosthesis or in large department stores. Your local unit of the American Cancer Society can usually supply you with a list of available styles. There is also a mail-order house which carries these suits: Cameo Stores, Inc., Rockwell & Hartel Avenues, Philadelphia, PA 19111.

The nurse insisted I look at my mastectomy scar and care for it before leaving the hospital. It's so disfiguring that I don't want to look at it again, and I don't want anyone else to see me, either. Why do the nurses do this?

The nurse was attempting to help you adjust to your loss. By showing you how to care for the incision, she was giving you an opportunity to take a first look at your scar. This is a difficult step for all mastectomy patients, but when the swelling goes down and the scar heals completely, you'll begin to feel better able to cope. Being able to talk about your feelings will help, too. Until you are able to accept yourself and the changes in your body, it may be difficult for you to resume sexual intimacy.

Since my mastectomy operation, I'm afraid to have my partner get near me for fear of pulling the incision. Is this a legitimate fear?

This is a natural fear. However, sexual relations can be resumed as soon as you feel ready. The body's ability to heal is quite rapid. Intimacy can help to make you feel better psychologically. A small, soft pillow to protect the scar may be helpful at first. You may need to experiment to find comfortable positions—such as side by side—that do not put pressure on the area where you had surgery. Be honest with your partner; explain your fears and enlist your partner's help.

Why is it that since my mastectomy I seem to be having difficulties with my partner—having sex less often and not enjoying it as much?

Several studies have shown that some, but certainly not all, women who have had a mastectomy may be faced with a problem involving their sexuality. There seem to be several parts to it:

- You may be afraid of showing your scars to your partner.
- You may be afraid of having your partner see you with only one breast.
- You may feel you will never be the same person sexually as you were before.
- Your partner may be afraid of causing you pain.
- Your partner may be upset with the change in your body.
- The emotional problems may be more involved than having the breast removed.

For some women, the loss is so great they cannot overcome it alone. If you are having problems of this kind, it is important for you to get some professional help.

I keep feeling as though my breast is still there even though it was removed. Is this a normal sensation?

The so-called phantom breast sensation is experienced by many women who have undergone mastectomy. It can also include the feeling of pain in the missing breast, numbness, or a pins-and-needles feeling and may last a few weeks to many years.

My whole perception of my body has changed since I had a mastectomy—and I'd like to do something positive to help work through the changes. Any suggestions?

Joining a support group can help you discuss your feelings with others who have shared your experience. A hospital social worker, your local American Cancer Society, or the Cancer Information Service 1-800-4-CANCER can put you in touch with a group in your area.

Physical exercise, such as tennis, swimming, dance classes, or exercise classes, can help to improve your feelings about yourself. Your sense of balance and grace can be enhanced through dance-exercise classes. Yoga has been recommended as a way of achieving a sense of wholeness about the body. Many persons have taken up such challenging new activities as skiing.

Others have returned to college and found a whole new sense of self-worth. Creative activities such as music, painting, sewing, needlepoint, and writing are excellent fields to explore to help to strengthen self-image. In addition, you may want to explore the possibility of breast reconstruction if you have not already done so.

Is there anything that a family member or a friend can do to help a woman who has had a mastectomy adjust to the loss of her breast?

Patients who have gone through the experience tell us that several things have been helpful to them. Of course, different things are beneficial to different people.

- Many women find that talking about the loss of the breast is very helpful.
- A husband who tells his wife that he still loves her and needs her and will help her through these difficult days and makes her feel worthwhile is of great reassurance to the patient. It helps if the husband can also talk about the loss of the breast with his wife.
- Friends and family members who are willing to talk and who are not afraid to bring up the subject make it easier for conversation to begin.
- Nurses who encourage the patient to look at the scar and who listen to what she has to say are helpful.
- People who are willing to go with the patient to buy her prosthesis are helpful.

There is also help from the American Cancer Society—the Reach to Recovery program and the support groups for cancer patients are designed to help. In some towns and cities, the YMCAs run programs of exercise and support for recent breast-cancer patients.

I have had a breast removed. I felt that I had faced this fact very honestly and well and had accepted the mastectomy. Now a few weeks have gone by and I feel very depressed and cheated. Is this a normal reaction?

Patients react to a mastectomy in very different ways. Much of the reaction, it has been found, depends upon the expectations you have and how you approached the operation.

It is not unusual for women to have emotional distress. It may be a feeling of panic. Some women cry. Others say they don't feel like eating. Some can't sleep or concentrate. Still others can't talk about the operation to others. Many women have a "why did this have to happen to me" feeling. These are normal kinds of feelings for mastectomy patients.

It is not abnormal to be afraid of what the disease will mean to the rest of your life. If you are married, you may be worried about your husband's attitude and what he will think about your scar. If you are not married, you might worry about what you might face with a mate in the future. You may be concerned about how you can face people when you return home or to work. Discuss these concerns if you can.

Don't be concerned about *when* you have these feelings; some people have them directly after the operation, others not until a month or several months have gone by. Just understand that they are normal reactions to losing an important part of your body and to the feeling of helplessness about it.

Most important, don't feel that you are strange because you have these feelings. It is normal to have them. Get some help. Sometimes you can talk with a member of your family or a good friend. Other people turn to the American Cancer Society or the Cancer Information Service to have someone to talk with. The American Cancer Society in some areas runs sessions where cancer patients can talk with each other. You may want to go back to the hospital and talk with the social worker or a nurse who was helpful to you during your admission. Or maybe your physician or your clergyman can help you.

Who will be responsible for my follow-up care?

You will want to discuss this with your surgeon. Some surgeons monitor patients themselves. Others, if there has been chemotherapy or radiation therapy used as a follow-up, may decide those physicians or a family doctor will be responsible for following your progress. During the first 3 years, you will be asked to see the doctor about every 3 to 6 months, then every 6 months to a year. Regular visits to a doctor following a mastectomy are important.

What will the doctor do during these follow-up visits?

The doctor will probably check your scar, the other breast, and the lymph nodes. He will tell you to make sure you are practicing breast self-examination on your other breast each month and make sure you know what you are looking for. He will answer any questions you might have about how you are feeling. At the annual visit, he will give you a physical examination, including a Pap smear. He will probably order blood tests, x-rays, a mammogram, and bone scans.

Should I be examining the side where my mastectomy was done?

Yes, you should be doing it each month as part of breast self-examination. Examine the scar from beginning to end, raising your arms as necessary to expose the scars in the underarm area. With your fingers together, place the tip of the middle finger directly over the beginning of the scar line. Press gently in small circular motions. Lift up and move on to the next section of the scar. Repeat until you have checked the entire length of the scar, feeling for any lumps, hard knots, or thickenings. Feel gently, carefully, and thoroughly. If you find something that is different for you, contact the doctor.

In front of a well-lighted mirror, check for swelling, lumps, redness, and/or color change. Redness may be caused by irritation from your prosthesis or bra, but if it persists, let your doctor check it. Make sure your doctor has taught you how to do breast self-examination in the other breast. If you have had both breasts removed, don't neglect the sides of the chest, the armpits, and particularly the scar examination. Be aware of any pain in your shoulder, hip, lower back or pelvis. Also note any unusual breast ache or pain that does not come and go with your menstrual cycle. Report any new pain to your doctor.

Is radiation used in treating breast cancer?

Yes. Radiation is often advised for lumpectomy or segmental mastectomy as well as when the lymph nodes under the armpit are involved or when the tumor is located in the center of the breast. In some cases of Stage III breast cancer, radiation is used before surgery. There are various sequences of radiation, surgery, and chemotherapy used in breast cancer treatment.

What additional treatment is given if there is cancer in the lymph nodes—that is, if the lymph nodes are positive?

If cancer is detected in the lymph nodes under the arm, there is a strong possibility that other microscopic cancer cells may be circulating somewhere else in the body. For this reason, chemotherapy may be used in addition to the surgery and radiation treatment. This is known as adjuvant chemotherapy.

How and when will the chemotherapy be given?

You may receive drugs by mouth or by injection on a daily, weekly, or monthly schedule. It may last from 6 months to more than a year. If you are getting radiation treatment, chemotherapy may be delayed until the radiation treatment is complete. Or, you may receive one course of chemotherapy first, followed by radiation therapy. Some current studies are experimenting with giving adjuvant chemotherapy before surgery is performed.

What drugs are used in adjuvant chemotherapy?

The drugs most commonly used to treat breast cancer include melphalan, cyclophosphamide, methotrexate, 5-fluorouracil, Adriamycin, vincristine, tomaxifen, and prednisone. You may receive two of these drugs or as many as five in combination.

Why is this adjuvant treatment given?

In several research studies, patients who had one or more positive lymph nodes and received chemotherapy after breast cancer surgery, lived longer and had a longer time without disease than those patients with positive nodes who were treated with surgery alone. These studies are continuing, researching many different combinations of drugs. The selection of a specific drug or a combination of drugs is something that will be discussed by your doctor.

When is the drug tamoxifen used?

Tamoxifen (Nolvadex) is a drug that changes a woman's estrogen level. It may be used, alone or in combination with other drugs, for post-menopausal women, if estrogen receptor tests show that the breast cancer relies on estrogen for growth.

How is the estrogen receptor test done?

Preparations for the test must be done before the tumor is removed, because it must be tested immediately after its removal from the breast. The doctor sends a sample of about 1 gram of the tumor to the laboratory to be measured for chemical marking called an estrogen receptor. It is best done before chemotherapy treatments are started, since chemotherapy may alter the test's accuracy.

What is a progesterone receptor test?

It is a similar test, measuring the progesterone receptors.

Why are these tests important?

They are a means of predicting which women will respond to hormone treatment. Hormone treatment, the use of hormone drugs, or removal of one of the hormone-secreting organs (such as the ovaries, adrenal glands, or pituitary gland) are among the treatments available to the doctor. Scientists believe that changing the normal hormonal environment may affect cancers, such as those in the breast, which may depend on the presence of hormones for their growth. Women who are estrogen receptor positive have a 50 to 60 percent chance of responding to hormonal therapy, and a patient who is both estrogen and progesterone receptor positive has nearly an 80 percent chance of responding.

Are there guidelines for follow-up treatment for breast cancer?

In September 1985, a panel of the National Institutes of Health, after three days of reviewing scientific evidence on drug treatment for breast cancer, issued a set of recommendations. The panel concluded that adjuvant chemotherapy and hormonal therapy are effective treatments for breast cancer patients, but that the *best* treatment for *all* stages for *all* patients cannot yet be defined. The following recommendations were issued by the consensus conference:

- For premenopausal women whose nearby lymph nodes are involved, regardless of hormone receptor status, treatment with established combination chemotherapy should become standard care.
- For premenopausal women whose lymph nodes are not involved, follow-up treatment is generally not recommended. For certain high-risk patients in this group, follow-up chemotherapy should be considered.
- For postmenopausal women whose lymph nodes are involved and whose tumors test positively for hormone receptors, tamoxifen is the treatment of choice.
- For postmenopausal women whose lymph nodes are involved and whose tumors test negative for hormone receptors, chemotherapy may be considered but cannot be recommended as standard practice.
- For postmenopausal women whose lymph nodes are not involved, there is no indication for routine follow-up treatment, regardless of the status of their hormone receptors. For certain high-risk patients in this group, follow-up treatment may be considered.

The panel urged that all patients and their physicians participate in controlled clinical trials.

Is the use of immunotherapy new in the treatment of breast cancer?

There are several experimental trials being done using chemotherapy and immunotherapy in combination.

Can a woman who has had breast cancer safely have a baby?

Most doctors discourage women from becoming pregnant for from 3 to 5 years following treatment for breast cancer, since recurrences most often happen during this period of time. Recent research has shown that pregnancy after breast cancer has no effect on survival rates. Statistics for women who have had breast cancer and become pregnant are at least as good as those of similar women who do not become pregnant.

What is the outlook for women who discover breast cancer during pregnancy?

About 7 percent of women who develop breast cancer happen to be pregnant at the time of diagnosis. The outlook for a pregnant woman is just as favorable as that for a nonpregnant woman of the same age with a similar stage of disease—provided that the cancer is diagnosed and treated promptly. When a suspicious lump is found, prompt biopsy is just as appropriate for a pregnant woman as for a nonpregnant woman. Biopsy can usually be performed on an outpatient basis, with little risk to the fetus. The types of biologic changes that occur during pregnancy—high output of hormones like estrogen and prolactin—are known to favor breast tumor growth. Nevertheless, termination of the pregnancy does not improve a woman's prognosis. Breast cancer has never been known to spread across the placenta to the fetus. Chemotherapy is hazardous to the development of the baby during the first 3 months. During the second and third trimesters, the drugs may not interfere with the development of the baby, but the long-range effects are uncertain. Radiation also poses hazards to the baby, and its use is discouraged during pregnancy.

I would like to have breast reconstruction after my surgery for breast cancer. Can this be done?

You should ask your surgeon for a consultation with a plastic surgeon before the mastectomy if possible. Depending on the individual, breast reconstruction is available to women who have had either a single or a double mastectomy. The results and the difficulty of the operation will vary with each individual case. Many women having mastectomies may be candidates for breast reconstruction if they and their surgeons know the facts about current techniques. In many cases, if arrangements are made before the operation, the plastic surgeon can be in the operating room at the time of the mastectomy.

Questions to Ask Your Plastic Surgeon Before Breast Reconstruction

- What type of surgery do you recommend for me? Why?
- What are the risks and benefits associated with it?
- What is your experience with this operation?
- Do you have any before-and-after pictures you can show me?
- May I talk with someone who has had the operation?
- What can I expect my new breast to look like? What will it feel like? Will it change in time?

Will the breast look as it did before the mastectomy?

You should not expect that it will. The new breast will probably look more flattened than tapered. It may not droop as much as your natural breast and may not match it. Under clothing, you can probably not notice the difference, and most patients are pleased with the results of the reconstruction. They say it makes them feel more like their old selves. Although the new breast will not be a perfect replica of the old one, most women who have the reconstruction surgery can wear a normal bra or a bikini. The plastic surgeon will talk to you about your expectations. If they are not realistic, he may suggest that you not have the reconstruction.

What is involved in breast reconstruction?

Breast reconstruction means a second operation, and sometimes even two or more additional operations. The plastic surgeon implants a silicone-rubber envelope (usually a half-moon of silicone gel which has been specially molded) under the skin. Unlike silicone injections which have been used to enlarge breasts (and are now banned in many states), the silicone implant appears to be entirely safe. This implant forms a breast mound.

Are there different types of surgery performed for breast reconstruction?

There are three types of surgery:
- Simple breast reconstruction
- Latissimus dorsi reconstruction
- Rectus abdominus reconstruction

What does simple breast reconstruction entail?

The surgeon makes a small incision along the lower part of the breast area, near the mastectomy scar, and puts the implant into a pocket created under the chest muscle. A drain may be put in to take away the fluid that may accumulate during the next few days, and then the incision is closed. The operation takes about 1 to 2 hours and is usually done under general anesthesia. Sometimes this operation is done as outpatient surgery.

What is latissimus dorsi reconstruction?

This operation is used when chest muscles have been removed and where there is too little skin to hold and cover an implant. The surgeon transfers skin, muscle, and other tissue from the back to the mastectomy site. To create a new muscle on the front of the chest, a broad flat muscle on the back below the shoulder blade—called the latissimus dorsi—is used. An implant is then placed under the new chest muscle. Drains may be put in and kept in place for several days after the surgery to remove fluid. This operation takes several hours, and patients stay in the hospital for about a week. You will have a scar on your back as well as on your chest.

What is rectus abdominus reconstruction?

This operation is also used when a lot of skin and muscle have been removed. The surgeon transfers one of the two abdominal muscles—the rectus abdominus—to the breast along with skin and fat from the abdomen. This flap of muscle, skin, and fat is shaped into the contour of a breast. If there is enough abdominal tissue available, no implant is needed. Transferring tissue in this way also results in tightening of the stomach, called a tummy tuck. You will have a horizontal scar across the lower abdomen plus the scar on your chest.

Will I be able to have a nipple as part of breast reconstruction?

If you wish to have one, it is usually possible. However, construction of the nipple and areola (the circle of dark-colored skin surrounding the nipple) may require another operation, usually lasting 1 or 2 hours.

How is the nipple reconstructed?

The nipple is usually reconstructed using tissue from the newly created mound or by grafting a piece from the opposite nipple. The areola is made by using skin from the upper inner thigh or skin from behind the ear. Skin from the vaginal lips can also be used to reconstruct the nipple and areola. If the reconstructed areola is not dark enough, ultraviolet light may be used to improve the color match.

Is it true that reconstruction can hide new cancer?

No. Doctors believe there is little or no difficulty in promptly finding a recurrence of cancer, either beneath or around an implant, using examination by hand or mammography. If cancer were to recur in the reconstructed breast, it would most likely be located just under the skin and easy to find.

When can breast reconstruction surgery be done?

It depends upon the kind of operation you have had, the extent of your cancer and the wishes of your plastic surgeon. If you have had a simple or modified radical mastectomy, you will probably have to wait for 3 to 6 months until the scar has healed, although some doctors say that patients with minimal disease can have reconstruction immediately following cancer surgery. In several major centers, breast reconstruction, including implanting the soft plastic artificial breast and reconstruction of the nipple, is being done at the same time as the mastectomy. If you are having chemotherapy or radiation treatments, most doctors prefer to wait until you have completed them. Most doctors wait another 3 months between the operation which creates the breast mound and the construction of the nipple.

I had my mastectomy more than 10 years ago. Can I still have breast reconstruction?

There are women who have had successful reconstructions with mastectomies over 20 years old. The fact that you had a mastectomy many years ago does not disqualify you as a candidate for the operation. Nor does your age.

I have had radiation treatments. Can I still have a breast reconstruction operation?

Probably. Almost any woman who has had a mastectomy for breast cancer can have her breast reconstructed. Radiation-damaged skin, grafted, thin, or tight skin or the absence of chest muscles are no longer obstacles to breast reconstruction.

My remaining breast is large. Can I have the reconstruction operation?

Yes. However, there is a limit to the size of the reconstructed breast. The limit is based on what the skin can support. Usually the surgeon will reduce the size of the remaining breast so that it will more nearly match the new breast. This operation may be done at the time of reconstruction or as a second operation. The operation to reduce the size of the remaining breast is called reduction mammoplasty.

Are there any complications from the surgery for breast reconstruction?

You must remember that there is always the possibility of complications from any surgery, even with the best surgeon. Sometimes, the body creates a firm, fibrous capsule around the implant to protect itself; this may be improved by the surgeon without an operation or may need to be surgically fixed. If an infection occurs at the breast site, the implant may need to be removed until the infection heals and then replaced. Sometimes the implant is temporarily removed if large areas of skin die. Part or all of a transferred muscle may fail to survive. You should also be aware that mastectomy and reconstruction scars are permanent, although the degree of scarring varies among individuals. You should not expect that reconstruction will restore the sensation lost through mastectomy. Discuss possible complications with your plastic surgeon before the operation, realizing that as with any type of plastic surgery, it is difficult to predict the overall results.

Will I have to do anything to my breast after reconstruction?

If an implant is used, after the operation you will be taught how to massage and exercise the muscles surrounding your implant. It will take a few months for the skin and muscle to stretch and for the reconstructed breast to take on a natural appearance.

How long is the recovery period?

It depends upon what operation you have had. Most women are able to resume normal activities in 2 to 3 weeks, although it is usually several more weeks before you can do strenuous exercises.

Do I need to do breast self-examination after I have had reconstruction?

Yes. Breast reconstruction does not cause cancer to come back, nor does it prevent recurrence. After reconstruction you will continue to have periodic examinations. In addition, you should examine both of your breasts monthly, following your doctor's instructions.

What if my doctor does not think I should have breast reconstruction?

This depends upon his reasons. If his decision is based on health reasons, you should probably abide by his judgment. However, you could ask to have his reasoning confirmed by a second opinion. If he simply has given you the feeling that breast reconstruction for cosmetic reasons is frivolous or unnecessary, and you would like to have breast reconstruction, you should arrange to talk with a plastic surgeon about your case.

What kind of doctor should perform the plastic surgery?

A board-certified plastic surgeon should do the breast reconstruction. Be sure that he is experienced with the operation. Ask him how many he does and what his results have been. Most doctors have before-and-after pictures they can show you. Ask your doctor to recommend someone for the consultation or call a teaching hospital in your community. There is also a society of reconstructive surgeons: American Society of Plastic and Reconstructive Surgeons, Suite 1900, 233 N. Michigan Ave. Chicago, IL 60601, or call its 24-hour patient referral service (312-856-1834).

Is it possible for me to talk with someone else who has had the operation?

You should ask your surgeon or plastic surgeon if he will allow you to talk with some of his patients. In addition, local units of the American Cancer Society may help introduce you to women who can describe their personal experiences. The organization RENU (Reconstruction Education for National Understanding) offers up-to-date information and support. There are active RENU programs in Philadelphia, Cleveland, and Washington, D.C.

How much does breast reconstruction cost?

The operations are expensive and depend upon the extent of the surgery as well as other factors. The surgeon's fee can run from $1,500 to over $4,000, with hospital costs ranging from $2,000 to $4,000. Almost all of the Blue Cross/Blue Shield plans and many of the private insurance plans now cover postmastectomy surgery. Some only cover the hospital costs, while others will also pay part or all of the plastic surgeon's cost. Be sure to know the cost and what your policy will cover before deciding on the operation.

chapter 12

Lung Cancer

Lung cancer develops slowly; it can be present for 10 to 20 years without causing noticeable symptoms. The most common symptoms—a cough, a wheeze, or an ache—are easy to ignore. It is especially easy for a heavy smoker to ignore them, since smoker's cough and shortness of breath are often a way of life for a long-time smoker. The cough is usually the result of a growing cancer blocking an airway and is the attempt of the body to get rid of a foreign object stuck in the lung. In some cases, the sputum coughed up contains streaks of blood. Chest pains, usually resulting in a persistent ache, can be early symptoms, as are recurring attacks of pneumonia or bronchitis. Persistent shoulder and arm pains can also sometimes signal the presence of lung cancer.

Those Most Likely to Get Lung Cancer

- Age 50–64 and live in a city
- Have smoked one or more packs a day for 20 years or longer and/or began to smoke before age 20 and still smoking
- Smoke and work in an industrial plant with high-risk materials (such as asbestos)
- Have a persistent or violent smoker's cough

- Don't smoke but have had a violent cough for more than 2 weeks
- Have a nagging chest pain unrelated to cough
- Breathe with a wheezing sound
- Have noticed blood in sputum—even once
- Have had a change in color or volume of sputum

Symptoms of Lung Cancer

- A smoker's cough which has become persistent or violent
- A nonsmoker whose cough hangs on for more than 2 weeks
- A chest pain that is persistent and unrelated to a cough
- A wheezing sound in your breathing
- Bloodstained sputum
- Change in color or volume of sputum

Questions to Ask Your Doctor

- What are my chances for cure?
- Is the operation worth the pain and discomfort?
- Has the cancer spread outside the lungs?
- If I am not operated on, what other treatment do you suggest?
- Is my other lung in good enough condition so that I can still function fairly normally after the diseased lung is removed?
- How limited will I be in my activity?
- Will I need radiation therapy?
- Will you prescribe chemotherapy?
- How long will it be before I regain my strength?
- Do I have small-cell (or oat-cell) carcinoma?

What kind of doctor should I see if I have symptoms of lung cancer?

Usually the internist or general physician will refer you to a surgeon. It is important that he be a thoracic surgeon and one who specializes in lung diseases.

Is the National Cancer Institute supporting any studies on lung cancer?

The National Cancer Institute's clinical cooperative groups are presently studying new treatment methods. (See Chapter 23.)

What are the lungs?

The lungs are two spongy, pinkish-gray organs that take up much of the room inside the chest. They enfold the other organs of the chest such as the heart, the large blood vessels entering and leaving the heart, and the esophagus (tube carrying food from mouth to stomach). The left lung has two lobes or sections. It is smaller than the right lung because the heart takes up some of the space on the left side of the chest. The right lung has three lobes and is a little bigger than the left one.

How does the air get into the lungs?

Air passes through the mouth or nose into the windpipe (trachea). The windpipe divides into two tubes called the left bronchus and the right bronchus. These large bronchi are about the size of a man's little finger. They divide into ever-smaller branched tubes like the branches of a tree and lead to the several lobes of the lungs. These air passages get smaller and smaller until they are only 1/100 inch across.

How do the lungs work?

The lungs bring needed oxygen into the body and expel carbon dioxide. The bloodstream brings the oxygen to the cells, which need it to carry out their work and stay alive. When we inhale, air enters the lungs through the bronchi. Cells of the lung are self-cleaning. Certain cells that line the bronchi produce mucus to wash out foreign materials. Other cells, which are equipped with tiny hairs, called cilia, sweep the mucus toward the throat. Impurities are carried away into the bloodstream or lymph system by other cells.

Where does lung cancer start?

Most lung cancers begin in the bronchi (the larger air tubes) or the bronchioles (the smaller tubes branching off the bron-

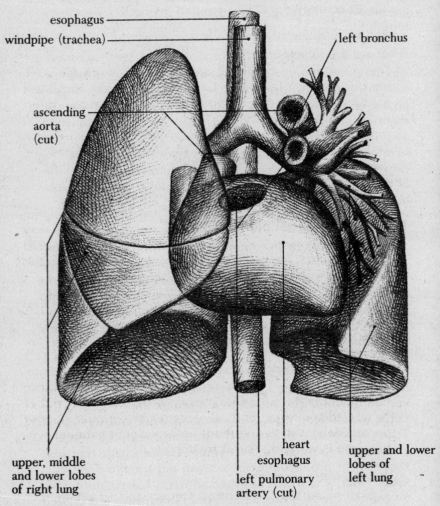

esophagus

windpipe (trachea)

left bronchus

ascending
aorta
(cut)

upper, middle
and lower lobes
of right lung

left pulmonary
artery (cut)

heart
esophagus

upper and lower
lobes of
left lung

Lungs

chi) in the moist mucous layer of the breathing tubes. Some cancer researchers think that 20 or more years may pass between the time someone is first exposed to a cancer-producing substance such as tobacco smoke and the time cancer actually develops.

Are there different kinds of lung cancer?

There are thirteen different kinds. The most common are squamous-cell (also known as epidermoid or spindle-cell), adenocarcinoma, large-cell, and adenosquamous. Small-cell carcinoma (also known as oat-cell) is usually treated differently from the other types. These types make up over 90 percent of all lung cancer. They are named for the different cell types found in the tumors when looked at under the microscope.

Are all kinds of lung cancer treated the same way?

No. There are different forms of treatment, depending on the cell type, on the extent of the disease, and on the way the disease responds to the treatment. Small-cell (oat-cell) carcinoma calls for a different form of treatment than do the other cell types.

What is small-cell or oat-cell cancer, and why is it treated differently?

Small-cell or oat-cell carcinoma is a very fast-growing variety of lung cancer. Major advances in treatment of this type of lung cancer have been made, using chemotherapy and radiotherapy. The tumor is highly sensitive to these treatments. If you have this type of cancer, you should either be treated at a major medical center or be certain that your doctor contacts someone at one of the cancer treatment centers who is using the latest treatments.

Is lung cancer common?

Cancer of the lung is the most common cancer among men in the United States and is on the increase among women. All cancers of the lung have a high degree of malignancy. When lung cancer is diagnosed in its earlier stages, of course, the chances of cure are much greater. Small epidermoid carcinomas, for example, can be cured in a large percentage

Tests for Lung Cancer

TEST	EXPLANATION
Physical exam and full health history	Important for doctor to know your health habits. Will listen to lungs to see if fluid has collected. Will check lymph nodes on neck to see if normal. Includes complete blood and liver-function tests.
Chest x-ray	A basic test. Detects tumors already about ½ inch in diameter. Can also show fluid or enlarged lymph nodes. X-ray useful in detecting changes in lung tissue. Should be part of regular checkup. Heavy smokers should have one every 6 months or on doctor's recommendation.
Sputum examination	Can detect abnormal cells in sputum. Sometimes used to tell what kind of cancer is present. Can sometimes detect cancer before large enough to appear on x-ray.
Bronchoscopy	Doctor looks into bronchial passages in search of tumor. Allows doctor to take cell samples. Performed under local anesthesia. Helps locate source of cancer cells found in sputum. Can use rigid or fiberoptic bronchoscope, depending on location.
Tomogram	Three-dimensional x-ray used to detect location and size of lump. Shows one thin layer of lung at a time. May show cancer not seen in regular x-ray. Also called laminagram. CT scan is a type of tomogram. CT scan also used to determine if cancer has spread to other sites such as brain or abdomen.
Bronchogram	Specialized x-ray exam using radio-opaque dye to better define area.
Pulmonary-function test	Uses radioactive materials plus camera or computer to measure breathing and evaluate patient's ability to get oxyen into blood.
Biopsy	All-inclusive term. There are different methods of obtaining tissue, but tissue examination is essential part of determining presence of cancer, cell type, and degree of malignancy.
Mediastinoscopy	Method of getting diagnosis. Also necessary to tell whether lung cancer has spread to lymph nodes behind breastbone (mediastinum). Doctor passes instrument through small incision in neck, taking lymph nodes for biopsy.

Tests for Lung Cancer

TEST	EXPLANATION
Bone scan, liver scan, brain scan, bone marrow biopsy	Also known as metastatic workup. Depending on results of other tests, one or more of these tests may be done. Scans are relatively painless, routine outpatient diagnostic procedures, similar to x-rays. Tests help determine whether cancer has spread to bones, liver, and brain. Bone marrow biopsy is done with needle on breastbone or hipbone.
Thoracentesis	Fluid examination used when there is fluid and other attempts to find cancer have failed. May be used to relieve pain or shortness of breath caused by fluid collection. Fluid is drawn by needle from space between lungs and chest wall and checked for cancer cells. Can be done in examining room or hospital.
Thoracoscopy	Helps pinpoint location of cancer. Done in operating room. Incision is made between two ribs, slender tubular instrument is inserted into lung cavity, lung is deflated, and instrument is used to examine entire surface of lung and chest wall for tumor. Tissue taken for examination. Lung reinflated.
Thoracotomy	Exploratory chest operation. Used as a diagnostic tool when other tests have failed to locate tumor. Question doctor carefully before submitting to this test to be certain that all other diagnostic tests available have been made. This is major surgery used to examine lung. If tumor is found, immediate testing is done and if cell type is favorable and there is no evidence of metastases outside lung (which normally should have been determined before this procedure was done), surgical removal of lung is usually performed at this time.

of patients. The other carcinomas are more difficult to cure. The survival rate is better for those persons whose lung cancer is found before it spreads outside the lung. Each year approximately 100,000 new cases of lung cancer are diagnosed in the United States.

What is the major cause of lung cancer?

The major cause of lung cancer is smoking. It is estimated that smoking causes 85 percent of all lung cancers.

Does nicotine chewing gum work in helping to stop smoking?

This chewing gum, which must be prescribed by a doctor, is designed for use by smokers who wish to stop smoking cigarettes. Smokers who have a high degree of nicotine dependence are most likely to benefit from its use, since it provides nicotine blood levels sufficient to alleviate withdrawal symptoms in smokers who want to stop smoking.

Can cigarette or cigar smoke harm the lungs of a non-smoker?

People who do not smoke, when they are in a smoke-filled atmosphere, inhale a good deal of smoke that is not drawn through the cigarette. Smoke exhaled by smokers is filtered by the lungs of the smoker. Undiluted smoke, on the other hand, contains much higher percentages of tar, nicotine and noxious gases than exhaled smoke.

The Environmental Protection Agency estimates that between 500 and 5,000 cases of lung cancer appear each year in non-smokers as a result of inhaling someone else's smoke. Some scientists question that statistic. Even though this issue has not yet been resolved, it is cause for concern.

Studies show that children in households where one or both parents smoke have double the amount of bronchitis or pneumonia during the first year of life as do children in non-smoking households. They also have more adenoid and tonsil operations than do children of parents who do not smoke.

Tobacco smoke is also dangerous to people with certain kinds of heart disease. It can cause breathing problems in some persons and can set off strong allergic reactions in others.

Once a person has smoked, can the damage be undone?

Once a person stops smoking, the body can clear the lungs and protect them from further damage as well as decrease the risk for lung cancer.

Is marijuana smoking harmful to the lungs?

There is some evidence that marijuana may have the same harmful, paralyzing effects on the cilia and on the mucus

production as cigarette smoke. Also, since marijuana cigarettes contain much more tar than do tobacco cigarettes,
they may be more harmful. Marijuana smokers inhale very
deeply and hold the smoke for a long time in their lungs.
They also smoke the cigarette down to the very end where
tar concentrations are the highest. The scientific evidence
is just beginning to be gathered but researchers are beginning to conclude that marijuana smoking may be a more
serious problem than was originally anticipated.

Is there any research being done on ways of preventing lung cancer?

There are several studies underway, trying to determine
whether modifying or adding to the diet can have an effect
on the risk of lung cancer. One study involves people who
are at high risk for lung cancer because they have been
exposed to asbestos at work. These people are taking beta-
carotene and retinol (substances from which vitamin A is
formed) daily. Another study involves cigarette smokers and
ex-smokers and is designed to determine the value of daily
oral vitamin A in preventing cancer.

Is the use of smokeless tobacco becoming more prevalent in the United States?

Yes. Smokeless tobacco—which includes snuff and chewing tobacco as well as the newer cloth pouches filled with
tobacco—is being advertised as a replacement for cigarettes. Users either put a pouch or a wad in the cheek and
suck, or place a pinch of snuff (finely cut tobacco) between
the lower lip and teeth, where it stimulates the flow of saliva
and mixes with it (called dipping). In both instances the
increased saliva must either be spit out or swallowed.

Is smokeless tobacco harmful?

Yes. It's tobacco and is habit forming. The nicotine in it lifts
up the person and then lets them down. This high-low effect
on the nervous system sets a person up for continued need.
Habitual use of chewing tobacco and snuff can lead to other
health hazards, including the following:
 • Leukoplakia, leathery white patches inside the mouth,
   are the result of direct contact with, and continued ir-

ritation by, tobacco juice. About 5 percent of cases of leukoplakia develop into oral cancer.

- The sense of taste and the ability to smell are lessened, which results in the need to add more salt and sugar to food.
- In addition to the bad breath and discolored teeth common to most tobacco users, dental problems can include receding gums, greater wear and tear on tooth enamel, and more tooth decay.
- Tobacco juices contain hundreds of chemicals which may delay wound healing.
- Nicotine also affects the heart and the rest of the circulatory system. As nicotine enters the bloodstream, the arteries tighten and become smaller, blood platelets clot, and the heartbeat increases, which may cause an increase in blood pressure.

What is sarcoidosis?

Sarcoidosis, a disease characterized by noncancerous growths called granulomas, can be very difficult to diagnose, since it closely resembles some cancers or tuberculosis. It is not cancer. It most often affects the lungs but can also be found in the skin, liver, spleen, eyes, and bones. The course of the disease varies with the patient and the form of sarcoidosis. There are two forms of this disease. The acute type is characterized by an abrupt onset and sometimes sudden disappearance of symptoms. The chronic form has a slow, poorly defined beginning. Persons with relatively mild symptoms often do not need treatment. Drug treatment can relieve symptoms but will not prevent the granulomas from forming and appearing in other locations. Symptoms may include enlarged lymph nodes in the neck plus lung problems. Fever (especially a fever up to 101° daily), weight loss, and tiredness are also symptoms of sarcoidosis.

What is histoplasmosis?

Histoplasmosis is a fungus infection most commonly found around the Ohio, Mississippi, and Missouri Valley areas. It is also found in the southeastern parts of the United States.

Farmers and cave explorers are the most usual victims. Often, exposed persons will develop a lung spot with calcium which can be seen on the x-ray. If the disease spreads throughout the lung, hospitalization may be necessary and antibiotics are administered. Histoplasmosis is not a form of cancer.

How does lung cancer spread?

Lung cancer usually begins as a tiny spot, most often on the inner lining of a bronchial tube. Lungs have a rich supply of blood and lymph vessels close to the cancer cells. If these cells get into the bloodstream or the lymph system, they can act as seeds and spread to other parts of the body. When this happens, it is called a metastasis. A metastasis (or "met," as it is sometimes called) is not a new kind of cancer, but is the lung cancer which has moved to another part of the body and begun to grow there. Therefore, even if it has spread to the bone, for example, it is not bone cancer but simply an extension or metastasis of the lung cancer. The metastasis looks and behaves in the same way as the original lung cancer, and therefore the same treatment which has been used to contain the lung tumor is likely to be used in treating the metastasis.

How does the original lung tumor affect the lung?

There can be several effects on the process of breathing. As the tumor on the lining of a bronchus or bronchiole grows, it may interfere with the flow of air through the breathing tube and cause a wheeze or whistling noise as the air passes through the narrowed part of the bronchus. Or the tumor may cause a cough as it obstructs the upward movement of mucus. Sometimes it makes an already existing cough worse or, because it is bleeding, produces blood-streaked sputum (mucus and/or pus coughed up from the bronchial tube).

Are tumors of the lung ever found to be benign?

Benign tumors (adenomas) do occur—but they are rare. Prior to surgery they are difficult to distinguish from cancerous tumors and are therefore treated in the same manner.

Are most cases of lung cancer operable?

No. About 50 percent of all cases of lung cancer are inoperable.

What if the tumor has spread outside the lung? How does it affect other parts of the body?

Sometimes fluid accumulates in the space between the lungs and the ribs. This can cause chest pain and make it hard to breathe. A tumor growing between the two lungs may press on the esophagus and make it hard to swallow. It may affect the nerves that go to the voice box and make you hoarse. When it grows in one of the smallest bronchial tubes, it may not have any effects that you notice.

When should I have a cough investigated to make certain it isn't something more serious?

It is wise to investigate the source of any cough that lasts for more than 2 or 3 weeks. This rule goes for the cough that hangs on after a chest cold or for the cough of chronic bronchitis—even though you have had it checked before. A cough, or a change in cough habit, is found in most lung cancer patients at some time during the course of the disease. The tumor seems to act like a foreign body or obstruction within the lung, and the cough represents the effort to expel it.

Are there any other symptoms I should be looking for?

Other signs which are fairly common in lung cancer are vague chest pains, a faint wheezing sound in breathing, or blood-streaked sputum. Chest pain is the second most common symptom. It is usually felt as a persistent ache unrelated to a cough and is commonly experienced on the side on which the tumor is located. Faint wheezing is fairly common at a relatively early stage. It is not necessarily constant. Blood-streaked sputum is a first symptom in a small percentage of cases. However, even small amounts of blood in the sputum—fine streaks, for instance—must be regarded seriously. Its appearance, even once, should always be reported to the doctor. Coughing up blood, either in flecks or streaks, occurs in over half the patients with lung cancer.

Can arm and shoulder pain be a symptom of lung cancer?

Yes. One type of lung cancer, known as a superior sulcus tumor, is sometimes incorrectly diagnosed as cervical arthritis or bursitis because of arm and shoulder pain symptoms. The tumor is located in the upper part of the chest and usually extends into the adjoining ribs and spine, producing shoulder and arm pain, sometimes extending to the forearm and the fourth and fifth fingers. An x-ray of the chest, with special attention to the superior sulcus area, helps to determine whether this tumor is the cause of shoulder and arm pain.

How much time does it take for symptoms of lung cancer to show up?

Lung cancer is fairly slow-growing and it ordinarily takes about 20 months from the time the tumor becomes visible on an x-ray to the appearance of the first symptom. And that symptom is usually a change in the character or severity of a chronic cough. Unfortunately, what happens all too often is that the patient usually waits 2 or 3 months before seeing a doctor—and then another 3 or 4 months go by before treatment is started, thus compounding the problem.

Who are the people most likely to get lung cancer?

People most likely to develop lung cancer are between 50 and 70 years old and have smoked almost all of their adult lives.

Is it true that lung cancer in women is on the increase?

Yes. With many more women smoking than ever before, the number of women with lung cancer has increased at an alarming rate, so that smoking is now responsible for 75 percent of all lung cancers in women. The cancer rate for female smokers is 67 percent higher than for nonsmokers.

Do industrial pollutants cause lung cancer?

Studies being supported by the National Cancer Institute show that occupations and environmental factors may play a role in the development of lung cancer. Persons who have been exposed frequently and for many years to irritating substances (such as asbestos, chromium compounds, radio-active ores, nickel, arsenic, and uranium) in the air they breathe in an industrial plant are thought to have a some-what greater chance of developing lung cancer. A worker in these kinds of industries who smokes faces an even greater risk. If you are over 40, smoke two packs a day, and/or are in an occupation that is thought to be cancer-producing, you should have frequent medical checkups.

How do I know if I have been exposed to asbestos?

If you have worked for any length of time in a shipyard building or repairing ships, in a factory manufacturing as-bestos materials, or as an insulation installer, a construction worker, or in automotive brake-lining repair, you may have been exposed to asbestos on the job. The National Cancer Institute and other governmental agencies are informing workers and their families that job-related exposures to as-bestos can result in certain diseases, particularly asbestosis and lung cancer.

What are the symptoms of the various asbestos-caused diseases?

Asbestosis is a chronic lung disease whose signs and symp-toms result from permanent changes in lung tissue. The earliest and most prominent sign is shortness of breath after exertion.

Lung cancer has a cough or change in cough habit as its most common symptom. Chest pain is the second most com-mon. Blood-streaked sputum, coughed up from the lungs, is the first symptom in a small number of cases.

What is mesothelioma?

Mesothelioma is a relatively rare cancer that affects the membrane lining the chest cavity (the pleura) or the mem-brane lining the abdominal cavity (the peritoneum). The most common first symptoms are shortness of breath, pain in the wall of the chest which is aggravated by deep breath-ing, or abdominal pain which may vary from vague discom-fort to severe spasms. Asbestos exposure is a risk factor— and workers in asbestos mines, asbestos mills, and factories, as well as installers of asbestos insulation, should be aware of the connection between mesothelioma and asbestos. Cigarette smoking increases the risk of lung cancer. Asbestos and cigarette smoking together increase lung cancer risk five-fold over the already high risk due to smoking alone.

How can I find out if I have medical problems resulting from asbestos exposure?

If you have been exposed to asbestos on the job you should tell your doctor so he can watch for signs or symptoms of asbestos-related diseases. Tests for asbestosis include a physical exam with x-rays and lung-function tests. Tests for cancer, if it is suspected by your doctor, are more extensive and depend on your specific symptoms.

How does smoking affect the lungs?

Constant irritation of the bronchial lining by cigarette smoke causes the tiny hairs (cilia) that line the bronchial lining to disappear. Without these tiny hairs to sweep it into the throat in the cleansing action, the mucus remains trapped and "smoker's cough" often results. Continued smoking can cause the cells to form abnormal growth patterns and eventually to turn into cancer. Some recent studies indicate that lung cancer could be cut by as much as 80 percent if all smoking ceased. When a person stops smoking, the lungs begin to cleanse and repair themselves.

What kinds of tests does the doctor do when he is looking for lung cancer?

Usually the doctor starts by getting a health history, which gives him important clues to the most likely diagnosis. Then he will do a physical exam, looking, for example, for a hard lump in the neck which would suggest that cancer may have spread from some nearby part of the body to the lymph nodes of the neck. He will order complete blood counts and tests to check the functioning of your liver. A chest x-ray is a very basic test for lung cancer. If it is present, it usually shows up as a shadow on the x-ray. However, the smallest tumor which can be seen on an x-ray of the chest is about ½ inch in diameter. At this time metastasis may already have occurred. The doctor may see fluid that is collected in the space between the lung and the chest wall. This fluid, called pleural effusion, can be seen on the x-ray film. Pleural effusion is not always a sign of lung cancer. Usually when the cancer is in the very small bronchial tubes or in the air sacs in the outer portions of the lung, it is easy to see on the x-ray. Cancers in the larger bronchi are less easy to see, but they frequently cause a change in the adjacent lung tissue, and that can be located through the x-ray. The chest x-ray might also show enlarged lymph nodes that have filled with cancer cells even when the original tumor cannot be seen in the lung. When this happens, the doctor must continue to look for the original site of the cancer, using other diagnostic tools.

Is the chest x-ray ever used when the doctor has already made the diagnosis of cancer with other tools?

The initial x-ray will give the doctor a basis with which he can compare later x-rays, following the patient's progress and watching for changes in the lung tissue by comparing the early chest x-rays with later ones.

What other diagnostic tools does the doctor use to detect lung cancer?

There are several other diagnostic tools which can be used. They include sputum examination, bronchoscopy, tomogram, bronchogram, pulmonary-function test, biopsy, mediastinoscopy, bone scan, liver scan, brain scan, bone-marrow biopsy, thoracentesis, thoracoscopy and thoractomy.

What is the sputum cytology test, and how is the sputum examination done?

There are several studies under way using sensitive diagnostic tests which can be done easily, accurately, and inexpensively on a large number of people, since if lung cancer is found in its earliest stages, cure is possible in many cases. One such test that has already shown some success is sputum examination. The patient is asked to cough up some sputum (material coughed up from the lungs). The sputum is examined under a microscope to see if there are cancer cells present which have been shed from the inner lining of the breathing passages. Abnormal cells in the sputum can indicate a hidden cancer too small to be seen in x-ray photographs. The tumor is then located by such techniques as flexible fiberoptic bronchoscopy—this is an important part of the test because the sputum examination by itself does not tell the doctor where the tumor is located in the bronchial tree.

How is the sputum cytology test done?

You will be asked not to have anything to eat or drink except water or tea without milk. The nurse will give you a specimen jar which contains 50 percent alcohol to act as a fixative. You must cough very deeply and spit into the specimen jar. If you are unable to cough deeply enough, the doctor will order a machine to assist in getting a good specimen.

What is a bronchoscopy?

A bronchoscopy is performed with the use of a rigid bronchoscope or a fiberoptic bronchoscope, depending on the location. The doctor using this instrument can look into the bronchial passages. The bronchoscope is a slender tube with a light at the far end which slides down the throat and into the bronchi.

Bronchoscopy sounds like a very uncomfortable procedure. Is it?

It doesn't need to be if you cooperate with your physician and the anesthesiologist. Local anesthesia is sprayed into the throat and bronchial tubes, making them feel numb. The bronchoscope is put into only one bronchus at a time, so you have no trouble breathing normally during the examination. You are relaxed and responsive to instructions and remain awake, although you will not remember much of the procedure afterward. Your head will be draped and your eyes covered. You will be asked to cough so that the doctor can obtain a good sample.

What does the doctor see during the bronchoscopy?

Looking through the bronchoscope, the doctor can illuminate the walls of the bronchi and examine the area. The development of new, flexible fiberoptic bronchoscopes means that the doctor can see around corners and into the inside of much smaller bronchial tubes. The flexibility of the instrument makes it possible for the doctor to take cell samples, using special attachments for biopsy, brushing, scraping, or washing.

How is that done?

Once the tumor is found, a small bit of liquid can be squirted through the bronchoscope onto the tumor and then withdrawn by suction. This liquid is then examined under the microscope for the presence of tumor cells, just as a sputum specimen might be. A slender cutting tool can be put through the bronchoscope. The doctor uses it to snip a small sample of tissue, which can then be examined under the microscope.

Are there any aftereffects of a bronchoscopy?

It is common for patients to cough up a small amount of blood after a specimen has been taken. This should be no cause for alarm. Some patients have a sore throat or hoarseness. Many people report no discomfort.

What is a tomogram? Is it related to a CT scan?

A tomogram or laminagram is a special chest x-ray. If the regular chest x-ray shows a shadow in the lungs, tomograms can tell the physician more about the size, shape, or other characteristics of the lump. It is a series of pictures of various sections of lung tissue which when put together give a three-dimensional picture of abnormal lung growth. In cases of benign lumps, the tomogram tells the doctor enough about the tumor so he can make the diagnosis based on the tomogram pictures alone. If the tomogram suggests that the lump is cancerous, more tests will be needed to narrow down the diagnosis. A CT scan—computerized tomography—is often taken.

What is a bronchogram?

A bronchogram is another specialized x-ray examination which is sometimes used. A small amount of radio-opaque dye is put into the bronchial tubes, and usually into the trachea after the area has been numbed. The patient is tilted into various positions to distribute the dye into the lungs and throughout the bronchi. X-rays are then taken.

What are pulmonary-function tests?

Pulmonary-function tests (also called lung-function tests) are given to measure your breathing and evaluate your ability to get oxygen into your blood. The tests measure the amount of air moving in and out of the lungs and indicate if there is an obstruction in the air passages. The tests give a baseline value of how well your lungs are presently functioning. The doctor will do these before the operation to be sure that your lungs are in good enough condition to keep you functioning even if a part of them is removed.

How are pulmonary-function tests done?

The test consists of various breathing exercises. It takes about 1 or 2 hours and will probably make you tired. You breathe pure oxygen. Then you have blood samples drawn. Cooperation is very important in this test, and you must follow the instructions closely. The tests themselves are painless but time-consuming. In some places, radioactive materials and a camera or a computer are used in performing these tests.

Is a biopsy a necessary test?

A biopsy is an *essential* test. It means obtaining and examining a piece of tissue under the microscope. The tissue can be obtained in many different ways, as discussed above. You should remember that not all spots on the lungs are cancerous. As a matter of fact, according to the Mayo Clinic, an estimated 50 to 60 percent of lung biopsies are benign or noncancerous, depending on age. If lung cancer has spread to the lymph nodes in the neck or to other body tissues, a specimen of these might be taken for biopsy. When the pathologist studies a biopsy specimen under the microscope, he can identify the cell type of lung cancer along with its degree of malignancy.

What is a mediastinoscopy?

This is a minor surgical procedure that tells whether lung cancer has spread to the lymph nodes behind the breastbone in the area called the mediastinum. It is common for lung cancer to spread here first. The doctor passes an instrument through a small incision in the neck. You are anesthetized and asleep at the time. The nodes that are taken out are looked at by the pathologist. If they contain cancer, surgery may not be done. Radiation may be given instead to try to diminish or shrink the tumor tissue in the chest.

What is mediastinotomy?

This procedure is similar to mediastinoscopy, except the incision is made either to the right or left side of the breastbone.

What is a sternotomy?

This operation requires the midline splitting of the sternum and is sometimes used for patients who have lung disease which has spread. Some doctors feel that this surgical approach allows them to see both sides of the chest during the operation so that any undetected cancer can be found. Doctors who use this procedure report that recovery is rapid, there may be fewer breathing problems, and there is less postoperative pain.

What is thoracentesis?

Fluid from the space between the lungs and the chest wall is removed by needle. A local anesthetic is applied to the skin where the needle will be inserted to minimize discomfort. Gentle suction draws the fluid through the needle into a syringe or bottle. There is then an examination of the fluid under the microscope to see if there are cancer cells. This test is usually used after other attempts to find cancer have failed. It can also be used to relieve pain or shortness of breath caused by the collection of fluid in the pleural space. This test can be done either in a hospital room or in an examining room.

What is a thorascopy?

This surgical procedure is used for diagnosing cancer in the lung. The patient is anesthetized and asleep in the operating room. A small incision is made between two ribs, and a slender tubular instrument is inserted into the space occupied by the lung. The instrument is much like a fiberoptic bronchoscope. When the instrument slips into the lung cavity, the lung is deflated and the thorascope can be used to examine the entire surface of the lung for tumor growth as well as the lining of the chest wall. Suspicious tissue is snipped, withdrawn through the thorascope, and given microscopic examination. The lung is reinflated at the end of the procedure. The lung not being examined remains expanded and able to function during the entire procedure.

Is magnetic resonance imaging being used to detect lung cancer?

Investigators are conducting studies to evaluate the usefulness of this technique in staging lung cancer.

This seems like a lot of tests. Are they all necessary?

Not all of the tests are done on all patients who are suspected of having lung cancer. However, it is important to have thorough testing and staging in lung cancer before any surgery is done. The time spent in doing diagnostic tests is time well spent. For example, if lung cancer has spread to the lymph nodes in the neck, to the opposite lung, or to other distant organs such as the liver or the brain, surgery alone will not cure it. Small-cell cancer of the lung is rarely cured by surgery. For it, other forms of treatment—chemotherapy and radiation—must be relied on. Operations for lung cancer (thoractomy with lobectomy or pneumonectomy) are major surgery and are usually not performed unless the patient stands a reasonable chance for cure.

Why would the doctor decide to give me radiation before he operates?

In some cases, depending on the size and the location of the tumor, radiation is given to shrink the size of the tumor. This can be done either in conjunction with the operation or in place of the operation, depending on the circumstances of the case.

Is radiation therapy sometimes used after surgery?

Yes. It can be used this way. About a month after the operation, when the chest tissues have had an opportunity to heal, radiation treatment may be started. Radiation is given to that part of the chest where metastases were found or

seemed likely to occur. For more information on x-ray therapy, see Chapter 7.

**Can x-ray therapy be given to the other lung if one has been
removed?**

Since radiotherapy to the lung can cause scar tissue to form,
making it difficult for the lung to function, radiotherapy is
usually not given to the opposite lung.

**How does the doctor determine the stage of lung cancer
when it is found?**

The staging will include three sets of letters and numbers.
The first two grade the tumor size, the second two indicate
the nodal involvement, and the third pair relate to whether
or not the tumor has metastasized. The general categories
of staging and more information on how it is done can be
found in Chapter 3.

Is surgery usually used for lung cancer?

Yes, in most cases. The doctor will usually operate if he
feels that the entire tumor can be removed or if the operation will remove a portion of the tumor and will help the
patient live with the disease better. If the cancer affects
only one lobe, it will be removed. If it affects both lobes
on the left side or all three lobes on the right side, the whole
lung on the involved side may be taken out. If the lymph
nodes involved are around the main bronchus and the large
blood vessels of the lungs or in the center of the chest, it
might be possible to remove all of the malignancy as long
as only one lung contains the cancer. The use of surgery
and the operation which will be performed depend upon
many factors. Surgery may or may not be used for small cell
lung cancer, depending on many factors.

What happens if the cancer has spread to the chest wall?

Again it depends upon the amount and location of the spread.
It is possible to treat with surgery if the cancer has grown
directly from the lung into a small area of the chest wall.
Then the involved part of the chest wall is taken out along
with the lung, and skin and muscle are used to cover the
part of the wall which has been removed.

The Stages of Non-small-Cell Lung Cancer

STAGE	OTHER CLASSIFICATIONS	EXPLANATION
Occult	TX, N0, M0	Indicates secretions containing malignant cells but without other evidence of tumor or metastasis.
Stage I	Tis, N0, M0 T1–2, N0, M0 T1, N1, M0	Includes carcinoma in situ or non-invasive cancer. This stage also includes tumors up to 3 centimeters in size which have metastasized only to nearby lymph nodes or tumors which may be larger but show no signs of metastasis.
Stage II	T2, N1, M0	A tumor larger than 3 centimeters with involvement of nearby lymph nodes.
Stage III	T3, any N, any M any T, N2, any M any T, any N, M1	The cancer extends to nearby organs or is involved with lymph nodes in the mediastinum or has spread to other parts of the body.

The Stages of Small-Cell Lung Cancer

STAGE	EXPLANATION
Limited stage	Tumor is in the lung where it began and in nearby lymph nodes.
Extensive stage	Tumor has spread to other, more distant parts of the body.

Treatment Choices for Non-Small-Cell Lung Cancer

STAGE	POSSIBLE TREATMENTS
Occult	• Usually surgery.
Stage I, II	• Surgery. • Radiation, if surgery not possible. • Investigational: radiation and/or chemotherapy after surgery.
Stage III	*Without Distant Metastasis:* • Surgery or radiation or a combination of the two. • Investigational: usually chemotherpy. *With Distant Metastasis:* • Radiation, for relief of pain or other symptoms. • Close watching and support, with treatment given when symptoms occur. • Investigational: chemotherapy and/or radiation.
Recurrent	• Radiation for relief of pain or other symptoms. • Investigational: chemotherapy and/or radiation.

Treatment Choices for Small-Cell Lung Cancer

STAGE	POSSIBLE TREATMENTS
Limited stage	• Combination chemotherapy, usually with three or more drugs, sometimes with radiation to brain. • Combination chemotherapy and radiation to chest, sometimes with radiation to brain. • Surgery (highly selected cases) followed by combination chemotherapy with or without radiation to the brain. • Investigational: combination chemotherapy and surgery or radiation.
Extensive stage	• Combination chemotherapy, usually with three or more drugs, sometimes with radiation to the brain. • Combination chemotherapy and radiation to chest, sometimes with radiation to the brain. • Radiation to other sites of metastasis. • Investigational: combination chemotherapy, sometimes with experimental agents, and surgery or radiation.
Recurrent	• Radiation for relief of pain or other symptoms. • Investigational: usually combination chemotherapy.

When is surgery not used?

Surgery usually is not the treatment—or not the only treatment—for lung cancer in which the tumor has grown directly into one or more of the important structures in the chest, such as the heart, the esophagus, large blood vessels, or windpipe, or if it has spread to the lymph nodes in the neck, to the opposite lung, or to other organs far from the lung, such as the liver, kidneys, or brain. When this happens, radiation and chemotherapy—alone, in combination, or with surgery—are used, depending upon the location and the extent of the disease.

Is the laser ever used for lung cancer?

Some investigational work is being done in this area, with mixed results. Laser surgery to enlarge the size of the tracheal opening has been helpful to some patients with shortness of breath.

What if I decide I don't want my lung removed?

If your general health is good and it seems that the cancer is confined to one lobe or one lung, the doctor will probably recommend removal of the entire tumor. If all the cancer is removed, statistics show there is an excellent chance for recovery. Radiation following surgery is not usually necessary in cases where the entire cancer is removed. If surgery is not recommended, radiation therapy can be used. However, radiation therapy may not be as successful a treatment as surgery. New combination programs employing chemotherapy, as well as radiation and/or immunotherapy, are being tested. Chemotherapy has been found to be successful in treatment of lung cancer of the small-cell (oat-cell) variety.

What is a coin lesion?

This is a term sometimes used to refer to a small tumor of the lung which is confined to the lung without extension to adjacent structures. It is often found as the result of a routine chest x-ray. A coin lesion is considered to be potentially curable.

Where does lung cancer spread to most often?

Unfortunately, distant metastases can spread to virtually any organ of the body—liver, skeleton, and other lung, for instance. One of the most common sites for metastases is the brain. Radiation of the sites is usually used for treatment in these cases.

What are the various types of lung operations called?

The three most common types of lung operations are thoracotomy, lobectomy, and pneumonectomy.

What is a thoracotomy?

This is a major operation used as a diagnostic tool when other diagnostic tests have failed to locate the tumor or to clarify the nature or extent of the tumor. The operation is performed in the operating room under anesthesia. It involves opening up the chest on one side and examining the lungs and nearby areas, such as lymph nodes. To perform the procedure, the doctor removes a rib or goes between two ribs, just below the shoulder blade. His cut follows the curve of the ribs, going from the back just under the shoulder blade around to the front of the chest. He spreads the ribs apart so he can see and work in the area of the lung. If a tumor is found, an immediate examination of it is made by the pathologist. If his report shows that the cell type of the tumor is favorable for operating, the surgical removal— lobectomy or pneumonectomy—is usually performed immediately.

What is a lobectomy?

A lobectomy involves the surgical removal of one lobe of the lung. The procedure for operating is similar to a thoracotomy.

What is a pneumonectomy?

A pneumonectomy is the removal of one lung. Again, this is a major operation done in an operating room with the patient under anesthesia and follows the same procedure as the thoracotomy.

Does the surgeon ever change his mind and not remove the lung?

If the surgeon finds that the cancer has spread too far for him to remove it all or is in an area where removal is impossible, he may leave the lung intact and close the incision. Then radiation and chemotherapy will be used to help shrink the tumor growth.

Will the surgeon ever remove the lung even though the cancer cannot be totally removed?

It depends on many conditions. If, for example, the tumor is causing serious bleeding and the patient is coughing up blood or if there is an infection with abscess formation, it may be necessary to remove the lung. X-ray therapy and chemotherapy will then be used to help reduce the remaining cancer.

How does the patient breathe during lung operations?

Special equipment is used to assist breathing. The other lung continues to breath while the surgeon is working on the diseased lung.

After a lung operation, what happens to the space that's left in the chest?

Like empty closets, the space manages to get filled up. Body fluid and scar tissue take up most of the room. Structures from the opposite side shift toward the side of the operation. The other lung expands a little. At the beginning there may be a feeling of one-sidedness or emptiness on the side of the operation.

Where are the incisions made for a lung operation?

They are made beneath and behind the shoulder blade, paralleling the ribs, and will not be visible unless the back is exposed, as in a bathing suit.

How long do most lung-cancer operations take to perform?

Approximately 2 to 5 hours.

When can I get out of bed?

You will be up in from 1 to 3 days, depending upon the extent of the operation and your physical condition.

Will breathing be painful?

Breathing may be painful for about a week after the operation.

Is the incision painful?

Most people experience no pain. However some find that scars are sensitive for several months.

Can a patient breathe and live normally after the removal of one or two lobes of the lung? After the entire lung is removed?

A patient can breathe and live normally after the removal of one or two lobes of the lung, except that there might be a slight restriction placed on strenuous physical exercise. Those with an entire lung removed tend to get short of breath when they exert themselves. However, at rest, they breathe normally. Therefore, it is necessary to restrict activity somewhat.

How long a hospital stay is necessary on the average?

Most doctors will send their patients home—barring complications—in about 10 to 14 days.

Why am I asked to cough after the operation?

Though it sounds cruel and though your entire insides hurt, coughing is necessary to dislodge secretions in the lungs. The nurse will explain just how it is done and will show you how to support the incision. Coughing is one of the most effective ways of keeping the lungs free of secretions and of avoiding complications. With any respiratory surgery done under general anesthesia, the area becomes dry and mucous plugs form at the lung bases. Coughing helps dislodge the mucus and helps prevent pneumonia.

Why are arm and leg exercises necessary following the operation?

Since the thoracotomy incision usually runs under one arm, there may be a tendency to favor that arm and hold it close to the body. To prevent the arm and shoulder from getting tight, you can exercise them by bringing the affected arm up slowly in front of the body to shoulder height and extending it out to the side to shoulder height. Simple leg exercises should be performed while in bed to help prevent phlebitis. You will probably be wearing elastic stockings to help decrease the possibility of phlebitis.

What should I know about the chest-drainage equipment?

The tube is there to permit drainage of any air or fluid that accumulates during surgery and will usually remain in place after surgery for 2 to 4 days. The first few days the tube will drain bloody fluid. This is normal. Each day, the amount of drainage will decrease and the color will get lighter. The tube is sutured to the skin and will not come out during deep breathing or coughing. In fact, you will be encouraged to get up, to take deep breaths, and to cough. This will help the lung to expand and will force out the air and fluid that has accumulated in the lung area. The only caution you must take is not to allow the tube to kink up or to fold over, since this can cause pressure to build up in the chest, resulting in pain or shortness of breath. Removal of the tube will probably not hurt.

Why does it hurt when I lift my arms or take a deep breath?

Sometimes this happens after lung surgery and is due to the surgery. Your nurse or doctor will instruct you in breathing deeply—you will be encouraged to breathe each time to the point of pain. Amazingly enough, the pain on breathing will go away more quickly if you breathe deeply than if you try to prevent the lung pain by shallow breathing.

Will I be needing intravenous fluids?

Probably, for at least 24 hours after the operation.

Can I catch lung cancer by kissing someone who has it?

There is no indication that cancer can be "caught" by kissing a person. There is also no evidence to suggest that living in the same household with a cancer patient, sharing his or her possessions, or being physically intimate over a long period of time will increase a person's chances of getting cancer. You should not be afraid that you will "catch" cancer.

I have recently had an operation in which one lung was removed. I am very depressed and tired. I can't even climb the stairs without being short of breath. Does that mean that my cancer is worse?

No. Many patients complain of fatigue after a lung operation. Remember that the body needs to repair itself after any operation—and surgery in which a lung is removed is a major operation. Take time and rest and do not worry. When your body gets adjusted to having only one lung, you will be able to climb stairs more easily.

chapter 13

Skin Cancers

Cancer of the skin is the most common kind of cancer—and, because it is visible, it is the most easily diagnosed and treated. It is estimated that between 300,000 and 600,000 such cancers are treated each year. With the exception of malignant melanoma, skin cancer is also the most curable of all cancers. Skin cancer can develop in almost any area of the skin. The face, neck, forearms, and backs of hands, because they are most exposed, are the most common sites. Long-term exposure to the sun is the most common cause of skin cancer.

Those Most Likely to Get Skin Cancer

- Light-skinned persons living in the southern part of the country
- Persons who have had excessive exposure to the sun without protection, such as farmers, seamen, ranchers, etc.
- Persons over 40 years of age, males more often than females
- Persons with fair complexions whose skin sunburns rather than tans
- Relatives of persons with basal-cell skin cancer
- Persons who have had excessive exposure to x-rays
- Persons whose families have a history of melanoma

Symptoms of Skin Cancer

- Any spot which forms a scab, rescabs, and fails to heal
- A scaly skin thickening which develops in a small area, usually on face, neck, or hands
- A molelike growth that increases in size, darkens, becomes ulcerated, bleeds easily
- A pearly or waxy growth
- Any sore, blister, patch, pimple, or other blemish that does not show signs of healing within 2 to 3 weeks

Tests for Skin Cancer

- Excisional biopsy for lesions of less than 2 centimeters
- Incisional biopsy for larger lesions
- If doctor suspects melanoma, electrocautery biopsy or electro-excision should *never* be performed. If there is any question, ask for a second pathologist's opinion.

What do I need to remember?

- Skin cancer is the most common kind of cancer, is the most easily diagnosed and treated, and is the most curable.
- Ninety-five percent of skin-cancer patients are free of their disease following medically approved treatment (usually surgery).
- Any sore, blister, patch, pimple, or other skin blemish that does not heal in 2 to 3 weeks should be seen by a doctor.

Questions to Ask Your Doctor About Skin Cancer

- What kind of skin cancer do I have?
- What kind of treatment will you give me? Why?
- What are the alternatives?
- Will I need a skin graft?
- Who will do it?
- How extensive will it be?

Skin Cancer

Type	Symptoms	Treatment	Remarks
Basal-cell	Raised lump usually small and nodular. Center sometimes a crusted sore. Skin covering looks tense and shiny, sometimes pearly-gray. Usually found on head or neck. Sometimes on face, nose, or upper lip. Rarely found on trunk or body.	Surgery, radiation, heat, freezing, chemotherapy drugs, immunotherapy	Most common form of skin cancer. Found in lowest skin layer. Grows slowly. Rarely metastasizes. Rarely spreads. Tends to run in families. Most common in men over 50.
Squamous-cell	Usually scaly without center ulcer. Lump may be raised from skin surface. Sometimes looks like wart. Found on neck, face, near lower lip, ear, on hands.	Same as basal-cell	Next most common form but seen much less frequently than basal-cell. More likely to spread than basal-cell. Can metastasize. Tends to occur on sun-exposed skin, and this type is less likely to metastasize. Generally seen in persons over 60.
Actinic keratosis	Rough red plaques barely raised from skin surface.	Topical fluorouracil, surgery, or cryosurgery	Premalignant stage of squamous-cell carcinoma. Usually seen on sun-exposed skin.
Malignant melanoma	Mole which changes in size or appearance. Red, white, or blue specks appear in long-standing moles. Moles that bleed, become darker in color, or have tiny dark spots appearing in skin around them.	Surgery, chemotherapy, radiation	Relatively rare. Much more serious than basal-cell and squamous-cell. Be sure to have qualified cancer specialist. Difficult to diagnose and treat.
Mycosis fungoides (not a true skin cancer but manifested first in skin tumors)	Reddish, plaquelike tumors of scaly, thickened skin. Itchy.	Chemotherapy drugs, radiation therapy	Thought to be related to Hodgkin's disease. Lymph-node involvement.

What kind of doctor should I see if I have symptoms of skin cancer?

You should see your own family doctor or a dermatologist. If you have malignant melanoma, a surgeon specializing in cancer treatment or an oncologist should be handling your case. If you need reconstructive work done as a result of some kind of skin cancer, a plastic surgeon, dermatologist, otolaryngologist, or maxillofacial surgeon would be the doctor of choice.

Is the National Cancer Institute supporting any studies on skin cancer?

The National Cancer Institute's Clinical Cooperative Groups are presently studying new treatment methods for malignant melanoma and mycosis fungoides, two types of skin cancer (see Chapter 23).

What is the skin?

The skin is one of the largest organs in the body. It has two main layers with several sublayers. The main top layer is called the epidermis, and the main underlying layer of connective tissue is called the dermis. The two skin layers, together with specialized structures (such as nerves, hair, nails, and various types of glands), protect the body from injury, receive sensory impulses, excrete waste products, and regulate body temperature. The skin in performing these functions is constantly exposed to the sun, wind, industrial elements, and other harsh external and internal stresses.

What results from these exposures?

What usually results are benign abnormalities. However, sometimes the results are malignant. When they are malignant, they develop as two main kinds of skin cancer, which are distinguished by the cell type: basal-cell cancer and squamous-cell cancer.

Is it true that skin cancer is the most common cancer?

Yes. Skin cancer is the most common form of cancer. Fortunately, it is also one of the easiest to diagnose and to detect at an early stage. It is estimated that 45 to 50 percent of all persons living to age 65 will have had at least one skin cancer.

Is skin cancer curable?

Yes. Today, 95 percent of skin cancer patients are free of their disease following medically approved treatment. If patients were to seek medical attention early enough, it is possible that the cure rate could be even higher—98 percent or even 100 percent. And most skin cancer can be treated either in an outpatient clinic or in a doctor's office.

What causes skin cancer?

Ultraviolet radiation from the sun or other sources is the leading cause of skin cancer in people.

Should I take precautions while sunbathing?

Yes, you should. Try to acquire your tan slowly in the early-morning or late-afternoon sun. Begin at 15 minutes per day and gradually work up to between 30 and 45 minutes. Avoid blistering sunburns. *Avoid* midday sun. Use a sunscreen, beginning with the highest sun protection factor (SPF) and gradually decreasing.

What does the term *sun protection factor* mean?

Sun protection factor indicates how long you can stay in the sun without burning. If a sunscreen has an SPF of 4, it means you can stay out in the sun four times longer than without the screen and not get burned. People with lighter skin need a higher SPF than those with darker skin.

What SPF gives the highest protection?

The SPF values range from 2 to 15. They are usually numbered 2, 4, 6, 8, 15. Some newer sunscreens have an SPF of 18 and above with the ability to stay on for many hours even when you are wet. Apply at least 30 minutes before going into the sun to allow for good penetration in the skin. You should reapply the screen every 2 hours or after swimming or showering.

What are the rating values?

- *SPFs 2 to 4* give minimal protection from sunburning and permit suntanning. They are recommended for people who rarely burn and who tan easily and deeply.

- *SPFs 4 to 6* give moderate protection from sunburning and permit some suntanning. They are recommended for people who tan well with minimal burning.
- SPFs 6 to 8 give extra protection from sunburning and permit limited suntanning. They are recommended for people who burn moderately and tan gradually.
- SPFs of 8 to under 15 give maximum protection from sunburning and permit little or no suntanning. They are recommended for people who always burn easily and tan minimally.
- SPFs of 15 or greater give ultra protection from sunburn and permit no suntanning. SPFs of 15 and higher are recommended for people who always burn easily and never tan.

What is the difference between a sunscreen and a sunblock?

Sunscreens selectively screen out redness-producing rays. Sunblocks screen out everything. If you are the kind of person who cannot tolerate any exposure at all, the best sunblock for you is zinc-oxide paste. You can buy this over the counter. If you need even more protection, use a sunscreen with PABA plus a titanium-dioxide paste. Your druggest can make this up for you.

Do the rays from sunlamps cause skin cancer?

Many sunlamps produce ultraviolet radiation that, like ultraviolet rays from the sun, can cause eye injuries, skin burns, and possibly even cancer. In addition, some sunlamps also give out ultraviolet rays of a short wavelength that can be dangerous to the cell structure of your body. Most of the time, the cells repair the damage. But sometimes this results in changes in cell character called mutations. Some mutations may be cancerous. The FDA is developing a performance standard for sunlamps, because they are potentially hazardous. The standard would require that sunlamps prominently display warning labels and that they have timers that shut them off automatically.

Are suntanning booths safe?

Early tanning booths used ultraviolet B (UVB) radiation (fluorescent sunlamps) in an attempt to mimic sunlight.

Newer booths and beds provide ultraviolet A (UVA) radiation. Ultraviolet B radiation is known to cause skin cancer. Ultraviolet A rays go deeper into the skin and may be more dangerous because they damage deeper lying cells. Long-term effects are unknown, but it is believed that damage is cumulative and the more exposure, the more harm which may be undetectable for many years. People with light skin who have difficulty tanning are particularly at risk and should avoid tanning salons. In addition, many prescription drugs—including sulfas and tetracyclines, medications for high blood pressure, tranquilizers, diuretics, some birth-control pills, and some oral medications used in treating diabetes—may make you painfully sensitive to the intense light in tanning booths.

I hear that when you are taking some kinds of medicine you get a worse sunburn. Is that true?

Yes, it is true. There are some substances that are photosensitizing—that is, when you are taking them you can get a bad sunburn from relatively little exposure. Among them are birth-control pills, diuretics (prescribed for high blood pressure), oral hypoglycemics (antidiabetic drugs), and phenothiazines (tranquilizers such as Thorazine), sulfa drugs (used for bacterial infections), and antibiotics ending with the suffix -cycline (including tetracycline sometimes prescribed for acne). Also watch out for saccharin, halogenated salicylanilides (the active ingredient in deodorant soap), oil of bergamot (used in most perfumes), and essences of lemon and lime (in many aftershave lotions and bath soaps). Persons taking some of the chemotherapeutic drugs or who have had radiation must be careful to protect their skins from sunburn.

I'm allergic to PABA. What can I use for sunburn protection?

PABA can cause an allergic skin reaction in some people, such as those who are allergic to anesthetics (benzocaine or procaine), antibiotics, diuretics or aniline dyes. Because most sunscreens contain a form of PABA, you will probably need to ask your pharmacist for help in finding a sunscreen without it. Two products which are PABA-free are TiScreen and Piz Buin Exclusiv Extrem.

Be careful when you're reading the labels because PABA comes in several forms. Some of the other names include para amino benzoic acid, glyceryl PABA, octyl dimethyl PABA, padimate O and padimate A. Any of these can irritate your skin if you are allergic to PABA.

I borrowed suntan lotion from a person who has skin cancer. Can I catch cancer from using the suntan lotion?

No. Cancer is not an illness which you can catch from someone else. Although the exact cause of many cancers is unknown, the results of many tests and studies show that cancer is not contagious in humans. Skin cancer is most often caused by overexposure to the sun. Using the same suntan lotions, swimming in pools where patients swim, or kissing a cancer patient in no way increases the risks of contracting cancer.

Do black people get skin cancer?

Most skin cancer is directly related to overexposure to the sun's damaging ultraviolet rays, and while black people do indeed develop skin cancer, they do so much less often than people with lighter skin. The pigmentation in their skin, a substance called melanin, protects them. Very fair people are most susceptible to skin cancer.

I've heard that arsenic causes skin cancer. Is that true?

Arsenic in the form of Fowler's solution was used to treat problems like asthma and psoriasis some 20 years ago. Doctors are reporting that some people who used arsenic for prolonged periods have developed skin cancer.

Are there different kinds of skin cancer?

Yes, there are two basic common kinds of skin cancer: basal-cell cancer and squamous-cell cancer. The overwhelming proportion of skin cancers are basal-cell cancer. Squamous-cell cancers are next most common but are seen much less frequently than basal-cell cancers. There are two other conditions which are quite uncommon, but which also appear on the skin. They are malignant melanoma and mycosis fungoides. These are not strictly classified as skin cancer because they are not confined to the skin, but they will be discussed later in this chapter.

What is basal-cell cancer?

Basal cells are spherical and are found in the lowest layer of the epidermis. The cancer involving these cells is the most common kind of skin cancer. You usually notice a lump that is about ¼ to ½ inch across. The edge of the lump is raised; sometimes the center is depressed and is an open sore. The skin covering it looks tense and shiny, even pearly. The lump enlarges at the point where it began. When it ulcerates in the middle, it becomes covered with a scab or crust. Basal-cell cancer grows slowly and rarely metastasizes, but if not treated for a long time, this slow-growing cancer penetrates the layers of tissue below the skin's surface and involves the bone.

Where is basal-cell cancer usually found on the body?

About 90 percent of these cancers are found on the neck and head. Many times they are found on the face, around the nose or upper lip. They are not usually found on the trunk. Basal-cell cancer rarely spreads to the lymph nodes, so usually a simple removal ensures a permanent cure. Since basal-cell cancer rarely metastasizes, it is the most curable skin cancer.

What is squamous-cell cancer?

Most of the epidermis is composed of squamous cells, which are flat. Squamous-cell cancer is less common than basal-cell but it is more serious, because it is more likely to spread to the lymph nodes and it metastasizes more often. Squamous-cell cancer grows more rapidly than does basal-cell cancer. As with basal-cell, you usually first notice it when the lump is about ¼ to ½ inch across. The lump is raised from the skin surface slightly, sometimes looking like a wart. It doesn't have the shiny surface of the basal-cell cancer. Instead it is usually scaly without a central pit or ulcer. Squamous-cell cancer metastasizes but usually not until the primary cancer has been present for a long time.

Can you really tell the difference between the two kinds by looking at them?

A skilled dermatologist or a doctor experienced in detecting skin cancer may be able to tell the difference by looking at the lump in question. However, sometimes the lumps look like benign growths and further tests are needed to determine whether they are cancerous.

What are the major things I should be checking?

You might notice a pimple or a small sore that hasn't healed or disappeared but instead is gradually growing bigger. Or you may have had a skin lesion for many years which has started to grow or become irritated. As noted before, any pale, waxy, pearly-looking lump which eventually becomes an open sore or any red, scaly, sharply outlined patches should be seen by a doctor.

Moles which change in appearance or size are especially important to watch. Go to the doctor at once if any red, white, or particularly blue specks appear in a long-standing mole. Moles that are a uniform bluish-black, bluish-gray, or of uneven surface also should be looked at by a doctor. If the mole begins to bleed, becomes darker in color, or has other tiny dark spots appearing in the skin around it, it may have become a malignant melanoma—a condition which will be discussed later in this chapter. You should remember that any sore, blister, patch, pimple, or other skin blemish that does not heal in 2 to 3 weeks should be seen by a doctor.

Can skin cancer spread to other parts of the body?

Yes, skin cancer is still cancer, and although it grows slowly and usually doesn't metastasize, if it does spread to the structures beneath it, extensive and sometimes disfiguring surgery may be necessary. As with all cancer, the best safeguard against it is early treatment.

What are precancers?

An abnormal skin condition that tends to become cancerous at a later date is referred to as precancer. The most common are senile or actinic (sun-ray) keratosis and hyperkeratosis. Since they tend to become malignant, these precancerous conditions should be checked regularly.

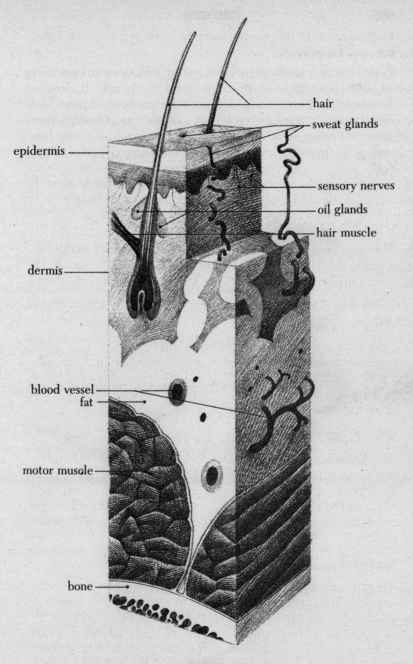

hair

sweat glands

epidermis

sensory nerves

oil glands

hair muscle

dermis

blood vessel

fat

motor musole

bone

Cross-section of skin (enlarged)

What is keratosis?

Keratosis is a scaly skin thickening which develops in a small area, usually on the face, neck, or hands. It usually develops in older persons whose skin has been exposed for many years to the ultraviolet rays of the sun. In older persons it is referred to as senile or actinic keratosis, and this variety frequently occurs on the unexposed parts of the body such as the chest, back, or arms. There are several varieties; some are benign, but some may become cancerous and should be checked by the doctor regularly.

What is leukoplakia?

This is a condition, resembling keratosis, which occurs as a white thickening on the lip or tongue or in the mouth. It frequently occurs in heavy pipe smokers and tobacco chewers.

What is hyperkeratosis?

This is a precancerous condition that appears as a scaly patch or small scab of the skin in a sharply limited, usually small area. Hyperkeratoses are usually caused by exposure to direct strong sunlight and to hot drying wind. They are nearly always found on the face, neck, and hands.

What is Bowen's disease? Is it a kind of skin cancer?

Yes. Bowen's disease is a rare form of skin cancer. It often occurs in several primary sites. The growth is reddish-pink and raised, with scaling. It usually occurs on the unexposed areas of the skin. Some doctors regard it as a precancerous condition. Sometimes it is associated with internal malignancies.

What is keratoacanthoma?

This is an unusual skin lesion which appears in a sun-exposed area and may grow rapidly to substantial size over a short period of time. It is usually a smooth, red nodule, sometimes with a central umbilical spot, which is often difficult to distinguish from other skin cancers. Keratoacanthomas do not metastasize, but careful diagnosis is important because they are similar in appearance to squamous cell carcinoma, which can metastasize. A biopsy is needed to determine the cell type.

What is sweat-gland cancer?

It is a very rare kind of cancer that may metastasize to the lymph nodes or to distant sites. It can originate from any gland but usually occurs near the anus, eyelids, ears, armpits, and scrotum.

What is xeroderma?

Xeroderma is an inherited condition. It is thought to be a precancerous disease. The skin is irregularly pigmented and scaly and later becomes thin, ulcerated, and scarred. It is strongly sensitized to sunlight, and cancer occurs on the areas which have been exposed to it, even briefly.

What is a lipoma?

Lipomas are not cancerous. They are soft, fatty tumors that lie directly beneath the skin. They are the most common tumor in the body. They can be small like a pea or as big as a grapefruit. You can find them almost anywhere on the body. Usually they are underneath the skin of the trunk or the neck or on the arms and legs. They feel soft and move freely under the skin. They are usually not firmly attached to surrounding structures. If they are somewhere where you can see them or if they show signs of growth, the doctor might remove them for cosmetic reasons. Removal is usually done in the hospital. However, they are usually not removed. They do not cause pain and rarely become cancerous. If they do become malignant, they will show rapid growth and the feel of the tissue will change.

Do warts ever turn into cancer?

No. Warts do not turn into cancer.

What are hemangiomas?

Hemangiomas are usually nonmalignant. They are blood-vessel tumors of the skin. They may appear at any time from birth to old age on any part of the body. They look like red spots on the skin and can be anywhere from the size of a pinhead to the size of a nickel. Sometimes they bleed if they are in an area which gets irritated, such as a man's face. Most of them are harmless and do not grow. They very rarely become malignant. Doctors usually do not remove them unless they are unsightly.

What is a ganglion?

A ganglion is not a cancer. It is a thin-walled cyst which appears in the tendons or joints. It is filled with a colorless, jellylike substance. Ganglions are usually seen on the inside wrists of children and young adults.

What is a sebaceous cyst?

Sebaceous cysts, or wens, are thin-walled sacs which contain a soft cheeselike material. The openings of the glands which secrete oils into the skin (sebaceous glands) get clogged and the cysts develop. They can be the size of a nut or get as big as a plum. Usually you find them on the scalp, on the upper back, behind the ear, or on the neck and face.

Do sebaceous cysts turn into cancer?

These cysts rarely turn into cancer. Those which are stable in size usually are left alone unless they are located in areas where there is constant or repeated irritation. When cysts increase in size over a period of weeks or months, they are usually removed. Sometimes they become infected and are treated with warm wet packs or antibiotics or, if needed, with incision and drainage. These cysts can be removed in the doctor's office or in the hospital.

What is a fibroma?

Skin fibromas very rarely become cancerous. They are small, hard lumps about the size of a cherry pit. They are quite common and sometimes are referred to as fibrous tumors. They are not usually removed. Another type, pedinculated fibromas, little tags that dangle on stalks from the skin, are common on necks and armpits and are usually treated by electrocautery.

Are there any other skin conditions which are not cancerous?

Yes, there are several others. Seborrheic keratoses (raised, warty-looking, appear to be stuck onto the skin's surface, easy to scrape off with a fingernail), skin tags (papilloma— little outpatchings of skin), syringomas (benign tumor caused by an enlarged sweat gland), histiocytomas (solitary, well-rounded firm nodule), senile lentigo (liver spots), and sebaceous hyperplasia (shiny, yellow, waxy-oily tumors) are skin conditions that are almost always benign and rarely turn into cancer.

Can a tattoo cause skin cancer?

No, a tattoo usually does not cause cancer. However, if there is itching or bubbling around the edges, it should be checked by a doctor.

How can I tell whether or not a growth is cancerous?

You cannot. You should bring any skin change to the attention of your doctor. Only a physician can determine the nature of an abnormal skin growth—whether it is benign, precancerous, or malignant.

Can a doctor tell just by looking whether or not a growth is cancerous?

An experienced doctor can tell when a growth looks suspicious and will order a biopsy to make a definite diagnosis. The doctor will take out the entire lesion if it is small, or if it is large he will take a small wedge of it for the biopsy. As with all cancers, the only way the doctor can be sure whether or not a growth is malignant is on the basis of a biopsy, in which the cells are examined under the microscope.

How does skin cancer spread?

Basal-cell and squamous-cell cancers typically spread by sending out tentacles through the surrounding tissues. Although these kinds of skin cancer may be destructive locally, they seldom metastasize or spread to bones, lungs, or other organs.

Should all growths on the skin be removed?

No, most growths on the skin need not be removed. They should be seen by a doctor if
- They show a change, such as increase in size
- They are painful
- They become infected
- They bleed
- They are being irritated by something such as a bra strap, a belt, shaving, etc.

Should all skin growths which are cancerous be removed?

Yes. They should be treated with some kind of therapy.

Are any tests other than a biopsy needed for skin cancer?

It depends on what the biopsy shows. If the biopsy shows squamous-cell cancer, a chest x-ray is usually taken, particularly if the growth is large. Although mestastases are rare, if they do occur, they are likely to be in the lung. Also if the biopsy shows squamous-cell cancer the physician is likely to check the lymph nodes in the area.

How is skin cancer treated?

There are several ways of treating skin cancer. The most common ones are surgery and radiation therapy. However, heat, freezing (cryosurgery), chemotherapy, and immunotherapy are all being used in some instances.

Treatment Choices for Skin Cancer

TYPE/STAGE	POSSIBLE TREATMENT
Basal-cell	Surgery; cryosurgery or radiation when excellent cosmetic result with surgery cannot be achieved; topical fluorouracil. Investigational: Other topical treatments.
Squamous-cell	Surgery or cryosurgery. Radiation is often used for lesions where a good cosmetic result may be difficult to achieve with surgery. Lymphandenectomy may be used when regional lymph nodes are involved.
Actinic keratosis	Topical fluorouracil or surgery.

What factors determine the treatment used?

The treatment depends upon many things: the type of growth, its location, its size, the rate of growth, the degree of extension and mestastasis, and whether or not it is a recurring growth. The doctor must also take into account the physical condition of the patient and how the person might respond to the various treatments. The treatment chosen should be the one which will give the best results both medically and cosmetically. The patient's preference should be taken into consideration.

When are surgery and radiation therapy used?

A small growth which is easily accessible is usually removed completely by surgery in the doctor's office. If the growth is large or is in a place where the surgery might leave a disfiguring scar, the procedure would be different. A biopsy would be done by removing a piece of the growth and having it checked microscopically to make sure it is cancer. If it is, there are several alternatives. Surgery would generally be used if it would leave a smaller and less visible scar. Radiation would be the treatment in areas where it gives better cosmetic results. For example, in an area such as the eyelids, where surgery would involve additional reconstructive work, radiation or one or more of the other treatments might be recommended.

When is a curette used?

A curette is a surgical instrument used to take out some lesions. Many of the skin tumors are scraped off the skin either with a scalpel blade or a curette—a stainless-steel hand tool. The open bottom has sharp edges which pry away a raised lesion.

When are heat or freezing used?

Electrocautery and the use of electric needles are sometimes used on small cancers. This treatment is usually performed in the office, and healing takes place in a week or two. Cryosurgery, in which the cancer is subjected to subzero temperatures without damage to underlying vital structures such as cartilage, is showing some promising results.

How does an electric needle work?

Sometimes the doctor uses an electric needle to take out the growth. He holds a stylus whose point is giving out raw cutting electricity. The amount of electricity is regulated with a foot pedal. Sometimes this treatment is called desiccation, which means "drying up."

When are chemotherapeutic drugs and immunotherapy used?

Chemotherapeutic drugs such as 5-FU in the form of ointment have been effective for both cancers and precancers of the skin. Chemotherapy and immunotherapy are used to treat melanoma and mycosis fungoides when these tumors have spread or to prevent spread.

Are the different treatments ever combined? Are the treatments for skin cancer usually repeated over a long period of time?

Sometimes one treatment is sufficient. In other circumstances, repeated treatments are necessary. In some cases, a combination of methods may be used. Again, it depends upon the individual case.

Does skin cancer recur?

Yes. Skin cancer is one of the most common recurrent cancers. A person with skin cancer has a 50 to 60 percent chance of having a second cancer, usually another skin cancer. Therefore, patients should have follow-up visits two to four times a year.

Is there any research under way using vitamin A to prevent the recurrence of basal cell cancer?

The National Cancer Institute is conducting a five-year study to test the effectiveness of a form of vitamin A—isotretinom—in slowing the development of new basal-cell skin cancers.

Skin cancer patients are randomly assigned to one of two groups and receive either the isotretinom or a placebo. Neither the patient nor the doctor knows which agent is being taken. When all patients have taken capsules for three years, researchers will compare the groups to see if those taking isotretinom have fewer basal cell cancers.

Among the institutions involved are Roswell Park Memorial Institute (Buffalo, New York), Brooke Army Medical Center (San Antonio, Texas), Portsmouth Naval Hospital (Portsmouth, Virginia), Walter Reed Army Medical Center (Washington, D.C.), Eisenhower Army Medical Center (Augusta, Georgia), Fitzsimmons Army Medical Center (Aurora, Colorado), University of Arkansas (Little Rock) and Northwestern University (Chicago, Illinois).

Are operations for removal of skin cancer, especially around the eyes and the mouth, disfiguring?

No, they need not be. Usually some kind of skin graft or other plastic surgery is done so that a person with these skin cancers on the face need not worry about disfigurement.

What is malignant melanoma?

Malignant melanoma is a less common form of skin cancer. When diagnosed early, it is easily cured. But if it is not found soon enough, it can be very difficult to treat. It is dangerous because, unlike the other skin cancers, it mestastasizes early and spreads quickly. It is one of the more uncontrollable cancers. The cell involved is the melanocyte, the cell which produces melanin, the dark protective pigment of the skin.

What is the difference between an ordinary mole and melanoma?

An ordinary mole is evenly colored, and either brown, tan or black. It may be flat or raised. It is round or oval and its edges are sharply defined. An ordinary mole is usually less than 6 millimeters in diameter—about the size of a pencil eraser. Ordinary moles may be present at birth. Sometimes several appear at the same time, usually on areas of the skin which have been exposed to the sun. Once the mole develops, it usually stays the same size, shape and color for many years. In older people, moles eventually fade away.

The moles that are melanoma, called unusual moles or dysplastic nevi, are more complicated. One half usually

Differences Between Ordinary Moles and Melanoma (Dysplastic Nevi)

	ORDINARY MOLES	UNUSUAL (DYSPLASTIC) MOLES
Color	Uniformly tan or brown. One mole looks much like all others.	Mixture of colors such as tan, brown, black, red/pink within a single mole. Moles may look very different from each other.
Shape	Round. Sharp, clear-cut border between mole and surrounding skin. May be flat or bumpy.	Irregular border. May have notches. May fade off into surrounding skin. Always a flat portion level with the skin, often occurring at edge of mole.
Size	Usually less than 6 millimeters in diameter (about the size of a pencil eraser).	Usually more than 6 millimeters, may be more than 10 millimeters.
Number	Typical adult has 10–40, scattered over body.	Usually more than 100, although some patients may *not* have an increased number of moles.
Location	Generally on sun-exposed surfaces above waist. Scalp, breasts, buttocks rarely involved.	Back most common site. May occur below waist and on scalp, breast, buttocks.

does not match the other half—that is, they are not round or oval. The color is not uniform. Shades of tan, brown and black, red and pink can be found within the same mole. The edges are ragged, notched or blurred, not clear and sharp. They are usually bigger than a pencil eraser. They usually appear on the back, although they may also be seen below the waist and on the scalp, breast and buttocks.

Are new techniques being used to detect melanoma?

There are some new techniques being used. One is an imaging technique called tomographic gallium scanning, which can be used to detect melanoma early. Another approach is the use of antibodies tagged with isotopes to locate the melanoma.

Should moles which do not show any change be removed ?

No. Moles are very common in various places on the body. It is estimated that most people have from fifteen to fifty of them on the body. Since melanoma is relatively rare—about one to two percent of all human cancers—the odds that any one mole will become malignant melanoma are less than one in several million. It would be impractical to recommend removal of all moles.

Are there any places on the body where moles should be removed?

Moles on the palms of the hands, the soles of the feet, or the genitalia are more apt to turn into malignant melanoma than are moles elsewhere. In addition, if you have a mole in a location that is likely to be repeatedly irritated, such as where a brassiere strap rubs, or where it might be nicked in shaving, it is wise to have it removed. You can have this done in a doctor's office or in an outpatient clinic in the hospital. Usually it will be examined under the microscope just to make certain it is not cancerous.

I am pregnant. The moles on my body are getting darker. Should I be worried about that?

No. Moles on a woman's body may become darker than usual during pregnancy. This is normal and not a sign of melanoma, but you should mention it to your obstetrician.

Is it true that a hair growing from a mole means that the mole is not malignant?

Most doctors agree that the presence of hair suggests that a mole is not malignant, but this is not a hard-and-fast rule. As with any other mole, any change in the color, size, or shape should be regarded as a symptom that should be investigated by the doctor.

Who usually gets melanoma?

Most often, malignant melanoma of the skin occurs in people with light complexions, sandy hair, with skins that burn and freckle easily. It is most commonly seen in younger people between 15 and 50 and is about evenly distributed between men and women. Persons with a family history of melanoma or those who have many moles or certain types of moles (dysplastic nevi) are at higher risk. It is now also believed that people who get blistering sunburns early in life are at more than average risk. Although rare in black persons, they can develop this cancer especially on the palms of the hand, the soles of the feet and under the nails. In whites, melanoma is usually found on the trunk area in men, on the lower legs in women. Other common sites are head, neck, and arms.

Is melanoma inherited?

There seems to be a predisposition of melanoma in some families. Studies have shown that dysplastic nevi carry with them a very high risk among persons with a family history of melanoma. Suspicious moles should be surgically removed as soon as possible.

Persons without a family history of melanoma may also get dysplastic nevi. The risk of melanoma is increased for these people but it is not as high as for those with a family history of the disease. Their moles should be watched carefully for any changes and removed if changes take place.

Are there any prevention guidelines for a person at high risk of developing melanoma?

People who are at high risk for developing melanoma should follow these guidelines:

- Do a monthly skin exam. Get familiar with your skin and the pattern of moles, freckles and beauty marks on it.
- If you see any changes in your skin, see the doctor right away.
- Find a doctor with experience in melanoma for your skin care. This doctor should know the importance of your family background and be willing to remove any changing skin lesions early.
- Spend as little time in the sun as you can. Ultraviolet (UV) radiation from the sun is the major known factor for causing melanoma. Avoid getting sunburned, and do not try to get a "good" tan. Use a 15 SPF-rated sunscreen,

especially from 10 A.M. to 3 P.M. Reapply the sunscreen after swimming or sweating. Remember that UV radiation can pass through clouds or be reflected from snow or water. Thus, sunscreens may be needed even on a cloudy or winter day.

- Avoid indoor sunlamps, tanning parlors or tanning pills.
- Pay extra-special attention to changes in skin moles during adolescence, pregnancy and menopause when hormonal changes take place in the body. Although the scientific evidence is not fully developed, there is enough to suggest that women at high risk should discuss the use of oral contraceptives, estrogens, and even the question of whether or not to get pregnant, with their specialists.

The most important point to remember is that for persons at high risk, careful, regular self-examination, combined with regular visits to a physician who specializes in melanoma will detect skin changes early when they can be carefully cared for.

How can I do a skin exam for melanoma?

The American Cancer Society suggests the following skin exam monthly, after a bath or a shower:

1. Use a full-length mirror and a hand mirror so you can check any moles, blemishes or birthmarks from the top of your head to your toes, noting anything new—a change in size, shape or color or a sore that does not heal.
2. Examine your body front and back in the mirror, then right and left sides, arms raised.
3. Bend elbows and look carefully at forearms and upper underarms and palms.
4. Sit, if that is more comfortable, to look at backs of the legs, feet and spaces between toes and soles.
5. Examine the back of your neck and scalp with the help of a hand mirror, part your hair (or use blow dryer) to lift it and give you a closer look at the scalp.
6. What you are looking for is something different and doing the exam regularly will help you to know what is normal for you and make you feel confident. If you find something, check with your doctor.

Where does malignant melanoma metastasize?

Malignant melanoma can metastasize to any part of the body but most commonly to the lungs, liver, and brain. The cells in malignant melanoma show a tendency to metastasize early, traveling through the lymph system and/or the blood system. The commonest route of spread is to the regional lymph nodes.

What kind of doctor treats melanomas?

Melanomas are usually found by dermatologists, who usually perform the biopsy, which is then read by a pathologist. If the lesion is found to be malignant, further treatment should be carried out by a specialist—either a surgeon who specializes in cancer or a medical oncologist.

Is there more than one kind of malignant melanoma?

There are four fairly distinct forms of primary (original-site) melanoma. They are superficial spreading melanoma, nodular melanoma, acral-lentiginous melanoma, and lentigo màligna melanoma. Superficial spreading melanoma and nodular melanoma start from a preexisting mole or as a new growth. Acral-lentiginous melanoma appears as a dark mark on the palms, soles, or around the nails. Lentigo maligna melanoma (also known as Hutchinson's melanotic freckle) is a relatively rare tissue abnormality which tends to occur on the face or in areas of the body exposed to the sun in light-skinned individuals.

What will the doctor do to a mole which has shown some change?

The doctor will arrange to have it removed for examination under the microscope. If it is small, he will take out the whole mole. If it is large, a partial biopsy will be done. It is generally considered wise for the doctor to take out the entire mole if possible, although there is no strong scientific evidence that a partial biopsy is harmful to the patient.

Is it easy for the pathologist to tell whether or not the mole is malignant melanoma?

Diagnosis of this kind calls for an experienced pathologist, since malignant melanoma is a very difficult cancer to diagnose correctly. If there is any doubt at all about the diagnosis, the slides should be reviewed by several pathologists before any decision about treatment is made.

After biopsy, what other tests are needed before treating malignant melanoma?

Usually, before any treatment is begun, patients with malignant melanoma undergo a complete evaluation. This usually includes a complete physical, documentation of the size and location of any tumor present and the site of primary origin, a history of past and current symptoms, complete blood count, a survey of blood chemistry, and a chest x-ray. In addition, if needed, a bone-marrow aspiration and biopsy, x-rays of the skull and lumbar spine, liver and spleen scans, an electroencephalogram and brain scan, and a stool examination for the presence of occult blood are done.

What is the treatment for malignant melanoma?

The treatment for malignant melanoma depends upon the location, extent, and stage of the disease. If the microscopic examination shows that the mole is a malignant melanoma, then further surgery is usually done. The doctor will remove some of the normal-appearing skin around the mole. Sometimes the nearby lymph glands are also removed.

Is chemotherapy ever used for malignant melanoma?

Sometimes single-drug or combination chemotherapy is used, usually in combination with surgery or immunotherapy. If a limited treatment of a single part or organ of the body is needed, chemotherapy in isolation perfusion (introducing the drug to an isolated part of the circulatory system) may be the treatment.

Is radiation treatment ever used for malignant melanoma?

Although surgery is generally considered the treatment of choice for malignant melanoma, radiation therapy is sometimes used for treatment, especially for those patients who cannot have an operation for some reason. Radiotherapy is used in certain eye tumors and is frequently used to control localized pain.

The Stages of Melanoma

STAGE	OTHER CLASSIFICATIONS	EXPLANATION
Stage IA	T1, N0, M0 (Clark's II)	Invasion of 0.75 mm thickness or less
Stage IB	T2, N0, M0 (Clark's III)	Invasion of 0.76 to 1.5 mm thickness
Stage IIA	T3, N0, M0 (Clark's IV)	Invasion of 1.51 to 4.0 mm
Stage IIB	T4, N0, M0 (Clark's V)	Invasion of 4.0 mm or greater
Stage III	any T, N1, M0	Any lesion with involvement of regional lymph nodes that are movable and not over 5 cm in diameter or the presence of less than five in-transit metastases beyond 2 cm from the original site
Stage IV	any T, N2, M0 any T, any N, M1 or M2	Invasions of 4.1 mm or greater thickness or satellites within 2 cm of original site

Clark's Classification determines the level of invasion. Breslow's Classification is also sometimes used to classify the thickness.

What is the role of immunotherapy in malignant melanoma?

There is a great amount of research now going on in the use of immunotherapy as an adjuvant therapy for malignant melanoma. Clinical trials are being conducted with immunostimulants such as BCG and monoclonal antibodies.

How are monoclonal antibodies used in treating melanoma?

In some centers, monoclonal antibodies are being used to see if the melanoma has spread anywhere else in the body.

Treatment Choices for Melanoma

TYPE/STAGE	POSSIBLE TREATMENT
Stage IA	Wide excision of primary tumor
Stage IB	Wide excision. May include lymph-node dissection.
Stage IIA	Wide excision. May include lymph-node dissection.
Stage IIB	Same as IIA Investigational: If primary tumor on extremity, regional chemotherapy. Isolation perfusion; adjuvant chemotherapy and/or biological therapy.
Stage III	Wide excision of primary tumor. Regional lymph-node dissection of clinically involved lymph nodes. Investigational: Isolation perfusion for control of primary and in-transit metastases; adjuvant chemotherapy or biological therapy.
Stage IV	Wide excision of tumor and regional lymph-node dissection. Surgery or radiation for metastasis. Investigational: Immunotherapy—such as BCG; isolation perfusion with chemotherpy; specific monoclonal antibodies.
Recurrent	Investigational: To distant lymph node areas: regional lymphadenectomy. Isolated metastases to GI tract, bone, brain: surgery or radiation. Chemotherapy, single drug or combination.

This is done by attaching radioactive material to monoclonal antibodies and, with x-rays, determining if the antibody shows up in any other part of the body.

There are also investigational treatments using monoclonal antibodies. In some centers, toxins are attached to the antibody with the substance given intravenously to the patients. Some patients with certain stages of melanoma are also being treated with interferon. Other treatments under discussion include using antibodies combined with interferon and the use of tumor necrosis factor, a natural substance which selectively kills tumor cells.

Will reconstructive surgery be needed in a person with malignant melanoma?

It depends upon the location and the extent of the operation. Patients with facial and neck areas involved usually need cosmetic surgery, either skin grafts or other plastic surgery.

What is a skin graft?

A portion of healthy skin is taken from one area of your body (called the donor site) and moved to another area (called the recipient site). In skin cancer, such grafts cover the areas that have been left bare by the surgical removal of portions of the skin. The skin is usually taken from the back or thigh or other part of the body and is stitched to the injured part. The graft is nourished by small arteries from the tissue surrounding the injured area.

Are there different ways of doing skin grafts?

There are several different ways:
- *Pinch grafts:* Small pieces, usually about ¼ inch in diameter, are taken from the uppermost layer of the skin and spaced in the area missing the skin. The small pieces grow in the new location and spread out to cover the bare area. This method is used usually in very small areas such as the eyelid.
- *Split-thickness grafts:* These are sheets of skin, sometimes measuring several inches in diameter, taken from the uppermost layer of flat surfaces such as the back, the thigh, or the stomach. This method is used when a larger area needs to be covered. Stitches are taken around the edges of the grafts and compression bandages are put on top.
- *Full-thickness grafts:* These contain all the layers of the skin but not the fat tissue which lies underneath. They are used in areas subject to friction or in weight-bearing areas. The grafts are cut so that they will exactly cover the bare area.
- *Pedicle grafts:* One portion of the skin remains attached to the donor site while the rest is transferred to a recipient site. These are used to cover defects on the face

when a wide area of skin has been removed along with the tumor or to cover a finger or hand with new skin.

Are skin-graft operations dangerous?

No. The doctor must be sure that both the donor site and the recipient site are free from infection. The graft must be evenly applied and held in place snugly.

Is it painful to have a skin graft?

No. There is usually only a little pain and a burning sensation in the area from which the skin has been taken and no pain at the site where it is applied.

What is used to cover the skin graft when it is done?

Firm bandages are used to keep the graft snugly applied to the area. The dressing is not changed for 1 or 2 weeks, until the grafted skin is living and growing in its new location.

Does the grafted skin look like the normal skin?

This depends upon where the graft is taken from. Sometimes it might be a different color and texture. The graft will develop sensation after a few months. The new skin can get sunburned but often it does not get as dark as the surrounding skin. The new skin will grow hair only if it grew hair in its original location.

What kind of doctor would do a skin graft?

It depends upon the size and the type of grafting which needs to be done. Facial procedures are done by dermatologists, otolaryngologists, maxillofacial surgeons, and plastic surgeons.

What is intraocular melanoma?

Intraocular melanoma is the most common form of eye cancer in adults. It is highly curable, and vision in the eye can be saved in some tumors which are small and localized to the eye.

How is intraocular melanoma treated?

The treatment of intraocular melanoma depends on the size and location of the tumor, the amount of damage that has occurred to the eye, the age of the patient, and whether the tumor has grown during a period when it was being closely watched. If the tumor extends beyond the white of the eye, radical surgery may be needed to remove the eye, the fat, and the muscle surrounding it.

What is mycosis fungoides?

Mycosis fungoides is an uncommon chronic type of malignancy which can last for many years. In its early stages it usually affects the skin and may stay confined to one area for years. The disease is slowly progressive, and patients live for many years with localized disease. Eventually the lymph nodes and internal organs may become involved.

Is mycosis fungoides some kind of fungus?

The disease was named several centuries ago when it was thought to be caused by some kind of fungus. It has long been recognized that it is a disease primarily affecting the reticuloendothelial system—cells scattered throughout the body which destroy other cells, bacteria, and fragments of foreign materials, form antibodies, and regulate the immune reaction and the formation of blood cells.

Is mycosis fungoides a form of leukemia?

Because it may arise simultaneously in many different areas of the skin, mycosis fungoides is considered to be a T-cell lymphoma related to Hodgkin's disease and leukemia, two other systemic cancers which affect the lymph and blood systems. However, mycosis fungoides has a tendency to remain confined to the skin for long periods of time, unlike Hodgkin's disease and leukemia, which spread rapidly if untreated.

What are the stages of mycosis fungoides?

There are three stages of the disease. The first is called the promycotic stage. Reddish plaquelike tumors of scaly, thickened skin develop. They itch and have a tendency to spread and ulcerate. The plaques, which may resemble eczema or psoriasis, may be found almost anywhere—on the back, arms, stomach, face, or scalp. This stage can persist for several years or longer without distinctive biopsy changes which would enable a positive diagnosis to be made.

The second stage is the infiltration stage. The lymph nodes may be enlarged. The skin becomes infiltrated with an overgrowth of the reticuloendothelial cells of several kinds. This allows a microscopic diagnosis to be made.

In the third stage, large tumors develop on the skin. They may become ulcerated, painful, and odoriferous. In the fourth stage, the lymph nodes, liver, or lung may be involved.

How is mycosis fungoides treated?

Entire-skin radiation therapy may be the treatment. Topical chemotherapy with compounds such as nitrogen mustard may be used. Ultraviolet light treatments may be used. Systemic chemotherapy may be prescribed as the disease progresses. Sometimes radiation treatment is added to the chemotherapy.

What is Sezary syndrome?

Sezary syndrome is a more advanced form of mycosis fungoides and is considered to be a T-cell lymphoma.

chapter 14

Adult Leukemia, Lymphoma, and Sarcoma

Adult leukemias and lymphomas are diseases that attack the blood and lymph nodes. Although most people consider leukemia to be a childhood cancer, the majority of those who are diagnosed with leukemia are adults. Improvements in treatments over the last decade have made it possible for physicians to treat the disease aggressively—and in some cases to cure it. There are several major types of the disease, each with its own set of symptoms and treatments.

Hodgkin's disease is a cancer of the lymph nodes. Once considered fatal, it is now usually curable. Other diseases of the lymph tissues include adult non-Hodgkin's lymphomas, some of which are slow-growing, while others progress rapidly. Careful planning is necessary to determine the best treatment in each individual case.

Sarcomas, cancers that begin in the body's connective tissue, are usually divided into two groups: bone cancers and soft-tissue sarcomas. Surgery, chemotherapy, and radiation are often used in the initial treatment of sarcoma. An expert staff and resources are needed for effective treatment from the very beginning in treating these cancers.

LEUKEMIA

THOSE MOST LIKELY TO GET LEUKEMIA

- Whites more often than blacks
- People of Jewish ancestry more often than other whites
- Males more often than females
- For acute leukemias, children and young adults more often than older adults
- For chronic lymphocytic leukemia (CLL), adults over age 50 more often than younger adults
- Those exposed to ionizing radiation
- Those with some genetic abnormalities, such as Down's and Bloom's syndromes and Philadelphia chromosome
- Those who have had long-term exposure to certain chemicals and drugs, such as benzene, chloramphenicol, and phenylbutazone, and chemotherapy drugs such as alkylating agents

Symptoms of Leukemia

- Fever and influenza-like symptoms
- Enlarged lymph nodes, spleen, and liver
- Bone or joint pain
- Paleness, weakness
- Tendency to bleed or bruise easily
- Frequent infections

Tests for Leukemia

- Blood tests
- Bone marrow biopsy
- Spinal test

What studies is the National Cancer Institute supporting on leukemia?

The National Cancer Institute's clinical cooperative groups are studying the various kinds of leukemia.

Adult Leukemia

Type	Other Names or Forms	Age	Symptoms	Treatments
CLL	Chronic lymphocytic Hairy cell Adult T-cell	Usually appears in later life, between 60 and 70. More common in males than females. Average age at onset is 60.	Often discovered on routine exam. General feeling of ill health, fatigue, lack of energy, fever, loss of appetite and weight, or night sweats. Enlarged lymph nodes in neck or groin. Anemia or infections.	Often no treatment necessary for early-stage disease. Chemotherapy and radiation therapy. Sometimes spleen is removed. Investigational treatments include biological response modifiers, whole body radiation, intensive combination chemotherapy.
CML	Chronic myelocytic Chronic granulocytic Chronic myelogenous Chronic myelosis	Seldom occurs before age 25, usually between 30 and 60. Average age is 40.	Increasing fatigue or weight loss. Sense of fullness or heaviness under left ribs. Anemia, abnormal perspiration, fever, bleeding, pain in spleen or attack of gout. Sometimes discovered accidentally in routine exam or blood tests.	Sometimes no treatment for chronic phase of disease. Chemotherapy. Removal of spleen in some patients. Investigational treatments include bone marrow transplant, biological response modifiers and combination chemotherapy.

ANLL	Acute nonlymphocytic Acute myelocytic Acute myelogenous Acute granulocytic Monocytic Promyelocytic Erythroleukemia Myelomonocytic	Seen at any age, but primarily in 20–55 age group.	Enlarged lymph nodes, spleen, or liver. Bone pain, paleness, tendency to bleed or bruise easily, frequent infections.	Combination chemotherapy plus radiation and/or chemotherapy if needed for central nervous system disease. Bone marrow transplants may be done on adults under 40.
ALL	Acute lymphocytic Acute lymphoblastic Acute lymphatic Childhood leukemia	Found in children and young adults, occasionally in older age groups.	Same as ANLL.	Combination chemotherapy plus radiation if needed for central nervous system disease. Bone marrow transplants may be done on adults under 40.

Questions to Ask Your Doctor If You Have Leukemia

- Exactly what type of leukemia do I have?
- Is it chronic or acute?
- Exactly which cells are affected?
- Can you explain my blood counts to me? What would you consider normal for me?
- Was my type of leukemia difficult to diagnose?
- Has the diagnosis been checked by a hematopathologist?
- What kind of treatment are you planning for me?
- How often will you want to see me?
- What is the usual prognosis for this kind of leukemia?
- Is there a leukemia specialist in the area?

What kind of doctor should I see if I have symptoms of leukemia, Hodgkin's disease, or non-Hodgkin's lymphoma?

Your internist or family physician will usually refer you to an oncologist if he finds evidence of these diseases. It is important that you be under the care of a physician who specializes in these diseases. A hematopathologist should be consulted to properly stage the disease if classification is difficult. If you have lymphoma and the necessary x-ray equipment or radiotherapeutic expertise is not available in your community, you should be referred to the nearest major medical center for high-dose, precision radiotherapy.

What is leukemia?

Leukemia is a cancer of the blood-forming tissues characterized primarily by uncontrolled multiplication and accumulation of abnormal white blood cells.

What causes leukemia?

The cause of leukemia is not known. Certain specific factors, such as excessive exposure to radiation and possibly to certain chemicals, such as benzene, and chemotherapy drugs, such as alkylating agents, have been identified as having some connection to the onset of leukemia. Certain viruses are known to cause leukemia in animals, but this has not been proved so in humans. Some genetic abnormalities, such as Down's syndrome, have also been implicated.

Isn't leukemia a children's disease?

Though it is thought of by many people as a disease that only strikes children, leukemia actually affects more adults than children. More than half of all leukemias occur in persons over 60 years of age. ALL is the type of leukemia that appears most often in children and young adults. (For information on ALL in children, see Chapter 20.)

Can you tell me more about blood to help me understand leukemia?

Blood is made up of cells and fluid. The three major types of cells in the blood are red blood cells, known as erythrocytes, white blood cells, known as leukocytes, and platelets, known as thrombocytes. All of these cells are produced in the bone marrow. After the red blood cells, white blood cells, and platelets are made, they remain inside the marrow until they mature and become adult cells. After maturing, the adult cells slowly leak into the blood vessels and become part of the blood. The bones which produce red blood cells include the ribs, the breastbone, the wide top portion of the hipbone, and the spinal vertebrae.

What is the function of red blood cells?

Red blood cells act as a transportation system. They carry oxygen from the lungs to the other cells of the body and bring back waste products or carbon dioxide. If there are too few red blood cells, anemia results and the body cannot get enough oxygen to do its work.

What do white blood cells do?

White blood cells defend your body against illness. They capture, destroy, and remove germs. They prevent infection. If you have too few white blood cells, you are more likely to develop an infection and less able to fight an infection. There are several kinds of white blood cells. Granulocytes fight infections by engulfing bacteria. Lymphocytes play a role in producing antibodies. *Leukocytes* is a general term used to include all white cells.

What is the role of platelets?

Platelets work by clotting your blood after an injury or cut. They act as "stoppers" which keep the blood from leaking out. If you have too few platelets, your blood clots more slowly and bleeding may be prolonged following an injury.

What are the symptoms of leukemia?

In some varieties of leukemia, there are no symptoms—and leukemia is found during the course of a routine physical examination, pointing up the need for physical examinations on a regularly scheduled basis. As with all other cancers, the earlier the illness is diagnosed, the better the chances of a cure. Fatigue, fever, weight loss, bone pain, easy bruising, or abdominal discomfort may indicate the presence of leukemia. In some forms of leukemia, patients will experience night sweats or abnormal perspiration.

Is leukemia difficult to diagnose?

While leukemia is usually not difficult to diagnose, certain preleukemic states and poorly defined types of leukemia may make it difficult for the doctor to classify the illness. The various classifications have been modified and renamed as greater understanding of leukemia has come about through the medical advances in the last 15 years. A blood picture resembling leukemia may appear with some infections such as mononucleosis, tuberculosis, and whooping cough.

How is leukemia classified?

Leukemia is classified as acute (progressing rapidly) or chronic (progressing slowly). In acute leukemia, there is abnormal growth of immature cells called blasts. In chronic leukemia, there are some abnormal immature cells but there are also some mature cells, indicating that some cells are still behaving normally. Leukemia is also classified according to the type of white cell that predominates in each form of the disease. Thus, a diagnosis of lymphocytic leukemia indicates that there are an excessive number of abnormal lymphocytes, the white blood cells formed in the lymph nodes. In granulocytic (myelocytic) leukemia, there are abnormal quantities of granulocytes, the white cells produced in the bone marrow.

What are the types of acute leukemia?

Acute leukemias are broken down into two categories: acute lymphocytic leukemia (ALL) and acute nonlymphocytic leukemia (ANLL).

What is ALL?

Persons with acute lymphocytic leukemia, or ALL, have an abnormal number of immature lymphocytes in their blood and bone marrow. This form of leukemia, which is also known as acute lymphoblastic leukemia, acute lymphatic leukemia, or childhood leukemia, accounts for 85 percent of leukemia in children and about 15 percent of leukemia in adults.

What is ANLL?

Other forms of acute leukemia are grouped under the heading *acute nonlymphocytic leukemia* (ANLL). The most common of these forms is acute myelocytic leukemia (AML), also called acute granulocytic leukemia or acute myelogenous leukemia. AML is the most common form of acute leukemia in adults. Other rare forms of acute nonlymphocytic leukemia include monocytic leukemia, promyelocytic leukemia, erythroleukemia, and myelomonocytic leukemia. Treatment for these forms of acute leukemia is similar to that for acute myelocytic leukemia.

What is smoldering leukemia or preleukemia?

Several bone marrow disorders, called preleukemia and smoldering leukemia, may, in a small percentage of cases, precede the onset of acute nonlymphocytic leukemia (ANLL) by months or years. Persons with preleukemia are generally older and have a deficiency of white cells, red cells, and platelets in their blood, with signs of red- and white-cell abnormalities. Smoldering leukemia is a form of acute myelocytic leukemia that begins slowly and, scientists believe, involves abnormal changes in more than one cell line. Generally, chemotherapy for these conditions is not begun until the disease begins to progress.

What are the types of chronic leukemia?

Chronic leukemias are also broken down into two categories: chronic lymphocytic leukemia (CLL) and chronic myelocytic leukemia (CML).

What is CLL?

CLL is the most common of the chronic leukemias. It is characterized by an abnormal increase in lymphocytes. Scientists think that the lymphocytes of CLL are produced in the lymph nodes and spleen rather than in the bone marrow. The average age of onset for CLL is 60.

Besides CLL, are there other forms of chronic leukemia that start in the lymphocytes?

Yes. There are several rare forms, including hairy cell leukemia and adult T-cell leukemia/lymphoma.

What is hairy cell leukemia?

Hairy cell leukemia is a rare form of chronic leukemia. It is called hairy cell because of the unique, hairy-like appearance of the leukemic cell under the microscope. Scientists believe that hairy cell leukemia originates in the B cells (the antibody-producing lymphocytes).

What is adult T-cell leukemia/lymphoma?

It is a rare human leukemia which is now known to be caused by a virus. This disease, which has a rapid clinical course, has been found in southern Japan, parts of the Caribbean, and the southeastern part of the United States as well as in other parts of the world. This human T-cell leukemia has no association with the more common, well-known types of leukemia. Instead, human T-cell leukemia more closely resembles rare T-cell cancers that begin in the skin such as mycosis fungoides and Sezary syndrome. In the human T-cell leukemia patients observed so far, the disease usually progresses rapidly and is often characterized by enlarged liver, spleen, and lymph nodes. Researchers believe the virus can only be spread by prolonged intimate contact and is not contagious like influenza or other common viral diseases. The virus, HTLV-I is believed to be distantly related to the HTLV-III virus that causes AIDS.

Who is at highest risk to get leukemia?

In the United States, there is slightly more leukemia among whites than among blacks, and there is a somewhat higher incidence among people of Jewish descent than among other groups. The male-to-female ratio overall is about 1.7 to 1, and men develop CLL almost two times more frequently than do women.

What causes leukemia?

The answer to that question is not fully known. The leukemias appear to be caused by a number of factors that act alone or in combination. Some are human factors such as genetic traits and immune status; others are environmental factors such as radiation, chemicals, or viruses. A number of family clusters of leukemia have been investigated at various times in this country, but so far there is very little clear evidence of a family predisposition for the disease. The near absence of CLL among Orientals, on the other hand, argues for a genetic resistance to it among them. Leukemias are associated in some instances with abnormal chromosome patterns, such as the so-called Philadelphia chromosome found in the bone marrow cells of persons with CML. Leukemia is also about twenty times more common than usual in persons with Down's syndrome. And it occurs more often in persons with rare conditions, some of them hereditary, that are characterized by increased chromosome breakage. In addition, some anticancer drugs are believed to cause leukemia.

What chemotherapy drugs used to treat other cancers cause leukemia?

Long-term exposure to certain chemicals and drugs has been linked with a higher risk of developing various forms of leukemia. Despite their effectiveness in treating cancer, some anticancer drugs are believed to be cancer-causing agents themselves. A number of studies have shown an association between some drugs used to treat cancer and the development of second cancers years later. For example, a class of anticancer drugs called alkylating agents has been linked with the later development of acute leukemia in some patients treated for Hodgkin's disease or ovarian cancer. The risk of leukemia, estimated by most studies at around 5 percent 10 years after treatment, seems highest in patients age 40 and over who have been treated with intensive chemotherapy alone or in combination with intensive radiotherapy. These findings do not suggest that patients should stop or avoid the use of alkylating agents or other chemotherapy treatments, since the benefits of drugs capable of curing .diseases that would otherwise be fatal, far exceed their risks. The findings do suggest caution in using chemotherapy for the treatment of cancer patients at low risk of relapse and for patients with noncancerous conditions.

Do cats get leukemia?

Yes, cats can get leukemia and can transmit it to other cats. There is no evidence that humans can develop leukemia from exposure to cat leukemia virus. This conclusion is based on National Cancer Institute studies of blood samples from pet owners, veterinarians, and research workers who handle the viruses, as well as cancer patients, and healthy humans. None has shown evidence of infection by cat leukemia virus. There is also a new vaccine to prevent leukemia and related fatal diseases in cats. The vaccine is not designed to treat or prevent leukemia in humans.

What is CML?

CML, also known as chronic granulocytic leukemia, chronic myelogenous leukemia, or chronic myelosis, is characterized by abnormal granulocytes which accumulate in the bone marrow and bloodstream. The average age of CML patients at diagnosis is 40 years.

What is the Philadelphia chromosome?

The Philadelphia chromosome is an abnormal chromosome. About 90 percent of patients with CML have the Philadelphia chromosome. The median age of onset for patients with chronic myelogenous leukemia with the Philadelphia chromosome is 40 to 45. For those without the Philadelphia chromosome, it is 50 to 65.

How is leukemia staged?

Staging systems differ among the different types of leukemia. Acute leukemia (ALL and ANLL) has three stages: untreated, in remission, and relapsed. CML can go through five phases: chronic, accelerated, blastic, meningeal and relapsed. CLL follows a regular staging system: Stage 0 through Stage IV.

The Stages of Acute Leukemia*

STAGE	EXPLANATION
Untreated	Newly diagnosed with no previous treatment. Abnormal blood counts, abnormal bone marrow with more than 5% blasts, and signs and symptoms of disease.
In remission	Normal blood counts, bone marrow with less than 5% blasts, and no signs or symptoms of disease.
Relapsed	Disease has progressed, recurred or relapsed.

*Adult acute lymphocytic (ALL) and adult acute nonlymphocytic (ANLL)

The Stages of Chronic Myelogenous Leukemia (CML)

STAGE	EXPLANATION
Chronic phase	More than 5% blasts and promyelocytes (large uninuclear cells in blood) in bone marrow.
Accelerated phase	5%–30% blasts in bone marrow.
Blastic phase	Less than 30% blasts in bone marrow. Fever, malaise, progressive involvement of spleen; occasionally involvement of lymph nodes.
Meningeal phase	Involvement of central nervous system during blast crisis.
Relapsed	Disease has progressed, recurred or relapsed.

The Stages of Chronic Lymphocytic Leukemia (CLL)

STAGE	OTHER CLASSIFICATION	EXPLANATION
Stage 0	Clinical Stage A	There is an increase in the number of lymphocytes.
Stage I	Clinical Stage A or B	Number of lymphocytes increases, and lymph nodes are affected.
Stage II	Clinical Stage A or B	Number of lymphocytes increases; lymph nodes affected; spleen or liver may be enlarged.
Stage III	Clinical Stage C	Number of lymphocytes increases and patient is anemic; lymph nodes, spleen, or liver may be affected.
Stage IV	Clinical Stage C	Lymphocytes increase, platelets decrease; lymph nodes, spleen, or liver may be affected; patient may be anemic.

The Clinical Stages of Chronic Lymphocytic Leukemia (CLL)

STAGE	EXPLANATION
Clinical Stage A	No anemia or lowered platelet count; fewer than three areas of nodal groups involved.
Clinical Stage B	No anemia or lowered platelet count; three or more areas of nodal groups involved.
Clinical Stage C	Anemia and lowered platelet count regardless of number of areas of nodal groups involved.

What kind of treatment is used in arresting leukemia?

Specific treatment varies depending on the type of leukemia diagnosed—so do not try to compare your treatment with that of another leukemia patient, since a great many factors enter into the type of treatment you will receive. Most acute leukemias (ALL or ANLL) are being treated with the administration of two or more drugs, although radiation therapy and bone marrow transplants may also be used. CML is most commonly treated with the drug bulsulfan in early stages of the disease. Other chemotherapy drugs as well as bone marrow transplants may also be used. CLL may be left untreated until there is evidence of further progression of the illness.

Just to give me some handle on what the doctor is talking about, what is the meaning of some of the tests he does?

The table on page 456 explains the terminology and some of the average values that the doctor uses as indicators. It is important to remember that averages mean that "normal" varies a great deal from person to person. The average ranges given here are broad. More important is *your* change from what is normal for you. If you wish to know, ask your doctor exactly what your counts are and how they relate to your case.

Why all the emphasis on blood tests?

When you have leukemia, blood tests become a part of your life. Since leukemia means that there is an abnormality in the production of blood, the blood counts tell the doctor about the state of your disease. His blood checks help him determine how you are progressing.

What are petechiae?

These are little spots on the skin due to tiny hemorrhages. The spots may form a red or brown rash. They are a result of a low platelet count and decreased clotting function. They should be reported to the doctor.

Blood Tests for Leukemia

TEST	MEANING	AVERAGE COUNT
WBC	White blood cell count	Averages 5,000–10,000 for adults
Differential count	Percent of white cells in peripheral blood	Based on 100-cell count
Hematocrit	Percentage volume of red cells to total blood	Average for men: 42–46 Average for women: 38–42
Hemoglobin	Amount of oxygen-carrying protein in known volume of peripheral blood	Male: 14–17 g/100ml Female: 12–15 g/100ml
Platelets	Also called thrombocytes. Microscopic estimate of number of platelets per cubic millimeter. Indicates blood-clotting condition.	Normal range 150,000–300,000 for most laboratories.
Granulocytes	Those white blood cells that have ability to fight infection.	Average between 2,000–4,000. Below 500 indicates body's ability to fight infection is limited.
Erythrocytes	Red cells. Carry oxygen from lung to other areas of body.	Average red cell count is 4.5–5 million.
Reticulocytes or "retic"	Count of young new red cells being manufactured	0.5–1.5 percent of red cells
Blasts	Abnormal cells found in marrow of blood	Less than 5 percent in normal marrow
Leukocytes	A general term used to include all white blood cells.	Normal 5,000–10,000

What is thrombocytopenia?

It is a decreased number of platelets (those substances that along with plasma help blood to clot). There are different causes of thrombocytopenia. Leukemia is one of them.

Is the white blood cell count always high in leukemia?

No. The white blood cell count may be high or low. The more reliable diagnostic indicator is the proportion of immature or leukemic white cells present.

What happens when the platelet count is low?

If there are too few platelets, your blood clots more slowly and bleeding may be prolonged following an injury. Blood may "leak" out of the small blood vessels near the skin and cause spots called petechiae. Extra care should be taken to avoid bleeding. Avoid situations where you might be injured. Use an electric razor rather than a blade for shaving. Use toothette swabs instead of a toothbrush for cleaning your teeth. Do not take aspirin at this time, because aspirin may increase your tendency to bleed. If you cut yourself or have to have an injection or shot while your platelet count is low, make sure pressure is applied for 5 or 10 minutes to stop the bleeding.

What is a remission?

A remission is the goal of therapy for acute leukemia. It means that the abnormal immature blood cells have disappeared from your bone marrow and bloodstream, allowing normal red blood cells, white blood cells, and platelets to form. Remissions can last for any length of time—from a few days to years. Remission, however, is not considered a cure. Rather, it is a healthy state brought about by treatment. A patient in remission can go about living his or her normal life, though it will be necessary for the doctor to continue to follow progress with regular blood and bone marrow testing.

What does the term *bone marrow depression* mean?

It refers to the inability of the bone marrow to produce a sufficient number of blood cells—often the result of treatment with medication for leukemia or other kinds of cancer.

What is the meaning of induction therapy?

Induction therapy is the initial aggressive course of chemotherapy which is designed to wipe out abnormal cells and allow the regrowth of normal cells. At the time of this initial treatment, the patient is extremely susceptible to infection, since normal cells which fight infection are destroyed along with the abnormal cells. Two or three courses of therapy may be necessary before a complete remission is obtained.

What is consolidation therapy?

This is the treatment given after remission has been obtained in an attempt to prolong the duration of remission. It is a slightly less intensive course of chemotherapy given after the initial induction has been achieved. It is used in hope of improving the results of maintenance therapy.

What is maintenance therapy?

It is an effort to keep the patient in remission, prevent the reappearance of leukemic cells, and maintain a normal bone marrow and blood picture.

How is a bone marrow aspiration done?

The bone marrow test may be done on the breastbone or hipbone. The breastbone test is done with the patient lying on his or her back. The patient usually lies on the stomach when it is done on the hipbone. The area is numbed and a tiny opening is made in the skin. The doctor will use a special two-part needle made up of a hollow tube with another solid tube fitted into it. When this has been inserted into the bone marrow, the solid tube is removed and an empty suction tube is attached to the opening of the needle. The doctor will pull some of the marrow out by pulling back on the plunger. You are likely to feel pressure, but it will hurt for just a few seconds. If the first attempt is not successful, the doctor will repeat the process. Sometimes it is difficult to obtain a bone marrow specimen and the doctor will try again. Sometimes when aspiration will not give adequate information, a bone marrow biopsy may be needed.

What is involved in a bone marrow biopsy?

A similar type of needle is used as for the bone marrow aspiration. The hollow needle is pressed farther into the bone so that it can pick up a piece of whole marrow and take it out so that a biopsy can be performed. Bone marrow biopsies are usually taken from the hipbone.

How long does it take to do a bone marrow test?

The whole procedure only takes 5 or 10 minutes, and complications are rare. You will be able to feel the needle, but the pain is minimal.

What is a bone marrow trephine?

This is a less commonly used procedure than the bone marrow aspiration or biopsy and involves taking a tiny piece of whole bone for examination. A larger needle than that used for an ordinary bone marrow test is usually used for this purpose.

When the doctor does my bone marrow test, he refers to spicules. What does that mean?

Spicules are bits of bone marrow with fat in them, which give a representative sample of marrow cells. Without spicules, it is impossible to make an accurate diagnosis of the bone marrow cells.

Does leukemia change the bones?

No. It does not change the shape or strength of the bones, but it does interfere with the work of the bone marrow. The red blood cells, along with the platelets and certain of the white blood cells, are formed primarily in the bone marrow and are then released into the bloodstream as they become mature.

The doctor talks about "blast" or "leukemic" cells. What does he mean?

Blasts or leukemic cells are immature white blood cells.

What complications are most common in leukemia patients?

Anemia (low red-cell count), thrombocytopenia (low platelet count), and infections are complications of the illness. You may have none, any, or all of these in your course of treatment—but it is important to be aware of them and report them to your doctor as soon as they occur. Your doctor will also be checking for bone pain, kidney problems, gonadal involvement, and central nervous system involvement.

Is it unusual for leukemia patients to stop passing urine?

If you have trouble passing urine, be sure to let your doctor know. When cells are dividing often or when the treatments are causing them to die in large numbers, it is more difficult for your body to dispose of wastes. The doctor will usually ask you to drink lots of fluid and to take pills if you have this problem.

What is plateletpheresis?

This is a process which makes it possible to get large numbers of platelets for transfusion by use of a continuous-flow centrifuge which removes platelets from the whole blood and returns red blood cells to the donor in a single operation. This technique permits donors to give platelets as often as twice in a single week for periods up to 3 months. Formerly, the limit was once in 6 to 8 weeks. Since transfusions of blood platelets are often effective in preventing or stopping hemorrhage, this advance is an important one for leukemia patients. Plateletpheresis enables a single adult donor to provide the major portion of the platelets required by a patient with leukemia.

Can this method be used for other types of blood cells?

Granulocytes can also be obtained by using a continuous-flow centrifuge. Leukopheresis is the donation of white blood cells through the same process.

How is leukopheresis used in leukemia patients?

Leukopheresis is a procedure in which the blood is withdrawn from the patient, about a pint at a time, and run through a sterile centrifuge. The centrifuge separates the blood into its component parts and can allow for the removal of a large percentage of life-threatening white blood cells. The process can be done at the patient's bedside, takes a few hours, and can be repeated daily until the blood cell level falls to a point where the patient is out of immediate danger.

What is the role of transfusions in treating leukemia?

Often different types of blood transfusions are used during treatment (particularly with patients who have AML) to help prevent infections and hemorrhaging. White blood cells, red blood cells, and platelets can all be transfused. It has been found, for example, that patients who are given transfusions of leukocytes and platelets early in their treatment may have fewer infections and less hemorrhaging. Since patients can become resistant to platelets from persons of different platelet types, platelets can be closely matched, if necessary, to the patient's own platelets through the same tissue-typing methods that are used in kidney and heart transplants.

What is the usual course for acute leukemia?

When acute leukemia is diagnosed, abnormal white blood cells usually make up 50 percent or more of the white cells in the bone marrow. Often there are signs of leukemic cells in the spleen, lymph nodes, liver, and other tissues. Blood samples show abnormally low levels of red cells, platelets, and mature white cells. Left untreated, acute leukemia leaves the body open to infection and bleeding and is rapidly fatal.

What treatments are used for acute leukemia?

Treatment with a combination of chemotherapy drugs begins with induction therapy, which usually lasts 4 to 6 weeks. This is the most intensive stage of treatment, since its purpose is to destroy as many abnormal white blood cells as possible. Induction therapy is followed by the second phase of treatment called consolidation therapy and the third called maintenance therapy.

Are the same drugs used for AML and for ANLL?

No. Treatment for AML differs from that for ANLL in both the combinations and the dosages of drugs used.

Is immunotherapy used for acute leukemias?

Not usually. Research has shown immunotherapy to be of little value against large numbers of leukemia cells. Its use

Treatment Choices for Adult Acute
Lymphocytic Leukemia (ALL)

STAGE	POSSIBLE TREATMENTS
Untreated	Combination chemotherapy plus radiation and/or chemotherapy if needed for central nervous system disease. Treatment should be by experienced physicians and provide effective supportive care.
In remission	Continued combination chemotherapy plus radiation and/or chemotherapy if needed for central nervous system disease. Investigational: combination chemotherapy. Bone marrow transplantation may be considered during the first remission for patients under 40 with suitable donor.
Relapsed	Dependent on specific cancer, prior treatment recurrence site, and individual patient considerations. Young adults with ALL may be eligible for selected protocols for childhood ALL.

has therefore been limited to patients in remission with the goal of prolonging the disease-free period. Intensive research continues on ways to stimulate the body's natural immune defenses against disease. So far, however, results of studies using immunotherapy have proved disappointing.

Who usually gets CLL?

Chronic lymphocytic leukemia (CLL) is a disease of old or middle age in which there is an abnormal increase in lymphocytes. The course of CLL varies a great deal from person to person. Generally, however, the disease begins slowly and progresses to an aggressive stage after a period of years. Scientists disagree on the best treatment for the early stage of CLL. Current thinking favors monitoring the patient and delaying anticancer treatment until symptoms, such as anemia or lymph-node enlargement, appear. Most patients respond well to moderate doses of chemotherapy. Radiation therapy also produces remission in a large number of pa-

Treatment Choices for Adult Acute Nonlymphocytic Leukemia (ANLL)

STAGE	POSSIBLE TREATMENTS
Untreated	Combination chemotherapy, plus chemotherapy if needed for central nervous system disease. Treatment should be by experienced physicians and provide effective supportive care.
In remission	Investigational: continued combination chemotherapy. Bone marrow transplantation may be considered during the first remission for patients under 40 with suitable donor.
Relapsed	Dependent on specific cancer, prior treatment, recurrence site, and individual patient considerations.

tients. Initially CLL responds well to treatment. In its later stages, however, leukemic cells develop resistance to therapy and most patients relapse. Various studies are under way, using experimental chemotherapies both as single or combination drugs, to overcome such drug resistance.

How is hairy cell leukemia treated?

At diagnosis, patients with hairy cell leukemia often have an enlarged spleen and a deficiency of red blood cells, white blood cells, and platelets. When these symptoms are present, most patients respond well to removal of the spleen. For patients who relapse or fail to respond to the spleen removal, treatment has usually consisted of low-dose chemotherapy. Recently the government approved the use of genetically-engineered alpha interferon as a general treatment for hairy cell leukemia.

How is CML treated?

Chronic myelocytic leukemia (CML) is a slow-growing form of leukemia found mainly in adults. It usually begins with a chronic, treatable stage of low-grade leukemia that may last for years before progressing to an acute phase of disease. During the first stage, practically all CML patients do well with chemotherapy, usually the drug called busulfan. CML becomes more resistant to treatment once it progresses to the next phase, where different anticancer drugs are used. Research is being done on the use of bone marrow transplants for the treatment of CML.

What do the doctors mean when they talk about DAT, VAPA, VP?

These abbreviations are shorthand to describe the various combinations of chemotherapy drugs which are used in

Treatment Choices for Chronic Lymphocytic Leukemia (CLL)

STAGE	POSSIBLE TREATMENTS
Stage 0	Stage 0 chronic lymphocytic leukemia is slow growing; there is usually no treatment
Stage I	Observation if there are no symptoms Local radiation treatment to local lymph nodes with symptoms Chemotherapy for patients with disease affecting the lymph nodes
Stage II	Chemotherapy Radiation therapy to the spleen Investigational treatments using biological response modifiers
Stage III	Chemotherapy Radiation therapy to the spleen Removal of spleen for selected patients Investigational protocols using intensive combination chemotherapy, whole-body radiation therapy, or biological response modifiers
Stage IV	Chemotherapy Radiation therapy to the spleen Removal of spleen for selected patients Investigational protocols using intensive combination chemotherapy, whole-body radiation therapy, or biological response modifiers
Relapsed	Investigational treatments are available

Treatment Choices for Chronic Myelogenous Leukemia (CML)

STAGE	POSSIBLE TREATMENTS
Chronic phase	No treatment if blood counts are near normal and stable Chemotherapy Removal of spleen for selected patients Investigational include: interferon and bone marrow transplant
Accelerated phase	Chemotherapy Investigational include: bone marrow transplant, biological response modifiers, and combination chemotherapy
Blastic phase	Chemotherapy Radiation treatment for bone lesions or pain Investigational include: bone marrow transplant, biological response modifiers, and combination chemotherapy
Meningeal	Chemotherapy with or without radiation treatment to the brain
Relapsed	Investigational treatments

treating the various kinds of cancer. Usually the abbreviation is derived from the initials of the drugs being used. For instance, DAT refers to the combination of daunorubicin (D), ara-C (A), and thioguanine (T).

What is the relationship of leukemia cells to the central nervous system?

Even after a remission has been achieved, studies of spinal fluid may reveal the presence of leukemic cells in the central nervous system of some patients. The fact that some leukemic cells have found a sanctuary in the central nervous system makes them a threat to the patient. Due to the properties of the capillary walls that prevent certain substances from passing from the blood to the central nervous system, these leukemic cells are not killed by the chemotherapeutic drugs. Radiation therapy and drugs administered directly into the spinal fluid are being used to help prevent and control central nervous system leukemia. This is more common with ALL than with other types of leukemia.

What is a bone marrow transplant?

Bone marrow transplantation is an approach used over the past 10 years for the treatment of acute leukemia and lymphoma. It is a complex procedure and should be undertaken only by physicians with the experience and resources needed to get the best results.

When is a bone marrow transplant used?

It may be used in some cases of several types of diseases — aplastic anemia (when patients do not have enough red cells to carry oxygen, enough white cells to fight bacteria, or enough platelets to help clotting), in some types of acute and chronic leukemia, for some lymphomas, for severe combined immunodeficiency syndrome, and for certain inherited blood disorders such as thalassemia. A bone marrow transplant replaces a patient's abnormal or diseased marrow with healthy marrow from a donor.

Can any leukemia patient undergo a bone marrow transplantation?

No. When patients and doctors consider the possibility of treatment with a bone marrow transplant, they must evaluate factors such as the patient's specific illness, age, and medical history; other treatments that might have been used earlier; and the possible risks and benefits of the transplant in the patient's particular case. Some types of leukemia and lymphoma, for example, are curable in many cases with anticancer drugs and/or radiation therapy. These treatments would be tried first, before bone marrow transplantation is considered.

When is bone marrow transplantation considered as a possible treatment?

Bone marrow transplants are sometimes suggested for patients whose leukemia has failed to respond to other methods of treatment, primarily chemotherapy, or who have forms of disease which have been identified as resistant to treatment. Patients with acute lymphocytic leukemia, acute myelogenous leukemia, chronic granulocytic leukemia, and resistant forms of leukemia and lymphoma may be candidates for bone marrow transplants. There are many considerations in determining if a patient might benefit from a transplant, including age of the patient (usually, but not always, under 45), general physical health, condition of organs such as the heart and liver, and prior treatment for blood-cell or other diseases.

What questions should I ask my doctor about bone marrow transplants?

- Is a bone marrow transplant the best option for treatment of my condition?
- What are the chances that the donated marrow will not grow in me?
- With my condition, what are my chances of being cured?
- What are the risks and possible side effects of a bone marrow transplant?
- What is the cost of a marrow transplant and how does it compare with the cost of other possible therapy?
- How long will I have to stay in the hospital?
- How long must I be treated as an outpatient?
- What are some of the risks and side effects of the radiation and chemotherapy used to prepare me for transplantation?
- How soon after the transplant will I be able to resume normal activity?
- If the transplant is done, will I need other treatment?
- What kind of complications occur?
- Because of the risk of infection, can friends and family visit me in the hospital?
- After the transplant, how often will I need medical checkups?

Who can donate bone marrow?

The ideal donor is an identical twin, because there is no risk that the patient will reject the graft. However, transplants are usually performed with marrow donated by other family members. Studies with animals have shown that a graft is more likely to take if certain proteins on the surface of white blood cells are the same for both the donor and the recipient. There is a 25 percent chance that any one brother or sister will have the same protein (HLA antigen) as the patient, since these proteins are inherited from the parents—one set from the mother and one from the father.

Are there different kinds of bone marrow grafts?

There are three different kinds. An *autologous* graft is taken from the patient's own marrow, removed before the patient is given chemotherapy or radiation. The marrow which is removed may be treated before it is retransplanted to the patient. A *syngeneic* graft comes from an identical twin. An *allogeneic* graft comes from a parent, brother, or sister.

How is the patient prepared for the graft?

The patient is usually given a treatment—radiation and a high dose of cyclophosphamide—to keep the immune system from rejecting the foreign marrow. In addition the patient is also given high-dose chemotherapy to destroy cancer cells in the marrow and elsewhere, plus radiation over the entire body to penetrate the bones and kill leukemia cells in the marrow.

How is the bone marrow taken from the donor and given to the recipient?

In an operating room, with the donor under general or spinal anesthesia, marrow is taken from the pelvic bone with a needle and syringe. The procedure takes about 3 hours. The marrow is passed through stainless-steel screens to break up particles and is then injected into the recipient. The marrow cells enter the general circulation and go through the blood to marrow cavities in the recipient's bones. The cells begin to grow in the marrow and produce new white blood cells, red blood cells, and platelets.

Is it painful to donate bone marrow?

The needle-puncture sites may be tender for up to a week. Some stiffness and difficulty in walking will last for a day or so, but the discomfort can be lessened through exercise. Donors are usually released the following day. Marrow cells are quickly produced by the body, and the amount removed will be replaced in 2 or 3 weeks.

How soon will the transplanted marrow begin to produce new blood cells?

The transplanted marrow may not begin producing new blood cells for 2 to 4 weeks or longer. The patient needs intensive supportive care. Infections must be prevented. Patients and visitors use face masks and hand washing to minimize exposure to bacteria. The patient is given antibiotics and sometimes is placed in the sterile environment of a laminar-air-flow room. The patient may receive granulocyte transfusions to help prevent infection and red blood cells to prevent anemia. Transfusions of platelets are often required to prevent uncontrolled internal or external bleeding. All blood products given to transplant patients are treated with radiation to inactivate lymphocytes from the donor which could cause an immune reaction against the patient. Adequate nutrition is another important factor, and many patients are given their nutrients through a feeding tube.

How do the doctors know if the graft has taken?

A rise in the number of granulocytes and platelets is usually a sign that the graft has taken. Gene markers in the blood and cytogenetic studies are among tests used to confirm that the donor marrow is growing. About 5 weeks after the actual transplant, the patient is allowed to leave the hospital if he is eating enough and has a normal temperature and satisfactory blood tests. Patients are not usually allowed to return to work or school for 6 to 9 months after the transplant, because the immune system needs that long to recover, and patients are especially susceptible to infections.

What research is being done in bone marrow transplants?

Many transplant teams around the world are investigating new techniques. They include using an unrelated donor, using specially prepared antibodies called monoclonal antibodies, using the patient's own bone marrow by first cleaning the removed bone marrow with monoclonal antibodies or anticancer drugs, and examining the possibility of establishing a donor bank to collect marrow samples from donors in the general population.

What is splenectomy?

This operation involves the removal of the spleen. It is sometimes used in the treatment of leukemia, especially CML, or in lymphomas when the spleen enlarges and is responsible for destroying large numbers of normal blood cells.

Spleen removal is performed under general anesthesia. The incision is usually made in the upper left abdomen and is about 8 inches long. Once removed, the spleen does not grow back, but since its normal functions are taken over by other body tissues, the absence of the spleen does not interfere with normal living. Cancer of the spleen is rare, but when it does occur a splenectomy is the usual treatment.

HODGKIN'S DISEASE AND NON-HODGKIN'S LYMPHOMA

Persons Most Likely to Get Hodgkin's Disease and Non-Hodgkin's Lymphona

- Hodgkin's disease:
  Peak ages: 20–25 and late 70s,
  mostly people between 15 and 34,
  more males than females.
- Non-Hodgkin's lymphomas:
  Peak age 55–70, very few under 50,
  more males than females,
  more whites than blacks.

Symptoms of Hodgkin's Disease

- Painless swelling of lymph nodes in neck, armpits, or groin
- Fever
- Persistent fatigue
- Weight loss
- Itching
- Night sweats

Types of Hodgkin's Disease

- Lymphocyte predominance
- Nodular sclerosis
- Mixed cellularity
- Lymphocyte depletion
- Unclassified

Symptoms of Non-Hodgkin's Lymphoma

- Painless swelling of lymph nodes in neck, groin, or armpit
- Small lumps in skin
- Skin rashes
- Enlarged tonsils
- Swelling in some part of abdomen
- Fever
- Feeling of weakness
- Bone pain
- Loss of appetite

Tests for Hodgkin's Disease and Non-Hodgkin's Lymphoma

- Complete history with special attention to unexplained fever, night sweats, or weight loss of more than 10 percent in prior 6 months
- Physical examination with particular attention to lymph nodes, liver, spleen, and bone tenderness
- Chest x-ray and/or whole-lung tomography and CT scans
- Blood and urine tests
- Bone marrow tests
- Lymphangiography

Depending on condition, these may also be needed:
- Liver, spleen, and bone scans
- Staging laparotomy (in selected patients)
- Splenectomy
- Liver biopsy
- Kidney tests

Careful and complete testing is of the essence before any treatment is given—so be patient. The initial treatment determines the course of the disease, so tests must be done in depth to assure the most effective treatment. (Of course, the extent of testing is determined by the age and state of health of the patient. In those whose age and medical problems limit therapy, less aggressive testing procedures are done.)

Questions to Ask Your Doctor If You Have Hodgkin's Disease or Non-Hodgkin's Lymphoma

- What have you found that makes you think I have Hodgkin's disease or non-Hodgkin's lymphoma?
- Is the disease confined to one area or more than one area?
- Can my case be discussed with someone at one of the cancer centers?
- Will my spleen have to be removed?
- Are you absolutely certain about the extent of the disease?
- Has a hematopathologist checked the pathology? I want to be certain that the diagnosis has been confirmed by someone else.
- Did the pathologist find Reed-Sternberg cells?
- Can you explain what cell type is involved and how my disease has been staged?
- What plans do you have for my treatment, and what alternatives do I have?
- How many cases like mine have you treated?

For female patients of childbearing age (or younger):
- Can I plan on being married and having children?
- If I am pregnant, will the pregnancy have to be terminated?
- Would you advise me not to have any more children?
- What effect would pregnancy have on me and the child?
- How long would I have to wait before I can think about becoming pregnant?

For young male patients:
- How will this affect my ability to father children?
- What can be done to avoid sterility?

What studies is the National Cancer Institute supporting on lymphomas?

The National Cancer Institute's clinical cooperative groups presently have studies covering all types of lymphoma including Hodgkin's disease and non-Hodgkin's lymphoma. (See Chapter 23)

What are lymphomas?

Lymphomas are cancers that affect the white blood cells of the immune system. They are characterized by the abnormal growth of lymphocytes, the infection-fighting cells in the lymph nodes, spleen, and thymus. The tonsils, stomach, small intestine, and skin may also be affected. Lymphomas are usually classified as Hodgkin's disease, the most common form, or non-Hodgkin's lymphoma. There are also other rare forms of the disease, such as mycosis fungoides, a primary skin lymphoma. Burkitt's lymphoma, rare in most of the world, is the most common childhood cancer in central Africa and is one of the fastest-growing human cancers.

What is the role of the lymph system in the body?

The lymph system is made up of nodes and thin-walled tubelike veins along which the nodes lie. Its job is to help fight diseases and infection, and it serves as part of the body's drainage system. Lymph nodes are usually very small and soft but become enlarged when there is an infection or disease present, such as mononucleosis or strep throat. Lymph glands are found throughout the body: behind the ears, in the groin, behind the knee, in front of the elbow, under the armpit, at the angle of the jaw, deep inside the abdominal cavity, at the junction of the right and left bronchi, and in many other areas. Lymphatic tissues include the tonsils, adenoids, and spleen. The lymph system is a sensitive indicator of illness in the body.

How is lymphoma diagnosed?

It is usually diagnosed by biopsy of a lymph node and the examination under the microscope by a hematopathologist.

How are lymphomas treated?

The treatment depends on where in the body the disease is found. Lymphomas differ from many other cancers in that they are not treated by surgery. However, lymphoma can be successfully treated by chemotherapy and/or radiation.

What is lymphangiography or a lymphangiogram?

A lymphangiogram is a test which shows where malignant lymph nodes are located in the abdomen. The procedure is done under local anesthesia, by injecting a special dye into the lymph vessels of the foot. The lymphatic system carries the dye to all lymph nodes. When the x-rays are taken, the dye outlines the lymphatic system. It shows the size of various lymph nodes, their shape, and even their internal structure. This allows the doctor to identify abnormal nodes. The patterns of lymph flow that show up on the x-rays are also important, because lymph does not pass easily through the nodes that are filled with cancerous cells, so abnormal patterns of lymph flow develop. From this x-ray, the doctor is able to identify involved nodes and to choose several lymph nodes to remove and examine. Because the dye remains in the lymph vessels for long periods of time after a lymphangiogram, x-rays can be taken during and after therapy to monitor the effects of treatment on the cancer.

When is a laparotomy used to diagnose lymphoma?

A laparotomy is a surgical operation to explore the entire abdomen. It allows the doctor to determine the extent of the disease and if it has spread to the abdomen. It was, in the past, a routine procedure for diagnosing lymphoma. Now it is performed only if the information gained will actually change the treatment to be given. Sometimes a simpler procedure is done, called a periotoneoscopy. This uses a much smaller incision in the abdomen through which a fiberoptic instrument, called a periotoneoscope, can be inserted to examine internal organs and take tissue samples. In most cases of non-Hodgkin's disease, laparotomy is not recommended for diagnostic purposes, since other clinical methods can be used to tell the extent of the disease ac-

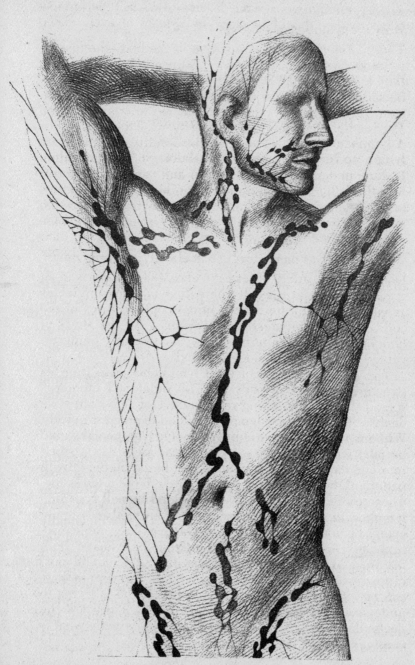

Lymph system

curately enough to stage the disease properly. If performed, a laparotomy should be done by a team of experienced surgeons.

Why is staging so important?

Because the symptoms, rate and pattern of spread, and treatment of lymphomas vary greatly, it is important that the disease be accurately diagnosed by an experienced pathologist who can recognize subtle cellular distinctions among the various lymphatic cancers. The nature and extent of your first treatment influences and can severely limit future treatments. Therefore it is important for the doctor to stage your condition correctly before beginning treatment. The staging procedure may take from 1 to 3 weeks.

What definitions do doctors use in classifying lymphomas?

Doctors use a variety of terms to classify lymphomas in an attempt to describe the cell where the lymphoma originates as well as to indicate certain microscopic features of the cells. So much progress has been made in the study of lymphomas that new terminology is constantly being invented and old terminology updated.

The unique features of each lymphoma arise from its structure and growth patterns. The indolent lymphomas spread slowly, often taking years to develop into aggressive disease. The aggressive lymphomas tend to progress quickly. Without treatment these rapidly growing lymphomas would be fatal within 6 months. Lymphomas are also classified into nodular and diffuse lymphomas, based on the growth pattern of the cancer cells as seen through the microscope. These categories are further subdivided by cell type into lymphocytic (cancer cells are small and resemble lymphocytes), histiocytic (cancer cells are large and resemble macrophages or histiocytes), and mixed (cells have both features). Most nodular lymphomas are indolent, and most diffuse lymphomas are aggressive. All of this terminology can be extremely confusing to a patient who is trying to understand the nature of his disease, but if you ask the doctor, he should be able to clarify for you exactly what is involved in your disease process.

Is pregnancy a problem for a woman with lymphoma?

Although pregnancy has no effect on the course of the illness, women with lymphoma should consult with their physicians about family planning. Treatment cannot be given during pregnancy, since drugs can be harmful to the fetus. Family planning is an important issue because it is difficult to predict when treatment may be needed. Men should also discuss the possible effects of changes in sperm due to drugs and radiation therapy. Some work has been done in the field of repositioning ovaries to sites that can be shielded when x-ray therapy is performed. The disease itself does not seem to have an adverse effect on fertility, the course of pregnancy, labor, or the baby. The treatment and its side effects, however, must be taken into consideration in making a judgment. If at all possible, a waiting period after remission is advised before becoming pregnant.

How does Hodgkin's disease differ from non-Hodgkin's lymphoma?

Hodgkin's disease has unique microscopic features that distinguish it from other lymphomas. Often, it is recognized by the presence of unique cells, called the Reed-Sternberg cells, in lymph tissue that has been removed by surgery for biopsy. Also, Hodgkin's disease tends to follow a more predictable pattern of spread and its spread is generally more limited than that of the non-Hodgkin's lymphomas. By contrast, the non-Hodgkin's lymphomas are more likely to begin in sites like the liver and bones than in the lymph nodes.

What is the most usual symptom of Hodgkin's disease?

The most common first sign is a swollen lymph gland, in the neck, armpit, or groin, caused by enlarged lymph nodes. Many doctors believe that Hodgkin's disease begins in one area of the lymph system and, if left unchecked, spreads throughout the system and later to other tissues and organs. Unexplained weight loss and unexplained fever and night sweats should all be reported to the doctor. An enlarged spleen or liver may be present in some instances. Skin rashes, itching, and weakness may occur. Anemia and reduced ability to fight infection may develop.

If I have an enlarged lymph node should I see a doctor immediately?

Lymph glands may be enlarged as a result of infections or other illnesses such as mononucleosis or rheumatoid arthritis—but any lymph gland in the neck, armpit, or groin that remains enlarged for 3 weeks or longer should be checked by your doctor.

Is itching a common symptom for those with Hodgkin's disease?

Itching—or pruritus, as it is sometimes referred to by the medical profession—is not unusual. It usually disappears with treatment of the disease, and some relief may be possible with antihistamines. It may reappear at a later time and should be reported to the physician if it occurs. This symptom is one of the most distressing and most difficult to cope with for many patients.

Is fever often a symptom of Hodgkin's disease?

A low-grade fever is not uncommon, though some patients may be unaware of it unless they experience night sweats. A pattern of high fever alternating with normal or subnormal temperature may also be seen.

Are there any other symptoms?

Some patients report that an alcoholic drink can induce pain in enlarged lymph nodes, sometimes accompanied by nausea and vomiting. This symptom occurs in less than 5 percent of all patients.

What causes lymphoma?

Though a great deal is known about lymphomas, their actual cause remains a mystery. Some researchers suspect a virus, but direct proof is lacking. Research has shown an increase in the rate of lymphomas among survivors of the atomic bomb in Hiroshima. Persons with damaged immune systems, caused either by immune disorders or immunosuppressive drugs, are also more susceptible to lymphoma. There does not seem to be a hereditary factor involved, although there are instances where more than one person in the family has had the disease. The incidence is higher among males than females.

Is there an association between Hodgkin's disease and mononucleosis?

It does not seem so. Epstein-Barr virus, a herpes virus, has been isolated from patients with Burkitt's lymphoma, the most common cancer among African children. This virus is also linked with one type of infectious mononucleosis. These observations led to a search for associations between mononucleosis and Hodgkin's disease. Most studies have found no convincing evidence of increased risk of Hodgkin's disease for people who have had infectious mononucleosis. Possible associations between Hodgkin's disease and tonsillectomy, polio, multiple sclerosis, and some other conditions have also been explored but without success.

What are Reed-Sternberg cells?

These are the abnormal cells that help confirm a diagnosis of Hodgkin's disease. They are named for the two scientists who first identified them. Reed-Sternberg cells alone are not sufficient for diagnosis of Hodgkin's disease, since similar cells have been described in mononucleosis and other diseases.

Why is it important to have Hodgkin's disease properly classified before treatment is started?

A complete evaluation before the start of treatment is necessary because the nature and extent of previous treatment influences and can severely limit future treatment.

How is Hodgkin's disease staged?

Hodgkin's disease is classified into four stages, depending on the extent of the disease. Stages I and II denote involvement of one or more lymph-node regions above or below the diaphragm. Stage III includes disease limited to the lymph nodes, but both above and below the diaphragm. Biopsy-proven involvement of the liver, bone marrow or other organs is defined as *Stage IV disease.*

The Stages of Hodgkin's Disease

STAGE	EXPLANATION
Stage I	Limited to one group of lymph nodes in one limited area of the body
Stage II	Involves two or more groups of lymph nodes but is entirely above or entirely below the diaphragm
Stage III	Involves lymph-node groups both above and below the diaphragm, and may or may not involve the spleen
Stage IV	Involves organs—such as the liver, lung, bone, and bone marrow—in addition to lymph nodes

Stages are also subclassified as A or B. B are those with any symptom such as unexplained loss of more than 10% of body weight in the 6 months before diagnosis, unexplained fever with temperatures above 38° C (100.4°), or night sweats. A are those without symptoms.

What is the usual treatment for Hodgkin's disease?

Treatment depends upon the stage of disease when the patient is diagnosed. The preferred treatment for early-stage Hodgkin's disease is high-intensity radiation of the lymph nodes. According to the National Cancer Institute, research has shown that radiation therapy to large fields at high doses is more effective at preventing relapse than radiation of the diseased nodes alone. If up-to-date radiation equipment or radiotherapeutic expertise is not available in your community, you should be referred to the nearest major medical center for this treatment. Modern radiation equipment, like the linear accelerator, is capable of quickly delivering high-intensity radiation to large areas with little scattered radiation beyond the targeted field. Combination chemotherapy pioneered by National Cancer Institute researchers is considered the most effective treatment for more advanced Hodgkin's disease (Stages III and IV). For Stages IIB and IIIA Hodgkin's, cancer researchers are still examining the comparative advantages of chemotherapy, radiotherapy, or a combination of the two.

Treatment Choices for Hodgkin's Disease

STAGE	POSSIBLE TREATMENTS
Stage IA	Radiation with linear accelerator Radiation with or without combination chemotherapy for selected children and adults
Stage IB	Radiation with linear accelerator Combination chemotherapy with or without radiation Radiation plus combination chemotherapy
Stage IIA	Radiation with linear accelerator Radiation plus combination chemotherapy
Stage IIB	Radiation with linear accelerator Combination chemotherapy with or without radiation
Stage IIIA	Combination chemotherapy Radiation Combination chemotherapy plus radiation
Stage IIIB	Combination chemotherapy Combination chemotherapy with radiation to areas of bulky disease
Stage IV	Combination chemotherapy Combination chemotherapy with radiation to areas of known disease involvement
Relapsed	Investigational treatments including chemotherapy and bone marrow transplants

Investigational treatments are available for all stages of Hodgkin's disease.

Is there any long-term danger to this intensive radiotherapy and chemotherapy?

Despite their effectiveness, some cancer treatments are suspected to be cancer-causing agents themselves. For example, several studies have shown an association between certain therapies and the development of leukemia many years later. The risk of leukemia, estimated at around 5 percent at 10 years by most studies, seems highest in patients aged 40 years and older who have been treated with both intensive radiotherapy and intensive chemotherapy.

What treatment is available to a patient who relapses after the first set of treatments?

It depends on the first treatment and also on the stage of the disease. If the treatment was radiation, chemotherapy may be administered. If chemotherapy had been given, another combination of drugs might be tried.

Is progress being made in the treatment of Hodgkin's disease?

Yes, definitely. Before 1970, few patients with advanced Hodgkin's disease recovered from their illness and most died within 2 years. Today, there is a far brighter outlook. Now, more than half of all patients with advanced Hodgkin's disease are disease-free for more than 10 years. For early-stage Hodgkin's patients, the news is even better. Due mainly to advances in radiotherapy, the cure rate for early Hodgkin's disease has soared to nearly 90 percent in some treatment centers. Scientists are continuing their search for safer and more effective drugs to combat Hodgkin's disease. Carefully controlled studies comparing established regimens with new and promising approaches using drugs, immunotherapy, and radiation are yielding steady progress in the treatment of Hodgkin's disease and other forms of lymphatic cancer.

What tests are usually required to diagnose non-Hodgkin's lymphoma?

Tests include blood tests, a biopsy, and test of kidney function. Bone marrow biopsy, as well as some of the more complicated tests used in diagnosing Hodgkin's disease, may be required.

What symptoms usually accompany non-Hodgkin's lymphoma?

The most common symptom of non-Hodgkin's lymphoma is painless swelling of lymph nodes in the neck, groin, or armpit. In about one-third of all cases of non-Hodgkin's lymphoma, enlarged lymph nodes are not the first symptom.

Instead, small lumps on the skin, skin rashes, enlarged tonsils, or a swelling in some part of the abdomen may be early signs. Other symptoms that sometimes occur are fever, a feeling of weakness, bone pain, and loss of appetite.

What is meant by indolent non-Hodgkin's lymphoma?

The indolent non-Hodgkin's lymphomas are said to have "favorable" histologies (growth patterns). They are slow-growing cancers affecting mainly adults over age 40. Many patients have no symptoms other than painless enlargement of lymph nodes in the neck, armpit, or groin. Five to 10 years after the disease begins, the cancer becomes more aggressive, causing fever, night sweats, and weight loss. At this time an indolent lymphoma may change to one of the aggressive forms. There are two schools of thought regarding treatment of the slow-growing lymphomas. One approach is not to treat patients who are relatively symptom-free. Another approach is to begin treatment at the time of diagnosis in an effort to achieve and maintain complete remission. Long-term studies comparing various approaches are helping scientists to identify the safest, most effective therapy for these diseases. Meanwhile, investigators are continuing their search for new ways to prevent recurrence and to bolster the body's own natural defenses against cancer. One substance under active study is interferon, which has shown some activity against nodular lymphoma in early clinical trials. Another promising area of research for some types of lymphoma is bone marrow transplants for patients who have had relapses.

What is aggressive non-Hodgkin's lymphoma?

Several forms of non-Hodgkin's lymphoma are aggressive cancers which, if left untreated, rapidly spread and become fatal. Approximately half of all patients with non-Hodgkin's lymphoma have this aggressive type, which includes nodular histiocytic lymphoma, diffuse histiocytic lymphoma, diffuse mixed lymphocytic-histiocytic lymphoma, diffuse undifferentiated lymphoma, and diffuse lymphoblastic lymphoma. Combination chemotherapy is the mainstay of treatment for patients with these lymphomas, since most already have disease in their systems or advanced disease at the time they are diagnosed. Most patients with aggressive lymphoma who achieve complete remission can live for a long time without any sign of disease. Moreover, scientists have observed that practically all patients with these lymphomas who survive the first 2 years without a relapse (instead of the usual 5-year measure) are permanently cured.

The Stages of Non-Hodgkin's Lymphoma*

STAGE	OTHER CLASSIFICATIONS	EXPLANATION
Indolent Stage I	Small lymphocytic Diffuse lymphocytic, well differentiated Follicular, small cleaved cell Nodular lymphocytic, poorly differentiated Follicular, mixed small cleaved and large cell Nodular mixed, lymphocytic and histiocytic Diffuse small cleaved cell Diffuse lymphocytic, poorly differentiated	Involves one group of lymph nodes in an area of the body or a single organ site without lymph-node involvement
Indolent Stage II	Same as Stage I	Involves more than one group of lymph nodes that are either all above or all below the diaphragm or a single organ and an adjacent group of lymph nodes on the same side of the diaphragm
Indolent Stage III	Same as Stage I	Involves the lymph nodes both above and below the diaphragm with or without involvement of the spleen
Indolent Stage IV	Same as Stage I	Widespread involvement of one or more organ sites with or without widespread involvement of the lymph nodes

The Stages of Non-Hodgkin's Lymphoma*

STAGE	OTHER CLASSIFICATIONS	EXPLANATION
Aggressive Stage I	Diffuse, mixed small and large cell Diffuse mixed, lymphocytic and histiocytic Diffuse large cell Diffuse histiocytic Follicular, large cell Nodular histiocytic Small noncleaved cell Diffuse undifferentiated, Burkitt's or non-Burkitt's†	Involves one group of lymph nodes in an area of the body or a single organ site without lymph-node involvement
Aggressive Stage II	Same as Stage I	Involves more than one group of lymph nodes that are either all above or all below the diaphragm or a single organ and an adjacent group of lymph nodes on the same side of the diaphragm
Aggressive Stage III	Same as Stage I	Involves lymph nodes both above and below the diaphragm with or without involvement of the spleen
Aggressive Stage IV	Same as Stage I	Widespread involvement of one or more organ sites with or without widespread involvement of lymph nodes

Stages of adult non-Hodgkin's disease may also be subclassified into A and B categories. A is for those without defined general symptoms, and B includes those with symptoms like unexplained loss of more than 10% of body weight in the 6 months before admission or unexplained fever with temperatures above 38°C (100.4°F).

Lymphoblastic lymphoma is not staged in the usual staging manner.
†Burkitt's lymphoma is presented with childhood non-Hodgkin's disease.

Treatment Choices for Non-Hodgkin's Lymphoma

STAGE	POSSIBLE TREATMENTS
Lymphoblastic lymphoma	Combination chemotherapy with or without radiation treatment to areas with disease
Indolent Stage I	Radiation therapy with linear accelerator Investigational treatments available
Indolent Stage II	Radiation therapy with linear accelerator Investigational treatments available
Indolent Stage III	Careful observation of patients without symptoms Radiation therapy with linear accelerator Combination chemotherapy Single-agent chemotherapy Investigational treatments including radiation therapy with combination chemotherapy
Indolent Stage IV	Careful observation of patients without symptoms Combination chemotherapy Single-agent chemotherapy Investigational treatments including radiation therapy with combination chemotherapy
Relapsed Indolent	Investigational treatments available
Aggressive Stage I	Radiation therapy with linear accelerator Radiation therapy plus chemotherapy Combination chemotherapy Investigational treatments available
Aggressive Stage II	Combination chemotherapy Combination chemotherapy plus radiation to involved sites Radiation therapy alone for selected patients Investigational treatments available
Aggressive Stage III	Combination chemotherapy Combination chemotherapy plus radiation to involved sites Investigational treatments available
Aggressive Stage IV	Combination chemotherapy Combination chemotherapy plus radiation to involved sites Combination chemotherapy plus treatment for central nervous system involvement Investigational treatments available

Treatment Choices for Non-Hodgkin's Lymphoma

STAGE	POSSIBLE TREATMENTS
Relapsed Aggressive	Investigational treatments available

What is Burkitt's lymphoma?

Burkitt's lymphoma, one of the fastest-growing human cancers, can be cured with chemotherapy alone. Although rare in the United States, it is a common childhood cancer in tropical Africa. In African children, Burkitt's lymphoma most often starts in the jaw, ovaries, and kidneys. However, in Americans, the lymph nodes of the neck and digestive system are the most common tumor sites. Because Burkitt's lymphoma is a fast-growing cancer, patients may need surgery or radiation to help reduce the size of the tumor.

What is myeloma?

This is a type of cancer in which abnormal plasma cells destroy normal bone tissue, causing the bones to become extremely fragile. It is often referred to as multiple myeloma, and in Europe is known as Kahler's disease.

Who usually gets multiple myeloma?

Multiple myeloma is most often seen in adults between the ages of 50 and 70. Statistics show that more men than women have multiple myeloma, and it is more common among black men.

What are the symptoms of multiple myeloma?

The main symptom is bone pain, which seems to worsen at night. Back pain is often present. Bone fractures may occur. Abnormal bleeding, difficulty in urination, anemia, a tired feeling, painful swelling on the ribs, and susceptibility to infections are all possible symptoms.

How does the doctor diagnose multiple myeloma?

X-rays may show destroyed patches of bone. Blood and urine tests can detect certain abnormal proteins which suggest the presence of the disease. (The term *Bence-Jones protein* is used in connection with multiple myeloma to identify a specific protein excretion which is used in diagnosing the condition.) A small-needle aspiration of bone marrow, made under local anesthesia, is needed to make a final diagnosis.

Are most myeloma patients anemic?

Since the bone marrow is producing fewer oxygen-carrying red blood cells and disease-fighting white blood cells, myeloma patients are often anemic and susceptible to infections such as pneumonia. As the plasma cells act against the bone tissue, calcium is released sometimes in amounts exceeding the kidney's capacity to dispose of it. The patient may become weak, nauseated, and disoriented.

Is exercise important to the myeloma patient?

Yes. Since immobilization can aggravate the imbalance of calcium, exercise and adequate fluid intake are important. Every effort is made to provide pain relief through radiation and chemotherapy so that the patient will be able to move around.

What treatments are prescribed for multiple myeloma?

Treatment depends upon the extent of the disease. Combination chemotherapy has been found to be effective in treating multiple myeloma. Radiation therapy may be used on specific parts of the back and neck to relieve pain and help repair bone damage. The tumor cells usually decrease in number at a rapid rate during the first few months of treatment, and the patient may go into remission. When a complete remission occurs, there is a complete return to a state of normal good health: The symptoms disappear, the physical findings become normal, and abnormal cells are no longer found in the bone marrow and blood. Sometimes the remission is only partial, and one or more signs of myeloma may not disappear completely. Examination of the blood, urine, and bone marrow at regular intervals allows the doctor to follow the course of the disease and to select the proper treatment. Back braces and pain-relieving medications may also be used to keep patients active.

Treatment Choices for Multiple Myeloma

STAGE	POSSIBLE TREATMENTS
Stage I	For patients without symptoms, careful observation with no immediate treatment Chemotherapy Radiation treatment for local symptoms Investigational treatments available, including biological response modifiers and multi-drug treatment
Stage II	Chemotherapy Radiation treatment for local symptoms Investigational treatments available, including biological response modifiers and multi-drug treatment
Stage III	Chemotherapy Radiation treatment for local symptoms Investigational treatments available, including biological response modifiers and multi-drug treatment

Is Sjögren's syndrome a form of cancer?

Sjögren's syndrome is a combination of symptoms associated with inflammation of the cornea and conjunctiva of the eye, enlargement of the parotid glands in the neck, and dryness of the mouth due to lack of normal secretions. The syndrome itself is not a form of cancer, but in some cases lymphoma later develops, and it is believed that there may be an association between the two diseases.

What is polycythemia vera?

Polycythemia vera is an illness in which all types of blood cells, especially red cells, are produced at a faster-than-normal rate. It is not cancer, although in its more advanced stage, some patients develop acute leukemia. Treatment may include removing excess blood cells, and sometimes chemotherapy or radiation therapy.

ADULT SARCOMAS

Persons Most Likely to Get Sarcomas

- Those persons exposed to heavy doses of radiation
- Those who have Paget's disease

Symptoms of Sarcomas

- Persistent ache, mostly in the knees, thighs, upper arms, ribs, pelvis
- Pain, especially if worse at night
- Swelling or fever
- Repeated, unexplained stumbling
- Unexpected fracture
- Inability to move a body part normally

What are sarcomas?

Sarcomas are cancers that begin in the body's connective tissues. They are usually divided into two groups: bone cancers and soft-tissue sarcomas.

Are there special physicians who treat sarcomas?

It is best for someone diagnosed with sarcoma to begin treatment in a hospital that has an expert staff and resources to apply all forms of effective treatment from the very beginning. Surgery, chemotherapy, and radiation are often used in the initial treatment of sarcoma. It is important for specialists in these fields to decide jointly on the treatment plan.

How are sarcomas diagnosed?

The doctor will ask questions about symptoms and past health problems and examine the affected site. X-rays are taken of the affected area of the body. If the doctor suspects bone or soft-tissue sarcoma, further tests—such as chest x-rays, laboratory analyses of urine and blood, tomograms, and CT scans—are done. Sometimes a scintigram—injecting a radioactive substance into a vein and scanning the skeleton with a special camera which shows whether there is radioactivity in the area of rapidly dividing cells—is done. A biopsy is the next step. For bone cancer it consists of cutting or punching a sample of tissue from what the radiographs show is the most typical part of the suspected area.

What is bone cancer?

Any malignant tumor developing in the skeletal system is known as bone cancer. It begins in the hard substance of the bone itself, a highly specialized connecting tissue which forms the rigid framework that bears body weight, provides fixed points for muscle action, and protects vital organs of the body. Bone cancer is relatively rare. About 1,900 new cases are diagnosed each year in the United States.

Who is at high risk for bone cancer?

Persons who have been exposed to heavy doses of radiation, such as radium workers, are at higher risk for bone cancer and soft-tissue sarcoma. In the future, the number of sarcoma cases caused by radiation is expected to be smaller due to the growing use of megavoltage radiotherapy, which spares bone and soft tissue from high doses.

Paget's disease, a noncancerous disorder resulting in bone deformity, leads to bone cancer in some cases.

Osteogenic sarcoma tends to arise in bones that grow very rapidly, with the peak occurrence among teenagers.

Are all bone tumors cancerous?

No. Many tumors of the bone are not cancerous.

What are the symptoms of bone cancer?

Pain is the most noticeable symptom in bone cancer, especially if the pain is worse at night. A persistent ache may develop anywhere in the skeleton, but most often in the knee, thigh, upper arm, ribs, and pelvis. There may be swelling or fever. There may be repeated, unexplained stumbling. In children, these symptoms are often dismissed as due to a sprain or growing pains until the size of the tumor and the amount of pain make its seriousness apparent. In older people, cancer may be discovered only when a weakened bone fractures or a tumor gets to be very large.

What are secondary bone cancers?

Secondary bone cancers are those that spread from other parts of the body to the bone. They are cancers that have metastasized, reaching the bone through the body's circulatory system or by extension from nearby tissues. Secondary bone cancers are much more common than cancers that start in the bone. Breast, lung, thyroid, and kidney cancers are those most likely to spread to the skeleton, particularly to the red marrow areas of the skull, spine, ribs, pelvis, shoulders, and upper thighs.

What are the major types of primary bone cancer?

The major types of primary bone cancer are osteogenic sarcoma, chondrosarcoma, Ewing's sarcoma, fibrosarcoma of the bone, malignant giant-cell tumor, chordoma, and parosteal osteosarcoma.

What is osteogenic sarcoma?

Osteogenic sarcoma is the most common form of bone cancer and develops in a leg or arm bone. It occurs mainly in teenagers. Information on osteogenic sarcoma is included in Chapter 20.

What is chondrosarcoma?

Chondrosarcoma occurs mainly in persons of middle age and usually begins in cartilage of a leg, hip, or rib. It causes tender masses, usually in the knee, trunk, or upper ends of the thighs or shoulders. It can also develop in children, usually in the knee bones. Generally it grows slowly and does not spread to other parts of the body for many years, if at all. Lung metastases are uncommon.

How is chondrosarcoma treated?

Chondrosarcoma is usually treated by surgery. Depending on the tumor's size and location, either part of the bone or the entire bone is removed. In many cases, adequate surgery requires amputation.

Major Types of Bone Cancer

Type	Usual Age Range	Ages of Peak Occurrence	Major Locations in the Body
Osteogenic sarcoma (also called osteosarcoma)	10–55	10–20	Bone of leg, arm, or hip
Chondrosarcoma	25–65	50–60	Cartilage of leg, hip, or rib
Ewing's sarcoma	10–30	10–20	Bone of leg, hip, or arm
Fibrosarcoma of bone	25–60	30–40	Bone of leg, arm, or hip
Malignant giant-cell tumor	40–60	40–55	Bone of leg or arm
Chordoma	40–70	55–65	Spinal column or skull
Parosteal osteosarcoma	20–45	30–40	Bone of leg or arm

What is Ewing's sarcoma?

Ewing's sarcoma begins in the marrow spaces inside the midshafts of bones. It usually starts in the bone of the leg, hip, rib, or arm. It is a fast-growing cancer that spreads quickly to the lungs and may also spread to other bones. It is usually a children's cancer. It is discussed in Chapter 20.

What is fibrosarcoma of the bone?

Fibrosarcoma of the bone is a very rare cancer that arises in the ends of major limb bones and spreads into soft tissue. It more often affects the middle-aged and the elderly. Like other adult sarcomas, it sometimes develops slowly in bones that have been x-rayed many times. In older patients, a usual site is the pelvis; in younger patients, the knee. Surgery is the usual treatment, with the affected bone being removed.

What is giant-cell tumor of the bone?

Giant-cell tumor of the bone is a benign tumor that sometimes becomes cancerous. Its most common location is in the thigh bone near the knee. It is one of the few bone tumors to which women are more susceptible than men. If the tumor is not cancerous, it and a margin of normal tissue are removed. If the tumor is cancerous, a wider margin of normal tissue must be taken out.

What is chordoma?

Chordoma is a very rare cancer which occurs in the spinal column or skull. It causes pain and constipation. If it affects the skull, it can affect vision. Chordoma grows slowly and is usually treated with radiation.

What is parosteal osteosarcoma?

Parosteal osteosarcoma is a very rare cancer involving both the outer part of a limb bone and the membrane which covers the bone. Patients are treated and usually cured by surgery that removes the tumor and a margin of healthy tissue.

What is soft-tissue sarcoma?

Soft-tissue sarcomas start in muscle, fat, fibrous tissue, blood vessels, or nerves or in other supporting tissue of the body. The term *soft tissue* refers to the connective tissues that support, surround, and connect the structures of the body. Soft-tissue sarcomas occur mostly in the trunk, head, neck, arms, and legs. They are usually aggressive, with a tendency to invade surrounding tissues and to spread to the lungs.

How are soft-tissue sarcomas treated?

Although there are many different types of soft-tissue sarcomas, to the doctor planning the treatment, the type is not as important as the cancer's location, and its stage, and whether the patient is an adult or a child.

How are soft-tissue sarcomas of the extremities treated?

Soft-tissue sarcomas of the extremities occur mainly in adults. Researchers at the National Cancer Institute have

Major Types of Soft-Tissue Sarcoma

Type	Usual Age Range	Ages of Peak Occurrence	Major Locations in the Body
Liposarcoma	25–79	60–74	Fat in extremities* or trunk*
Fibrosarcoma of soft tissue	25–79	55–69	Fibrous tissue of extremities or trunk
Leiomyosarcoma	40–79	45–54	Smooth muscle of uterus or digestive tract
Rhabdomyosarcoma Embryonal rhabdomyosarcoma	30–84 0–19	55–69 0–4	Muscle of extremities Muscle of head and neck area or genitourinary tract
Blood vessel sarcoma	20–84	70–74	Blood vessels of extremities or trunk
Synovial sarcoma	15–69	15–24	Tissue near joints of extremities
Mesenchymoma	10–74	60–69	Mixed tissue of extremities

*The word extremities *refers to legs, feet, arms, and hands. The word* trunk *refers to the body apart from the head and extremities.*

found that surgery which saves the limb plus radiation treatment can be offered to most patients instead of amputation. The use of chemotherapy immediately after surgery often leads to marked improvement in freedom from disease recurrence and in possible cure of these patients.

How are soft-tissue sarcomas in the trunk of adults treated?

These sarcomas are usually treated with surgery and postoperative radiation therapy. There are studies under way using chemotherapy in various combinations.

The Stages of Adult Soft-Tissue Sarcoma

STAGE	OTHER CLASSIFICATION	EXPLANATION
Stage I	G1, T1–2, N0, M0	Well-differentiated tumors which have not spread to the surrounding lymph nodes or to other sites
Stage II	G2, T1–2, N0, M0	Moderately well differentiated tumors which have not spread either to lymph nodes or to other sites
Stage III	G3, T1–2, N0, M0 Any G, T1–2, N1, M0	Poorly differentiated tumors which have not spread to distant sites
Stage IVA	Any G, T3, any N, M0	Tumors of any grade or size which invade bone, a major vessel, or a major nerve, but have not spread to lymph nodes or distant sites
Stage IVB	Any G, any T, any N, M1	Tumors which have spread to distant sites beyond the lymph nodes draining the area of cancer

Stages I, II, and III are also subdivided. A includes tumors less than 5 cm in diameter, and B includes tumors greater than 5 cm in diameter. Stage IIIC are tumors of any grade or size which have spread to surrounding lymph nodes but not to distant sites.

What is synovial sarcoma?

Synovial sarcomas usually arise from the synovial tissue of the joints, tendon sheaths, and bursa—the fluid-filled sac-like cavities in tissues that prevent friction from occurring. This type of cancer is rare and occurs in young adults more often than in other age groups. It is usually in the lower extremities, but may be found in other parts of the body. Synovial sarcoma, also known as synovioma, varies greatly in its rate of growth. It sometimes remains in the original

Treatment Choices for Adult Soft-Tissue Sarcoma

STAGE	POSSIBLE TREATMENTS
Stage I	Surgery, either limb sparing or amputation, depending on local factors Surgery plus radiation therapy, depending on primary site; radiation can be before or after operation High-dose radiation therapy Investigational treatments available
Stage II	Surgery, either limb sparing or amputation, depending on site Surgery plus radiation therapy, before or after operation, with or without regional chemotherapy. High-dose radiation therapy Surgery plus chemotherapy Surgery plus radiation therapy followed by combination chemotherapy Radiation therapy plus chemotherapy, if location does not allow cancer to be removed by surgery Investigational treatments available
Stage III	Surgery, either limb sparing or amputation, depending on site Surgery plus radiation therapy, before or after operation, with or without regional chemotherapy High-dose radiation therapy Surgery plus chemotherapy Surgery plus radiation therapy plus chemotherapy Radiation therapy plus chemotherapy, if location does not allow cancer to be removed by surgery Investigational treatments available
Stage IV	Surgery plus radiation therapy and chemotherapy Radiation therapy and chemotherapy, if location does not allow cancer to be removed by surgery High-dose radiation therapy Investigational treatments available, including use of chemotherapy, biological therapy, and adjuvant chemotherapy

area for a long time, without spreading. In some patients, secondary tumors may develop in the lungs. The treatment is usually surgery. Radiation may be added. The tumor may return after surgery. Chemotherapy, together with surgery and radiation, may be used for synovial sarcomas that are found in the extremities.

chapter 15

Gastrointestinal Cancers: Colon-Rectal, Bladder, Kidney, Stomach, Liver, Pancreas

After lung and skin cancers, colon and rectal cancers are the most common form of cancer among Americans. The disease affects men and women equally and is most prevalent in people over the age of 40. There appears to be little difference in incidence rates among black and white persons. The outcome for patients with colon and rectal cancer varies, depending on the stage at which the disease is detected and treated.

Cancer of the colon is highly treatable and often curable when confined to the colon and its lymph nodes. The type of treatment depends on how far the cancer has spread from its original location. For more extensive disease, many investigational treatments—such as the use of monoclonal antibodies as well as radiotherapy and chemotherapy, sometimes given through an infusional pump—are being used.

Rectal cancer is also a highly treatable and often curable disease. The type of treatment depends on how far the disease has spread from its original location. It is important to know the initial stage before determining treatment.

Bladder cancer can be of a slow-growing type which can be cured with proper treatment. Other types of bladder cancer are more aggressive and, although sometimes curable, are more likely to spread to other organs.

Cancer of the kidney, which is also referred to as renal cell carcinoma, is a curable disease if diagnosed and treated early. The majority of patients are diagnosed when the tumor is still in a localized stage.

Stomach, liver, and pancreatic cancers are more difficult to cure, and the stage at which they are discovered is, of course, important.

Those Most Likely to Get Gastrointestinal Cancer

- Age 50–74
- Personal or family history of rectal polyps
- History of ulcerative colitis
- History of stomach cancer among close relatives
- History of chronic liver disease (hepatitis)
- Diet heavy in smoked, pickled, or salted foods

Symptoms of Gastrointestinal Cancer

- Signs of blood in stool or urine (this is always a warning—must see doctor immediately)
- Change in bowel habits, increased use of laxatives, change in stool size
- Sense of incomplete evacuation
- Gas pains or cramps
- Constant indigestion or heartburn
- Abdominal pain or distended feeling
- Burning sensation when urinating
- Need for frequent urination
- Vomiting
- Feeling of lump or mass in abdomen

Tests for Gastrointestinal Cancer

- Health history and physical exam
- Digital rectal examination
- Endoscopy, proctosigmoidoscopy, or colonoscopy
- Barium enema, barium swallow (GI series)
- Stool blood test (hemocult, stool-guaiac test, occult blood test)

- Intravenous pyelogram
- Hematologic studies
- Blood-chemistry studies
- Cytology
- Liver biopsy (if there is suspicion of liver metastases)

Questions to Ask the Doctor Before an Operation

- Where exactly is the cancer located?
- Do you have any evidence that the cancer has spread?
- Who will be performing the surgery? How often does he do this operation?
- What kind of anesthesia will be used?
- Is there a patient who has had the operation who could talk with me about it?
- Will I need to have an opening outside the body?
- If the answer to the preceding question is yes: Can you show me exactly where the opening will be? Will the opening be permanent, or is there a chance that it would be reconnected? Can I try on the appliance so that I can be sure that the opening will be comfortable?
- Will the operation change my eating habits?
- Will I still be able to have sexual relations?
- Will I be scheduled for radiation therapy? (If yes, be sure to read Chapter 7.)
- Will I be scheduled for chemotherapy? (If yes, be sure to read Chapter 8.)
- Can immunotherapy be used in my case?

What kind of doctor should I see if I have symptoms of gastrointestinal cancer?

The specialists who deal in this area include gastroenterologists (who treat diseases of the GI tract from mouth to anus, including the stomach, liver, pancreas, and intestines), endocrinologists (who treat diseases of the organs which secrete hormones in the bloodstream, such as the pancreas), nephrologists (who treat diseases of kidneys), proctologists (who treat colon and rectal conditions), and urologists (surgeons who treat the urinary system).

Abdominal Cancer

Type	Symptoms	Diagnostic Tests	Treatment
Colon-rectal	Rectal bleeding, blood in stool, jet-black stool, change in bowel habits, alternating constipation/diarrhea, crampy abdominal pain, weakness, loss of weight, loss of appetite	Digital exam, sigmoidoscopy or proctosigmoidoscopy, barium enema, colonoscopy, CEA	Surgery (can range from snipping of polyps in doctor's office to colostomy or ileostomy); chemotherapy and/or radiation therapy is being tested on an investigational basis.
Bladder	Bloody urine, change in bladder habits, increase in urination, retention of urine, incontinence	Cystoscopy, cystogram, intravenous pyelogram, cytology	Surgery, radiation, radium implant, chemotherapy, immunotherapy
Kidney	Back or side pain, blood in urine, abdominal mass, fever, weight loss	Intravenous pyelogram, blood studies, urinalysis, renal arteriography, scans	Surgery, radiation, chemotherapy, biological therapy
Stomach	Indigestion, dark stools, vomiting, weight loss, early fullness	Barium x-rays, gastroscopy, cytology (gastric washing), CEA	Surgery, chemotherapy, radiation therapy
Liver	Discomfort in upper abdomen on right side (more acute with deep breathing), hard lump, pain in right shoulder, jaundice	Needle biopsy, radiography, angiography, tomograms, liver scans	Surgery, regional chemotherapy
Pancreas	Jaundice, itching of skin, abdominal pain and discomfort, nausea, diarrhea, belching, feeling of fullness, intolerance of fatty foods, weight loss, loss of energy and strength, clay-colored stools, severe back pain	Barium x-rays, liver-function tests, angiography, ultrasound, CEA, CT scan	Surgery, chemotherapy, radiation therapy

Is the National Cancer Institute supporting any studies on gastrointestinal cancer?

Yes, the National Cancer Institute's clinical cooperative groups are presently conducting studies on colon-rectal, bladder, stomach, pancreas, and kidney cancers as well as on general genitourinary tumors. (See Chapter 23.)

COLON-RECTAL CANCER

What is the colon?

The colon, also called the large intestine or bowel, is the final 5 to 7 feet of the intestinal tract. It starts at the right lower part of the abdomen and, defying the laws of gravity, continues upward on the right side of the abdomen, close to the liver under the ribs (this section is known as the ascending colon). It makes a left turn and crosses to the left portion of the abdomen (this 2-to-2½-foot portion is known as the transverse colon). The next portion heads down the left side of the abdomen to the pelvis (called the descending colon). The final section, which is S-shaped (the sigmoid colon), and the final 8 or 10 inches located in the pelvis behind the urinary bladder, are known as the rectum, with the final 2 inches being referred to as the anal region. The colon joins the small intestines to the rectum. The colon and rectum form the lower end of the digestive tract.

What is the small intestine?

The small intestine, or bowel, is part of the digestive tract and consists of three parts. At the lower end of the stomach it is called the duodenum. The jejunum is the portion between the duodenum and the ilium. The ilium joins the large intestine (or colon) in the lower right side of the abdomen, just above the appendix. The small intestine is longer than the large intestine—about 20 feet in length— but is narrower in width.

What kind of tumors develop in the colon?

There are two kinds, primarily—benign growths such as adenomas or polyps, and malignant growths, which are cancer.

What tests should I have regularly to assure that any cancers of the colon or rectum are discovered early?

The following three tests are valuable aids in detecting colon and rectal cancer early in people without symptoms:

1. A digital rectal examination every year after age 40.
2. The stool-blood slide test (stool-guaiac test), which can be done at home and returned to the doctor's office, hospital, or clinic for examination. This should be done every year after age 50.
3. The proctosigmoidoscopy, known as the "procto," should be performed every 3 to 5 years after the age of 50, following two annual exams with negative results.

Many doctors feel these tests should be done up to the age of 75.

What is a polyp?

A polyp is a growth originating from the mucous membranes of the colon (polyps also occur in the bladder, uterus, nose, etc.). They are very common, occurring in 10 to 15 percent of all adults. Usually they cause few symptoms and are most often found during routine intestinal examinations. Cure, through removal, entails little surgical risk. If cancer is found in the polyp, the area surrounding it is removed. Painless rectal bleeding is the most frequent symptom of a polyp. Because some polyps have a tendency to become cancerous, their removal is recommended by many doctors.

How does the doctor remove a polyp?

This depends on where the polyp is located. If it is within 8 inches of the rectal opening, it can be removed with a sigmoidoscope through the rectum—either burned off or clipped and removed through the rectum. With improved techniques of colonoscopy almost any polyp with a "stalk" can be removed through a colonoscope. Some will still require surgery if they are large or flat. The incision is made at the area of the polyp, the colon is opened, and the polyp

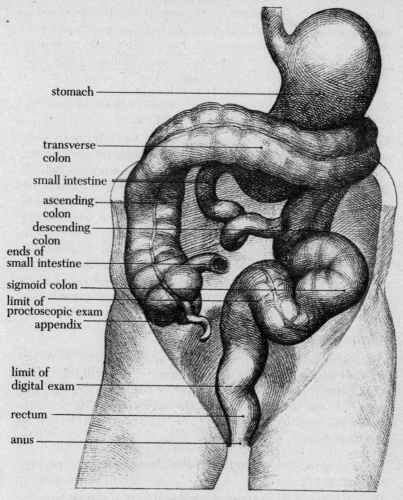

stomach

transverse colon

small intestine

ascending colon

descending colon

ends of small intestine

sigmoid colon

limit of proctoscopic exam

appendix

limit of digital exam

rectum

anus

Colon-rectal area

is removed. The polyp will be carefully examined to make sure that it is not cancerous. If cancer is found, the segment of the bowel where it grew must be removed.

What is familial polyopsis?

Familial polyopsis is an inherited condition, which means that if members of your family have developed large numbers of polyps in the intestine, you are more likely to develop these lumps. They grow in the mucous membrane and may become cancerous. People at high risk can protect themselves by getting regular checkups that include a proctosigmoidoscopy, and by seeing a doctor immediately if they have any symptoms of bowel disease.

What is a sigmoidoscope?

This is an instrument which enables the doctor to view about 12 inches of the intestinal tract through the rectum. This is the area where polyps and cancers are most usually found. Small polyps can be removed with this instrument in the doctor's office with general or local anesthetics. The sigmoidoscope also allows a small portion of tissue to be extracted from the wall of the colon for laboratory testing. The procedure using the sigmoidoscope is called a sigmoidoscopy or proctosigmoidoscopy and should be included by your doctor as part of your annual physical exam if you are over 40 years of age, or earlier if you have a family history of colon cancer.

What causes tumors to form in the colon?

The causes are unknown, but it is suspected that heredity as well as diet may play a role in some cancers of the colon. Conditions such as polyps, ulcerative colitis, and colitis also may be causes. Periodic checkups with a rectal examination make it possible for tumors to be discovered before they become dangerous.

What is involved when the doctor does a digital rectal examination?

With a gloved finger, the doctor will probe the rectum for lesions. This examination will detect the presence of any masses in the lowest 4 inches of the rectum. The portion of stool on the gloved finger may be tested for blood.

How do I prepare for a proctosigmoidoscopy?

Usually the doctor will instruct you to have a tap-water enema the night before or the morning of the examination. The conventional instrument he uses is a sigmoidoscope, which allows him to view the last 12 inches of the colon.

Some doctors prefer a flexible fiberoptic sigmoidoscope, which allows viewing higher into the colon. If bleeding, obstruction, or diarrhea is present, the doctor will suggest a less vigorous bowel cleansing.

Is a proctosigmoidoscopy dangerous?

No. Complications from this examination are rare—but an inexperienced doctor could perforate the bowel, causing serious problems. This procedure is best done by a proctologist, a gastroenterologist or a physician who is trained to do this procedure.

What is the stool-guaiac test?

The guaiac (pronounced *gwi-yak*) test (also called occult stool or stool blood test) is a simple, inexpensive method of testing stools for traces of blood. Usually stool samples are taken of three consecutive bowel movements so that if there is intermittent bleeding, this can be discovered. To increase the accuracy of the stool analysis, the doctor may ask you to start a meat-free, high-fiber diet 48 hours before the collection of the first stool specimen and continuing through the next 3 days. Vitamin C, iron and aspirin should be avoided during this time to ensure that the test is accurate.

Do hemorrhoids (piles) usually turn into cancer?

No. However, hemorrhoids may exist along with cancer. Any rectal bleeding should be followed by an examination by the doctor to determine its cause. Do not assume that all bleeding is caused by hemorrhoids, because one of the symptoms of cancer of the colon or rectum is bright-red blood in the stools.

What is the CEA test?

Research is under way to discover specific antigens, or biological markers, that might indicate the presence of colorectal cancer. One of these antigens, carcinoembroyonic antigen or CEA, may be found in greater amounts in the blood of patients with colorectal cancer. It has been suggested that this marker may be useful in showing at an early stage whether the cancer has recurred in some patients who had been treated for colorectal cancer previously. However, this test cannot be used alone in diagnosing colorectal cancer.

What are some of the symptoms of a tumor in the rectum or colon?

Rectal bleeding, red blood in the stool, jet-black stools, a change in bowel habits or the size of the stool, alternating constipation and diarrhea, crampy abdominal pains, weakness, loss of weight, and loss of appetite. Sometimes you will see a streak of blood in the stool only once. It is important that any sign be checked by a doctor.

If tumors are found, must they always be removed?

Yes. Most doctors agree that even benign tumors (adenomas or polyps) should be removed, because they may eventually develop into cancer.

How serious is the surgery for tumors of the colon and rectum?

The operation varies depending on the location, kind, and size of the tumor. Polyps near the rectum can often be removed through the rectum without anesthesia in a surgeon's office, on an outpatient basis in a hospital, or during an overnight hospital stay. For any benign tumor, the procedure is simple removal of the tumor at its base. If the tumor is cancerous, the tumor as well as a generous portion of the colon above and below is removed.

What preparations are necessary before surgery of the colon?

Usually the patient is required to enter the hospital several days before surgery. Medication with antibiotic drugs and low-residue or liquid diets will be prescribed. Blood transfusions may be necessary if you are anemic, as well as vitamin, mineral, and glucose feedings by vein. If there is an obstruction, an attempt may be made to overcome it by passing a tube into the small intestine.

What kind of anesthesia is used?

General anesthesia is usually preferred. Spinal is sometimes used.

What do Dukes and Astler-Coller have to do with colon-rectal cancer?

These are two different methods which doctors sometimes refer to in accurately staging colon and rectal cancers and determining treatments to be given. They correlate with the staging that is referred to in the charts.

The Stages of Colon-Rectal Cancer

Stage	Other Classifications	Explanation
Stage 0	T1S, N0, M0	Carcinoma in situ as demonstrated by biopsy. Early cancer that hasn't spread beyond limiting membrane of first layer of colon-rectal tissue.
Stage IA	T1, N0, M0 (Dukes' A, Astler-Coller A)	Tumor confined to mucosa or submucosa. No evidence of regional or distant metastases.
Stage IB	T2, N0, M0 (Dukes' B1, Astler-Coller B1)	Tumor involves muscularis propria but not beyond. No evidence of regional or distant metastases.
Stage II	T3, N0, M0 (Dukes' B2, Astler-Coller B2)	Tumor has spread through the wall of the intestine but not to lymph nodes or immediately adjacent organs.
Stage III	Any T, N1–N3, M0 or T4, N0, M0 (Dukes' C, Astler-Coller B3, C1, C2)	Cancer has spread outside intestine to lymph nodes or beyond the wall or immediately adjacent organs.
Stage IV	Any T, any N, M1 (Dukes' D, Astler-Coller D)	Tumor has spread outside intestine to other distant sites or organs in the body, such as the liver.

Treatment Choices for Colon Cancer

STAGE	POSSIBLE TREATMENT
Stage 0	Limited surgery
Stages IA, IB	Surgery to remove tumor and a portion of the colon
Stage II	Surgery to remove a portion of the colon Investigational: radiation therapy before surgery, chemotherapy or biological therapy
Stage III	Surgery to remove tumor and portion of colon Investigational: radiation therapy before surgery, with or without chemotherapy or biological therapy
Stage IV	Surgery in selected cases. Possible surgery for limited liver metastasis Radiation, chemotherapy for symptoms Investigational: biologicals or chemotherapy
Recurrent	Depends on original treatment and sites of recurrence. If in liver, may include removal of metastases or intra-arterial chemotherapy with infusion pump. Investigational treatments include biologicals, single and combination chemotherapy

Treatment Choices for Rectal Cancer

STAGE	POSSIBLE TREATMENTS
Stage 0	Limited surgery Investigational: electrocoagulation or radiation
Stage I	Surgery Radiation within the rectum for selected patients Investigational: radiation immediately before, during, or after surgery; electrocoagulation
Stage II	Surgery Investigational: radiation immediately before, during, or after surgery, chemotherapy, biological therapies and chemotherapy with radiation therapy
Stage III	Surgery Investigational: radiation therapy and chemotherapy

Treatment Choices for Rectal Cancer

STAGE	POSSIBLE TREATMENT
Stage IV	Surgery, chemotherapy, and radiation delayed until needed for symptoms Possible surgery for single liver or lung metastasis Investigational: biologicals and new chemotherapy treatments should be considered
Recurrent	Treatments depend on original treatment. For local recurrence, radiation is recommended if surgery alone was first treatment. Surgical removal of single metastasis to liver or other organs Investigational: hepatic artery infusion, anti-tumor agents, biologicals

What kind of operation is necessary for cancerous growths in the colon or rectum?

Again, this depends on the kind, size, and location of the tumor. In all cases, the surgeon removes the tumor. If enough normal colon remains, he will rejoin the healthy pieces so that the patient can function in a normal manner. This happens in about 80 percent of all cases. When this is not possible, then an artificial opening, called a stoma, is made on the abdominal wall. Only about 20 percent of patients have a permanent opening (stoma) as a result of cancer.

What is a stoma?

A stoma is an opening or hole made in the skin for the end of the small or large intestine in cases where it must be brought through the abdominal wall. The end of the intestine is fastened at the skin level so that it cannot slip back. The diameter of the opening may vary from ½ inch to 3 inches or more.

What is the name of the operation used to create a stoma?

This surgery is an ostomy. Whether permanent or temporary, it takes the name of the area where it is performed. If in the colon, it is called a colostomy. Following colostomy, bowel movements are received in a pouch placed over the stoma.

Are all colostomies permanent?

No, many of them are temporary—that is, after a certain period of time, in a second operation, the colon is rejoined and the hole in the abdomen is closed up. These operations are often referred to as two-stage procedures. The first operation is a temporary colostomy. The second is an operation to rejoin the colon and close the colostomy. The number of patients who require colostomies has been reduced, thanks to new surgical techniques and materials. Often the doctor is able to perform a one-stage operation, bringing together the healthy sections of the colon after the tumor has been removed.

When is a permanent colostomy necessary?

Permanent colostomies are usually necessary when the growth is in the region of the lower rectum. In this case, the rectum is removed and the upper portion of the colon is brought out onto the abdominal wall in the form of a permanent colostomy.

What are temporary colostomies called?

There are several different kinds, each of which requires two-stage operations: double-barrel colostomy, transverse-loop colostomy, and cecostomy. Each of these requires the temporary use of an appliance outside the body to collect body wastes. Each, however, can later be repaired by the surgeon so that the colon is rejoined and the use of an appliance is no longer necessary.

Is a colostomy always due to cancer?

No. There are about twenty other diseases and conditions which lead to the need for this operation.

What is an ileostomy?

The ileum is a portion of the small intestine. When disease necessitates its removal, an ileostomy is created. This is usually, but not always, a permanent arrangement, depending upon whether the rectum remains healthy or must be removed as well.

What is the difference between a colostomy and an ileostomy?

A person with a colostomy usually has had a portion of the colon and the rectum removed. A person with an ileostomy usually has had the entire colon plus a portion of the small intestine removed as well. The word *ostomy* means a surgical procedure that creates a stoma (an artificial opening). A person who has had this kind of surgery is known as an ostomate.

What is a total colectomy?

This is when the surgeon removes the entire large intestine and rectum.

A stoma sounds uncomfortable. Is it?

A well-cared-for, healthy stoma is comfortable and painless and does not interfere with physical activity. However, much of the success with which a patient is able to handle the stoma is determined by the way in which the surgery is carried out, as well as the attitude of the patient.

How can I be sure that mine will be a stoma that is easily manageable?

That is a hard question—but a very important one. First of all, make certain that your surgeon is someone who specializes in this particular type of operation. Some surgeons undertake these operations without the benefit of repeated experience, and though they provide a stoma which is surgically correct, the stoma may not be functional from the patient's point of view. So, be warned. Ask the doctor how often he has performed this surgery. Ask if he examines the ostomy each time the patient visits him. Ask him what kind of long-term routine supervision he is prepared to give you or can suggest for you. You might even ask him if he has a patient who has had this operation who would be willing to talk with you. Be absolutely certain that the doctor has located a suitable site for the stoma before you are on the operating table. He will undoubtedly ask you to stand, sit, and lie down as he notes your body so he can determine the best site for stoma placement. Stomas situated in scars, in the navel, or where you wear your belt (particularly if you are a man) can be quite unmanageable. Proximity to bony prominences, or the waistline, or interference by rolls of fat—all can interfere with the use of ostomy appliances. These problems cause soiling and often make it difficult for the patient to make a good recovery. So be sure the doctor discusses with you the actual location of the opening. The type of ostomy you have determines where the stoma will be to some extent and the nature of the discharge you will have. Ask the doctor to show you on a diagram what portion of your colon he will remove and where the stoma will be.

How long do I have to stay in the hospital for a colostomy?

The time varies according to the type of surgery. A simple operation for the removal of polyps through the rectum may require only 1 or 2 days of hospitalization, or may even be done in the surgeon's office. A tumor removed through the abdomen may require a week to 10 days in the hospital. As with any surgery, complications can extend this time period. In the case of operations which are done in several stages, the patient may have to plan on several hospitalizations, each requiring a varying amount of time—from 10 days to several weeks—in the hospital.

How does a colostomy affect my general health?

You will probably be healthier than ever. The problem area has been removed and the intestine that remains is perfectly able to take care of the absorption of food elements.

Can the body function without a large portion of the intestines?

A person has about 20 feet of small intestine and 5 feet of large intestine (the large intestine is larger in diameter than the small intestine, thus its name). He can live quite well without a portion of his small intestine and without his entire large intestine (colon). Most digestion actually takes place before food reaches the colon. The colon's function is to absorb the water from the already digested material and to transport waste through its length and store it until it is ready to be expelled from the body. The remaining portions of the colon learn to assume some of the water-absorption role of the intestine that was removed. Even though to a layman the removal of a portion of the small intestine or even all of the colon and rectum sounds as though it would make it impossible for the body to function, the fact is that after successful surgery the body adjusts to the loss of the large or small intestine and rectum with very little effect. The patient will usually be able to eat what he likes and function in exactly the same way—usually feeling better than he did before.

What happens to bowel movements if the colon and rectum are removed?

A permanent abdominal opening (stoma) through which the bowels will be evacuated must be created by means of a colostomy operation.

The thought of living with a permanent bowel opening is repulsive to me.

Better techniques and methods of caring for colostomies have really made care a routine and fairly simple matter. It will become a part of your regular routine. Many patients who at first thought they would not be able to care for their stomas are after a short time able to live a perfectly normal life. Hundreds of thousands of people are doing this and are in no way disabled.

Will I have to worry about my diet?

No special diet is needed. Your body will tell you which foods are best for you. You should be careful about eating highly laxative foods or foods which are "gassy"—such as beans, nuts, onions, cabbage. Just be sure you eat a complete and well-balanced diet.

Will I have the colostomy bag on when I return from the operating room?

Usually, patients who have had ileostomies will return from surgery with a temporary ostomy bag in place. A patient who has had a colostomy will not have fecal drainage until he begins to eat again a few days or a week after the operation. He will return from surgery with dressings but with no ostomy bag. When fecal matter begins to be expelled, a temporary colostomy bag will be applied. Because this is a temporary appliance, it may not work as well as the permanent one. Furthermore, the process is more complicated because you have so recently had the operation. Don't be dismayed by the whole procedure. It will become a simple, routine matter for you when you return home. Thousands of people from every walk of life have had colostomies and are able to attend to their businesses and their homes, marry, have babies, play golf or tennis, swim, dance, go to the movies—in other words, live perfectly normal lives.

How long will it take me to get adjusted to the bag and using it?

A lot depends on your attitude. There will be mental as well as physical adjustments for you to make. It is not an easy adjustment, but a positive attitude helps a great deal. Usually, after a few months' time, you will be accustomed to the routine and it will be a regular part of your daily life. The sooner you accept the fact that your stoma is a part of you, the sooner this adjustment will take place.

Will having an ostomy affect my having sexual relations?

It depends upon a lot of factors—your sex, the extent of the surgery, your attitude, and your age, to mention a few. This is a topic you should discuss with your doctor before you have the operation. There are also three good booklets which are published by the United Ostomy Association, Inc. (2001 West Beverly Boulevard, Los Angeles, CA 90057; telephone 213 413-5510): "Sex, Courtship and the Single Ostomate," "Sex and the Male Ostomate," and "Sex, Pregnancy and the Female Ostomate."

Can I get any other information on ostomies?

The United Ostomy Association is a remarkable and active organization. Its entire reason for existence is to help people who have had ostomies. You can check your local telephone-directory yellow pages under "Associations" or "Social Service Organizations" for a local chapter of the United

Ostomy Association, or call the American Cancer Society in your area and ask them where the nearest chapter is located. If you are not able to locate a local ostomy group, write to the United Ostomy Association (address given in the preceding answer). The association has helpful literature about caring for your ostomy and information on the manufacturers of equipment which you will find most helpful. The American Cancer Society also has literature on this subject and often sponsors ostomy group meetings. Be sure to avail yourself of this help.

Will Medicare pay for my colostomy supplies?

Medicare will pay for colostomy equipment and other prosthetic devices to replace internal organs if you have taken the supplemental benefits under medical insurance, Part B.

Is chemotherapy or radiation therapy ever used in treating colon-rectal cancer?

There are some studies being carried out in which chemotherapy or radiation and chemotherapy are being used in treating colon-rectal cancer. Usually these treatments are used following surgery.

Is cancer of the small intestine common?

Cancer of the small intestine is much less common than those of the nearby organs: esophagus, stomach, pancreas, and colon. Cancers of the small intestine are almost always treatable and sometimes curable.

How are cancers of the small intestine staged?

There is no specific staging system for this kind of cancer. Cell type is a major factor in determining treatment.

What are the cell types of cancer of the small intestine?

There are three major types:
* Adenocarcinoma is the most common and usually produces symptoms of obstruction of the bowel.
* Lymphomas also produce symptoms of bowel obstruction as well as bleeding. The majority of these tumors are non-Hodgkin's lymphomas.

- Leiomyosarcomas may reach large size before diagnosis. Symptoms include bleeding and obstruction as well as weight loss, fever, and abdominal pain.

How is cancer of the small intestine treated?

Cancer of the small intestine is treated with surgery in most cases. Small-intestine lymphoma may be treated with surgery, radiation, or chemotherapy, mainly following the treatment used for lymphoma. If surgery is not feasible, small-intestine adenocarcinoma and leiomyosarcoma are treated with radiation therapy. Investigational treatments are available for cancer of the small intestine.

How is cancer of the anus treated?

Cancer of the anus is a highly treatable, often curable cancer. Its treatment depends on the stage of the disease. Stages of anal cancer describe whether the cancer has remained within the anus, has spread to lymph nodes near the anus, or has spread to other sites or organs. The stage of anal cancer is important in determining the first treatment. Surgery and radiation therapy are the primary treatments. Chemotherapy is also used, usually as an investigational treatment. Since cancer of the anus is uncommon, most physicians have limited experience with this tumor.

BLADDER CANCER

What is the function of the bladder?

The urinary bladder is the reservoir for the urine. It is located in the front part of the pelvic cavity. It is elastic and increases in size as the urine accumulates. It is the seat of many disorders, including bladder stones, tumors, infections (or cystitis), obstruction, and paralysis.

What are the symptoms of bladder cancer?

Bloody urine is often a first sign, although bloody urine can also be the sign of many other urinary problems. The color can range from a smoky shade to deep red. There is usually no accompanying pain, and the amount of blood does not usually relate to the size of the tumor. Any sign of blood in the urine, even if it happens only once, is a warning to see your doctor immediately so that whatever condition is present can be treated. Bloody urine can also be a sign of conditions such as tumors, infections, or bladder stones. Other symptoms of bladder cancer include a change in bladder habits with an increase in the frequency of urination and, rarely, retention of urine or incontinence.

Who is most likely to get bladder cancer?

Bladder cancer occurs most frequently in persons between 50 and 70 years of age. Four of every five patients are men. There are two main types of cancer of the bladder—papillary and transitional-cell carcinoma. Less frequently found are squamous-cell carcinoma and adenocarcinoma.

What is papillary cancer of the bladder?

This is the most common type and the most easily cured. It starts on the bladder wall but grows into the bladder cavity and remains attached to the bladder wall by a mushroomlike stem. This type of tumor may be single or multiple, pea-sized or large enough to occupy the entire bladder. The tumor cells appear to be almost normal.

Are most bladder tumors found to be cancerous?

No. Many bladder tumors are found to be benign. However, benign tumors may become malignant. The doctor can often detect the change of a lesion by doing a cystoscopy. When seen with the cystoscope, the growths may appear to be like a series of warts, with the larger ones taking on a cauliflower appearance.

Is bladder cancer likely to metastasize to other parts of the body?

Fortunately most bladder cancers are slow-growing and do not tend to spread to other parts of the body as do other cancers. Metastases usually are found first in the pelvic lymph nodes and usually remain localized there for a long time. Early detection and removal is the easiest and surest cure, since bladder cancer can spread to the lung, bones, and liver.

Is it unusual for bladder tumors to recur?

There is a great tendency for bladder tumors to recur either in the same location or in some other part of the bladder. Most of these growths are noncancerous, and many that are malignant are slow-growing. Most recurrences can be treated easily and successfully.

How is a diagnosis of bladder cancer made?

A urologist usually performs an examination with a cystoscope, which allows him to inspect the lining of the urinary bladder. If any suspicious-looking areas or growths are observed, a piece of tissue is removed for microscopic examination without major surgery. The examination involves little time or discomfort. Cystograms, made after filling the bladder with an opaque solution, give further information about the size of the tumor and the width of its base. Intravenous pyelograms can be done to outline the ureters and upper urinary tract. Microscopic study (cytology) of the urine for presence of cancer cells sloughed off by the bladder is routine.

How is bladder cancer treated?

There are so many different types and stages of bladder cancer that therapy varies widely among individual patients. A single papillary tumor may be successfully treated by electrically destroying the tissue. When the tumor is malignant and extensive, it may be necessary to remove the entire bladder. Multiple tumors, even at an early stage, are usually treated by surgical removal of the tumors themselves as well as surrounding tissue. Following surgery, a solution containing an anticancer drug may be instilled into the bladder to decrease the chance of the tumors recurring. If surgery is not available, radiation therapy can be used to destroy the cancer. Tumor-killing doses of radiation can be delivered to the bladder without excessive damage to overlying tissues, permitting the cure of some advanced tumors not suited to surgical removal. Radioisotopes and chemotherapy are also used in the treatment of bladder cancer. Sometimes radiation is used before the operation in bladder cancer.

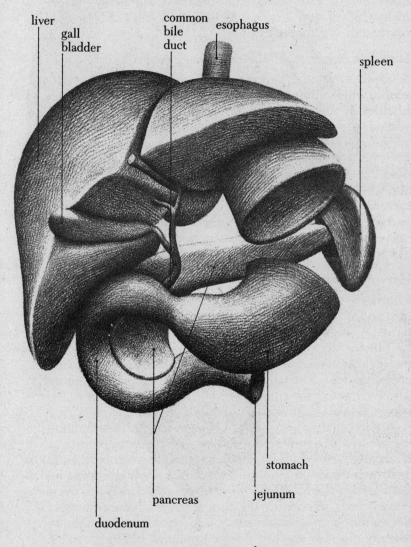

liver

gall
bladder

common
bile
duct

esophagus

spleen

duodenum

pancreas

stomach

jejunum

Front view, major internal organs

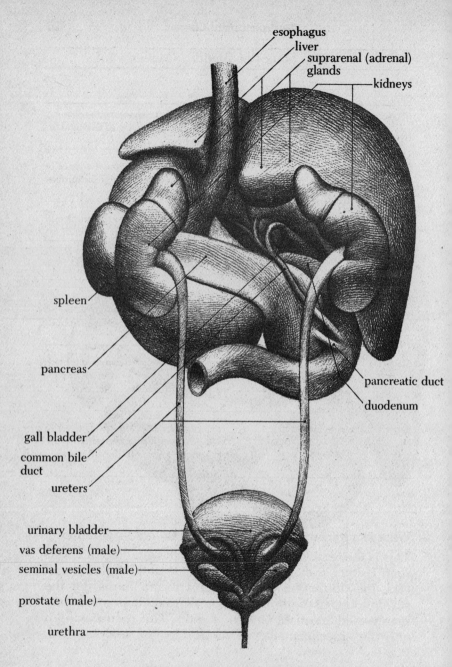

esophagus
liver
suprarenal (adrenal) glands
kidneys

spleen

pancreas

pancreatic duct

duodenum

gall bladder

common bile duct

ureters

urinary bladder

vas deferens (male)

seminal vesicles (male)

prostate (male)

urethra

Rear view, major internal organs

The Stages of Bladder Cancer

STAGE		EXPLANATION
Stage 0		Carcinoma in situ, representing changes in cells on the surface of the bladder wall
Stage A	Stage I T1, N0, M0	Tumor shows microscopic evidence of minimum invasion beyond the surface of the bladder wall.
Stage B1	Stage II T2, N0, M0	Tumor has invaded into the surface of the muscle of the bladder wall.
Stage B2	Stage III T3a, N0, M0	Tumor has invaded into the deep segments of muscle of the bladder wall.
Stage C	Stage III T3b, N0, M0	Tumor has invaded throughout the entire thickness of the bladder wall and beyond the wall into the fat surrounding the bladder.
Stage D1	Stage IV T4, N0, M0 Any T, N1–3, M0 Any T, any N, M1	Tumor has invaded through the bladder wall to nearby organs or has involved lymph nodes in the pelvis.
Stage D2	See above	Tumor has spread from the bladder to tissues beyond the pelvis into the upper abdomen or more distant parts.

What is a transurethral resection (TUR) and fulguration?

This is the removal of a bladder growth with electrical current. Using a cystoscope, which is passed through the urethra, the doctor removes the growth and burns out the surrounding tissue with electric current. It is most commonly used on small, benign growths. This is successful if only the superficial layer of the bladder has been invaded.

Treatment Choices for Cancer of the Bladder

STAGE	POSSIBLE TREATMENTS
Stage 0	Surgery, with or without chemotherapy or immunotherapy within the bladder Chemotherapy alone within the bladder Radiation therapy for selected patients Investigational treatments available
Stage A	Surgery, with or without chemotherapy or immunotherapy within the bladder Radium implant, with or without radiation therapy Chemotherapy alone within the bladder Radiation therapy for selected patients Investigational treatments available
Stage B1	Surgery Radiation before surgery Radium implant and/or radiation therapy for selected patients Investigational treatment available
Stage B2	Surgery with or without radiation before operation Radiation therapy for selected patients Radium implants in selected patients, usually with radiation treatment Investigational treatments, including chemotherapy, available
Stage C	Surgery with or without radiation before operation Radiation therapy for selected patients Radium implants in selected patients, usually with radiation treatment Investigational treatments including chemotherapy available
Stage D1	Surgery with or without radiation before operation Radiation treatment Chemotherapy alone or in addition to other treatments Investigational treatments available
Stage D2	Radiation treatment for symptoms Surgery for symptoms Chemotherapy alone or with other treatments Investigational treatments available
Recurrent bladder cancer	Investigational treatments available

After this treatment your doctor will ask you to return every 3 to 4 months, because new tumors have been known to grow in the same vicinity in about one-quarter of all cases. If no recurrences are found after a year, the intervals between examinations may be lengthened gradually.

What surgical procedures are used if the cancer is more extensive?

Depending on where the cancer is located and how far it has advanced, the doctor will perform either a segmental resection or a cystectomy.

What is involved in a segmental resection?

A segmental resection is used only if the tumor is localized in one area of the bladder with an adequate margin of tissue that can be removed from around the tumor. This operation is performed through a lower-abdominal incision and, when complete, the patient is left with a portion of the bladder and therefore can maintain urinary control. When this is not possible, then a cystectomy is necessary.

What is a cystectomy?

The operation for removal of the bladder is called a cystectomy. In order to remove all the tissue containing the cancer safely and completely, it is sometimes necessary also to operate on other nearby parts of the body. In women, this may mean the removal of the ovaries, fallopian tubes, and uterus, as well as a portion of the vagina which contains the urethra. In men, the prostate and seminal vesicles may also be removed. If the tumor is near the opening of the bladder neck or involves areas of the bladder lining, the urethra may also be removed. A cystectomy is a major operation, but with modern surgical techniques and anesthetics, it can be carried out successfully.

Is radiation sometimes used before surgery?

Preoperative radiotherapy has been found to produce partial or even complete destruction of tumors of the bladder and is sometimes used before a cystectomy is performed.

How long will I remain in the hospital after my cystectomy?

Usually the recovery period lasts 2 or 3 weeks.

What anesthesia is used for bladder operation?

Usually spinal anesthesia is used. General anesthesia may also be recommended.

Where is the incision?

The incision begins in the midline, above the navel, and extends to the level of the pubic bone.

How long does the operation take?

This is a complicated operation which takes between 5 and 6 hours to perform.

How long will the stomach tube remain in place after surgery?

This tube, placed through your nose and into your stomach to drain the gastric juices and prevent accumulation of air and fluid in your stomach, usually remains in place after surgery for 5 to 7 days, until your bowels have regained normal activity. This will allow your stomach and bowels to rest and give the connection time to heal.

What special preparations are made before surgery?

Usually, you are admitted to the hospital a few days before the scheduled surgery. Daily enemas and laxatives will be given to you. In addition, you may be given antibiotics to reduce the amount of bacteria in your system. A special diet and vitamin supplements will be ordered for you. Your doctor or nurse may ask you to test a sample appliance to ensure that the area chosen for your stoma is on the flattest possible surface and provides maximum comfort for your various normal activities.

How is urine stored and emptied when one has had a cystectomy?

The surgeon removes a small section of the small intestine and converts it into a conduit, or pipeline, for urine. The ureters—tubes that carry urine from each kidney to the bladder—are joined to one end of the segment. The other end is brought out through the wall of the abdomen, near the navel, where it forms an opening called a stoma. A flat

bag is placed over the opening to collect the urine. The bag
is held to the body with a special type of glue.

**Does this mean I'll have to wear a bag outside my body to
collect the urine?**

Yes. Though this is a large change in lifestyle, most patients
find that they can adjust to the change once they understand
that the existence of a stoma on the abdomen and a collection device over it need not be limiting or disabling.
Hundreds of patients of all ages have had to face this adjustment and have found that they can handle it and resume
normal activities.

Can I have a say in where the opening is placed?

Your doctor will usually discuss this with you, since the site
should be determined before the operation. Generally it is
located either in the right lower or upper abdomen. It should
be placed where, when the collection appliance is attached,
movements such as sitting, standing, twisting, and bending
will not pull the appliance loose. It should not be located
near an old scar or attached near rolls of fat. This should
all be discussed with your doctor before the operation.

**Will I be rigged to a urine-collection device when I leave
the operating room?**

The temporary appliance will be placed over your stoma
in the recovery room. This appliance will be connected to
a continuous drainage bag that will be emptied of urine by
one of the nurses or nurse's aides. For the first few days
someone else will take care of you and your stoma. As you
gain strength you will be taught how to do this yourself. It
is important that you learn to care for your appliance and
have confidence in it before you leave the hospital.

**Is there any way I can try the appliance out before the
operation?**

Yes. The nurse can help you try out the appliance. She can
apply it and put water in the pouch to simulate the weight
of the urine. You can dress yourself and try doing some of
your normal activities. This trial is a good way to eliminate
your own anxieties about wearing the appliance. Keep in

mind that there are many different types of appliances and many different solutions. You may need to try several before you find one that suits you. The United Ostomy Association (2001 West Beverly Boulevard, Los Angeles, CA 90057; tel. 213-413-5510) publishes several helpful booklets listed on page 516.

How often should the appliance be emptied?

About every 2 hours.

What happens to the appliance during sleep?

Usually during sleep the appliance is connected to drainage tubing attached to a bottle placed on the floor beside the bed. Running the tubing under the leg allows greater freedom of movement. Most patients find they can sleep in any position once they are accustomed to wearing their appliances.

Does the urine look the same as before?

It does not look exactly the same as urine from the bladder, since the conduit through which it passes is made from a segment of the small intestine, which secretes mucus. This mucous membrane is sensitive, and urination can cause mucus as well as slight amounts of blood to appear in the urine. Check with your doctor if there are changes in the consistency or color of the urine or a decrease in the amount of drainage.

Should I get a spare appliance?

Yes. It is a good idea to have one to wear and one to keep ready for use. This ensures that the one to be applied will be well dried and aired. You'll find you need a new appliance about every 6 months.

Can I bathe and shower as usual?

Yes. You can bathe and shower with or without the appliance. If the stoma seems irritated, remove the appliance and soak yourself in a tub of warm water.

How does a cystectomy affect a man's ability to function sexually?

It depends upon the extent of the operation. Sometimes sexual function may be impaired even though the penis is left intact. You should discuss this point with your doctor before he performs the operation so that you will know how extensive the surgery will be.

Are women still able to function sexually?

Sexual activity may be possible, but it could be impaired if a portion of the vagina is removed. Again, this is a topic which you should discuss with your doctor before the operation is performed.

Is it usual for a patient to be depressed after this kind of operation?

It is not unusual to feel depressed. As a result of the depression, the patient's attention span may be short, and he or she may have difficulty in concentrating and be irritable. It is important for the family and friends to realize that this is a temporary but normal feeling. An inability to cope with the new way the body functions may reinforce the thought that the person may never be able to cope with anything again. The depression is usually short-lived and subsides when the patient finds that family and friends accept him or her and that he or she can return to a normal way of life.

KIDNEY CANCER

What is the function of the kidneys?

There are two kidneys, one on each side of the back portion of the abdomen, located rather high in the loin. Their function is to filter waste products from the blood, returning to the circulating blood those substances that are necessary for normal chemical balance. The central portion of each kidney is hollow and receives the body fluids. The urine leaves the kidney and passes down its ureter—a long tubular structure—which connects with the bladder.

What are the symptoms of kidney tumors?

Four symptoms can warn the patient of the possibility of kidney tumors: persistent pain in the area over the kidneys, either in the back or along the side of the body; blood in the urine; a feeling of a lump or mass in the kidney region; and fever or weight loss.

Are all kidney tumors cancerous?

No. Many are benign. The benign growths often are filled with fluid and can be classified as cysts. They vary in size. However, malignancy cannot always be determined without surgery.

How is cancer of the kidney diagnosed?

The doctor will usually assess kidney and bladder function with an intravenous pyelogram. Blood studies will be made to reveal the presence of anemia. Urinalysis, renal arteriography, and scans are sometimes recommended. Because cancer of the kidney is difficult to diagnose, it has been labeled the "internist's tumor."

The Stages of Cancer of the Kidney

STAGE	OTHER CLASSIFICATIONS	EXPLANATION
Stage I	T1, N0, M0	Cancer is confined to the kidney.
Stage II	T2, N0, M0	Cancer has spread into the fat surrounding the kidney and/or other tissues but not to the nearby lymph nodes or blood vessels.
Stage III	T1–T2, N1, M0 T3a, N0, M0 T3b–c, N1, M0	Cancer has spread from the kidney into surrounding tissue and has involved the renal vein, other vessels, or the nearby lymph nodes.
Stage IV	Any T, any N, M1 T4, any N, M0	Cancer has invaded surrounding organs or has spread to distant sites.

Treatment Choices for Cancer of the Kidney

STAGE	POSSIBLE TREATMENTS
Stage I	Surgery Radiation treatment if surgery is not done Investigational treatments available
Stage II	Surgery Radiation therapy before or after operation for selected patients Radiation treatment if surgery is not done Investigational treatments available
Stage III	Surgery with or without radiation therapy Radiation therapy for symptoms Investigational treatments available
Stage IV	Surgery Radiation therapy for symptoms Investigational treatments, including new chemotherapy drugs and biologicals such as interferon
Recurrent	Investigational treatments, including new chemotherapy drugs or biological agents

What symptoms are indicative of tumors of the ureter?

Usually blood in the urine, pain in the flank, and finally obstruction to the flow of urine to the bladder. This is an uncommon form of cancer and usually necessitates the removal of the kidney on the same side as the affected ureter.

Can one live normally if a kidney is removed?

Fortunately, people can live perfectly normal lives with only one healthy kidney.

What is kidney removal called?

The medical term is *nephrectomy*, and it is considered a major operation.

Are nephrectomies done only for cancer?

No.

What kind of incision is made for this operation?

The incision extends from the loin, just below the last rib and above the hipbone, around onto the abdomen.

What anesthesia is usually used?

General anesthesia is usually used for this operation.

Are other treatments besides surgery ever used for cancer of the kidney?

Sometimes, a course of radiotherapy will be done before surgery. Postoperative radiotherapy, chemotherapy, and immunotherapy are being used in some hospitals in addition to surgery. The use of a biological response modifier, called interleukin-2, to activate killer white cells has shown some response in people with renal cell cancer. This investigational treatment is presently in preliminary trials.

What is adrenocortical cancer?

It is cancer of the outer layer of the adrenal glands, which are located near the kidneys. This rare cancer usually occurs in adults and is often curable when detected at an early stage. Since the majority of adrenocortical tumors do not secrete steroid and/or sex hormones, tests for hormone levels play an important role in diagnosis, treatment, and follow-up. Treatment consists of surgery followed by hormonal treatments. Sometimes chemotherapy is given for more extensive disease.

STOMACH CANCER

Where is the stomach located?

The stomach is a pouchlike organ which makes up a relatively small part of the intestinal tract. It lies below the diaphragm in the left upper part of the abdomen, crossing over to the right below the liver. The stomach hangs comparatively free in the abdominal cavity and moves with breathing.

What symptoms indicate the possibility of stomach cancer?

Unfortunately, the symptoms of stomach cancer are often vague and nonspecific. The most common symptom of stomach cancer is indigestion. This may consist of a sense of discomfort or mild pain, fullness or bloating, burping, slight nausea, heartburn, or loss of appetite. Of course these are signs which we find easy to ignore, but if they persist— even intermittently—for a period of 2 weeks, your doctor should be consulted. Later signs might include blood in the stools or vomiting, rapid weight loss, and severe pain. These symptoms may also indicate the presence of an ulcer.

How is the diagnosis made?

A careful history and physical and rectal examination come first. Laboratory tests such as red and white blood cell count and analysis of the acidity of stomach contents will be or-

The General Stages of Cancer of the Stomach

STAGE	OTHER CLASSIFICATIONS	EXPLANATION
Stage I	T1, N0, M0	Tumor is confined to the lining and connective tissue of the stomach. There is no regional or distant metastasis.
Stage II	T2, N0, M0 T3, N0, M0	Tumor involves the stomach wall but has not penetrated through it. There are no regional or distant metastases.
Stage III	T1–3, N1–2, M0 T4a, N0–2, M0	Tumor has penetrated the stomach wall and invaded nearby structures. There is no distant metastasis. There may be regional metastasis.
Stage IV	T1–3, N3, M0 T4b, any N, M0 Any T and N, M1	The tumor has penetrated the stomach wall and invaded nearby structures and spread to liver and other organs.

dered. The most important of all diagnostic methods is the x-ray examination, with the radiologist observing the flow of barium under the fluoroscope with x-rays of various areas of the stomach taken from different angles with the patient in various positions. Gastroscopy, in which a flexible instrument is passed into the stomach for viewing, along with a diagnostic procedure known as exfoliate cytology, is sometimes used. Cytology allows the examination through a microscope of cells shed by the lining of the stomach. In order to collect the cells, a gastric washing is done. An abrasive brush or balloon is introduced into the stomach and the stomach lining is gently scraped. The material collected is studied by a pathologist to determine if malignant cells are present.

How is cancer of the stomach usually treated?

The usual treatment for cancer of the stomach is prompt surgical removal of the malignant tumor. The operation usually involves the removal of a part or all of the stomach, depending on the location of the malignancy. Sometimes parts of other abdominal organs, such as spleen and pancreas, are removed if they are in the area of the tumor and are believed to be affected.

Is any other treatment recommended?

It depends upon the location and extent of the tumor. Sometimes chemotherapy is used following surgery. Some experimental work is being done with implantation of radioactive sources into the malignant stomach tumor to give relief from pain in patients whose cancers are inoperable. Stomach cancers usually are considered resistant to x-rays, since a radiation dose safe for the surrounding normal tissues is not strong enough to destroy the cancer.

Do doctors sometimes suspect cancer of the stomach and find a benign tumor?

Yes. Preoperative x-ray examinations cannot always distinguish a malignant tumor from a harmless benign tumor. Furthermore, x-rays occasionally will give the appearance of a tumor but an ulcer may be discovered at surgery.

Is the same operation performed for ulcer of the stomach and stomach cancer?

This depends on the extent of the stomach cancer. The same procedure—removal of the stomach—is usually performed for either condition.

Do stomach ulcers lead to stomach cancer?

This is a question over which there has been much speculation. Most doctors feel that the danger of stomach ulcers rests not so much in the possibility that an ulcer may lead to malignancy, but rather that it may be cancerous even while being treated as an ulcer.

What is the difference in the usual treatment between a stomach ulcer and a duodenal ulcer?

A duodenal ulcer can be treated conservatively for long periods of time without the fear of cancer. A stomach ulcer must be followed closely. A patient is usually put on a strict diet, given appropriate medication, and subjected to further x-ray examination every 2 to 4 weeks. If a clean x-ray picture does not result from this treatment within a few weeks, an exploratory operation is usually performed to determine whether there is a malignancy.

How can a person live without a stomach?

Quite successfully. Sometimes, only a section of the stomach is removed. However, when necessary, the entire stomach is removed. The patient is required to eat smaller, more frequent meals—perhaps half as much food at each meal as previously. The patient learns to eat more often and more slowly and adjusts to this way of life quite easily.

What must be done to prepare for stomach surgery?

Patients are usually admitted to the hospital a few days before the scheduled operation. They are put on a liquid diet and the stomach is washed out with a stomach tube once or twice daily. Often intravenous medications, vitamins, and blood transfusions are given prior to the operation.

Can the doctor tell immediately if there is a malignancy?

It is usually necessary to wait several days for the pathological examination of the stomach to determine if cancer is present.

Is the postoperative period for a stomach operation uncomfortable?

There is likely to be discomfort caused by the use of stomach tubes, intravenous feedings, and injections. Food and drink is usually withheld for 2 to 4 days. For at least the first 3 to 4 months, small, frequent feedings are recommended. The patient can then gradually return to a normal diet of bland foods. Spicy foods and alcohol should be avoided. The doctor may prescribe the addition of iron and liver extract to the diet.

What is the dumping syndrome?

Following gastrectomy, some patients develop what is known as the "dumping syndrome"—weakness, dizziness, sweating, nausea, vomiting, palpitation—which occurs when the remnant of the stomach empties itself of food too quickly. This can usually be controlled by frequent small feedings and by a high-protein diet with the addition of dry foods and fluids between feedings.

How long is the convalescence period following extensive stomach surgery?

The patient will usually be able to return to normal activity after about 2 months.

Treatment Choices for Stomach Cancer

STAGE	POSSIBLE TREATMENTS
Stage 0	Surgical removal of all or part of the stomach
Stage I	Surgical removal of all or part of the stomach Investigational treatments available
Stage II	Surgical removal of all or part of the stomach Investigational treatment with adjuvant chemotherapy available

Treatment Choices for Stomach Cancer

STAGE	POSSIBLE TREATMENTS
Stage III	Radical surgery unless nodal involvement is confined to the immediate vicinity of the tumor Investigational chemotherapy and radiation therapy
Stage IV	Surgery to remove obstruction or to reduce the risk of bleeding Investigational chemotherapy
Recurrent	Investigational studies testing new anticancer drugs and biologicals

LIVER CANCER

What does the liver do?

The liver performs more complex functions than any other organ of the body except the brain. It breaks down worn-out red blood cells and converts them into bile. It produces proteins essential to proper blood clotting. It regulates the level of many hormones. It stores sugar and regulates the amount which circulates in the blood. It controls the metabolism of cholesterol. It stores vitamins A, D, E, and K. In fact, the functions of the liver are so many and varied that it is almost impossible to test them all in the clinical laboratory.

Where is the liver located?

It fills the upper right side of the diaphragm and is protected on both the right and left sides by the rib cage.

Can one function without a liver?

No, it is not possible to function without any liver. However, one can live normally with as little as 15 to 20 percent of the normal liver. The liver's powers of recuperation are truly amazing.

Can cysts on the liver be removed?

Yes, most cysts can be successfully removed.

Are all tumors of the liver cancerous?

Tumors of the liver may be malignant or benign. Cancer of the liver itself is rare in the United States; the cancer usually has started elsewhere in the body and spread to the liver. Benign tumors are usually small, produce no symptoms, and may be discovered only during the course of another operation. Such tumors are usually not removed. Suspected malignant cancer of the liver alerts the doctor to the possibility of cancer elsewhere in the body. Cancers of the lung, breast, or gastrointestinal system can spread to the liver.

Is cancer of the liver and cancer which has spread to the liver treated in the same way?

No. They are two very different problems. Cancer of the breast which has spread to the liver is treated in the same way as breast cancer with metastases would be treated. Liver cancer—that is, cancer which has started in the liver and not metastasized there from some other organ—is treated as liver cancer. Many people whose cancer has spread to the liver from some other place think they also have liver cancer. This is not true.

What symptoms alert the doctor to the possibility of liver problems?

Vague discomfort in the upper abdomen on the right side, which becomes more acute with deep breathing, is one possible symptom. Sometimes an enlarged liver can be felt as a hard lump just below the rib cage on the right side. If the tumor is located under the diaphragm, pain can sometimes be felt around the right shoulder blade. Jaundice, which produces a yellowish look to the skin, may develop.

Will cirrhosis of the liver turn to cancer?

No. Cirrhosis of the liver will often be found in patients who have cancer of the liver. However, only about 4 percent of the patients who have cirrhosis of the liver later develop cancer. In cirrhosis of the liver, the liver may be badly scarred or swollen. Cirrhosis of the liver may be the result of a severe case of hepatitis, or may be caused by heavy drinking or by drugs such as carbon tetrachloride (cleaning fluid), chlorpromazine (a tranquilizer), or isoniazid (a tu-berculosis drug). Damage leads to an obstruction of the liver, which prevents the normal rate of flow of blood through the liver. Surgery can help by lessening the quantity of blood delivered through the liver. Relief of the blood load often permits the liver to recover its normal function.

How is cancer of the liver diagnosed?

A needle biopsy is sometimes used to determine whether the liver is cancerous. A careful history and physical examination, radiography, endoscopy, angiography, tomograms, biochemical tests of the liver, liver scans—all can be employed in making a diagnosis.

Will the doctor attempt to remove the primary growth if he finds metastases to the liver?

It depends on the location of the primary tumor and the condition of the patient. Extensive surgery may be too debilitating when metastases have spread to other parts of the body.

What treatment is possible if a cancer is found in the liver?

If cancer is confined to a segment or a lobe, surgical removal may be indicated.

What other forms of treatment may be recommended?

Regional chemotherapy—that is, chemicals introduced directly into the arteries which are supplying the tumor—is sometimes used successfully to deprive the tumor-bearing area of oxygen and some of its nutrient supply. The chemotherapy may be put into a "pump" which is implanted in the body.

CANCER OF THE PANCREAS

What is the pancreas?

It is a pulpy, flat gland about 5 inches long by a few inches high, which lies far back on the rear wall of the upper abdominal cavity. The part it plays in the body is a vital and specialized one. It manufactures digestive juices which are passed through the pancreatic duct into the intestine for digestion of proteins, fats, and carbohydrates. Insulin, which is essential for the utilization of sugar, is manufactured in the pancreas and deposited directly into the bloodstream. A duct, called the pancreatic duct, runs through the entire length of the pancreas. The pancreas is often referred to as having a head, a body, and a tail. The head fits into the curve of the duodenum on the right, close to the common bile duct, and the tail curves up toward the spleen. At the head of the pancreas there is often a branching of the main pancreatic duct. These ducts are responsible for collecting the digestive juices manufactured by the gland and depositing them through their openings into the small intestine.

What are the symptoms of cancer of the pancreas?

A variety of symptoms that can also be the signals of diseases other than cancer of the pancreas, as well as the hidden location of the pancreas, combine to make cancer difficult to diagnose. For this reason, pancreatic cancer is often advanced before it is detected. Cancer in the head of the pancreas, because it involves the common bile duct, usually causes jaundice, and often there is intense itching of the skin. There may be some abdominal pain and discomfort, nausea, diarrhea, belching, a feeling of fullness, and intolerance of fatty foods. Weight loss, loss of appetite, and loss of strength or energy may be other symptoms. The color of the bowel movement may be affected, being foamy, clay-colored, or, more rarely, silvery in color. All of these symptoms might also be present when there are cysts or benign tumors in the pancreas. Another set of symptoms can present themselves in cases where the tumor is located in the body portion of the pancreas. Severe back pain may be present as the result of the size of the tumor. The pain may worsen after eating or when lying down and be slightly relieved when bending forward or sitting. The disease is so difficult to diagnose that the majority of patients are treated for 3 to 6 months for other causes before actual diagnosis of the pancreatic cancer is made.

What tests will the doctor need?

The doctor will usually order barium x-rays, liver-function studies, and angiography to determine more clearly where the tumor is located.

Can cysts in the pancreas turn into cancer?

Rarely will a cyst in the pancreas become cancerous. Usually, cysts can be removed successfully with a good chance of recovery. If allowed to remain they can continue to grow and cause serious problems in pancreatic activity. It is important to remember that all cysts, tumors, or inflammations of the pancreas do not indicate the presence of cancer.

Can the doctor tell whether or not the condition of the pancreas is cancerous before he operates?

Usually he cannot. Benign tumors and growths often grow in the pancreas, causing the cells that produce insulin to overproduce, causing symptoms that include intense hunger, trembling, fainting, confusion, or convulsions. The operation to remove a cyst is a low-risk one. However, if the presence of cancerous cells is found, it may be necessary to operate so as to bypass the obstruction or to remove the entire gland. Then it becomes a complicated operation.

What kinds of cancer of the pancreas are there?

There are two kinds of cancer of the pancreas: islet-cell carcinoma of the endocrine pancreas and adenocarcinoma of the exocrine pancreas. Cancer of the endocrine pancreas is a highly treatable and often curable collection of tumors. Cancer of the exocrine pancreas, on the other hand, is much more difficult to treat and is not often curable.

How does the doctor decide if there is cancer in the pancreas?

The only certain way at present is through a biopsy—which in this case requires a laparotomy. However, many experimental programs are under way to help aid better diagnosis, such as endoscopy, ultrasound, CT scans, and CEA. Doctors agree that ultrasound looks promising in diagnosing small pancreatic cancers earlier.

What is a laparotomy?

A laparotomy is a surgical operation to open the abdominal cavity either to make an inspection or to perform surgery.

What does the incision look like, and where is it?

The incision for a laparotomy is about 4 or 5 inches long and is located in the upper abdomen.

The doctor says I'll need more than one operation. Why?

Sometimes operations for cancer of the pancreas are done in several steps.

How long does the operation take?

The operation to remove a localized tumor or cyst of the pancreas takes 1 to 3 hours. If the entire pancreas is to be removed, the operation can take anywhere from 3 to 6 hours.

What happens when the entire gland is removed?

The operation to remove the entire gland and the adjacent duodenum, called a pancreaticoduodenectomy, is one of the most extensive in all surgery. The bile duct and the stomach are both reconnected into the small intestine. This is a high-risk operation, not often performed. It can be successful in those cases in which the tumor has not spread to other organs.

Can a person live with only part of the pancreas or without the pancreas?

Yes, an active, comfortable existence is possible when medicines are prescribed to substitute for the function of the pancreas.

What happens if the cancer has spread beyond the pancreas?

If the cancer has spread and is in places where it cannot be removed, the prognosis is very serious.

Would the doctor advise against surgery?

Since this cancer is so difficult to diagnose, surgery is usually a necessity. If cancer is not the cause, the surgery will determine this happy diagnosis. If cancer is the cause, the doctor can at least relieve the jaundice and the exasperating itching through surgery, even when the cancer cannot be removed. Sometimes, when the patient is elderly or has other health problems which put him in a high-risk category, surgery will not be attempted.

What sort of operation is performed?

If possible, the tumor of the pancreas, the surrounding bile duct, and part of the stomach and intestine are removed, and everything is rejoined. If that is not possible, a new opening is made for the bile, to relieve the jaundice and help in the digestive process.

What are the chances for cure of exocrine cancer of the pancreas?

Of course it depends upon many factors. However, it is important for the patient with exocrine pancreatic cancer to understand the seriousness of the condition and the risks. Because it is usually found late and has frequently spread to nearby organs, the five-year survival rate at the present time is only 2 percent.

The Stages of Adenocarcinoma of Exocrine Pancreas

STAGE	OTHER CLASSIFICATIONS	EXPLANATION
Stage I	T1-2, N0, M0	Cancer is entirely confined to the pancreas or has directly spread to involve nearby organs, but in either case can be removed by surgery
Stage II	T3, N0, M0	Cancer has directly spread further to involve nearby organs but it cannot be removed by surgery
Stage III	T1-2, N1, M0	Cancer involves regional lymph nodes
Stage IV	T1-3, N0-1, M1	Cancer has spread to the extent that it cannot be treated entirely by surgery or radiotherapy. It has usually spread to the liver, peritoneum or other sites.

Treatment of Adenocarcinoma of Exocrine Pancreas

STAGE	POSSIBLE TREATMENT
Stage I	Radical surgery
	Investigational: surgery followed by radiation therapy, surgery and radiation therapy during operation, surgery followed by radiation therapy and chemotherapy
Stage II	Surgery for symptoms followed by radiation therapy with or without chemotherapy
	Investigational: radiation therapy with radiosensitizers, radiation therapy during operation or implanting radioactive material, radiation therapy alone, chemotherapy alone
Stage III	Surgery or radiation for symptoms with or without chemotherapy
	Investigational: radiation therapy with or without radiosensitizers, chemotherapy, radiation during operation
Stage IV	Surgery or radiation for symptoms
	Investigational: New anticancer agents or biologicals

Will I need transfusions and other intravenous medication?

Yes. This is an extremely serious operation. Blood transfusions may be needed during and after the operation. Intravenous feedings, medications, and special drugs will be used to help speed recovery. You will usually not be allowed out of bed until several days after the operation.

What are the aftereffects when the pancreas is removed?

The recovery period will be a long one, and a permanent low-sugar, low-fat diet will be essential. Vitamin K will probably be prescribed. Because of the restricted diet, it is very difficult to gain weight, which makes recovery slower than usual.

When will I be able to get back to work?

Convalescence will take from 2 to 6 months. Physical exercise should be postponed for 4 to 6 months. About 2 months after the wound is completely healed, you will be able to resume some of your normal activities.

Will radiation therapy or chemotherapy be prescribed?

Sometimes radiation therapy is used after surgery. In other cases chemotherapy is used, either alone or in combination with the radiation therapy. The drug 5-Fluorouracil has been used with some success; other drugs are being evaluated.

Are most doctors qualified to diagnose and operate for pancreatic cancer?

This is a difficult diagnosis and a very specialized area. Major medical centers, especially those specializing in cancer treatment, have had more experience than smaller local hospitals. You should ask your doctor to check with the clinical cooperative groups in your area for information on new treatments or to see if you can be admitted into one of the controlled studies being conducted on pancreatic cancer. (See Chapter 23.)

chapter 16

Cancer of the Female Reproductive Organs

The entire female reproductive system is still a mystery to many women, even though we are reminded of its existence by monthly menstrual periods. Cancer can occur in a number of different areas in the reproductive system, and each type of cancer has different symptoms, different stages, and a different set of attendant problems. It is important for you to know exactly where the tumor is located, what the surgery will involve, and what treatment is being planned.

Cancer of the vulva includes that of the labia majora, the labia minora, and clitoris. Although it has been predominantly a disease of elderly women, it has recently become more common in women below the age of 40.

Because of its location, cancer of the vagina is often diagnosed early. If discovered and treated in its early stages, this cancer is often curable. The type of treatment given depends on the stage of the disease and how far it has spread from its original location.

Cervical cancer is a highly treatable, usually curable cancer. The regular use of Pap smears has helped to detect cancer of the cervix earlier, so that the cure rate has improved.

The lining of the uterus, called the endometrium, is a common site for cancer, accounting for 13 percent of all cancers in women. If diagnosed in the early stages, it is highly curable.

Because ovarian cancer is difficult to diagnose early and the symptoms may be overlooked, the disease may be well advanced before it is detected, making it more difficult to cure. It is especially important that staging and treatment of ovarian cancer be under the care of a gynecologic oncologist.

In whatever part of the reproductive system the cancer is located, it is helpful to learn exactly what the extent of the operation will be and what plans the physician has for treatment.

Questions to Ask Your Doctor Before Any Operation on the Female Reproductive Organs

- What size is the tumor and where is it located?
- Is it a cancerous tumor or is it benign?
- Has there been any spread?
- Will the ovaries be removed?
- Will this operation impair my ability to have a baby?
- Is there any chance that the ovaries can be saved?
- Will this operation impair my urinary function or control?
- Is the operation really necessary or is it elective?
- Is there an alternative way of treating this condition? Radiotherapy? Implant? Chemotherapy?
- Where will the scar be—and will it be horizontal or vertical?
- Will you show me on the diagram exactly where the problem is and what you are planning to remove?
- Will I still be able to have sexual intercourse?

Is the National Cancer Institute supporting any studies on cancer of the female reproductive organs?

The National Cancer Institute's clinical cooperative groups are presently conducting studies of new treatment methods for all female cancers. (See Chapter 23)

What kind of doctor should I see if I have cancer of the female reproductive organs?

Either a gynecologist or a surgeon whose specialty is in the area of gynecological cancer should be responsible for the primary treatment of your case; sometimes the specialist will be a gynecologic oncologist. If you will have a radium implant or radiation therapy, a therapeutic radiologist will also be involved. If you are being treated with chemotherapy, you will probably be referred to an oncologist or hematologist.

Which organs are involved in cancer of the female reproductive system?

The main organs involved in cancer of the female reproductive system are the following:
- Vulva
- Vagina
- Cervix (neck of uterus)
- Womb or endometrium (body of uterus)
- Ovaries and fallopian tubes

What is the vulva?

The vulva is the external fatty tissue around the outside of the vagina. It is made up of several structures, including the clitoris, the labia, and the hymen.

What is the vagina?

The vagina is the barrel-shaped female organ through which a woman has babies. It is also known as the birth canal.

What are the cervix and the endometrium?

The cervix and the endometrium are both part of the uterus, which is a hollow, pear-shaped muscular organ in which the fertilized egg attaches itself and develops during pregnancy. It is also called the womb. The cervix is the lower part of the uterus, located at the top of the vagina. It is the mouth of the womb. The endometrium is the lining of the body of the uterus.

What are the ovaries?

The ovaries are two almond-shaped female organs that produce estrogen and that once a month release an egg during ovulation.

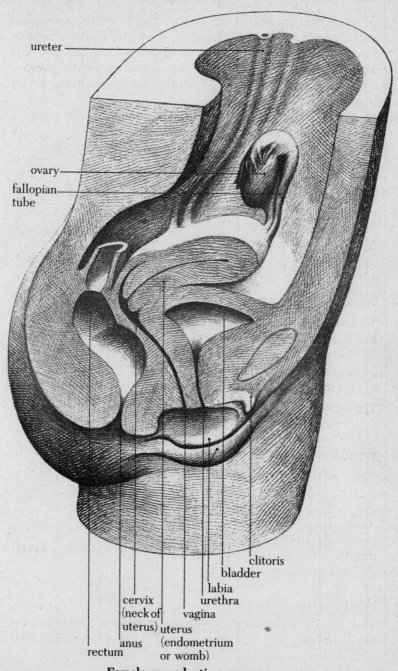

ureter

ovary

fallopian
tube

clitoris

bladder

labia
urethra

cervix
(neck of
uterus)

vagina

anus

rectum

uterus
(endometrium
or womb)

Female reproductive organs

Cancer of the Female Reproductive Organs

Type	High Risk	Symptoms	Diagnostic Tests	Treatments
Vulva	55–65 age group	Itching, burning, pain, bleeding	Pap smear, simple biopsy, colposcopy, dermatologic punch	Removal of skin of vulva, wide excision, laser beam therapy, radical vulvectomy and/or surgical removal of inguinal lymph nodes, radiation therapy
Vagina	50–70 age group; young women whose mothers took DES	Painless bleeding following intercourse or exam, bladder pain, frequent urination	Pap smear, colposcopy, iodine or Schiller's test, biopsy	Radiation, radium implant, surgery, laser
Cervix or neck of uterus (cervix, cervical canal, or entrance to womb)	40–49 age group; more than 5 pregnancies; early intercourse; multiple sex partners; young women whose mothers took DES	Unusual bleeding or discharge; pelvic pain	Pap smear, colposcopy, biopsy, conization. *Note:* Pap smear 97% accurate for this type of cancer.	Radiotherapy, surgery, chemotherapy and hormones, cryotherapy, laser
Body of uterus or womb (endometrium)	60–70 age group; women with diabetes or high blood pressure; overweight; Jewish women; few or no children; women who take replacement estrogen.	Unusual bleeding especially if past menopause; lower abdominal and back pain. *Note::* Fibroids and other nonmalignant conditions may cause same symptoms.	Vaginal pool smear, aspiration curettage, D&C. *Note:* Pap smear only 50% accurate for this type. Diagnostic results unreliable in menopausal women using estrogen.	Hysterectomy or preoperative radiation followed by hysterectomy and oophorectomy. Hormone therapy with surgery.

Fallopian tubes (uterine tubes)	Extremely rare	Profuse, intermittent watery discharge or bleeding	Diagnosis difficult. Positive Pap smear; usually requires operation to identify.	Hysterectomy and bilateral oophorectomy, radiation, and chemotherapy
Ovary	40–70 age group; history of ovarian imbalance or malfunction; no pregnancies; history of breast cancer	No symptoms except vague abdominal discomfort or indigestion. Advanced symptoms: abdominal pain and swelling.	Diagnosis difficult. Physical exam only method for detection. Positive diagnosis requires exploratory laparotomy. Ultrasound has been used in experimental studies in London.	Hysterectomy and oophorectomy. Important to be treated by gynecologic oncologist. Best results in university hospitals. Radiation sometimes used. Chemotherapy used following surgery. Difficult to cure.
Choriocarcinoma	Asian women, women over 40	Abnormal vaginal bleeding following abortion or childbirth. Uterus size out of proportion for pregnancy stage.	Biopsy, ultrasound, isotope scan, HCG tests	Chemotherapy or hysterectomy, depending on future fertility desires

Operations for Cancer of the Female Reproductive Organs

OPERATION	PROCEDURE	YOU SHOULD KNOW
Surgical conization or cold-knife conization	Removal of localized preinvasive lesion	More extensive than simple biopsy; performed under general anesthesia. May be done instead of hysterectomy. Pregnancy possible but should be discussed.
Subtotal or supracervical hysterectomy	Uterus is removed, but cervix remains	Will be unable to bear children. Normal sexual relations.
Vaginal hysterectomy	Uterus removed through vagina	Not advisable if uterus is enlarged or not fully movable. More difficult to perform than hysterectomy.
Total hysterectomy	Removal of cervix and uterus	Unable to bear children. Will not menstruate. Normal sexual relations.
Radical hysterectomy, also called Wertheim's operation	Removal of uterus, fallopian tubes, and ovaries as well as much of tissue surrounding uterus, regional lymph nodes, and part of vagina	Because of extent of operation, greater chance of postoperative complications. If done on premenopausal woman, causes abrupt menopause. Will be unable to bear children. Sexual relations still possible.
Myomectomy	Fibroid tumors removed from wall of uterus but uterus left intact	Usually recommended for younger women with fibroid tumors who wish to retain ability to become pregnant.
Oophorectomy, also called ovariectomy	Removal of one or both ovaries	Abrupt menopause if both ovaries removed. If only one ovary removed, may still become pregnant; may continue to menstruate. Normal sexual relations.

Salpingectomy or bilateral salpingo oophorectomy	Removal of both fallopian tubes and ovaries	Menstruation ceases. Unable to reproduce. Normal sexual relations.
Simple vulvectomy	Removal of skin of major and minor lips of vulva and clitoris	Sexual relations still possible.
Radical vulvectomy	Removal of vaginal lips, clitoris, skin surrounding vulva, and lymph glands	Preoperative radiotherapy often prescribed prior to operation. Sexual relations still possible.
Vaginectomy	Removal of vagina	Vagina may be smaller or shorter after surgery. Plastic surgery may be necessary.
Pelvic exenteration	Radical hysterectomy plus removal of rectum and bladder	For very advanced cancer of cervix. Leaves patient with both bowel and urinary openings on abdomen. Very extreme operation.

What are the fallopian tubes?

The fallopian tubes, also called uterine tubes, run from the ovaries to the womb. The fallopian tubes transport the egg from the ovaries to the uterus.

What is the most common place for cancer cells to grow in the reproductive organs?

The most common place is in the cervix. If the cancer starting there is not found or is not treated, it can grow and spread to other reproductive organs and to other body organs.

Can cancer be treated during pregnancy?

Yes. Some cancers which occur during pregnancy include cancers of the breast, uterine cervix, ovary, lymphomas, and colon and rectal cancers. Most experts feel that cancers that occur during pregnancy should be diagnosed and treated without delay. At this time, it is not believed that pregnancy influences the growth and spread of the tumors, or that there is any risk that the cancer will spread to the fetus.

Are lasers being used to treat gynecological cancer?

Yes. Several institutions report good results with laser treatments for dysplasia, endometriosis, and in-situ cancers of the cervix and vulva. Carbon dioxide laser treatments are being used. The laser targets continuous high-powered waves at the malignancy, vaporizing the cancer.

CANCER OF THE VULVA

Who is at risk for cancer of the vulva?

Usually women with cancer of the vulva fall into the 60-to-80-year-old age group, though it can occur in premenopausal women. It is a fairly uncommon disease. Vulvular cancer which has not metastasized to other parts of the body is highly curable.

What are some of the symptoms?

Common symptoms include itching, burning, pain, and bleeding. A Pap smear and a biopsy are necessary to help diagnose whether these symptoms indicate cancer or whether an infection is present which may be causing the same symptoms.

How is a biopsy taken in the vulvular area?

The doctor will give a simple injection of local anesthetic. A small dermatologic punch is usually used to obtain a biopsy. The procedure is simple and almost painless. The doctor may use a colposcope in his routine checking of a suspicious growth in this area. This allows him to have a photographic recording of the site for future reference.

What are the doctor's considerations in deciding how to treat cancer of the vulva?

The physician must tailor treatment to the individual patient. He considers the size of the growth, whether it has spread from the original site, whether radical surgery is practical for the patient on the basis of her age and health, or whether radiotherapy is feasible.

What is leukoplakia of the vulva?

Leukoplakia is *not* a cancerous condition, though it may be a precancerous condition. Leukoplakia can appear in various parts of the body with mucous-membrane lining—such as the inside of the mouth, the anal region, and the genital areas. It is characterized by moist white patches that are raised and may contain grooves or clefts and have sharply defined edges. In the vulva, leukoplakia can cause itching. Because it can progress through the formation of fissures to a cancerous condition, it should be watched carefully by the physician and removed surgically if it does not disappear.

What operations are performed for leukoplakia of the vulva?

If a biopsy indicates leukoplakia (a condition which usually causes intense itching), a simple vulvectomy may be performed.

The Stages of Cancer of the Vulva

STAGE	OTHER CLASSIFICATIONS	EXPLANATION
Stage 0	TIS, N0, M0	Small area of cancer without evidence of invasion or spread
Stage I	T1, N0, M0	Cancer is confined to the vulva, is less than 2 cm in diameter, and has not spread to the lymph nodes.
Stage II	T2, N0, M0	Cancer is confined to the vulva, is larger than 2 cm in diameter, and has not spread to the lymph nodes.
Stage III	T3, N0, M0 T1–2, N1–2, M0	Cancer has spread to nearby tissues such as the urethra, vagina, and anus or has spread to the lymph nodes.
Stage IV	T4, any N, M0 Any T, N3, M0 Any T, any N, M1	Cancer has invaded the bladder or rectum or has spread to more remote areas such as the lungs.

What is a simple vulvectomy?

This operation includes the removal of the skin of the major and minor lips of the vulva and the clitoris. New skin will grow in the area to replace the skin removed by the surgery, or skin may be grafted. X-ray treatments may be given in conjunction with the surgery.

What is a radical vulvectomy?

This operation is performed when the biopsy shows that cancer has invaded the skin of the vulva. The operation includes the removal of the vaginal lips, clitoris, skin surrounding the vulva, and the lymph glands. Separate incisions are usually made in both groins to remove lymph glands.

Can cancer of the vulva be treated with radiation?

Yes. However, surgery is the preferred treatment, since tissues in the area are sensitive to radiation. The radiation is uncomfortable, and the area is difficult to treat with radiation. Radiotherapy is sometimes used prior to or following the operation.

Are any other treatments used for cancer of the vulva?

Surgery is the preferred method of treatment, as indicated by the excellent survival rates when this method is followed—as high as 85 to 95 percent, even in Stage II disease. However, if the cancer has metastasized beyond the regional lymph nodes, radiation therapy is usually used.

In early cancer of the vulva, can a chemotherapeutic ointment be used instead of surgery?

The use of topical fluorouracil (a chemotherapeutic ointment) is not the recommended first choice for stage 0 (in situ) cancer of the vulva. Surgical removal of the skin of the vulva, with or without grafting, is usually the preferred

Treatment Choices for Cancer of the Vulva

STAGE	POSSIBLE TREATMENT
Stage 0	Wide local excision or laser beam therapy Removal of skin of vulva with or without grafting
Stage I	Radical vulvectomy with node dissection Radical local excision for small lesions
Stage II	Radical vulvectomy with node dissection
Stage III	Radical vulvectomy with node dissection, sometimes with radiation therapy Investigational treatments available
Stage IV	Radical vulvectomy and pelvic exenteration Surgery plus radiation therapy Radiation plus radical surgery Investigational treatments available
Recurrent	Radiation for symptoms Surgery or radiation for local recurrence Radical vulvectomy and pelvic exenteration Investigational treatments available

treatment. Depending on the extent of the disease, in selected circumstances, wide local surgery or laser beam therapy is used. These treatments are recommended only for stage 0 or in situ cancers of the vulva.

What type of anesthesia is used for a vulvectomy?

Usually a general anesthesia or a spinal.

How long must the patient remain in bed after a vulvectomy?

Usually the patient will remain in bed for 2 days, depending on the extent of the surgery.

Are there any complications that one should be alerted to following vulvectomy?

In a radical vulvectomy, because of the removal of a large number of lymph nodes, fluid collects under the skin and may be a problem for quite some time following the operation until other lymph channels have become established. It is extremely important for the patient to start on deep-breathing, coughing, and leg exercises immediately after surgery to reduce the possibility of complications such as infections, pneumonia, leg edema, or lung problems. Usually, the doctor will leave orders for the patient to be turned frequently, and for pillows to be placed so as to lessen tension on the incision. Frequent irrigations with sterile saline solution, heat lamp treatments, and sitz baths may be used to promote healing of the wound.

Can a woman become pregnant after having a vulvectomy?

Yes, a patient who has had a vulvectomy can become pregnant. Delivery might be a problem, and a cesarean section would probably be done. However, since most of the people who require this operation are in the older age group, the problem does not arise often.

Is sexual intercourse possible after vulvectomy?

Yes, intercourse is still possible, because the vagina is still present. You may have to change position or technique. For example, the woman may have to keep her thighs close together to lengthen the distance from the vaginal cavity so that although the penetration is not as deep, it can still be satisfying.

Removal of the vulva may cause the remaining vaginal tissues to become tight—making intercourse and physical examination difficult. Intercourse and/or stretching of your vagina right after the operation is important to make sure that the tissues will remain supple and elastic. Check with your surgeon to determine if your clitoris was removed during surgery. Loss of your clitoris does not mean that you will no longer be able to experience orgasm. With an open, understanding relationship between you and your partner, and the guidance of an interested and informed health-care provider (nurse, counselor, physician, sex therapist), you can become orgasmic through stimulation of your nipples, the inner parts of your thighs, and virtually any other part of your body. Most important is whether or not the two people care enough about each other to work at finding new ways to satisfy each other.

Are cancer of the vulva and cancer of the vagina common?

Neither cancer of the vulva nor cancer of the vagina is a common cancer. Most frequently they appear in women over the age of 65. In the past few years, it has been found that some teenage girls were developing cancer of the vagina. The drug DES (diethylstilbestrol) given to pregnant women between 1945 and 1970 has been suspected of causing abnormalities in this area.

CANCER OF THE VAGINA

How is cancer of the vagina diagnosed?

Pelvic exams, Pap smears, colposcopy, and iodine or Schiller's tests are used to diagnose cancer of the vagina. Women who have previously had either in situ or invasive carcinoma of the cervix are likely to develop premalignant conditions of the vagina. Leukoplakia of the vagina is usually regarded as a precancerous condition.

Are biopsies usually performed to diagnose cancer of the vagina?

Yes. Biopsy is always necessary to confirm a diagnosis of cancer. Careful diagnosis is important in vaginal cancer, since a biopsy sometimes shows the condition to be a metastasis from another kind of cancer. A biopsy is also important because treatment for each stage of vaginal cancer varies.

What are the treatments for vaginal cancer?

The treatments are surgical, either removing the cancerous areas or doing a total hysterectomy and/or a total vaginectomy and vulvectomy, depending on the stage of the cancer and its location. Sometimes radiation therapy—both external and radiation implants in the vaginal cavity—is used.

What is the treatment for cancer in situ of the vagina?

The cancer is either removed surgically or treated with laser or chemotherapy.

The Stages of Cancer of the Vagina

STAGE	OTHER CLASSIFICATIONS	EXPLANATION
Stage 0	TIS, N0, M0	Carcinoma in situ. Tumor is confined to vaginal mucosa without evidence of invasion.
Stage I	T1, N0, M0	Tumor is limited to vaginal wall.
Stage II	T2, N0, M0	Tumor has spread to tissues surrounding vagina but not to wall of pelvis.
Stage III	T3, N0, M0	Cancer has spread to pelvic wall.
Stage IVA	T4, any N, M0	Cancer has spread outside pelvis or into bladder or rectum.
Stage IVB	T4, any N, M1	Cancer has spread outside pelvis to distant areas such as the lungs.

Treatment Choices for Cancer of the Vagina

STAGE	POSSIBLE TREATMENTS
Stage 0	Local surgery, with or without skin grafting Laser therapy Intravaginal chemotherapy
Stage I	Radiation implants Local surgery or total vaginectomy with skin-graft reconstitution
Stage II	Radiation therapy and implants Surgery plus radiation in selected patients
Stage III	Radiation therapy and implants Surgery plus radiation in selected patients
Stage IVA	Radiation therapy and implants, sometimes with surgery added Investigational treatments available
Stage IVB	Investigational treatments available Radiation therapy for symptoms
Recurrent	Pelvic exenteration for selected patients Investigational treatments available

Is there any special care which must be taken when having a radiation implant in the vagina?

Description of the procedure for radiation implants is given in Chapter 7. However, there are a few points which must be remembered if you are having vaginal radiation-implant treatments. For 2 weeks following the implant, you should not use tampons, should not have intercourse, and should not douche or take tub baths. After the 2-week period, it is necessary, in the interest of proper healing, for you to either use a dilator or to have intercourse in order to prevent the vaginal cavity from closing and/or forming adhesions.

Does a radium implant in the vagina cause problems with intercourse?

Following a radium implant, scar tissue will form in the vagina, unless the vagina is kept open. This can be done in several ways: sexual intercourse, the use of a dilator, or a combination of both. Most doctors suggest that you resume intercourse 3 weeks after leaving the hospital. Since the implant often causes vaginal dryness, use of a water-soluble lubricant may make intercourse more comfortable. It is advised that you have intercourse twice a week or use a dilator to help the tissues begin to stretch. Some degree of discomfort and perhaps a little bleeding may be noticed.

How is a dilator used?

A dilator is used to keep the vaginal opening from closing. Apply a water-soluble lubricant to the rounded end of the dilator. Lie on your back in bed with your knees bent and slightly apart. Insert the rounded end of the dilator into the vagina gently and as deeply as you can without causing discomfort. Let it stay in place for 10 minutes. Withdraw and clean the dilator with hot, soapy water, rinsing it well. Do this twice a week. Do not be alarmed if slight bleeding or spotting occurs following dilator use. If you are unable to insert the dilator easily, check with your nurse or doctor.

I tighten up when my partner wants to have sexual relations with me ever since I had a cancer operation in the vaginal area. Why am I so afraid of being hurt?

After vaginal surgery, this reaction is fairly normal. As you have probably guessed, the cause may be a combination of physical and psychological factors. You should first find out whether there are physical problems that need correcting. An important ingredient in success of sexual rehabilitation is acknowledgment of the problem by you, your partner, and your health-care provider. Honest, open communication must exist before counseling and alternative techniques can be successful. The use of medicine, including antispasmodics and analgesics, may be advised to help you to relax before intercourse and prevent a tightening of your pelvic muscles, which makes intercourse uncomfortable. Touching and exploring the vaginal area with your fingers may help you gain confidence. Short-term behavioral sex therapy, with instruction in relaxation and desensitization techniques, may also be helpful. Consultation with a sex therapist may be useful.

What suggestions are there for someone who cannot have intercourse because of extensive vaginal surgery—but still would like sexual contact with her partner?

There are many ways other than intercourse to have sexual contact with your partner, such as hugging, kissing, and oral and manual stimulation of the clitoris or penis. If surgery has been extensive and placement of the penis in the vagina is impossible, there are several alternatives you can try. Consultation with your health-care team or a sex therapist would be helpful.

Can reconstructive surgery be performed following surgery for a cancer condition in the vagina, and is sexual intercourse possible?

Just as women who have undergone mastectomies may have breast reconstruction, women who have vaginectomies (or colpectomies) may have plastic surgery to reconstruct the vagina. Women who have had vaginal reconstruction say it is possible to regain former sensations and feelings. Partners report pleasurable, successful sexual relations following this surgery. Reconstruction is often done in stages, and may involve several separate surgeries done several weeks or months apart. Consultation with a reputable plastic surgeon, who will do the reconstruction, as well as with the surgeon who performs the vaginectomy, is necessary. If possible, plans for reconstruction should be made *before* the original surgery.

CANCER OF THE CERVIX

Who is at greater risk of developing cervical cancer?

At greater risk of developing cervical cancer are women who have had sex at an early age, have had sex with many partners, and have had more than five pregnancies.

Is cancer of the cervix easy to detect?

Yes. Cancer of the cervix is detected through a Pap smear, which is a very simple examination. Cancer of the cervix is virtually 100 percent curable in its earliest stages.

How is the Pap test done?

Living cells are collected from the vaginal fluid by gently scraping the surface of the cervix. These cells are preserved with fixative solution, stained, and put on a microscope slide to be read by a pathologist. The test is done by a gynecologist or another physician in his office, or it can be done at a clinic.

Is it necessary to have a Pap test every year?

The American Cancer Society offers the following guidelines for women without symptoms:
* Women between the ages of 20 and 40 should have a pelvic exam every 3 years and a Pap test *at least* every 3 years after two initial negative tests 1 year apart. These guidelines are also for women under 20 if sexually active.
* Women 40 and over should have a pelvic exam every year and a Pap test *at least* every 3 years after two initial negative tests 1 year apart.

When should the first Pap test be done?

The recommendation of the National Institute of Health is that all women who have had sexual intercourse should begin a regular screening program for cervical cancer.

Should older women continue to have Pap smears?

The National Cancer Institute's Conference panel noted that if two negative Pap smears are obtained after the age of 60, further smears do not appear to be needed. Some doctors recommend Pap tests regularly up to the age of 65 and every three to five years beyond 65.

Besides the Pap test, how else can cervical cancer be detected?

There are usually no visible symptoms or signs in the early stages of cancer of the cervix. As the cancer grows, there may be unusual bleeding or discharge. You may have a longer menstrual period than usual, a heavier flow, bleeding between periods or after intercourse, or bleeding after menopause. The bleeding is usually described as bright red and unpredictable as to time, amount, or duration. Although these symptoms may not be cancer they should be checked by a doctor.

At what age is a woman most likely to get cervical cancer?

The age varies, with the peak for cancer in situ being between 30 and 40 and for invasive cancer between 40 and 50. However, cervical cancer may occur at any age. About 15 percent is seen before the age of 30. Statistics indicate that there is an increasing number of patients diagnosed at the age of 20 years or below. Women who have had first intercourse at an early age and women who have multiple sex partners are at higher risk for cervical cancer.

Is the papilloma virus linked to cervical cancer?

There is suspicion of a connection. Scientists are finding some strong evidence linking viruses in the papilloma family to cancers of the cervix and vulva. The National Cancer Institute has set up a special laboratory to study the links between some of the viruses and cancer. If the evidence continues in the same trend, efforts will be made to develop a vaccine for the future.

Isn't the cervix part of the uterus?

It is. The cervix is the lower part or neck of the uterus. It protrudes into the vagina and is the segment of the uterus which can be seen by the doctor during a pelvic examination. Cancer of the neck of the uterus or cervix and cancer of the body of the uterus (endometrium) present two very different sorts of problems, so it is important for you to ask the doctor exactly where the problem lies.

Can a Pap smear detect cancer of the uterus?

A Pap smear can accurately detect cancer of the cervix, but it is substantially less accurate for detecting cancer of the body of the uterus (endometrium), the fallopian tubes, or the ovaries. In cases where these types of cancer are discovered through a Pap smear it is because the cancer cells have passed down through the tube into the cavity of the uterus and continued out through the cervix and into the vaginal discharge.

In other words, the Pap test is really designed only to detect cervical cancer?

That is correct. Regular Pap smears help make cervical cancer a preventable disease. Since cells from the cervix are continually being sloughed off into the normal discharge from the cervix and vagina, the Pap smear makes it possible for most cervical cancer to be detected before it has had an opportunity to invade or spread. The use of the Pap smear has helped to drop the death rate for women with cervical cancer by 60 percent in the last 30 years.

Is it painful to have a Pap smear?

No. There is little or no discomfort—and most doctors include it as a part of the regular pelvic examination. It is a good idea for all women over the age of 20—and most especially for women of menopausal age—to have regular Pap smears. If you have a special, high-risk situation, your physician may require a smear to be taken more often than once a year.

How can I be sure I'm getting an accurate Pap smear?

The accuracy of your Pap smear depends on the quality of the laboratory interpreting the glass slide which is sent by the doctor—and so it is important to have a doctor who is fussy about the lab he uses. However, women themselves can ensure a more accurate reading if they follow these suggestions:

- Don't douche for at least 3 days before your Pap test. If you do, there won't be enough loose cells in your vaginal fluid for an accurate test.
- Use shower instead of tub bath for at least 48 hours before the test.
- Don't use tampons or birth-control foams or jellies for 5 days before your appointment.
- Try to arrange your appointment between days 15 and 20 of your menstrual cycle.

Is it necessary to have a Pap smear after a woman has had a hysterectomy?

That depends upon why the hysterectomy was done and what was removed. If the cervix is still present, Pap tests are necessary. If the hysterectomy was done because of cancer, it is absolutely necessary to have a regular Pap test. You should discuss this with your doctor.

I usually douche before going to the doctor for a gynecological exam. Is this wise?

No, it is not. Since the Pap smear is based on an examination of the actual vaginal discharge, a smear would not be accurate if you have douched during the few days prior to the examination. You should not douche for at least 3 days prior to the day of your examination, because a douche washes away the vaginal discharge which is examined in the Pap smear.

What do the different classes of Pap test mean?

Pap test results are usually assigned numbers from 1 to 5, although some laboratories use slightly different systems. The usual meaning of the tests is as follows:

- *Class 1:* Smear completely normal. No abnormal cells.
- *Class 2:* Some atypical cells present but none suggest cancer. May be due to an inflammation and/or possible infection. Usually no treatment is prescribed because many of the abnormalities return to normal without any treatment. Pap test should be repeated between 3 and 6 months.
- *Class 3:* Some abnormal cells present, suggesting but not confirming the presence of cancer. Referred to as dysplasia. The degree and kind of abnormality is greater than Class 2 test. Follow-up smear and biopsy may be needed.
- *Class 4:* Smear contains some cells that appear to be cancerous. There are signs of early cancer. Follow-up smear and biopsy needed.
- *Class 5:* Smear contains cells that are more cancerous than Class 4. Immediate treatment necessary.

What does the doctor do if I have a Class 2 Pap smear?

It depends on other conditions. A Class 2 Pap smear can be the result of a bacterial infection or inflammation, for example. If there is some evidence of inflammation, the doctor would probably treat you for that condition and then repeat the smear.

What does the doctor do about a Class 3 Pap test?

It depends upon what else the pathologist told the doctor about his findings. If no lesion is seen, usually a Class 3 would call for another Pap smear test. If the second test was also a Class 3, a biopsy would probably be performed. Sometimes the Class 3 level is referred to as dysplasia, which is still a noncancerous condition. The relationship between cancer and dysplasia is not entirely clear. Class 3 cells can return to normal cells for no obvious reason and without treatment.

What would the doctor do about a Class 4 or a Class 5 test?

In both cases, a biopsy would be done. Class 4 means the degree of abnormality has reached the level at which a biopsy should be taken to determine whether or not cancer is present. Class 5 means that the cells appear to be even more bizarre and are apt to be associated with a more aggressive and more widely spread tumor. Remember, as noted before, the classification of the Pap test may vary from one laboratory to another. Normally, your physician would discuss the findings with you. Rarely would you be given a numerical classification without an explanation.

What is the Schiller test?

The Schiller test, which is usually done in the doctor's office, is the staining of cervical cells on the cervix in order to locate possible cancerous cells.

Why must a biopsy be done? Doesn't the Pap smear indicate whether or not I have cancer?

The Pap smear is only a screening tool. Although it is very accurate as a screening device, a biopsy must be done to give a definite diagnosis of cancer. The biopsy also is essential for staging the disease. If the cell samples from the Pap smear show abnormality, additional diagnostic tests are performed. They may include colposcopy or conization.

What do the terms *dysplasia* and *hyperplasia* mean when used in reference to cancer of the uterus.

Dysplasia is a term used in describing a condition in the cervix. The cells covering the cervix usually go through mild to severe changes before becoming cancer. These changes are called dysplasia. Similar changes in the tissue lining the uterus are called hyperplasia. Dysplasia develops most often in women between the ages of 25 and 35, but it may also develop in women in their late teens or early twenties.

Does dysplasia or hyperplasia always lead to cancer?

No. These precancerous conditions do not necessarily lead to cancer. It is important, however, that any woman with such a condition be treated and then examined by a physician at regular intervals.

What is carcinoma in situ?

Carcinoma in situ is the earliest stage of cancer. It means that the cancer is confined to its original site. If not detected and treated properly, the cancer cells go into deeper layers of the uterus, then spread to neighboring organs such as the vagina, bladder, or rectum, and eventually metastasize to other parts of the body.

Does carcinoma in situ of the cervix usually become invasive cancer?

Usually the process of carcinoma in situ becoming invasive cervical cancer is very slow. Some studies have shown that between 30 and 70 percent of in situ carcinomas will develop into invasive cancer over a period of 10 to 12 years. However, in a small percentage of patients, the in situ cancer can develop into invasive cancer of the cervix in under a year. Invasive cancer of the cervix may be preceded by early cervical conditions that usually don't cause symptoms.

In fact, cervical cells may go through a series of changes—from normal to abnormal (dysplasia) to very early cancer (cancer in situ) to invasive cancer.

Is there any way the doctor can examine the cervix, the vulva, and the vagina without an operation?

Yes. The colposcope allows the doctor to look into parts of a woman's reproductive system—the cervix, vulva, and vagina—without operating. The colposcope is basically a microscope on a stand. It gives a lighted, magnified view showing greater detail than can be seen by the naked eye. Since using the colposcope properly requires special training, many doctors refer their patients to physicians who are specialized in this technique. Doctors can also biopsy the organs with this technique. No anesthesia is needed. The procedure usually takes only 10 or 15 minutes.

How is the colposcopy done?

In doing a colposcopy, the doctor proceeds with the usual pelvic examination. With the speculum (the instrument used to separate the walls of the vagina to expose the cervix) inserted into the vagina, the doctor points the magnifying lens and a powerful light at the opening of the vagina and looks through an eyepiece. The cervix and/or vagina are swabbed with a special solution. The solution, along with a green lens placed on the colposcope, makes the abnormal area appear as whitish spots. Biopsies of these white spots or any abnormal areas are usually taken for examination. The sensation of a biopsy is similar to a mild menstrual cramp. A TV attachment on the side of the colposcope beams a picture to a nearby monitor. If he wishes, the doctor can make videotapes of the cells to study changes over a period of time. No part of the instrument is inserted into the vagina.

When is a colposcopy done?

Sometimes a colposcopy is done when you have had an abnormal Pap smear. With the colposcope the doctor can see if there is an abnormal pattern to the blood vessels in your cervix and whether there is a lesion there. Using the colposcope, the doctor can very often identify the abnormal tissue from which abnormal cells on the Pap smear have been scraped. In many instances such abnormal tissue may then be destroyed or removed painlessly in the office, often avoiding other surgical procedures.

Is a colposcopy painful? Will it affect my ability to have children?

No, the colposcopy is neither painful nor will it affect your ability to bear children.

Will I have a discharge after I have a colposcopic examination?

Sometimes. The biopsied area is usually swabbed with a brown solution to prevent bleeding. This solution can cause a slight brownish vaginal discharge for 1 to 2 days. The solution may be irritating to your partner, so the doctor will usually advise you to abstain from intercourse for a day or two.

Is the colposcope used for DES daughters?

Yes, the colposcope is also used as an examining tool for girls whose mothers took DES during pregnancy.

What is conization?

Conization is a surgical procedure to remove a cone-shaped specimen of tissue from the cervical canal. It provides a larger tissue sample than is removed for a biopsy. It is used sometimes when the area causing the abnormal Pap smear is a large one or if it extends into the cervical opening. Conization involves removing the central portion of the cervix and its other opening. The amount of tissue removed depends on the size and location of the abnormal area.

Is conization used instead of colposcopy?

Before the colposcope, conization was used to do a biopsy of the cervix. Today, colposcopy is the preferred method, because conization is more expensive and takes more time. Conization can also cause difficulty with future pregnancies. However, conization is used as a diagnostic tool if colposcopy fails to determine the source of the abnormal Pap smear.

The General Stages of Cancer of the Cervix

Stage	Other Classifications	Explanation
Stage 0	TIS	Carcinoma in situ as diagnosed by Pap smear and confirmed by biopsy. Has not spread below lining of first layer of cervical tissue.
Stage I	T1, N0, M0	Tumor confined to cervix.
Stage II	T2, N0, M0	Extends outside cervix but not to walls of pelvis or lower third of vagina.
Stage III	T3, N0–N1, M0	Tumor has extended out to walls of pelvis or to lower third of vagina or has blocked ureters.
Stage IV	T4, NX–N1, M0 or any T, any N, M1	Tumor has spread to the bladder or rectum or there are distant metastases.

Treatment Choices for Cancer of the Cervix

Stage	Possible Treatments
Stage 0	Conization (squamous cell) Hysterectomy Radiation therapy, cryosurgery and laser surgery
Stage I	Hysterectomy Radiation therapy and/or implant
Stage II	Radiation therapy and/or implant Hysterectomy Investigational treatments available
Stage III	Radiation therapy
Stage IV	Radiation therapy Investigational chemotherapy, single or combination
Recurrent	Investigational chemotherapy combinations and new anticancer agents available Surgery for locally recurrent disease

If the biopsy shows that I have cancer of the cervix, what other tests will the doctor perform before he begins the treatment?

Before treatment is started, the doctor will usually perform a cystogram, an intravenous pyelogram, and barium-enema examination. Depending upon the stage of the disease, he might also perform some body scans to check for involvement in the bone or liver or a lymphangiogram to look for lymph-node involvement. The stage of the tumor is the principal factor in determining the particular treatment which will be used, so the tests the physician performs are very important.

What kind of treatment is used for cervical cancer in situ?

The treatments used for cervical cancer in situ include minor surgery such as conization, cryosurgery (freezing), laser surgery, or sometimes removal of the uterus. The important point is that cancer of the cervix is 100 percent curable if discovered early. In some early cases, childbearing function can be maintained.

What are the treatments for Stages I through IV cancer of the cervix?

In its early stages, cervical cancer is usually treated with surgery or radiation or a combination of the two. Chemotherapy is often recommended for later stages of the disease.

Stage I cervical cancer is usually treated with either surgery or radiation therapy. Surgery is often selected in younger women because it preserves the reproductive and hormone-producing activities of the ovaries. In older women radiation may be selected because it is more easily tolerated than surgery, particularly if other medical problems are present. Surgery may be combined with radiotherapy if the shape of the tumor in the cervix makes insertion of radioactive implants difficult.

Most patients with cervical cancer Stages II through IV are treated with radiation therapy alone, although for some younger patients with early Stage II disease, surgery may be the treatment of choice. Radiation is usually a combination of external and internal radiation.

If the cancer has spread extensively or has reappeared after initial treatments with surgery or radiation, chemotherapy may be used.

Investigational treatments include using various combination of chemotherapy drugs, immunotherapy agents such as C. parvum, and radiation sensitizers (drugs such as misonidazole and hydroxyurea, which are given before radiation therapy to make the cancer cells more sensitive to the radiation).

Is cryosurgery often used in place of conization?

It depends upon the extent of the abnormality. Cryosurgery is effective in eliminating abnormal cells in carefully selected patients. If the abnormal area is large or goes into the cervical opening, then conization is usually used. Sometimes, if cryosurgery does not eliminate all the abnormal cells, conization will be done.

Is the conization used for treating early cervical cancer the same procedure that is used in diagnosing it?

Yes. A conization takes a cone-shaped piece of tissue and involves removing the central portion of the cervix and its outer opening. The amount of tissue removed depends on the size and location of the abnormal area.

Will a conization mean that I can no longer have a baby?

This will depend upon the amount of tissue removed and on the future progress of the disease. The conization alone usually does not rule out future pregnancy. This is a question you should definitely raise with your doctor so he can discuss it with you in relation to your particular case.

When is cryosurgery used?

Cryosurgery is often recommended to treat abnormal Pap smears due to early changes in cell structure called dysplasia. The procedure is often done in the doctor's office. It takes about 15 minutes to perform the treatment, no medication is needed, and it can be done with an IUD in place.

How is cryosurgery done?

After you are positioned on the examining table, the doctor will use a speculum to expose the cervix. A probe is used to transmit the gas used for freezing from the tank to the cervix. The gas, usually nitrous oxide or carbon dioxide, is applied for 3 minutes or longer while an ice ball forms.

Will I feel anything during the procedure?

You might feel some cramping, like mild menstrual cramps. After the procedure is finished you might feel "weak in the knees."

Will I have any kind of discharge after the cryosurgery?

You will probably have a heavy, watery discharge for 2 to 4 weeks. It might be blood-tinged, be irritating to the skin, and have an odor. If you wish, you can wear a sanitary pad to absorb the fluid. Do not use tampons. You may take warm tub baths as often as you like to relieve the irritation. The mild cramps may also continue for a few hours or a few days. The doctor will probably prescribe medication to relieve the discomfort.

Will there be a change in my periods because of the cryosurgery?

You might experience a temporary change in the pattern of your periods—they might be early or late. Bleeding may be heavier or lighter than normal.

Are there any side effects of the cryosurgery I should report to the doctor?

There are some side effects you should call to the attention of the doctor immediately:
 • Fever and chills
 • Heavy vaginal bleeding with clots
 • Extreme pain in the lower abdomen or back

Can I have intercourse after cryosurgery?

You cannot have intercourse for 10 days after cryosurgery, since the treatment has temporarily injured the cervix. You must be careful in order to protect yourself against infection and bleeding. During those 10 days you should not douche or use tampons.

Can the cryosurgery be done while I have my menstrual period?

No, it cannot. It is best done within 1 week after your menstrual period ends.

What follow-up is necessary after cryosurgery?

You should have a Pap smear done about 3 months after the cryosurgery and again in 3 more months. Then, if the smears are normal, you will probably have pap smears every 6 months from then on.

What happens when cervical cancer is discovered in a pregnant woman?

The treatment depends upon the extent of the cancer and upon how pregnant the woman is when it is discovered. A punch biopsy can be taken at any time during pregnancy if there is a lesion on the cervix. If no lesion is present but the smear is suspicious, most doctors wait until the end of the third month to carry out a conization, thus reducing the risk of abortion. If a Class 3 smear is discovered late in pregnancy, a vaginal delivery may be possible with delay of conization until several weeks after the birth. If a Class 4 or Class 5 smear is discovered, conization is usually postponed, an early cesarean birth is planned, and conization or hysterectomy is performed several weeks later, followed by radiation therapy.

How is cancer of the endometrium detected?

The Pap test is less than 50 percent effective in detecting endometrial cancer—that is, cancer in the womb or lining of the body of the uterus. Two other techniques are used in diagnosing this cancer: dilation and curettage (D&C) and aspiration curettage.

How is dilation and curettage (D&C) performed?

After the patient is anesthetized, usually with light general anesthesia, the doctor gently stretches the cervix and inserts an instrument called a curette, which he uses to scrape the wall of the uterus. Tissue samples are removed for study under the microscope. The procedure is usually done on an outpatient basis.

What is aspiration curettage?

The doctor, in his office, takes a tissue specimen from the lining of the uterus. A device, called an endometrial aspirator, consists of a disposable tube connected to a syringe. The tube is inserted through the cervix into the uterus and scrapes a piece of tissue from the uterine lining. The tissue samples are then studied under the microscope for abnormal cell changes.

What do the results from the aspiration curettage show?

If analysis of the tissue shows endometrial hyperplasia (an overgrowth of lining cells), the doctor usually advises the patient to have a D&C to help prevent future problems. If there is a history of uterine cancer in your family, or if you are overweight, have high blood pressure, have been on estrogen replacement therapy, and/or are going through the menopause, ask your doctor about having this kind of analysis.

What is endometriosis?

Endometriosis is a condition in which the kind of tissue which normally lines the uterus is found in abnormal places, such as on the surface of the ovaries, the outside of the uterus, in operation scars in the lower abdomen, in tissue between the vagina and rectum, etc. It is not a cancerous condition, but it does cause painful menstrual periods, abnormal bleeding, and general discomfort. Surgery is usually required.

What is hyperplasia?

Endometrial hyperplasia is an overabundance of cells lining the uterus. It is generally considered a precancerous condition. Severe hyperplasia is often called in situ cancer of the endometrium. Though every case of hyperplasia does not develop into cancer, uterine cancer always goes through a hyperplastic stage before becoming cancerous. Therefore, hyperplasia is a warning that cancer may develop.

What are the symptoms of hyperplasia?

If the uterus is hyperplastic, bleeding will occur. In addition to heavy menstrual periods, there will be bleeding at irregular intervals.

What is the treatment for hyperplasia?

Treatment of endometrial hyperplasia depends largely on the stage of the disease and the age of the patient. In young women, endometrial hyperplasia is often associated with irregular menstrual cycles. These women are usually given female hormones to try to regulate the cycles, and the tissue of the endometrium is sampled often to check the success of the treatment. In women who are near their menopause, the conditon is treated with progesterone, if it is not severe. In severe cases and for postmenopausal women, a hysterectomy is the usual treatment.

What causes bleeding between periods?

Bleeding between periods can be caused by many different conditions: polyps in the cervix or uterus, fibroid tumors, overactivity of the endometrial lining, and vaginitis in which the skin of the vagina thins and bleeds easily, to name just a few. Bleeding between periods is *abnormal* and indicates that you should be examined to determine the cause. Any bleeding that occurs 6 months or more after your period has stopped should be investigated by your doctor.

Is it normal to have heavy clotting during premenopause?

Heavy bleeding and clotting are very common during premenopause. As the ovarian function decreases, the pituitary gland attempts to make the ovaries respond and a large amount of estrogen is produced by the body. The endometrium becomes filled with tissue, and when the buildup starts to shed, heavy clotting and bleeding result.

Why does the doctor prescribe progesterone when I have heavy bleeding and clotting?

He does this to test the reason for the heavy bleeding and clotting. After you have taken progesterone for 1 week, the uterus can usually be stimulated to return to a more normal menstrual rhythm. If normal periods return, the doctor knows that the heavy periods were caused by a lack of ovulation and progesterone. If the heavy bleeding and clotting continue, further investigation is necessary.

What is the treatment for cancer of the endometrium?

Cancer of the endometrium or uterine cancer is generally treated by surgery or radiation therapy or implant or by a combination of the two. In the precancerous stages, endometrial changes may be treated with the hormone progesterone. It is important for the doctor to assess the extent of the disease before treatment begins, since treatment differs depending upon the stage of the cancer.

What is a hysterectomy?

Technically, hysterectomy means only the removal of the uterus. It does not refer to the removal of ovaries or fallopian tubes, which are sometimes removed at the same time.

The General Stages of Cancer of the Endometrium or Uterus

STAGE	OTHER CLASSIFICATIONS	EXPLANATION
Stage 0	TIS	Carcinoma in situ, limited to lining of uterus
Stage I	T1, T1a, T1b, N0, M0	Confined to the uterus
Stage II	T2, N0, M0	Extends to the cervix
Stage III	T3, N0, M0 T1–3, N1, M0	Has extended outside uterus but not outside true pelvis
Stage IV	T4, N0, N1, M0 or any T, any N, M1	Extension beyond pelvis or invading bladder or rectum or distant metastases

Stage I may also have a G rating—GI highly differentiated; GII moderately differentiated; GIII undifferentiated.

Treatment Choices for Cancer of the Uterus or Endometrium

STAGE	POSSIBLE TREATMENT
Stage 0	D & C plus progesterone Hysterectomy
Stage I	Hysterectomy with removal of ovary Possible radiation therapy or implant
Stage II	Radium implant and radiation therapy followed by hysterectomy with removal of ovary Investigational: combinations of radiation and surgery
Stage III	Radium implant and radiation therapy, sometimes followed by surgery
Stage IV	Radiation therapy or implant Hormonal therapy Chemotherapy Investigational: new anticancer drugs, biological agents, hormones, new combinations
Recurrent	Radiation therapy Investigational treatments available

However, most women use the term vaguely, and many do not know exactly what was removed. You should be sure to ask your doctor to explain exactly what he is planning to remove and why. In cancer of the endometrium, the surgery usually includes removal of the uterus, ovaries, and fallopian tubes.

Are most hysterectomies performed because cancer is present?

No. Most hysterectomies are performed because of fibroids and hyperplasia.

What is a fibroid tumor?

A fibroid tumor is a noncancerous growth composed mostly of muscle and fibrous connective tissue. Fibrous tumors are most common among women who are over 35 years of age, and are not usually dangerous unless they grow very large. It is estimated that about 40 percent of women over 50 have fibroid tumors. Most fibroid tumors shrink after menopause. If a fibroid tumor grows large, it will usually cause bleeding and may cause pressure on the bladder, rectum, or ureter. Estrogen replacement may cause them to continue to grow. If you have fibroid tumors, they should be checked by your gynecologist. However, unless they are causing problems, they do not need to be removed. Only about three cases of fibroid tumors in every thousand become cancerous.

What kind of tests are done before a hysterectomy is performed?

A complete blood count, urine analysis, electrocardiogram, and x-rays of the chest are done before a hysterectomy is performed. Usually an intravenous pyelogram and a barium enema are used as part of the preparation tests.

What kinds of problems do doctors run into in making a diagnosis about hysterectomy?

Because it is difficult to examine the entire area fully, diagnosis is often complicated. Fibroids, for instance, can completely fill the uterus. They can be quite solid, but if they begin to degenerate, they become soft. X-rays will detect a large mass, but cannot differentiate between a large fibroid and an ovarian cyst.

What is a vaginal hysterectomy?

That is when the doctor performs the operation through the vagina, so that no incision is necessary.

Will I have menstrual periods after the hysterectomy?

No. After a hysterectomy, you will not have any more menstrual periods, nor will you be able to become pregnant.

How long does it usually take to perform a hysterectomy?

It usually takes between 45 and 90 minutes to perform a hysterectomy.

What type of anesthesia is usually used?

General anesthesia is usually used, but spinal anesthesia may be recommended.

Will I have problems with urination or bowel movements following the operation?

As with most abdominal surgery, patients find it difficult to urinate at first following the operation. It will be several days before the bowels resume their normal functioning.

Can I expect to have vaginal discharge and bleeding following the operation?

Do not be alarmed if there is vaginal discharge or bleeding following your operation, but be sure to report it to your doctor. The discharge or bleeding is usually a part of the healing process.

How soon can I take a tub bath?

It is usually wise to wait for about a month after the operation before taking a tub bath, but it is safe to take a shower once the abdominal incision has healed.

What kind of incision is made for a hysterectomy?

Usually a 4-to-8-inch incision is make in the lower abdomen below the navel. Some surgeons place the incision vertically; others do a horizontal incision. If you have a preference in this matter, you should mention it to your doctor so you can discuss it with him. Some hysterectomy procedures, especially when vaginal repair is necessary, are performed through the vagina so that no incision is required.

Is a catheter used following hysterectomy?

Yes. A catheter to empty the bladder is usually used for several days following either abdominal or vaginal removal of the uterus. If stretched muscles of the bladder and rectum are tightened at the time of the hysterectomy, a catheter may be left for as long as 6 to 8 days.

How will a total hysterectomy affect my lovemaking abilities?

Some women relax more and enjoy better orgasms because they no longer fear becoming pregnant. They report that lovemaking becomes more spontaneous and pleasurable. Other women have vaginal dryness associated with hormonal changes. This can often be corrected with water-soluble lubricants, estrogen creams, or estrogen supplements. The loss of ovarian androgens, affecting the supply of testosterone (the sexuality hormone), and/or the loss of the cervix and uterus (important in the sexual response of some, but not all, women) can also cause changes in sexual response. Although for many women the clitoris is more vital to female orgasm than the cervix and uterus, it is now known that for some women, the quality of the orgasm seems to be related to the movement of the cervix and uterus and may be altered when these structures are removed.

What happens to me sexually when the ovaries are removed?

As far as your ability to engage in sexual activity is concerned, there are no physical reasons why you cannot continue in your usual manner, though a decrease in vaginal lubrication may make it necessary to use extra lubrication during intercourse. Because the ovaries are not the only production site for estrogens (the adrenal glands also produce androgens, which govern sexual desire), there should be no change in your sexual desires. When the ovaries are removed or destroyed, either by surgery or radiation, menopause occurs, often bringing with it hot flashes or other symptoms which may be more severe than those that accompany naturally-occurring menopause. For women of childbearing age, this can be an emotionally difficult time, for they must come to grips with the fact that they can no longer have children.

I've had radiation treatments for cervical cancer and find that vaginal dryness is making sex uncomfortable. What's the solution?

This is a common problem following radiation of tissues in the reproductive area. The side effect may develop as early as 2 to 3 weeks after the start of treatment—that is, following the first dose of external radiation or implant therapy—or it may develop as long as 6 to 8 months after treatment.

A lessening in vaginal lubrication results from changes in the tissues lining the vagina. Vaginal dryness may cause itching and/or tightness in the vagina and make intercourse uncomfortable. For relief, use a water-soluble lubricant (such as K-Y Jelly) before intercourse. Your doctor may prescribe estrogen supplements or estrogen cream to help keep the vagina moist and supple.

Will removal of the uterus mean that I'll gain weight?

No. There is no evidence that there is any change in metabolism because of the removal of the uterus.

What happens to the body when both ovaries are removed?

When both ovaries are removed, as part of a hysterectomy, symptoms of the menopause develop.

What happens when one ovary is removed?

There are no noticeable effects when only one ovary is removed.

When cancer is found in one ovary, can the other ovary be saved?

In some cases only one ovary is removed. It depends on the stage of disease, the age of the patient and other factors.

Is radiation ever used before a hysterectomy to treat cancer?

In some cases, radiation treatment is done before the operation to try to shrink the tumor or to contain it. Radiation is also sometimes used after surgery. It may be external radiation or an implant.

What is the treatment for endometrial cancer if it has spread?

The hormonal drug progesterone is the usual treatment for endometrial cancer that has spread. Chemotherapy drugs are also being used on an investigational basis for this cancer.

What is choriocarcinoma?

This is a rare type of cancer of the placenta, sometimes preceded by the appearance of a hydatidiform mole, which usually occurs during childbearing years. A microscopically similar cancer can occur as testicular cancer in men. It spreads very rapidly, metastasizes, to other parts of the body—particularly to the lungs—and until 10 years ago was considered fatal. It was, however, the first malignancy

---

Stages and Possible Treatments for Choriocarcinoma*

STAGE	EXPLANATION	POSSIBLE TREATMENTS
Hydatidiform mole (molar pregnancy)	Disease is limited to uterine cavity.	Dilation, suction evacuation, and curettage Hysterectomy
Choriocarcinoma Stage I	Tumor has invaded body of uterus but has not spread beyond it.	Chemotherapy Investigational treatments available, including new combinations of chemotherapy
Stage II	Tumor has spread beyond the uterus to the vagina but is limited to the genital structure.	Chemotherapy Investigational treatments available, including new combinations of chemotherapy
Stage III	Disease has spread to the lungs, with or without involvement of genital tract	Chemotherapy Investigational treatments available, including new combinations of chemotherapy
Stage IV	Disease has spread to involve other sites.	Chemotherapy Investigational treatments available, including new combinations of chemotherapy

---

*Gestational trophoblastic neoplasm, hydatidiform mole

which proved to be curable by chemotherapy after it had metastasized. Today, thanks to the use of chemotherapy, these cancers are considered to be highly curable. However, since it is a rare disease, very few doctors outside treatment centers have had the opportunity to treat this type of cancer, and it is recommended that treatment be sought through a large medical center to ensure that the necessary expertise is available to handle the treatment. The cancer may start early in pregnancy, result in a miscarriage, and be followed by the development of a tumor. It may also occur after the delivery of a normal child. Physicians are able to cure between 95 and 100 percent of women in whom the disease is detected in an early stage and 75 percent of women with advanced choriocarcinoma.

Who gets cancer of the fallopian tube?

Primary cancer of the fallopian tube is the rarest cancer of the female genital tract. Usually the patient is between 50 and 60—but the range is 18 to 80 years. Symptoms can include excessive bleeding, vaginal discharge, or pains in the abdomen or pelvis.

What is the treatment for cancer of the fallopian tube?

Where the cancer is localized, hysterectomy and removal of the ovaries and fallopian tubes are usually recommended. Radiotherapy usually follows the operation. Chemotherapy is also sometimes used.

CANCER OF THE OVARY

What is an ovarian cyst?

An ovarian cyst is a hollow swelling containing fluid which grows in the region of the ovary.

Is an ovarian cyst often cancerous?

Most ovarian cysts—especially in younger women—are found to be benign. Cancer of the ovary is infrequent in patients under the age of 35; it is most frequent between ages 50 and 59. However, ovarian cancer develops silently, with no symptoms until it is often so far advanced that it is difficult to remove it successfully. The risk of having ovarian cancer is higher if close relatives have had it.

How can the doctor tell there is a cyst on the ovary?

Most ovarian cysts are first found by the doctor during a routine pelvic examination—and this is a very good reason for having a routine internal examination each year.

What symptoms make the doctor suspect an ovarian cyst?

Cysts of the ovary are quite common. The majority of them are benign, but some are cancerous. Cysts appear to grow quickly and often cause the abdomen to become distended. The patient may notice that she needs to urinate frequently or may complain of constipation or swelling in the legs. Interestingly enough, ovarian cysts often grow to the size of an orange or grapefruit before they are discovered. The ovaries are normally shaped like almonds; they are attached loosely to the undersurface of the fallopian tubes and have space around them, so a benign cyst of a fairly good size can be present for years without the woman being aware of its presence. When it starts to increase in size, it pushes the loose, flexible bowel away and fills in the space around it, causing a sensation of fullness or heaviness in the lower pelvic area.

Do ovarian cysts ever disappear?

Sometimes they do. Called physiological cysts because they are involved with the menstrual cycle, these cysts can some-times cause the patient to miss a period. Normally, the sac that contains the egg ruptures about halfway between periods. If the sac fails to rupture, it begins to swell and fill with a clear liquid or jellylike material and increase to the size of an egg or even larger. That is why the doctor will sometimes wait for a few weeks before suggesting surgery. If the cyst fails to disappear, then surgery will be recommended.

What if the cyst does not disappear?

If the cyst does not disappear, or is very large and is causing other problems, surgery will be necessary. A benign cyst in a woman under 30 is often treated in a different way than one in a middle-aged woman or an older woman. If the cyst has not destroyed the ovary, the doctor can remove the cyst and leave the part of the ovary not affected by the cyst. There are important decisions that need to be made and options that need to be discussed before going into surgery. Studies have shown that there are significant differences in treatment by physicians and hospitals, with gynecologic oncologists and university hospitals more accurately evaluating patients. It is important that appropriate examinations and procedures be carried out to determine the proper staging and treatment of the disease.

Ask these questions of yourself:
* Do I want the doctor to remove the uterus and other ovary if he finds nothing wrong with them?
* Since the operation is being done, do I prefer to have a hysterectomy at this stage in my life even if it is not necessary?
* Do I want the other ovary left if it is healthy so that I can have a normal menopause and avoid the need for taking hormones? (Hysterectomy does not cause you to have instant menopause unless both ovaries have been removed.)

What operation is performed if the cyst is cancerous?

If the ovarian cyst is cancerous, regardless of the patient's age, a hysterectomy with removal of one or both ovaries is usually performed. If only one ovary is removed, the second ovary needs to be biopsied to determine whether or not there are any cancer cells. Sometimes radiation therapy or chemotherapy will follow the operation.

The Stages of Cancer of the Ovary

STAGE	OTHER CLASSIFICATIONS	EXPLANATION
Stage I	T1, N0, M0	Cancer is limited to one or both ovaries.
Stage II	T1, N0, M0	Cancer involves one or both ovaries and uterus, fallopian tubes, or other structures within pelvic area.
Stage III	T3, N0, M0 T1–3, N1, M0	Cancer involves one or both ovaries and has spread to regional lymph nodes in abdomen or to surface of organs inside abdomen such as liver or intestine.
Stage IV	Any T, any N, M1	Cancer has spread outside abdomen or has invaded the liver.

Treatment Choices for Cancer of the Ovary

STAGE	POSSIBLE TREATMENTS
Stage I	Surgery alone (hysterectomy and removal of cancerous ovary) Surgery with radiation therapy or radioisotopes Surgery with adjuvant chemotherapy Investigational treatments available
Stage II	Surgery plus radiation therapy or radioisotopes Surgery plus combination chemotherapy Investigational treatments available
Stage III	Surgery plus radiation therapy Surgery plus radiation therapy plus chemotherapy Surgery plus combination chemotherapy Investigational treatments available
Stage IV	Combination chemotherapy Investigational treatments available
Recurrent	Investigational treatments testing new anticancer drugs and biologicals Surgery for symptoms Combination chemotherapy

Why are ovaries removed?

Ovaries are removed surgically because they are diseased or not functioning properly. Ovaries may also be removed in patients with breast cancer if the cancer has been found to be estrogen-dependent. Sometimes the ovaries are treated by radiation as an alternative to surgery. Some physicians remove healthy ovaries as a preventive measure against ovarian cancer while doing hysterectomies if the woman is past menopause.

What happens when the ovaries are removed?

When the ovaries are destroyed—either surgically or by radiation—the body no longer produces estrogen. The result is that menopause occurs, bringing with it sudden and severe symptoms, usually more severe than would have happened if menopause occurred naturally. Most premenopausal women who have an oophorectomy (removal of both ovaries) are given estrogen replacement therapy to help avoid severe menopausal symptoms.

Would the doctor prescribe estrogen if my ovaries were removed because of cancer?

No. If there is any sign of a cancerous condition, estrogen would probably not be prescribed.

What is the estrogen controversy?

Estrogen is a female hormone produced by the ovaries. Scientists have also developed chemical estrogen. Both regulate the development of female sexual characteristics. For a number of years, estrogens have been prescribed for women during and after menopause to make up for the decline in this hormone normally produced by the ovaries. Estrogen has been found helpful in relieving symptoms associated with menopause, such as hot flashes, in overcoming drying of vaginal tissues and in retarding osteoporosis (thinning of bones). However, the use of estrogen during and after menopause has been linked to an increase in endometrial cancer (cancer of the lining of the uterus), and it may be linked to other cancers as well. At this time, scientists do not agree about whether the risks of taking estrogen outweigh its benefits.

If the doctor prescribes estrogen therapy for my postmenopausal symptoms, should I expect to continue taking estrogen forever?

No. Patients who are using estrogen therapy should have a thorough physical checkup, including breast and pelvic examinations, before starting estrogen therapy and every 6 months thereafter. You should also examine your breasts monthly for lumps or changes in appearance that may be warning signs of cancer. You should be sure to ask the doctor to reevaluate the situation at each examination. The doctor will probably have you take estrogen for part of the cycle and progestin for the remainder. The lowest dose possible is usually prescribed, depending on the circumstances of each individual case.

What are the risks of taking estrogen?

Studies have shown that women taking estrogen for menopausal symptoms have roughly a 2 to 8 times higher risk of developing endometrial cancer than women who do not take estrogens. The risk increases after 2 to 4 years of use and seems to be greatest when large doses are taken. Therefore, it may not be wise for women who have already had endometrial cancer to take estrogen.

If I have had my uterus removed, am I still at high risk for developing uterine cancer?

No. A woman who has had her uterus *completely* removed—that is, someone who has had a total hysterectomy—is in no danger of developing uterine cancer.

Is there any link between estrogens and breast cancer?

There is conflicting evidence on this question at this time. Some studies have suggested that use of estrogen, either during or after menopause, may increase breast cancer risk for some groups of women, but other studies do not show such a relationship. Women who are already at high risk for breast cancer for other reasons may further increase their

risk of developing it if they take estrogens. In addition, any
woman who has had cancer of the breast should not take
estrogen for menopausal symptons.

**Are there problems with using vaginal estrogen cream? I
am using it to relieve vaginal dryness that has accompanied
my menopause.**

The warning about the increased risk of uterine cancer related to the use of postmenopausal estrogens for prolonged
periods does include the vaginal creams as well as the estrogens taken by mouth or injection. Estrogens are manufactured in several forms, including tablets for oral
application, liquids for intravenous and intramuscular injection, and vaginal creams for external application. They
can be manufactured synthetically in the laboratory or derived from animal sources. Estrogens, whether naturally
occurring, animal-derived, or man-made, presumably have
similar benefits, side effects, and risks associated with their
use. You should discuss the questions of estrogen replacement with your doctor. The two of you can decide whether
continued use of the cream is advisable in your particular
situation. Your doctor will probably advise you to take the
lowest dose that will control the symptoms and attempt to
discontinue the medication or decrease it at designated intervals.

Does a face cream that contains estrogen cause cancer?

Hormone creams have to be carefully used, and your own
individual situation should be discussed with your doctor.
Estrogen in the cream can be absorbed into your body. The
action once in the body is the same as if you had swallowed
a pill by mouth. Use of this kind of cream is not advised
for anyone with a history of cancer.

Aren't estrogens good for preventing bone loss?

There is evidence that estrogens prevent bone loss—and
perhaps fractures—in postmenopausal women. Some doctors feel that women who are at high risk for bone loss
should be given estrogens as preventive medicine. The individual doctor and patient must weigh the risks against
the benefits.

Is it true that the FDA has put warnings on estrogen products?

Because estrogen has been associated with endometrial cancer, the Food and Drug Administration (FDA) requires that a special brochure about the drug accompany each prescription for it, with the following warnings:

- There is probably an increased risk of cancer of the uterus if a woman uses estrogens for more than a year in treating symptoms of menopause.
- Patients should have their estrogen treatment reevaluated every 6 months.
- Estrogens should not be taken by women who have cancer of the breast or of the uterus, who have undiagnosed abnormal vaginal bleeding, or who have clotting in the legs or lungs.
- Estrogens should not be used in treating simple nervousness or depression during menopause, because it has not been proved effective for those purposes. Nor has it been proved that estrogens keep the skin soft or help a woman feel young.

The brochure also recommends that users of menopausal estrogen be monitored closely by their doctors, that they use estrogen for only as long as necessary, and that they take the lowest dose that will control symptoms.

Do oral contraceptives cause breast cancer?

A new major study of over 10,000 women between the ages of 20 and 54 has found that birth control pills do not appear to increase a woman's chances of developing breast cancer, regardless of the type of pill she uses or whether the disease runs in her family. The researchers studied more than 30 forms of oral contraceptives and found no indication that they increased the chances of developing breast cancer even among women who had a previous experience of benign breast disease, had a history of breast cancer in their family or who started using the pill before their first pregnancy. The study involved 5,000 women who had been diagnosed with breast cancer for the first time and compared them with 5,000 women who did not have breast cancer. The women in the study had used contraceptives for up to 15 years.

Do oral contraceptives offer protection against any types of cancer?

Some studies have shown that oral contraceptives appear to reduce the risks of cancer of the uterus and ovary. There was some indication in the new study that certain types of birth control pills actually provided a protective effect against breast cancer, but the findings were too small to be considered statistically significant, according to the researchers. It is clear that oral contraceptives will be studied for additional risks and benefits and for the effects of long-term use.

When did we discover that the estrogen drug DES might cause problems?

It was in 1971 that doctors discovered a link between DES (diethylstilbestrol) and cancer of the female reproductive system. Clear-cell adenocarcinoma of the vagina or cervix was found in a very small number of young women whose mothers had taken DES-type drugs during pregnancy.

What was the purpose of giving the drug to pregnant women?

During the 1940s and on into the 1960s the drug was given to women to prevent miscarriage. It was one of the first synthetic estrogen-type hormones developed that was inexpensive and could be given by mouth. Many of the women who took it had lost babies, were spotting or bleeding, or had other complications such as diabetes.

What are the DES-type drugs that may have been prescribed for pregnant women?

There are a good many, including the following:

Nonsteroidal Estrogens

Benzestrol	DesPlex	Diethylstilbestrol-diphosphate
Chlorotrianisene	Diestryl	
Comestrol	Dibestil	Diethylstilbestrol-dipropionate
Cyren A.	Dienestrol	
Cyren B.	Dienoestrol	Diethylstilbenediol
Delvinal	Diethylstilbestrol-dipalmitate	Digestil
DES		Domestrol

Estilben
Estrobene
Estrobene DP.
Estrosyn
Fonatol
Gynben
Gyneben
Hexestrol
Hexoestrol
Hi-Bestrol
Menocrin
Meprane
Mestilbol
Methallenestril
Microest
Mikarol
Mikarol forti
Milestrol
Monomestrol
Neo-Oestranol I
Neo-Oestranol II

Nulabort
Oestrogenine
Oestromenin
Oestromon
Orestol
Pabestrol D.
Palestrol
Restrol
Stil-Rol
Stibal
Stilbestrol
Stilbestronate
Stilbetin
Stilbinol
Stilboestroform
Stilboestrol
Stilboestrol DP.
Stilestrate
Stilpalmitate
Stilphostrol
Stilronate

Stilrone
Stils
Synestrin
Synestrol
Synthoestrin
Tace
Vallestril
Willestrol

Nonsteroidal Estrogen-Androgen Combinations

Amperone
Di-Erone
Estan

Metystil
Teserene

Tylandril
Tylosterone

Nonsteroidal Estrogen-Progesterone Combination

Progravidium

Vaginal Cream—Suppositories with Nonsteroidal Estrogens

AVC cream with
  Dienestrol
Dienestrol cream

Does the risk of cancer depend upon the amount of the DES-type drug taken during pregnancy?

The amount does not seem to be the important factor. The exposure during the first 5 months of pregnancy seems to be more of a determining factor than the amount.

What does research show was the most dangerous time for taking DES?

If DES or other hormones were taken before the eighth week, some effects may show up, but most probably will not be of a serious nature. The most critical time is when hormones were given between the eighth and eighteenth weeks. These are the cases where vaginal abnormalities are more likely. If taken after the eighteenth week, defects are extremely rare.

What are some of the problems the doctors have found in DES daughters?

There have been changes in the lining or wall of the vagina. Normally, the uterus is lined with a red (vascular) and moist (glandular) tissue that meets the pink, drier tissue of the vagina at the outer opening of the cervix. In DES daughters, this red tissue frequently extends into the cervix and is called eversion. Some DES daughters have spots of the red moist tissue on the walls of the vagina as well. Other DES daughters have an extra rim of tissue around the cervix. Depending on whether this rim is partial or complete, it might be referred to as a rooster's comb, cock's comb hood, collar, or pseudo-polyp.

Are the DES daughters being followed to determine what the long-term consequences of the drug will be?

A project funded by the National Cancer Institute and conducted by the Mayo Clinic is maintaining contact with a group of nearly 4,000 DES-exposed daughters as well as over 1,000 women whose mothers did not take DES. The project gets information each year from these women through questionnaires sent through the mail. There have also been investigations reviewing some 1,300 daughters identified through a review of their mothers' medical records and who were most representative of the total population of women exposed to DES before birth.

Have cancers been found in the DES daughters?

An unusual cancer of the vagina or cervix—called clear-cell adenocarcinoma—has been found in a small number of young women whose mothers had taken DES. Four cases have been reported among the DES daughters in the study, far fewer than had originally been anticipated. In addition, women 26 years of age and older had changes in the vagina less often than did younger women, suggesting that some effects of DES exposure may be lessened as women grow older. In a 5-year study of DES daughters, the two most common abnormalities—the presence of glandular tissue on the cervix, called cervical ectopy, and the presence of a ridge of tissue encircling the cervix—had diminished in more than half the women and had entirely disappeared in about a quarter of them.

Are DES daughters at higher risk for other cervical cancers?

It is now felt that DES daughters may also be at higher risk for developing the most common form of cervical cancer. A study shows that DES daughters are twice as likely to develop early cellular changes—called dysplasia—that *might* lead to cervical cancer. Only further study will tell whether these early cellular changes do indeed lead to a higher rate of cervical cancer in women exposed to DES. Dysplasia is the presence of abnormal but not cancerous cells. The study also notes that dysplasia rarely occurs in women who have never had sexual intercourse and that there was a definite connection between dysplasia and an early age of first intercourse (before 20), multiple sex partners, multiple pregnancies, and exposure to a male sexual partner who had had several sexual partners. It also discovered that genital herpes occurred twice as often in DES-exposed daughters, but the reason was not known. Barrier-type contraceptives, such as diaphragms and condoms, are a method of preventing contact with viruses that might further increase the risk for developing cervical cancer.

What kind of cancer could dysplasia lead to?

Dysplasia does not always go on to develop into cancer. In some women, however, dysplasia does go through a series of changes and then develops into cancer if it is not treated. Squamous-cell cancer is the form associated with dysplasia. Women generally do not get such cancers until they are around 35 to 40 years old. The majority of the DES daughters are still too young to develop this type of cancer.

Are there risks in DES daughters becoming pregnant?

Studies show that DES daughters have no problem becoming pregnant. And most—80 percent—carried the babies successfully to full term. Of the daughters who have had problems, premature births, miscarriages, and stillbirths were the major difficulties. Many of the women in the study project are just entering their childbearing years, so it will take many more years before all the information on this subject has been accumulated.

Are DES sons affected?

Early studies found that DES-exposed males more often had underdeveloped or undescended testes and other abnormalities such as cysts, low sperm counts, and possibly abnormal sperm forms. Later studies contradict this information and do not find any increase in risks of abnormalities in the genitourinary tract.

Do the mothers who took DES have problems?

There have been several studies and extensive followup among women who used DES during pregnancy. Those who took DES have an increased risk for breast cancer; they develop it almost one and one-half times more often than those who did not take DES. However, the scientists could not tell whether it was the DES itself or something else that accounted for the increase in breast cancer. The risk seems to become more pronounced with time. Until about 22 years after exposure, the risk is about the same for both groups. Later, the women who took DES are at a progressively greater risk, with highest risk at age 60 or older.

Are there any symptoms that DES-exposed daughters should be aware of?

The only symptom which is occasionally seen is an increase in vaginal discharge due to adenosis. Although this symptom is also found in women not exposed before birth to DES-type drugs, in DES-exposed daughters there seems to be more than the usual amount of tissue and more than the usual amount of vaginal discharge.

When should someone whose mother took DES during pregnancy be examined by a gynecologist?

A DES daughter should go to a doctor or a clinic with experience in DES screening. It is recommended that examinations be started. The time to go is:
- After she has started her first period
- If she is 14 years old or older and has not had her first period
- If she has any unusual vaginal discharge or irregular bleeding.

What kind of examination will the doctor do?

Make sure you are going to a doctor who is working with other DES daughters, because some DES-caused changes may not show up in the usual examinations or Pap smears given by most doctors. The special techniques are quick, inexpensive, and not painful. The examination should consist of the following:
- A medical history, including information about any illnesses, hospitalizations, or pregnancies. It is useful for you to give the doctor information about what kind of DES your mother took, when, and for how long. The doctor will ask what medicine you are now taking, including birth-control pills; the pattern of your menstrual periods; and information about your sexual activity.
- A complete physical examination including breast exam
- A careful inspection of the vagina and cervix, looking for physical differences
- A gentle examination to feel the walls of the vagina
- A four-sided Pap test, called a quadrant Pap test, lightly scraping the walls of the vagina to get cells which will be studied under the microscope
- Staining the vagina and cervix with iodine. Normal tissue stains brown; tissue with adenosis does not.
- Breast exam, using current guidelines for early detection of breast cancer.

What if the doctor finds abnormal tissue in the vaginal lining?

The doctor may do further tests or send you to a special clinic for more tests. They may include

- Looking at the tissue of the vagina with a colposcope. Photographs of abnormal tissue can be taken, and changes can be watched over a period of time.
- Taking tiny samples of tissue from the vagina as a biopsy to be sent to the laboratory and viewed under a microscope. This can be done in the doctor's office and involves little pain. You may have some slight bleeding.

What kind of treatment will usually be necessary?

If the pathologist finds no clear-cut cancer (and, as explained previously, chances of his finding it are slight) but only finds tissue abnormalities as noted earlier (eversion, adenosis, or rooster's comb), no treatment will be necessary.

How often does a DES daughter have to visit the doctor?

If the doctor has seen any changes after doing the examinations, she may be asked to come back every 3 to 6 months. Some or all of the examinations done at the first visit may have to be repeated. Usually the doctor will photograph or note any changes and will discuss any changes as they occur.

What if the doctor recommends preventive surgery for adenosis due to DES exposure?

If the physician's examination shows that the DES daughter is free from cancer, but he suggests surgery for preventive reasons, without question you should get another opinion. Preventive surgery in these cases has been practiced in some areas, but doctors who have treated many DES patients feel that this surgery is unnecessary unless it is proved that cancer is present. This is particularly true since it now seems that adenosis and other benign abnormalities are diminishing with maturity.

What is the treatment if cancer is found in a DES daughter?

Removal by surgery or radiation therapy is the usual treatment—depending, naturally, upon where the cancer is situated. Cancer of the vagina or cervix is not a happy prospect for anyone, and especially not for a young woman when it may mean that she will not be able to bear children. However, the cancer may be cured, especially if detected early. All efforts should be made in such cases to find the most experienced doctor for this surgery.

Should the mothers who took DES take any special precautions?

Yes. They should have an annual pelvic examination including a Pap smear. The examination should also include breast palpation. In addition, monthly breast self-examination should be practiced by the DES-exposed mothers and any abnormal findings reported promptly to the doctor, since DES-exposed mothers appear to be at an increased risk of breast cancer.

Should a DES-exposed mother have routine mammograms?

If there are no symptoms of breast cancer, mammography is not recommended under the age of 35 even for DES-exposed mothers. (It is suggested only for women between 35 and 39 who have a personal history of breast cancer or immediate relatives with a history of breast cancer.) For women over 40, mammography should be considered, using current guidelines for early detection of breast cancer.

Should a DES mother take estrogens?

Before taking any estrogens such as birth-control pills, the morning-after pill, or estrogens for menopausal symptoms, a DES mother should discuss the risks and the benefits with her doctor. Taking more estrogen in any form may add to the risk of cancer.

Can a DES daughter safely take estrogen?

Many doctors feel that DES daughters should not take any estrogens, either in pills or shots, because they might be harmful. Estrogen is contained in most birth-control pills and morning-after pills. Studies are under way on whether birth-control pills increase the risk of cancer in DES daughters. You should discuss this with your doctor. Many believe that DES daughters should use other contraceptive methods.

What recommendations are there for examinations for DES-exposed sons?

- Young boys and men exposed to DES should be advised to have a physical examination by a urologist to tell whether they have any abnormalities associated with DES exposure, such as underdeveloped or undescended testes.
- Underdeveloped or undescended testes need to be treated. Even in men who have not been exposed to DES, these conditions are well recognized as being associated with testicular cancer.

chapter 17

Cancer of the Male Reproductive Organs

Most men associate pride and ego with their sexuality and their reproductive organs—so any threat to this area causes psychological problems as well as physical ones. Many men do not like to talk about or think about cancer of the reproductive organs, but early detection and knowledge of the symptoms are important factors in curing cancer in these organs.

Cancer of the prostate usually occurs in older men. It may be cured when it is found early and can respond very well to treatment even when it is widespread. The rate of tumor growth can vary widely from patient to patient. Some men can live for many years even after the cancer has spread to the bone. Because this cancer occurs most often in older men, many of them die of other causes without ever suffering any discomfort from their prostate cancer.

Cancer of the testicle is a highly treatable, usually curable cancer which develops in young and middle-aged men. Testicular cancer does not affect male potency or virility.

Cancer of the penis is a rare disease in the United States. When diagnosed early, cancer of the penis is highly curable. The treatment is dependent on the size, location, and stage of the tumor.

Symptoms of Prostate Cancer

- Urination problems
- Blood in urine
- Pain in back, pelvis, hips

Symptoms of Cancer of the Testicle

- Small hard lump about size of pea
- Enlargement or change in testicles
- Dull ache in abdomen
- Dragging or heaviness
- Enlargement of breast; tender nipples

Symptoms of Cancer of the Penis

- A sore, nodule, pimple, wart, ulcer, etc., on penis
- Bleeding associated with erection
- Erection without sexual desire

Tests for Prostate Cancer

- Rectal examination
- Urine studies
- Blood studies (especially acid phosphatase)
- X-rays
- Needle biopsy
- Kidney-function tests
- EKG
- Ultrasound
- Bone scan
- Intravenous pyelogram (IVP)
- Lymphography

Cancer of the Male Reproductive Organs

Type	High Risk	Symptoms	Treatment	Remarks
Prostate	Over 55, black males, married	Urination problems, blood in urine, pain in back, pelvis, hips	Surgery, radiation, radiation implant, chemotherapy. Injection of female hormones sometimes used to suppress male hormones.	Most tumors found in prostate are *not* cancerous.
Testicle	Age 20–35, white males, those with undescended testicles	Small, hard lump; enlargement or change in consistency of testicles; dull ache in abdomen, dragging or heaviness; enlargement of breast, tender nipples	Depends on cell type. Removal of testicle. Follow-up treatment may be radiation therapy, chemotherapy or both.	Fast-growing tumor; often metastasizes while original growth is still small. Immediate attention imperative. *Do not allow investigative biopsy.* Extremely important before treatment to be certain doctor has latest information on treatment.
Penis	Uncircumcised males, ages 50–70	Pimple, sore, nodule, wart, ulcer, etc., on penis, usually tip. Bleeding associated with erection. Erection without sexual desire.	Surgical removal of tumor; radiation not usually effective except for very small tumors.	Very rare. Curable in early stages.

Tests for Cancer of the Testicle

Note: Investigative biopsy prior to removal of affected testicle should *never* be done. The tests that are done include:
- Physical examination—with careful attention to testes with patient in standing position, neck, breasts, abdomen, and groin
- Blood studies (especially alpha-fetoprotein and human chorionic gonadotropin)
- Intravenous pyelogram (IVP)
- Lymphangiogram
- CT scans
- Ultrasound

Questions to Ask Your Doctor Before Treatment for Prostate Cancer

- What type of treatment do you suggest?
- Is there treatment other than surgery that would be possible for me?
- Could I be treated with radium implants or radiation?
- Are you planning hormone therapy?
- Can I be treated with chemotherapy?
- If surgery, ask
  - Do you ever use treatment other than surgery?
  - How often do you do this type of surgery?
  - How extensive do you expect the surgery to be?
  - Where will the scar be?
  - Will the surgery leave me impotent? Can the surgery be done so it will not leave me impotent?
- If the scar is to be behind the scrotum, ask
  - Why are you planning to make the incision in that area?
  - Can you cut through the abdominal wall instead?

Questions to Ask Your Doctor Before Treatment for Cancer of the Testicle

- Are you planning to do a needle or simple biopsy? (*If answer is yes, see another doctor.*)
- Will only one testicle be removed?
- Is the tumor confined to one testicle?
- What is the cell type—seminoma or nonseminoma?
- Will this operation leave me sterile?
- Will you make arrangements for sperm to be collected for a sperm bank for me just in case I become sterile?
- Can an artificial testicle be implanted during surgery?
- Are you planning to follow the operation with chemotherapy or radiation therapy?

Is the National Cancer Institute supporting any studies on cancer of the male organs?

Yes, there are studies being conducted on cancer of the male organs. Most are involved with the use of chemotherapy and radiation for prostate and testicular cancers (see Chapter 23).

What are the most common cancers of the male reproductive organs?

Cancer of the prostate is the most common cancer of the male reproductive organs. Next to lung cancer, cancer of the prostate has the highest incidence of any form of male cancer. After age 75, it is the main cause of cancer deaths among men. Cancer of the testicles is one of the most common cancers in males between 20 and 40. Cancer of the penis occurs infrequently, and usually in uncircumcised males in the 50-to-70-year-old group.

PROSTATE CANCER

Who usually gets cancer of the prostate?

The risk of developing cancer of the prostate increases with age. Cancer of the prostate is primarily a disease of older men and occurs most often in those over 55 years of age. After age

Treatments for Cancer of the Prostate and Testicle

Treatment	Procedure	Results	Remarks
Transurethral resection (TUR)	Does not require external incision. Used only for very small tumors. Requires very skilled surgeon.	Does not reduce sexual potency.	No incision.
Suprapubic prostatectomy	Bladder neck is cut to reach prostate. Catheter and drain left in place for about 10 days. Vasectomy usually performed at same time.	Most uncomplicated from surgeon's viewpoint, allows correction of any bladder problems. Produces infertility but no loss of potency.	Incision is made above pubic bone.
Retropubic prostatectomy	Bladder neck and nerve and muscle attachments left intact. Catheter to bladder for about 10 days.	Less cutting, less surgical shock, more difficult to perform, takes longer than suprapubic. Usually no loss of potency.	Incision is below pubic bone over penis.
Perineal prostatectomy	Between legs, through surface separating the scrotum and anus, operation similar to retropubic.	Difficult for surgeon to perform. Patient lies with legs in stirrups, knees above waist, placing weight upon chest, creating breathing difficulties. Nerves involving erection often severed.	Little postoperative discomfort; incision is usually half-circle around inner side of anus.

Total prostatectomy	Removal of prostate	Suprapubic, retropubic, or perineal method is used. Newer method avoiding pelvic plexus retains erection ability.	Nerve and muscle connections between gland, bladder, neck, and urethra removed. Impotency results unless newer method used.
Radiation	Linear accelerator or cobalt 60 directed directly at prostate.	Often used in early stages; useful in shrinking tumors in later stages.	If carefully given should not affect fertility. May cause side effects.
Radium implants	Pellets inserted into prostate.	Used for small cancers or to reduce size of tumor and relieve pain.	Requires major abdominal surgery.
Chemotherapy	May be hospitalized during early stages of treatment.	Experiments still being conducted to determine most effective dosages. Several drugs, including 5-FU and Cytoxan, effective in relieving painful symptoms of advanced prostate cancer.	Usual side effects.
Cryosurgery	Catheterlike probe destroys cells through freezing.	Destroys malignant tissue, may develop antibodies against cancer. May be repeated.	Still experimental.

Treatments for Cancer of the Prostate and Testicle

TREATMENT	PROCEDURE	RESULTS	REMARKS
Hormone and drug treatment	Variety of by-mouth treatments, including estrogen, DES, cortisone, stilbestrol, and L-Dopa, being used.	Discrepancies in effect on different patients.	Not ordinarily used as primary treatment.
Hypophysectomy	Removal of pituitary gland	Reduces production of male hormone.	Used on patients who have shown previous response to estrogen therapy.
Adrenalectomy	Removal of adrenal glands	Reduces production of male hormone.	Used on patients who have shown previous response to estrogen therapy.
Orchiectomy	Removal of one or both testicles	If both removed, patient will be sterile, but not impotent.	Used in testicle cancer; plastic replacement of testicle is possible.
Bilateral orchiectomy	Removal of both testicles	Patient will be sterile, but not impotent.	Done to control hormone production in prostate cancer.

75, prostate cancer is the main cause of cancer death among men. Black men have two times more cancer of the prostate than white men. In the United States, black men have the highest rate of prostate cancer in the world.

How can I protect myself against cancer of the prostate?

Studies suggest that environmental factors, such as diet and other aspects of lifestyle, play an important role in developing prostate cancer. Workplace exposure to cadmium may increase the risk of prostate cancer. The specific causes are still unclear. Early detection is essential. Every man over 40 should have a rectal exam as part of his regular yearly checkup in order to detect the disease at an early curable stage.

What is the prostate and what does it do?

The prostate, a gland a bit smaller than a golf ball, weighs about ¾ ounce, is located at the base of the penis, just below the bladder and above the rectum. Physicians, in referring to the prostate, separate it into five lobes. The posterior lobe, the one which is felt when the doctor does a rectal exam, is the one which seems to be the most susceptible to cancer. Its main purpose is to secrete the fluid in which the sperm cells are ejaculated. Not all the gland's functions are fully understood, but it is sometimes possible to slow growth of the cancer through some variety of hormone therapy.

Are most prostate tumors cancerous?

No. The most common tumors found in the prostate are *not* cancerous. The most common prostate problem is called benign prostatic hypertrophy (BPH). More than half the men in the United States over 50 suffer from this enlargement.

What are the symptoms of cancer of the prostate?

Symptoms which should not be ignored include a weak or interrupted flow of urine, inability to urinate or difficulty in starting urination, need to urinate frequently (especially at night), blood in the urine, urine flow that is not easily stopped, painful or burning urination, and continuing pain

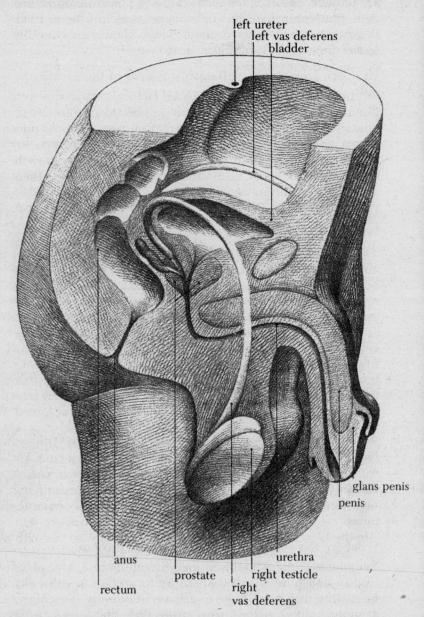

left ureter
left vas deferens
bladder

glans penis
penis

anus

prostate

right testicle

urethra

rectum

right
vas deferens

Male reproductive organs

in the back, pelvis, or hips. These symptoms are often the same symptoms that indicate other prostatic problems such as BPH, but they are symptoms which should be checked by the doctor who can detect the difference between a cancerous and noncancerous enlargement of the prostate.

How does the doctor check the prostate?

The initial step is through a digital examination of the gland through the rectum. The doctor inserts a gloved finger into the rectum and feels the gland. It often can enlarge to the size of an orange. The doctor suspects a cancerous growth if the gland is stony and hard to the touch, rather than rubbery. If there is an enlargement of the prostate gland, the doctor will usually order urine and blood analyses and x-ray.

Do most prostate glands enlarge as a man gets older?

This happens to the majority of men, beginning in the 40s and increasing in each subsequent decade of life. The enlargement itself becomes a problem only if it produces serious side effects, obstructing the flow of urine, but it should be checked yearly by the doctor. Surgery is necessary only in those whose symptoms become acute or where cancer is present.

How is cancer of the prostate diagnosed?

The presence of cancer can be confirmed by the removal of a small piece of prostate tissue for microscopic examination. Often a needle biopsy is used. In other cases, biopsy can be obtained during surgical procedures required for dealing with complications caused by the enlargement of the prostate. Blood tests are also important in diagnosis, since prostatic cancer cells secrete a chemical substance known as prostatic acid phosphatase, which finds its way into the bloodstream. In a large percentage of patients with prostate cancer, the level of acid phosphatase rises above normal when the tumor tissue has spread outside the prostate. However, the acid phosphatase test alone is not a definitive test and must be used with other indicators to determine diagnosis. This is because the rise in acid phosphatase is sometimes seen in people who do not have cancer. And it is often not detectable in people who do have cancer of the prostate.

Are new tests being developed to routinely discover prostate cancer?

A major effort of the National Cancer Institute and the National Prostatic Cancer Project is to develop and refine sensitive chemical tests that will permit the use of prostatic acid phosphatase as a more precise tool. A new method is a simple test called immunoenzyme assay (IEA) which seems to be as reliable as the tests in use now and costs less. Two other tests under study are the solid-phase fluorescent immunoassay (SPIF) and the counterimmunoelectrophoresis (CIEP). All of these tests are based on immune reactions of antibodies with a phosphatase enzyme. Scientists are continuing to isolate other biochemical changes, called markers, that are associated with cancer of the prostate.

Is ultrasound used to diagnose prostate cancer?

Some preliminary studies using ultrasound show some promise that this method of detection may improve the rate of finding prostate cancer early.

How is cancer of the prostate treated?

It depends on the patient's medical history, age, and stage of disease. Stage A disease usually requires either no treatment, removal of the prostate (prostatectomy), or radiotherapy, depending upon the number of sites in which the cancer cells are found. Stage B tumors are treated with either radiation therapy or surgery; both seem to have the same results. Stage C disease is treated with surgery, radiation therapy, or a combination of the two. Stage D disease may be treated with some form of hormone therapy, usually used when symptoms such as bone pain or bladder obstruction occur.

What is a prostatectomy?

A prostatectomy is the surgical removal of all or part of the prostate. A total prostactectomy is the removal of the entire prostate.

The Stages of Cancer of the Prostate

STAGE	OTHER CLASSIFICATIONS	EXPLANATION
Stage A*	T1, N0, M0	Tumor cannot be detected by any routine examination or tests but is found at surgery.
Stage B	T2b, N0, M0	Tumor can be felt within the prostate by rectal examination, but no spread can be detected.
Stage C	T3, N0, M0 Any T, N1, M0	Tumor has spread outside the prostate on rectal examination, but no further spread beyond the area and seminal vesicles can be detected.
Stage D	T4, N0, M0 Any T, N2–3, M0 Any T, any N, M1	Tumor has spread to lymph nodes in pelvis or to distant parts of body, most commonly the bones.

*Stage A is subdivided into Stage A1 (well-differentiated focal cancer) and Stage A2 (poorly differentiated, diffuse cancer).

What is a retropubic prostatectomy?

Retropubic prostatectomy is the removal of all or part of the prostate when the incision is made from the navel to the pubic bone to remove the gland and permit sampling of the pelvic lymph nodes. The surgeon performs the operation without opening the bladder.

What is a perineal prostatectomy?

It is similar to the retropubic procedure, with the incision a half-circle around the inner side of the anus.

What is a transurethral resection or TUR?

This operation permits removal of a tumor without an incision. It is usually used only for very small tumors or to treat benign disease. This approach is accomplished by inserting a special instrument through the penis to remove the tumor. Because it requires tremendous skill and ex-

Treatment Choices for Cancer of the Prostate

STAGE	POSSIBLE TREATMENTS
Stage A1	Careful observation following surgery; no further immediate treatment
Stage A2	Radiation treatment Radiation implant, sometimes with lymph-node removal Radical prostatectomy Investigational treatment available
Stage B	Radiation treatment Radiation implant, sometimes with lymph-node removal Radical prostatectomy Careful observation without further treatment for selected patients Investigational: radical prostatectomy avoiding the pelvic plexus to preserve potency. Other investigational treatments available.
Stage C	Radiation treatment Radiation implant, sometimes with lymph-node removal Radical prostatectomy in highly selected patients Careful observation without immediate therapy in selected patients with other serious medical problems Investigational protocols evaluating chemotherapy in conjunction with radiation therapy or newer forms of hormonal treatment
Stage D	Hormonal treatment Radiation treatment Careful observation without immediate treatment for patients without symptoms Investigational treatments evaluating chemotherapy and new forms of hormonal treatment Surgery and radiation for symptoms
Recurrent	Hormonal therapy Investigational treatments, including new chemotherapy agents or biologicals

pertise, this procedure should be done only by a urologist who is skillful in its use.

What are the aftereffects of total prostatectomy?

Although the cancer may be controlled, there are three consequences you should be aware of:
- Since the prostate gland produces most of the fluid released at the time of sexual intercourse and climax, most patients are sterile following this operation, just as they would be following a vasectomy.
- Many of the nerves that are involved with sexual function may be damaged, so that following surgery, many patients will no longer be able to have an erection. New investigational surgery avoiding the pelvic plexus is being done by selected doctors to avoid this problem.
- Some patients find that the operation causes them to lose their ability to control urine. Strengthening of muscles through simple exercise during recovery can sometimes help to return control. Urinary sphincter implants are possible to help control incontinence.

Is it true that after prostatectomy I will no longer ejaculate?

Yes. After prostatectomy, the ability to ejaculate through the penis is lost. What happens is that ejaculation occurs but it is directed backward into the bladder, rather than forward through the urethra. The semen remains in the bladder until urination, and is carried out via that route. The man who ejaculates in this manner has the very same sensations during sex that he had before except that there is no discharge through the penis.

Can a total prostatectomy be done without impairing the ability to have an erection?

Dr. Patrick C. Walsh, a surgeon at Johns Hopkins University Hospital in Baltimore, Maryland, has developed a way of removing the prostate which preserves potency by bypassing the intricate nerve branches of the pelvic plexus. This technique is now being adopted by many surgeons for patients with early-stage prostate cancer. Until the advent of this type of surgery, 90 percent of those having prostatectomies lost their sexual ability, and 2 to 5 percent became incontinent as well. It is important to discuss the expected results of prostatectomy with your doctor *before* surgery.

If I can no longer have an erection, can I have a penile prosthesis implanted?

Yes, it is possible to have a penile prosthesis implanted which will allow you to have an erection. There are several different kinds of implants. They are discussed on pages 632–633.

Even though the doctor says my prostate surgery was successful and that I should have the same sexual response as before treatment, why do I have problems having an erection?

There are many reasons for a man to lose his ability to have an erection. It happens to everyone—even to those who don't have cancer. The emotional stress of having cancer—depression, being tired, trying too hard, worry, alcohol—all can result in erection problems. Any signs of an erection will give you proof that your body is cooperating—but the psyche is so sensitive that it may take quite a long time for you to feel certain enough of your masculinity for you to resume normal intercourse. Perhaps this is a good time for you to experiment with other pleasuring techniques. If the doctor says there is no physical reason, perhaps the problem is psychological, due to pressure you feel about getting an erection. An appointment with a sex therapist or reading a self-help book such as *Male Sexuality* (Bernie Zilbergeld, Bantam Books, 1979) may be helpful.

If I ejaculate less fluid when I have an erection because of surgery, does that mean that I will be unable to father children?

As long as sperm is intact, the *amount* of fluid is not the determining factor. The sperm count makes a difference, but even the production of less sperm does not mean that you will be unable to father children. As far as your sexual enjoyment is concerned, the amount of fluid ejaculated should not cause noticeable changes for you and your partner.

Can I still have children even though I've had a transure-thral resection (TUR) for a prostate problem?

As many as three-quarters of the men who have had this type of surgery notice a decrease in the amount of fluid emitted at ejaculation. This is most likely due to unavoidable damage to the neck of the bladder during surgery. At ejaculation and orgasm, some or all of the seminal fluid backs up into the bladder (retrograde ejaculation) instead of being forced down and out of the penis. Nothing can be done to change this condition. But even if a smaller number of sperm are ejaculated, potency is not necessarily diminished and conception could result. In older patients who are not concerned about fathering children, a decrease in the amount of ejaculate should not cause a problem to patient or partner. If you are interested in having children, it is wise to have a complete fertility workup by a urologist or fertility specialist.

What types of radiation treatments are used for prostate cancer?

Either external and/or internal (implant) radiation can be used. The basic principle of radiation therapy is to bombard the cancer with rays at doses which damage or destroy the cancer yet produce only a minimum of damage to the surrounding normal tissues.

What type of external radiation is used?

External radiation employs either a linear accelerator or a cobalt-60 source to pinpoint the delivery of the radiation dosage. Some doctors use radiation as the primary treatment for prostate cancers in early stages. Others use it as additional therapy for some patients with later-stage disease. Radiation is usually given four or five times a week over a period of 6 or 7 weeks. It is important that the patient be in good enough general physical condition to tolerate this heavy concentration of high-energy radiation.

How are radium implants used in prostatic cancer?

Radioactive gold (Au^{198}), iodine (I^{125}), or iridium (Ir^{192}) is implanted directly into the tumor. With the patient anesthetized, a physician inserts thin metal tubes through the pubic region into the prostate. Then, through these tubes, he inserts the radioactive pellets, which remain in the patient's prostate. This procedure requires major abdominal surgery, often including examination of nearby lymph nodes. After the initial hospitalization, this type of radium implant is not considered dangerous in any way. Even in the hospital, forceps, linens, bandages, and so on are handled in the normal way. The patient does not endanger others and is advised that he may resume his normal living habits, having normal sexual relations, and that he can be near children and pregnant women without any fear for their health or safety due to potential contamination. Radium implants are sometimes combined with external radiation. The advantages and disadvantages of each kind of cancer therapy will become clearer as researchers monitor patients' progress over long periods.

Is chemotherapy used in treating prostate cancer?

Chemotherapy may be used alone or in combination with surgery or radiation especially for treatment of late stage cancer of the prostate as an investigational treatment.

What are the advantages of radiation therapy and radiation implants over prostatectomy?

Both kinds of radiation therapy are being used to treat some prostate cancers and the success rates indicate that these treatments are as effective or more effective than radical surgery, depending upon the spread of the disease. Since potency is maintained in 75 percent of patients following radiation, this is a consideration, particularly in men who are still sexually active. It is important that you discuss this question with the doctor before undergoing treatment.

When is an orchiectomy used for prostate cancer?

This procedure is sometimes used in the treatment of prostate cancer which has spread or when cancer recurs. Doctors have found that the spread of cancer can often be controlled for years by removing the testicles—man's natural source of the male sex hormone. An orchiectomy is the removal of the testicle. Removal of both testicles is a bilateral orchiectomy.

Isn't an orchiectomy the same as castration?

Some men have the mistaken belief that removal of the testicles will leave them with feminine voices and enlarged breasts. This is simply not so if the man has passed puberty. If both testicles are removed, orchiectomy does leave the patient sterile—but usually he does not lose his ability to have an erection.

Aren't sterility, impotency, and the lack of ability to ejaculate the same thing?

Sterility is the opposite of fertility and means that you are no longer able to father a child. Men who have had a vasectomy are sterile but are still potent and can ejaculate. Impotency refers to the inability to achieve erection. Prostatectomy may or may not leave a man impotent, depending upon whether the nerves governing erection are severed. Prostatectomy will often leave a man incapable of ejaculating, as the seminal fluids are forced backward into the bladder, from which they subsequently are excreted in the urine. If both vas are also severed, he will also be sterile.

What type of hormones are used in treating prostate cancer?

In late stage prostate cancer, instead of removing the testes, the administration of estrogen may be used. The female hormone counteracts or neutralizes the effects of testosterone. Among the hormones that may be prescribed are DES, E Stinyl, TACE, and flutamide.

Can hormone treatment cure cancer of the prostate?

No. Hormone treatment does not cure cancer of the prostate but is often used to control the activity of the disease and to lessen the pain. Many patients also recover appetite, gain weight, and return to normal activities as a result of hormone treatment. The tumor often shrinks, as well. However, in some patients, for reasons as yet not understood, the hormones may lose their effectiveness and the original symptoms may return.

What is LHRH?

These initials stand for leutenizing-hormone-releasing hormone, a hypothalamic hormone that controls sex hormones in men and women. A compound that is structurally similar to LHRH, known as LHRH agonist, when given on a long-term basis, suppresses the production of the male hormone testosterone and may be as effective as estrogen therapy or orchiectomy in blocking the production of male hormones, but without the cardiovascular and psychological side effects associated with conventional hormone treatment. In other investigational treatments, LHRH agonists have been combined with flutamide, a pure anti-androgen drug, in an attempt to suppress all male hormones, including the low levels of androgen produced by the adrenal glands. The FDA has approved the LHRH agonist leuprolide as a treatment for advanced prostate cancer. It is being marketed by TAP Pharmaceuticals under the brand name Lupron. The drug's only major side effect appears to be hot flashes.

Is the pituitary gland sometimes removed in treatment of prostate cancer?

Yes. Some research has indicated that the removal of the pituitary gland, called a transphenoidal hypophysectomy, can arrest the spread of prostate cancer in 50 percent of patients. Thanks to a relatively new operation, developed because of the high risk of previous pituitary surgery, which required opening the skull to reach the pituitary gland, removal has been simplified. The pituitary gland is removed by an operation performed through the upper gum and into the nasal passage to the pituitary below the brain. An unexpected result of the surgery is the disappearance of pain in about 75 percent of patients. The pain disappearance usually occurs within 48 hours and is usually permanent.

If a man has undergone surgery for a tumor of the prostate, does this mean he can no longer have prostate cancer?

No. Most operations performed for prostate problems other than cancer do not remove the whole prostate. Unless a man has undergone a total prostatectomy, he should remember that it is still possible for him to develop prostate cancer. Remaining prostatic tissue should be examined as part of every annual physical examination.

Are blood transfusions needed during prostate operations?

It depends upon the surgery. For most operations, there is considerable blood loss, which is replaced by blood transfusion.

Is pain very great after prostatectomy?

Usually, moderate pain is felt.

How is the urine drained after the operation?

Usually by a catheter placed in the urethra or bladder.

CANCER OF THE TESTICLE

What are the testes and how do they function?

The testes are egg-shaped glands situated in the scrotum. They produce spermatozoa. The sperm is collected at the back of the testicles in a maze of coiled tubes called the epididymis. It then travels up toward the seminal vesicles and prostate through a long tube known as the vas deferens.

How is testicular cancer usually discovered?

Most testicular cancers are discovered by patients themselves, by accident or by practicing a simple exam known as TSE or testicular self-examination. TSE is usually done once a month, during or soon after a warm bath or shower. While standing, the man gently rolls one testicle between his thumb and fingers, checking for lumps, swelling or other changes. The process is repeated for the other testicle.

Is testicular cancer a common type of cancer?

No, it is not. Testicular cancer actually accounts for only 1 percent of all cancer in males and about 3 percent of cancer of the male urogenital organs. However, in the age group where it occurs—in white men from 20 to 34—it is the most common cancer, accounting for 22 percent of all cancers for this age group. It is also the second most common cancer in men from ages 35 to 39 and the third most common from 15 to 19. Thanks to treatment advances in the last 10 years, testicular cancer is considered a highly curable cancer. Young men whose brothers or fathers had testicular cancer are more likely to have it.

Is testicular cancer more common in those who have undescended testicles?

Yes. In the male fetus, the testes are formed farther up in the body, near the kidneys, and, in normal development, descend to the scrotum shortly after birth. If they never make this descent or descend after the age of 6, the chances of testicular cancer developing in later years is forty times more likely than if they properly enter the scrotum.

What are the symptoms of testicular cancer?

The first sign is usually a small, hard lump, about the size of a pea or a slight enlargement or change in the consistency of the testes. There may be a dull ache in the lower abdomen and groin, accompanied by a sensation of dragging or heaviness. If the tumor is growing rapidly and hemorrhage is present, there may be sharp testicular pain. Enlargement of the breast or tenderness of the nipples may also be noticed.

How is cancer of the testicle diagnosed?

First, infection and other diseases are ruled out by physical examination and medical tests. Because most tumors in the testes are cancerous rather than non-cancerous, the standard procedure for a suspicious lump in the scrotum is surgical removal of the entire affected testicle. This is done through an incision in the groin. The operation is necessary to get the diagnosis. However, it also prevents further growth of the tumor and, if done at an early stage, may stop the spread of the cancer to other parts of the body. *A biopsy is not performed for testicular cancer* because it would need to cut through the fibrous outer capsule of the testis and could contribute to the spread of cancer cells.

Are there different kinds of testicular cancer?

Yes. Actually, there are many different kinds, but they are generally placed in two broad types of germ cell cancers: seminomas and nonseminomas. Seminomas account for 40 percent of all testicular germ cell cancers.

Are different treatments recommended for the different types of testicular cancer?

Yes. Surgery—the removal of the suspected testicle—is usually the first step. Treatment of the affected lymph nodes varies according to the type of cells found in the tumor.

Can I go to my local doctor for treatment of testicular cancer?

Since this is a rare form of cancer, the patient with suspected testicular cancer would be well advised to seek out a urologist specializing in cancer in one of the large medical centers to be certain that he receives the optimal treatment for this disease. Close cooperation and exchange of information among surgeon, radiotherapist, and medical oncologist is a must to ensure the successful outcome of this type of cancer.

The Stages of Cancer of the Testicle

STAGE	OTHER CLASSIFICATIONS	EXPLANATION
Stage I	T1–3, N0, M0	Tumor is limited to testis.
Stage II	T4, N0, M0 Any T, N1, M0	Tumor is limited to testis and the abdominal lymph nodes.
Stage III*	Any T, N2, M0	Cancer has spread beyond abdominal lymph nodes, based on physical examination, x-rays, and/or blood tests

Divided into non-bulky Stage III (metastases limited to lymph nodes and the lung with no mass larger than 2 cm in diameter) and bulky Stage III (includes retroperitoneal nodal involvement lung masses greater then 2 cm in diameter or spread to other organs such as liver or brain).

Treatment Choices for Cancer of the Testicle

STAGE	POSSIBLE TREATMENT
Stage I: Seminoma	Removal of testicle followed by radiation therapy to lymph nodes.
Stage I: Nonseminoma	Removal of testicle followed by removal of lymph nodes. Surgical technique can spare fertility. Monthly or bimonthly testing of serum markers and chest x-rays for 2 years. Chemotherapy at first evidence of recurrance. Investigational: radical orchiectomy.
Stage II: Seminoma	Bulky disease: radical orchiectomy followed by combination chemotherapy, possibly with radiation to lymph nodes. Non-bulky disease: radical orchiectomy followed by radiation to lymph nodes.
Stage II: Nonseminoma	Removal of testicle followed by removal of lymph nodes. Surgical technique can spare fertility. Monthly testing of serum markers and chest x-rays for 2 years. Chemotherapy for patients with non-normal markers. Removal of testicle followed by removal of lymph nodes, followed by chemotherapy. Monthly testing of serum markers and chest x-rays for 2 years. Removal of testicle followed by chemotherapy followed by monthly checkups. Investigational treatments are also available.
Stage III: Seminoma	Removal of testicle followed by multi-drug chemotherapy, possibly with radiation therapy.
Stage III: Nonseminoma	Combination chemotherapy, possibly with surgery. Investigational: Intensive chemotherapy for high-risk patients with bulky disease. Less toxic chemotherapy for patients with non-bulky disease.
Recurrent	Combination chemotherapy. Investigational treatments available.

Is a biopsy usually done before a testicle is removed?

No. This is one of the cases where the usual simple biopsy is not used for diagnosis. Doctors are warned against using needle aspiration or cutting into the tumor. In most cases, the doctor will schedule you for an operation to remove the testicle. Further therapy is based on results of a permanent section biopsy—not on a frozen-section examination.

Are any blood tests used in testicular cancer?

Two serum markers—blood proteins that often become elevated in cancer patients—have greatly helped in staging testicular cancers, monitoring how well the treatment is working, and detecting early relapse. The markers are AFP (alpha-fetoprotein) and HCG (the beta subunit of human chorionic gonadotropin). The markers are measured before and after surgery to help determine if any cancer cells remain.

Does removal of one testicle affect potency or fertility?

No, providing the remaining testicle is normal.

After removal of a testicle (orchiectomy) and x-ray therapy, is it still possible for a man to father a child?

If the radiation can be calculated to pinpoint the specific site without damaging surrounding tissues or organs, it may be possible to avoid sterility. Sperm can also be frozen and stored in a sperm bank for later use in case the patient does become sterile. Be sure to thoroughly discuss with your doctor before treatment the entire question of fertility, radiation, and sperm storage.

What is the role of chemotherapy in testicular cancer which has metastasized?

Chemotherapy was first found potentially curative for testicular cancer in the late 1950s. Many trials and protocols have been tested in the past 30 years—and it is important that your doctor be aware of the latest treatments being used. Several drugs have been found to be effective, and some patients with metastatic testicular cancer can now be cured with combination chemotherapy. The treatment is difficult, however, and requires an experienced medical oncologist to administer it.

Why are the abdominal lymph nodes removed in testicular cancer?

Surgery to remove the abdominal lymph nodes may be necessary in some patients in order to stage the disease accurately. Since cancer of the testicle spreads first to the retroperitoneal lymph nodes (the nodes deep in the abdomen below the diaphragm), this surgery may also help control the disease by taking out any nodes which are involved.

What kind of follow-up therapy is needed after treatment for testicular cancer?

Testicular cancer patients need continuing medical follow-up, including regular x-rays with CT scans of the lungs and abdomen and monthly checks of serum-marker levels for one to two years. After that, checkups are scheduled once or twice a year. If there is evidence that some cancer remains or that the cancer has spread or recurred, maintenance chemotherapy may also be necessary.

Is testicular cancer usually curable?

Today, cancer of the testicle is considered a highly treatable, usually curable cancer. The outlook for patients, of course, varies depending upon the extent of the disease when diagnosed, the tumor cell type, and the growth rate.

Do operations performed when cancer is found in the testicle have an effect on sexual ability or fertility?

Treatment for testicular cancer, if the cancer is localized in the testicle and is found to be of the seminoma type, usually requires that the testicle and the other surrounding glandular structures be removed. If cells other than seminoma cells are found, more extensive surgery is required to help prevent spread of the cancer into the lymph nodes that drain fluids from the pelvic area. A gel-filled implant, which has the weight, shape and texture of a normal testicle can be inserted surgically, either at the time of the original operation or later, to restore normal appearance. Since cancer of the testicle rarely involves more than one testicle, erection is usually still possible. There may be a decrease in ejaculate, but the remaining testicle should produce enough sperm for a man to be able to father children.

What technique can be used to increase fertility for men who have had testicular surgery?

This surgery may cause a decrease in ejaculation because nerves are cut during surgery and may result in infertility. However, there is a chance you may still have the ability to father children, even though you may be producing less semen. A study by a German doctor, since confirmed by patients at Memorial Sloan-Kettering Cancer Center Hospital in New York City, shows that some men who wish to father children may be able to raise their sperm counts by having intercourse on a full bladder, standing up, if possible, to force the fluid to be deposited properly.

How can I make arrangements to store my sperm so that I can father children if I become sterile because of my operation or radiation?

It may be possible for sperm to be frozen and stored in a sperm bank for later use in case you become sterile. However, many men with testicular cancer are ineligible for sperm-banking because their sperm production may be impaired as a result of the disease itself. It is important to discuss with your doctor *before* treatment the entire question of sterility, radiation, and sperm storage.

How do sperm banks work?

Sperm banks usually provide indefinite storage of sperm for cancer patients, pre-vasectomy patients, and others. Usually, enough semen is collected and frozen to provide an adequate amount to be used for a 6-month period. An analysis of the semen is done to assess the quality and assure that it can be banked satisfactorily. Usually, the first sample is used to assess the quality, then a 48-hour trial freezing is done and the quality is tested again. In order to ensure an adequate amount of semen, the patient is asked to come to the lab with a semen sample every 48 hours for several weeks, until enough semen has been provided. It is essential that the specimen be delivered within a half hour after ejaculation to ensure potency. The patient is asked to sign a consent form to allow the sperm to be stored. Sperm banks are available in various areas in the United States. Your doctor or the Cancer Information Service (1-800-4-CANCER) can provide you with a listing of the locations.

Does chemotherapy for testicular cancer affect fertility?

While some types of chemotherapy can cause impaired fertility, a recent study showed that fertility can return in some patients 2 to 3 years after treatment.

What is the effect of radiation of lymph nodes on fertility and sexual function in testicular cancer?

Radiation therapy of the lymph nodes, with proper shielding of the normal testicle, and proper shielding of other organs, usually does not affect fertility or sexual function.

CANCER OF THE PENIS

Does cancer of the penis ever occur?

Cancer of the penis is quite rare. It usually occurs on the tip of the penis and is almost exclusively found in uncircumcised males between the ages of 50 and 70. In others, cancer of the penis is found to be a metastasis from the bladder, prostate, lung, pancreas, kidney, testicle, or ureter.

What symptoms should alert a man to the possibility of cancer of the penis?

A pimple or sore, small nodule, white thickened patches, raised, velvety patch, wart or ulcer—especially a painless ulcer—are all suspicious symptoms. Bleeding associated with erection or intercourse, persistent abnormal erection without sexual desire, foul-smelling discharge, or a lump in the groin should all be carefully investigated.

What is the usual treatment for cancer of the penis?

The usual treatment is surgery. Approximately 90 percent of patients with cancer of the penis, if it is found in the early stages, will be cured through the surgical removal of the tumor. If the cancer has spread to the groin, nodes in the groin will usually be removed. Chemotherapy and radiation therapy are also used in some cases.

The Stages of Cancer of the Penis

STAGE	EXPLANATION
Stage I	Tumor is limited to the glans and foreskin and does not involve the shaft of the penis.
Stage II	Tumor has invaded the shaft of the penis but has not spread to lymph nodes.
Stage III	Tumor has spread to regional lymph nodes in groin.
Stage IV	Invasive tumor has caused extensive involvement of lymph nodes in groin and/or distant metastases.

Treatment Choices for Cancer of the Penis

STAGE	POSSIBLE TREATMENTS
Stage I	Circumcision for tumors limited to foreskin Topical chemotherapy (fluorouracil) for in situ cancer of the glans Radiation therapy Penile amputation Microscopically controlled surgery
Stage II	Penile amputation: partial, total, or radical Investigational: lymph-node removal with penile amputation
Stage III	Penile amputation with removal of lymph nodes Investigational: radiosensitizers or chemotherapy
Stage IV	Surgery or radiation therapy for symptoms Investigational: chemotherapy with surgery or radiation
Recurrent	Surgery or radiation therapy Investigational: new biologicals and chemotherapy agents

What sexual problems can I expect as a result of surgery on the penis?

It depends on the extent of the surgery. If only part of the penis has been removed, you may still be able to achieve erection and have the ability to perform penile-vaginal intercourse to the point of ejaculation. You may also be able to achieve orgasm and ejaculation by stimulation of the remaining part of your penis through masturbation or by your partner's manual or oral stimulation.

How can I have an active sex life if I am unable to have intercourse?

Your sex life will probably not be the same as before, but there are ways for you to have an active sex life and sexual enjoyment.
- Many men continue to be good lovers by using their hands or mouth to stimulate their partners.
- You may still be able to ejaculate with a non-erect penis or may learn to experience orgasms in other ways.
- There are several prosthetic devices which can be inserted surgically in the penis to make intercourse possible.

How do prosthetic devices for the penis work?

There are several kinds of penile prostheses that may be implanted in the penis to make intercourse possible. The device is placed inside the corpora cavernosa, two structures within the penis resembling long balloons that normally fill with blood during an erection. The prosthetic devices are either inflatable or semi-rigid. There are advantages and disadvantages to each type of prosthesis, which you will want to discuss with your doctor and your partner.

The inflatable prosthesis gives a natural-looking appearance. A pump placed in the scrotum allows the man to transfer fluid from a reservoir which is placed in the abdomen to two inflatable balloons that go in the penis. There are tubings from the pump to the reservoir and to the two inflatable balloons. When deflation is desired, he presses a valve on the side of the pump to release the fluid back into the reservoir. This type of prosthesis requires an ex-

tensive operation and, because it is mechanically complicated, some 40 to 50 percent of patients need to have it
repaired at some time. Correction of problems require another operation.

Another type of prosthesis is a semi-rigid device made
of silicone. Although it is easier to insert and hardly ever
malfunctions, it is less satisfactory because once it is inserted, the penis remains in the erect position. The penis
can be placed either up against the abdominal wall, into
the groin crease, or bent along the leg.

A third type is the rubber rod prosthesis, which has more
positions than the semi-rigid prosthesis and can be manually rotated.

Your doctor will be able to advise you where you can get
information about penile prostheses and may also be able
to help you contact others who have had the operation.

**What is the treatment for a metastasis that appears on the
penis?**

The treatment in this case would usually involve surgical
removal of the tumor followed by radiation to relieve the
pain which this type of metastasis usually causes.

chapter 18

Cancers of the Head and Neck

Cancers of the head and neck are those that affect any part of the oral cavity: lip, tongue, mouth, ear, and throat, as well as the sinuses and sometimes muscles in the neck and upper back. Reconstructive surgery is a recent blessing for those who have cancers in any of these areas, for defects in the various facial structures—such as eyes, ears, nose, mouth, lips, cheek and neck—can be minimized by the plastic surgeon.

Since cancers of the head and neck are quite rare, and the problems individualized, it is crucial that, if there is to be extensive surgery, treatment be sought at a center where there is a well-integrated team of maxillofacial specialists who can deliver the best possible techniques, management, and knowledge.

Thyroid cancer is a highly curable form of cancer. It affects women more commonly than men and the majority of cases occur between the ages of 25 and 65. Treatment depends on cell type and stage of disease.

Cancer of the larnyx can be cured if it is found early. One of the most common early symptoms is hoarseness that lasts for more than three weeks.

Cancer of the esophagus is a treatable and sometimes curable cancer. It is relatively rare and is seen more often in black than in white men. It is usually treated by radiation alone or combined with surgery, with surgery and chemotherapy or with chemotherapy alone.

Questions to Ask Your Doctor Before Agreeing to Any Treatment

- Who will be performing surgery?
- Where will the incision be and what will the scar look like?
- How disfiguring will the surgery be?
- What will I look like?
- Will I still be able to eat, talk, and swallow after the surgery?
- Can radiation or radium implant be used instead of the surgery?
- Will radiation or chemotherapy be used in addition to the surgery?
- What kind of reconstructive surgery can be done?
- How many operations will that entail?
- What are the effects?
- How long will it all take?
- Will it cure me?
- How expensive will it be?
- Who else will be on the treatment team?
- Can I talk with them before I have any operation?
- How many patients with head and neck cancer are you treating?

What kind of doctor should I see if I have symptoms of head and neck cancer?

The doctors who usually specialize in the treatment of head and neck cancer include otolaryngologists (ENT—doctors who treat ear, nose, and throat, air tubes to the lung, and neck regions), plastic surgeons (who do operations involving skin grafts, facial injuries, and tendon and nerve repair), and some general surgeons. Depending upon the type of cancer, the oral surgeon, maxillofacial prosthodontist (who specializes in replacing lost facial features), speech therapist, radiotherapist, and medical oncologist are ideally part of the team.

Can I go to my local doctor for the treatment of head and neck cancer?

The treatment of head and neck cancer often requires a team approach. It is important that your treatment not be decided on by an individual specialist because the diagnosis, evaluation of the extent of the disease, choice of primary treatment, and effective rehabilitation require special talents that cross over conventional lines. There are several doctors who have special interest and training in the management of head and neck cancer problems—the general surgeon, otorhinolaryngologist, plastic surgeon, oral surgeon, radiotherapist, and oncologist. The total care requires collaboration among these specialists as well as with the neurosurgeon, prosthodontist, speech therapist, and other allied health personnel.

Is the National Cancer Institute supporting any studies on head and neck cancer?

Yes. There are many clinical cooperative group studies being conducted by the National Cancer Institute on head and neck tumors. A variety of different trials, most of them involving radiation therapy or chemotherapy, either alone or in combination and either with or without surgery, as well as immunotherapy and neutron radiotherapy, are in progress (see Chapter 23).

What is head and neck cancer?

Cancer of the head and neck is a catchall phrase for an assortment of cancers which occur above the collarbone. It usually includes cancer in the ears, salivary glands, eye, upper airway and food passages, nose, paranasal sinuses, nasopharynx, lips, oral cavity, tongue, tonsils, pharynx, hypopharynx, larynx and cervical esophagus, neck, and thyroid and parathyroid glands.

What are the most common sites of head and neck cancer?

The most common sites of head and neck cancer (excluding the skin) are in the mouth (oral cavity), pharynx (throat), larynx (voice box), thyroid, and sinuses.

What are the most common symptoms of head and neck cancer?

The symptoms differ depending upon the site. A small ulcer in the mouth is one symptom. It may first appear somewhere on the tongue, around the tonsils, or along the edges of the upper and lower gums. It may look like a cold sore. It is usually painless and unlike a cold sore it does not heal by itself. Difficulty in swallowing, continued hoarseness, a sore throat that persists, neck swelling, and a lump on the side of the neck are all symptoms which, if they last for more than 2 weeks, should be checked by a doctor.

Are cancers of the head and neck common?

Head and neck cancers constitute only about 5 percent of all cancers. They are not common cancers, especially in comparison with cancers of the breast, lung, or colon-rectal areas. However, since they are difficult to manage and the team approach is most important in treating them, we discuss the major types of head and neck cancer in some detail in this book.

Do cancers of the head and neck metastasize to other parts of the body?

Unlike many other types of tumor, tumors in the head and neck usually remain confined to that area. They do not tend to metastasize to distant parts of the body. However, they do tend to spread to lymph nodes in the area.

What kind of treatment is used in head and neck cancer?

As is true with most other types of cancer, treatment includes all three disciplines: surgery, radiotherapy, and chemotherapy. Surgery is the treatment most often used. Usually early tumors are treated by surgery with adjoining tissue taken out. If the neck nodes are involved, a radical neck dissection may be done. Radiation therapy is used either before or after surgery. Sometimes chemotherapy is combined with immunotherapy in treating patients with head and neck cancer.

Is reconstructive surgery usually necessary for head and neck cancer?

It depends upon the kind of cancer, the extent of the tumor, and the kind of surgery which is performed. In many cases of cancer of the head and neck, reconstructive surgery is not necessary. However, where needed, skillful skin and bone grafting allows persons who have had radical surgery

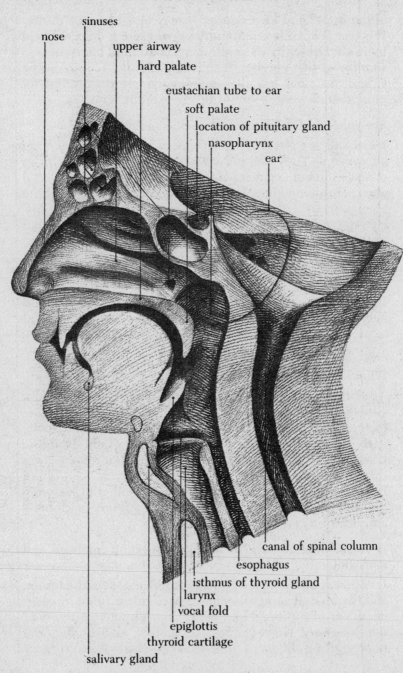

nose

sinuses

upper airway

hard palate

eustachian tube to ear

soft palate

location of pituitary gland

nasopharynx

ear

canal of spinal column

esophagus

isthmus of thyroid gland

larynx

vocal fold

epiglottis

thyroid cartilage

salivary gland

Head and neck

Head and Neck Cancer

Type	Symptoms	Diagnostic Tests	Treatment
Nose (including sinus, naso-pharynx)	Reddish, easily bleeding mass in nasal passage or cheek. If in paranasal sinuses, pain or swelling of cheek, inability to wear dentures	Head and neck examination, x-rays, biopsy	Surgery, preceded or followed by radiation. Nasopharyngeal radiation may be followed by surgery. Reconstructive surgery.
Salivary glands (including parotid gland)	Lump below ear and jaw; occasionally pain or tenderness, hard consistency, facial palsy	Manual examination, x-rays, biopsy	Surgery to remove tumor. Radical neck dissection if lymph nodes involved. Surgery may involve facial nerve. Reconstructive surgery. Radiation. Investigational: chemotherapy.
Mouth (including tongue, gums, floor of mouth, lip, cheek)	A lump in the cheek that can be felt by the tongue, white patches, sore that does not heal, lump or thickening, bleeding, difficulty in chewing or swallowing food, restricted movement of tongue or jaw, discomfort in wearing dentures	Manual examination by doctor and dentist, x-rays, biopsy	Surgery, radiation, radium implants, alone or in combination. Chemotherapy may be used as an investigational treatment. Reconstructive surgery.

Head and Neck Cancer

TYPE	SYMPTOMS	DIAGNOSTIC TESTS	TREATMENT
Oropharynx (including soft palate, tonsil, walls of pharynx and back of tongue)	Mild sore throat, lump in back of tongue, velvety red patches, open sores in mouth, earaches, lump in neck	Manual examination, x-rays, laryngoscopy, biopsy	Radiation, surgery, alone or in combination. Chemotherapy may be used. Reconstructive surgery.
Hypopharynx (lower pharynx)	Difficulty in swallowing, lumps in neck, difficulty in breathing, earaches, cough, bad breath	Manual examination, laryngoscopy, biopsy	Radiation, surgery, alone or in combination. Reconstructive surgery.
Thyroid	Lump in neck, persistent hoarseness, difficulty in swallowing	Thyroid scan, fine needle biopsy	Surgery, radiation, postoperative hormone treatment, and/or radioactive iodine
Larynx	Hoarseness, lump in throat, difficult or painful swallowing, pain in ear, shortness of breath, harsh and noisy breathing	Indirect laryngoscopy, laryngogram, direct laryngoscopy, biopsy, diagnostic x-rays	Surgery and/or radiation. Chemotherapy may be used for advanced cancers as an investigational treatment
Esophagus	Difficulty in swallowing, pressure, burning or pain in middle chest	Barium swallow, x-rays, esophagoscopy	Surgery, radiation

to return to as normal an appearance and function as possible.

Can a person develop head and neck cancer from smoking or chewing tobacco?

Cancer of the lip, tongue, mouth, and pharynx (the space behind the nose and mouth) do occur more often in people who smoke, chew tobacco, or use snuff. Snuff, particularly when used in the form of a pellet and held for long periods of time between the gum and the cheek, frequently causes irritation and may eventually produce cancer at the spot. Chewing tobacco has also been linked to the development of cancer of the mouth.

Are there any new treatments being tried for head and neck cancer?

There are several new treatments being tested, especially for large tumors of the head and neck region or tumors that have spread beyond the area. Chemotherapy, immunotherapy, a combination of the two treatments, chemotherapy used before surgery to shrink the tumor, chemotherapy and/ or radiotherapy after surgery, chemotherapy followed by radiation therapy are all being tried with some success. Radium implants are being used in the treatment of mouth cancer.

Is cancer of the eye a common tumor?

No. Cancer of the eye is quite rare. The most common form of eye cancer in adults is intraocular melanoma, which is highly curable and preservation of vision is possible in some tumors which are small and local to the eye.

Do children get eye cancer?

Yes, there is a type of eye cancer, called retinoblastoma which affects children. Information on this cancer is found in Chapter 20.

How is intraocular melanoma treated?

The treatment depends on the size and location of the tumor, the amount of eye damage which has occurred, the age of the patient, and whether the tumor grows quickly. If the tumor is extensive, it may be necessary to remove the eye and the muscle and fat surrounding it.

Are any new techniques being used in the treatment of eye cancer?

An experimental laser technique called photoradiation therapy (PRT) has been successfully used to treat patients with some types of melanoma of the eye and of retinoblastoma. The patient is injected with a chemical that washes through normal tissue but collects in cancer cells and renders them very light-sensitive. When exposed to the red light of a laser beam, the cancer cells are destroyed, while surrounding normal tissue is unharmed. This is the same type of laser used in cancers of the lung, stomach, bladder, and throat. The treatment does not expose the eye to radiation that might cause cataracts or damage the retina.

What is a radical neck dissection?

The surgeon removes a block of tissue from the collarbone to the jaw and from the front to the back of the neck. The large muscle on the side of the neck that is used for rotating, flexing or extending the neck is also taken out, along with the major vein on the side of the neck. Sometimes, a less drastic operation, called a supraomohyoid neck dissection is done. This takes out only the lymph nodes, the tissue surrounding the nodes and a muscle at the front of the neck. Another technique, called a functional neck dissection, saves the muscles of the neck, taking out only the lymph nodes and tissues surrounding them.

What kind of incision is made with a radical neck dissection?

The incision depends upon what the surgery is for. It can run from below the ear to the collarbone. Everything in the front of the neck on one side or on both sides may be removed. This may include the lymph nodes, blood vessels, nerves, and the salivary gland under the jawbone.

When is a radical neck dissection performed?

A radical neck dissection is performed to remove the tumor and the lymph nodes in the neck. Cancers such as those of the lips, tongue, and larynx sometimes spread to the lymph nodes, requiring them to be removed.

Is a tracheostomy done as part of the operation for radical neck dissection?

A tracheostomy (opening made in the windpipe) is usually necessary if the doctor is going to perform a radical neck dissection. After a few days the tube will be taken out and the opening will close.

Is a radical neck dissection a major operation?

Yes, it is. It may require up to 5 or 6 hours to perform when it is done along with the removal of the primary cancer.

Why is it important to exercise after I have had radical neck dissection?

In a radical neck dissection, the nerve responsible mainly for arm motion, which connects with one of the most important muscles in your neck and upper back, is cut. It makes it harder for you to raise your arm over your head or out to your side. If the surgery is on both sides of your neck, you will probably have some trouble raising both arms. However, there are special exercises which will help you get some of the strength back again.

How will I know what exercises to do?

Don't do any exercises until your doctor or your physical therapist tells you to. You may need to be seen by a physical therapist, who will determine your condition and give you exercises which will help your particular case. He or she will show you how to do them and tell you how often they should be done. It is important to make sure you do these exercises regularly. If they are not done, you may find the shoulder on the operated side will fall forward and look lower than the one on the other side. And if the surgery was on both sides of the neck, you might find that both shoulders are falling forward and you will be standing and sitting in an uncomfortable, slumped-over position which may cause shoulder pain.

Will I have trouble eating or swallowing after head and neck surgery?

You may have trouble in chewing, swallowing and speaking. You may also find your appearance has changed. Rehabilitation is a very important part of your treatment and may include plastic surgery.

What kinds of facial defects might a patient with head and neck cancer have?

Patients with head and neck cancer may be left with defects of various facial structures, including eyes, ears, nose, mouth, lips, cheek, and neck.

What kind of work is done to correct these facial defects?

The defects are corrected either by reconstructive surgery or with the use of maxillofacial prosthetics.

How will the decision be made as to what will be done?

The choice of methods depends upon the kind of defect which needs to be corrected, and discussion between the patient and the doctors involved.

What is reconstructive surgery?

Reconstructive surgery is the reconstruction of features from the patient's own tissue. A plastic surgeon does reconstructive surgery.

What does the reconstructive surgeon do?

The reconstructive surgeon usually has two roles: He attempts to minimize the deformity which results from the treatment of the tumor, and he initiates and coordinates an overall rehabilitation program.

What techniques can the reconstructive surgeon use?

The reconstructive surgeon must be familiar with the use of skin, cartilage, and bone grafts. He must be able to transfer tissue from a distant site to the tumor area. He helps people who have limited ability to speak, hear, see, eat, or even move, live more normal lives.

What are maxillofacial prosthetics?

The field of maxillofacial prosthetics grew out of prosthetic dentistry. It means using an artificial part to correct a defect in the body. The new plastics, plastic and silicone rubber, are used to make parts to replace what is taken out in the surgical operation. There are some specialized centers in the United States which have the facilities to construct these prosthetics for the rehabilitation of patients with facial defects.

What kind of doctors create maxillofacial prosthodontics?

Doctors who specialize in this field belong to the American Academy of Maxillofacial Prosthetics.

What does a maxillofacial prosthodontist do?

The job of the maxillofacial prosthodontist is to restore the patient's appearance and function. He uses the remaining tissues that the patient has to support the prosthesis. He manages the dental and paradental structures to prevent loss of the supporting tissues. You may need a maxillofacial prosthesis to speak or eat or swallow. Or it may be necessary because you have lost an eye, your nose, or some portion of your face.

When does the maxillofacial prosthodontist see me?

Many times the prosthodontist will be part of the team you see before surgery or radiation therapy. Sometimes, after surgery the prosthodontist will not see you until the sixth or seventh day. He may give you a temporary prosthesis for use until the permanent prosthesis is fitted and made.

What is an obturator?

An obturator is a "cork" which plugs a hole or seals off an opening. It is the basis of most prostheses. It fits into the defect which was made by the surgery. It may help make a part function naturally or may help build out the face cosmetically when some parts have been removed.

When is an obturator put in?

Sometimes the obturator is inserted at the time of surgery, sometimes about a week after.

If I am missing part of the face, how is the prosthesis made?

If you need to replace a missing part of the face such as the nose, eye, ear, or a combination of these, the missing or defect areas are sculpted in clay or wax on casts of the defect. Molds are then made, and the prosthesis is created of a flexible plastic from the mold. The prostheses are tinted to match your skin. If you wish, you can have more than one prosthesis made—tinted to match the skin color at different seasons.

Must I wear the obturator all the time?

It depends upon where the surgery is performed. If you have had oral surgery, the doctor will tell you to try to wear the obturator most of the time, even at night, and remove it only for cleaning the mouth. The obturator allows you to eat, speak, and swallow, and will keep the wound from contracting.

Do most head and neck patients need dental prostheses?

It is estimated that more than half the head and neck patients will need some kind of dental care—some form of prosthesis to restore function or appearance or both.

What kinds of areas can be fitted with prostheses?

There are several areas in the head and neck region where prostheses are used. For instance,
- An ear can be replaced by plastic material.
- An eye and even portions of the cheek can be replaced.
- Parts of the nose or the complete nose can be made either with a graft or with a prosthesis.
- Parts of the mouth and lip can be reconstructed.
- Teeth and parts of the palate are filled by prostheses which allow the patient to eat and to talk.

The doctors can simulate skin tones, ruddy complexions, freckles, and veins. They can fit parts which remain permanently in place. They use lightweight materials which are easily cleaned, durable, and compatible with the nearby tissue.

Is it true that many patients with head and neck cancer get very depressed and discouraged?

Again, it depends upon the site of the cancer and the attitude of the patient. Many patients whose operation has caused facial disfigurement or a great change such as a laryngectomy naturally go through some depressed periods. However, when they find out that they can live their lives in much the same fashion as they did before—with reconstructive surgery and help in learning to speak—most head and neck patients find that life is still worth living. However, most people need support and help from family and friends to get through the difficult period of adjustment.

What kinds of cancers are found in the mouth?

The cancers of the mouth (oral cavity) include the lip, tongue, floor of the mouth, cheeks (buccal mucosa), and gums (gingivae).

Who is at high risk to get cancer of the mouth?

This cancer is predominantly found in men between the ages of 60 and 70. People who are heavy smokers (more than a pack a day), drink alcohol heavily, are over 45, and have a family history of this kind of cancer are at a higher risk to develop cancers of the oral cavity, the mouth, and the throat.

Is cancer of the mouth easy to detect?

Yes, it is usually discovered early, since it can be seen easily. White patches (leukoplakia), velvety red spots (erythroplasia), or dark patches are symptoms which should be seen by a doctor, who will do a biopsy of them. Many cancers of the mouth are first discovered by dentists.

What are the symptoms of oral cancer?

The warning signs of oral cancer are as follows:
- A lump in the cheek that can be felt with the tongue
- Sore spot or ulceration of lips, tongue, or other area inside the mouth that does not heal in 2 weeks

- White scaly area inside the mouth
- Swelling of the lips, gums, or other area inside the mouth, with or without pain
- Repeated bleeding in the mouth with no apparent cause
- Numbness or loss of feeling in any part of the mouth

What is leukoplakia?

Leukoplakia is a fairly common condition among people who smoke. It is not cancerous, but it can become cancerous especially if it is continually irritated, as by smoking. It occurs as a white thickening or patches on the lip, on the tongue, or in the mouth. It replaces the normal, pink mucous membrane of the mouth. It may be flat or elevated and its edges may be sharply outlined or poorly defined. It may be found in one small area of the mouth or in several parts. Sometimes it is called smoker's tongue or smoker's patches. Poorly fitted dentures can also be irritating to leukoplakia. If you have this problem, it is important to have the dental defect taken care of.

Are the white patches usually removed?

It depends upon the extent of the patches. The patches may be removed with an electric needle, using local anesthesia. If there are many of them, you will need several treatments to take them all out. You can also have them removed surgically or with cryosurgery. They usually require either local or general anesthesia and an overnight stay in the hospital.

What is Plummer-Vinson syndrome?

Plummer-Vinson syndrome is a wasting away of mucous membranes of the mouth, pharynx, and esophagus caused by deficiencies in the diet. It is a noncancerous condition that tends to become malignant. It frequently precedes mouth cancer.

What is torus palatinus?

Torus palatinus is a bony growth in the middle of the hard palate in the roof of the mouth. It is a benign tumor which can grow to an inch or more in diameter. It grows slowly and you may not notice it. Unless you are having some problem with it, such as in fitting dentures, it is usually left alone. If necessary, it can be surgically removed. The operation can be done under local anesthesia. The membrane of the palate will be opened, the excess bone chiseled away, and the membrane stitched together.

Is bleeding in the mouth a sign of cancer?

Repeated bleeding of the mouth without cause is a sign of some kind of problem. If it has been going on for 2 weeks, you should have it checked by a doctor or a dentist. Most cases of bleeding in the mouth are not cancerous.

Can I examine myself for oral cancer?

Yes, it is possible for you to examine yourself for oral cancer.

There are six areas of the mouth—lips, cheeks, gums, tongue, roof, and floor—which should be examined. A well-lit mirror, a gauze pad or handkerchief, and clean hands are all that are needed.

- Check your lips, cheeks, and gums, looking for changes in the normal color. Look for areas of red, white, or blue. See if there are any scabs, cracks, ulcers, or areas of swelling or bleeding. You should feel for sore spots, numbness, bumps, or thickening within the tissues of your lips and cheeks. Feel your gums to see if there is any swelling, numbness, soreness, or a loose tooth.
- Look at your tongue. Stick it out as far as you can. Examine the tip, the top, the bottom, and edges. You are looking for white patches, velvety-red spots, ulcers, or swelling. Feel the tongue to see if there are any lumps, sore spots, or lack of movement. Extend the tongue in all directions by grasping it with the gauze pad or handkerchief.
- Check both the floor and the roof of your mouth. Look for lumps, swellings, or soreness. Feel along the sides and as far back as you can go. Tilt your head back and look at the front and back of the roof of your mouth in the mirror. If you have any problems that last for more than 2 weeks, you should see your doctor or your dentist. Although these signs don't always mean cancer is present, they are warning signals.

Will habitual biting of the inside of my cheek cause cancer?

No one really knows. Regular irritation has been suspected as a possible cause of cancer. Maybe the dentist can help with suggestions for stopping this habit. Sometimes chewing gum can help. If there are white, red, or darkened patches inside the cheek, see the doctor.

How does the doctor diagnose cancer of the mouth?

The physician or dentist will first carefully examine your mouth. He will also compare both sides of your neck to find differences in its shape. Next he will feel the inside of the mouth and neck, paying special attention to any areas that did not seem normal on the outside. The lymph nodes in the front and back of the neck will be checked for swelling or changes in the way they feel. Mouth cancer, like most other cancer, needs to be biopsied for a definitive diagnosis. The doctor will take a piece of the suspicious area or take out the entire area. Sometimes a needle biopsy may be used for lumps in the neck. X-rays of the skull and chest, endoscopy and liver and bone scans may also be done.

How is cancer of the mouth treated?

Surgery and radiation are the principal methods for treating cancer of the mouth, depending on the site and stage of the disease. Sometimes radiation is used to shrink tumors of the cheek or floor of the mouth before surgery. Radioactive implants are also used in treating some mouth cancers; they may be implanted for cancer of the upper lip, tongue, cheek, or floor of the mouth. Sometimes external radiation is used before the radium implant. The use of chemotherapy together with radiation therapy is also being tested.

Is radical neck dissection used for treating mouth cancer?

If involvement of lymph nodes in the neck is suspected, a radical neck dissection is sometimes performed.

Does plastic reconstructive surgery usually accompany an operation for mouth cancer?

It depends upon the extent of the surgery. Sometimes, to make sure all the malignant tissue is taken out, extensive surgery may be necessary. Although such procedures are sometimes disfiguring, highly developed techniques of reconstructive surgery can be used to rebuild or repair facial features or other affected areas. If a complete reconstructive procedure is not advisable at the time of cancer surgery, temporary artificial devices of a cosmetic nature can be used.

Are most tumors of the lip cancerous?

No, most tumors on the lips are benign. They are usually warty growths or tumors of the blood vessels. Most of these can be cured by one of several methods: cutting them out and stitching the cut edges together, burning them with an electric needle, freezing them, or treating them with x-ray.

The Stages of Cancer of the Mouth

STAGE	OTHER CLASSIFICATIONS	EXPLANATION
Stage I	T1, N0, M0	Tumor is 2 cm or less and has not spread to lymph nodes or other parts of the body.
Stage II	T2, N0, M0	Tumor is larger than 2 cm, but not more than 4 cm. It has not spread to lymph nodes or other parts of the body.
Stage III	T3, N0, M0 or T1–3, N1, M0	Tumor is larger than 4 cm and has not spread to lymph nodes or tumor is of any size (except massive) and involves a single lymph node less than 3 cm located on the same side of the neck as the tumor.
Stage IV	T4, N0–1, M0 Any T, N2 or N3, M0 Any T, any N, M1	Tumor measures more than 4 cm and deeply invades surrounding tissue or tumor involves one lymph node larger than 3 cm, one lymph node on the opposite side of the neck from the tumor or multiple nodes; or tumor has spread to distant parts of the body.

Do benign lip tumors ever turn into cancer?

Sometimes. Warty growths have a tendency to become cancerous and should be removed.

Where does cancer of the lip occur most commonly?

Lip cancer usually occurs on the lower lip, in men between the ages of 60 and 70. Chapping, overexposure to sunburn, and smoking (especially pipe smoking) are thought to be factors in developing this cancer. Cancer of the lip is fairly common and usually highly curable, especially if there is no involvement with the lymph nodes in the neck.

How is lip cancer treated?

Sometimes surgery is used, usually a procedure called a V-lip excision. Sometimes radiation therapy is used, especially for larger cancers. Very large lip cancers are usually treated with radiation therapy because major reconstructive work would be necessary after surgery.

Lip cancer, because it is slow-growing and visible, is usually discovered in the early stages. It often takes lip cancer months to spread to the lymph nodes in the neck.

Will I have disfiguring scars after a partial removal of the lip?

The lip regains almost normal appearance, even after large sections of it have been taken out.

How is the reconstruction done if surgery is performed on a large lip cancer?

Usually the reconstruction is done with the use of a skin graft taken from the forehead.

What is a lip shave?

A lip shave removes the mucous membrane on the lip. It is usually performed as a preventive measure for persons who have extensive leukoplakia (white patches) on the lower lip—even if the patches are not cancerous.

Is neck dissection done with lip cancer?

If the biopsy shows that the lymph nodes are involved, a neck dissection may be performed on the involved side.

Does lip cancer metastasize?

Lip cancer rarely metastasizes. When it does, it goes to the lymph nodes in the region. However, swollen lymph nodes can be an inflammatory reaction to lip surgery.

Who is at high risk to get cancer of the tongue?

Cancer of the tongue appears mostly in men who are over 40 although the proportion of women with tongue cancer is increasing, probably because of increased alcohol and tobacco use.

Where does most tongue cancer occur?

Most cancer of the tongue is situated at the tip or along the side of the tongue. It can usually be discovered early.

What are the symptoms of tongue cancer?

You might see deep-red patches. Sometimes there are white patches. Sometimes the deep-red patches turn bluish-white. This is called leukoplakia, which represents an overgrowth of cells. There may be only a few spots or they may be on the whole tongue. Sometimes they will not hurt. They may be irritating and uncomfortable. The greatest danger of these patches is that if they are not treated, some of the area might turn into cancer. Some people complain of pain, which they usually think is a sore throat. It gets worse when they talk and swallow. Sometimes the pain goes to the side of the head or the ear.

Can the red or white patches on the tongue be removed?

They can be removed with an electric needle or by surgery. They are thought to be caused by tobacco smoking, alcohol, sharp-edged or diseased teeth, and faulty-fitting or sharp-edged dentures.

Can these patches recur? Do they turn into tongue cancer?

Leukoplakia has a tendency to recur, and the recurrent areas can be retreated. The appearance of an ulcer or hard growth in one of these patches often indicates a cancerous change. An ulcer or cracking or peeling develops in the leukoplakic area, and the surrounding region becomes firm and hard. The doctor will take a biopsy of these tissues.

What does cancer of the tongue look like?

Cancer of the tongue usually appears as a painless, thickened, ulcerated area along the margin of the tongue. As it gets bigger, it may be swollen and tender and may bleed occasionally.

Does tongue cancer tend to spread?

Tongue cancer does not tend to spread rapidly. Although most tongue cancer remains confined for months to the original site before spreading to the lymph nodes of the neck, symptoms should not be ignored. If the cancer is toward the back of the tongue, it may spread to lymph nodes on both sides of the neck.

How can tongue cancer be treated?

Usually surgery is used to remove the tumor. Sometimes radiation—external beam, implant, or a combination—will be used. For large tumors, neck dissection may be required.

What operations are performed for cancer of the tongue?

Cancers located on the side of the tongue are usually treated by either removing a wedge or half the tongue (hemiglossectomy). If the cancer is on the top of the tongue or in the middle forward portion of it, the doctor will usually remove the front two-thirds of it. Cancers of the base of the tongue are almost always treated with radium and x-ray treatments. If the tongue cancer has spread to the lymph nodes, neck dissection will be needed to take out the nodes in the neck. If it has spread to the floor of the mouth, the areas under the tongue which have been affected will be removed. Sometimes the jawbone will be involved. If so, it may be replaced with a bone graft or a metal splint.

Is one treatment preferred above the others?

It depends upon the size of the tumor, the extent of the cancer, and the patient's and doctor's preference. Some cancers can be removed by taking out a wedge of the tongue. Another treatment involves inserting radium needles into the tongue. You should discuss with your doctor the advantages and disadvantages of all treatments before any decision is made.

Will I be able to swallow, speak, and eat normally if I have parts of my tongue removed?

It depends upon the extent of the operation. If a large portion of your tongue is taken out, swallowing can become awkward, but you can still do it. Speech may also be slightly impaired. If 75 percent of the tongue is removed, chewing may become very difficult, making it necessary for you to live on a soft diet. Again, speech may be impaired.

What kind of anesthesia is used for a tongue operation?

General anesthesia is usually used. A tube is placed in the trachea. Often there is a need for blood transfusions for this operation. Special nurses may be needed.

When will I be able to eat after the operation?

You will be on fluids, given through the tube placed in the nose and extending to the stomach, for the first few days. Then you will be able to eat soft foods.

Will I be able to speak if I have a part of my tongue taken out?

Yes, you will still be able to speak. If you have a small wedge taken out, the deformity is not great. If you have a larger cancer which might remove as much as one-third of the tongue from the tip back, your speech will be changed but will remain understandable. With training, many patients, even when more than half the tongue has been removed, learn to talk again. Radium implants or x-ray treatments, if they can be done for your type and stage of cancer, do not ordinarily involve any speech deformity.

Will I have a large scar after tongue surgery?

If you have had neck dissection along with the tongue operation, part of the jawbone and the glands in the neck are removed, leaving a visible scar.

How is cancer of the floor of the mouth diagnosed?

The doctor will look at and feel the tumor. He will take x-rays and do a biopsy to confirm the diagnosis.

Does cancer of the floor of the mouth metastasize?

Yes. This is one of the oral cancers which metastasizes to the lymph nodes in the neck in a good number of patients.

What treatment is used for cancer of the floor of the mouth?

In early-stage cancers, the treatment is usually radiation or surgery. Cancers that are more advanced are usually treated with surgery followed by radiation and sometimes chemotherapy.

Who is at high risk for cancer of the cheek?

Cancer of the inside of the cheek (sometimes referred to by doctors as buccal mucosa) occurs more often in males over the age of 55. It is believed that persons who chew tobacco and betel nuts or who bite their cheeks are at a higher risk of getting cancer of the cheek.

What are the symptoms?

The symptoms include a sore inside the cheek which does not heal, bloody saliva, and white patches inside the cheek. There is usually no pain.

Does cancer of the cheek metastasize?

Cancer of the cheek is usually slow-growing. It also has a relatively low rate of metastasis.

How is cancer of the cheek diagnosed?

It is diagnosed by direct inspection and feeling by the doctor. Final diagnosis is by biopsy.

How is cancer of the cheek treated?

Early stages of cancer of the cheek are treated with radiation or by surgery. Advanced cancer of the cheek is treated by surgery, followed by radiation and sometimes chemotherapy.

Who is at high risk for cancer of the gums (gingivae) and hard palate?

Women are at a higher risk for cancer of the gums and hard palate. The average age for this cancer is 60. Most cancers occur in the lower gums.

What are the symptoms of cancer of the gums?

The symptoms are painful ulceration and difficulty in wearing dentures.

What is the treatment method for cancer of the gums?

Early stages are treated by radiation or by surgery. Late stages are treated by surgery, followed by radiation and sometimes chemotherapy.

What are the parts of the nose?

The nose is made up of connective tissue (cartilage) and bone. It contains two cavities, which are separated in the middle by a septum. The nose serves as the organ of smell and is the airway for breathing. It filters, warms, and moistens the air which is breathed in.

What are the sinuses?

The sinuses are air spaces within the bones of the face and the skull. They connect through small openings (ostia) into the air passages in the nose. The soft, moist mucous lining which coats the inside of the nose extends into the sinuses. There are four types of sinus: frontal (within the bone just above and behind the eyebrows), maxillary (in the bones of the cheeks beneath the eyes), ethmoid (near the side of the nose and inner part of the eyes and going back into the skull), and sphenoid (in the skull above the level of the nose).

Is cancer of the sinuses common?

No. Cancer of the sinuses is very rare. Most often it is the maxillary sinus that is involved in the disease.

What are the cancers of this area called?

The cancers in the nose area are called cancer of the nasal fossa (nasal cavity), paranasal sinuses (sinus), and naso-pharynx (tube which connects the mouth and nose with the esophagus).

What are the symptoms of cancer of the nasal area?

One symptom is a reddish, easily bleeding mass in the nasal passage. Sometimes paranasal sinuses will produce pain and pressure in the cheek, a toothache, or persistent drain-ing of the sinus after tooth extraction, a nasal quality to the voice, a lump in the cheek, or bloodstained discharge from the nose.

How is this tumor diagnosed?

The doctor uses a head light and a small mirror or a naso-pharyngoscope (a flexible optical instrument) to look in the passages. He may also order x-rays of the facial bone. He can take a biopsy or a brush scraping with the nasopha-ryngoscope.

What is nasopharyngeal fibroma?

This is a tumor of the nasopharynx which is found mainly in youngsters. It is a benign tumor but may destroy bone and soft tissue about it as it enlarges. It should be diagnosed early. It is curable, but sometimes several operations are needed. Sometimes radium implant, radiation, or cryosur-gery is used to remove these tumors.

Are the tumors in the area of the nose and sinuses always malignant?

No. There are many noncancerous tumors in the area of the nose and the sinuses. Warts, polyps, and small blood-vessel tumors are often found and are usually nonmalignant.

How is cancer of the nose and sinuses treated?

Surgery and radiation therapy are the treatments, depending on the site of the tumor and the extent of it. Sometimes sections of the nose, the roof of the mouth, the floor of the eye socket, or the face and the cheek must be excised. Radiation can be used before or after surgery.

Why is such drastic surgery performed?

The main goal is to get beyond the cancer. Many lives have been saved with this kind of surgery, and the advances in plastic surgery mean that people can be restored to normal appearance.

How is cancer of the nasopharynx treated?

Cancer of the nasopharynx is usually treated with radiation therapy or with surgery or both, depending upon the extent of the disease.

What is cancer of the oropharynx?

Cancer of the region of the oropharynx includes the soft palate, tonsil, walls of the pharynx, and back third of the tongue. The most common site for this cancer is on the tonsil.

How is cancer of the oropharynx diagnosed?

The doctor will diagnose it by looking at it and feeling it if it is in an area that can be reached. In other areas he will use laryngoscopy. As with other cancers, biopsy is essential for a definite diagnosis.

What are the symptoms of cancer of the oropharynx?

The symptoms include a mild sore throat, lump in the back of the tongue and velvety red patches appear. Some are open sores. There is usually little or no pain associated with them. Some people complain of difficulty in swallowing, lumps in the neck, difficulty in breathing, and earaches.

What is the treatment for cancer of the oropharynx?

Primary treatment for this cancer is radiation therapy in most cases. Sometimes surgery is necessary—a neck dissection may need to be done.

What is cancer of the hypopharynx?

Cancers of the hypopharynx are tumors of the lower pharynx. They are found mostly in males from the ages of 49 to 60.

What are the symptoms of cancer of the hypopharynx?

The symptoms include difficulty in swallowing, lumps in the neck, difficulty in breathing, earaches, cough, and bad breath.

How does the doctor detect cancer of the hypopharynx?

He looks at it and feels it if it is in an area that can be reached. He will probably use a nasopharyngeal mirror or a laryngoscope (flexible optical instruments which allow him to look into the lower pharynx). He will do a biopsy to get a final diagnosis.

How is cancer of the hypopharynx treated?

Radiation therapy is used sometimes alone, sometimes followed by surgery. Part of the pharynx and/or part of the larynx may be removed.

Where are the salivary glands?

The major salivary glands are in the sides of the face, in front of and slightly below the ears. These salivary glands are also known as parotid glands. The saliva gets from these glands to the mouth through parotid ducts, which open on the inner surfaces of the cheeks. There is also a pair of glands in the lower jaws (submandibular glands) and under the tongue (sublingual glands). The ducts from these glands open into the floor of the mouth underneath the tongue.

Where are tumors of the salivary glands found?

Tumors of the salivary glands are most often found in the parotid glands. Most often these tumors are not malignant.

They are either on the outer surface of the parotid gland, which is near the ear, or in the inner surface, which is in the mouth. Benign parotid-gland tumors are usually painless and slow-growing. Malignant tumors of the parotid tend to grow rapidly. Sometimes a tumor seems to be benign for many years and then suddenly becomes malignant. Tumors of the parotid gland are relatively rare. Of those tumors that are found, 80 percent are benign. If a person has a lump in the neck which does not quickly disappear, or which grows, he should go to a doctor. A second opinion by a doctor specializing in head and neck surgery should also be sought.

What are the symptoms of cancer in the parotid gland?

Usually the most common complaint is the presence of a slowly growing lump in the cheek next to the ear. Sometimes there is a rather dull and indefinite but progressive pain and facial-nerve paralysis.

How does the doctor operate on the salivary-gland tumors?

He makes an incision running from in front of the ear to the neck. The doctor must be sure the incision is long enough to let him carefully separate the gland from the facial nerve so that the nerve is not cut. If the nerve is cut, distortion and paralysis of that side of the face may occur. Sometimes, such as when the tumor is malignant, the nerve must be cut. In many cases the treatment for cancer of the salivary glands is removal of the complete gland, the affected area around it, and sometimes the facial nerve.

Is there a long recovery after an operation on the salivary glands?

The doctor will leave the drain in for a few days after the operation. You will probably be out of bed the day after that and home in a week or less. You may have to remain on a fluid diet for several days because it may be painful to chew solid foods, but after that you will have an unrestricted diet. Usually the scar heals in about 10 days, but you may experience some facial nerve paralysis which may last for several months.

Where are the incisions made in operations on the salivary glands?

The incision placement depends upon which glands the doctor is operating on. If it is a parotid-gland operation, the incision is made in front of the ear and along the angle of the jaw. If it is the submaxillary gland, it is made parallel to and along the undersurface of the lower jaw. The incision for the sublingual gland is in the mouth or in the skin just below the chin.

Does the doctor take out the whole gland?

Again it depends upon the gland and on the problem. Usually if cancer is present, the whole gland is taken out. If the parotid tumor is benign, and can be completely taken out, the rest of the gland will be left.

Is radiotherapy used in treating cancer of the salivary glands?

Sometimes radiation is used in this type of cancer. It may be given to persons who cannot be operated on or to reduce the size of the tumor. Sometimes it is used after the operation on a portion of the facial nerve.

Can the facial nerve be replaced?

Yes, it can. However, some return of facial-nerve function has been seen in patients without a nerve graft. If the paralysis is due to the shock of the operation, the function usually returns within 6 to 8 weeks.

Will my hair be shaved for an operation on the parotid tumor?

Yes. Because of the location of the parotid gland, the hair around the ear must be shaved. Sometimes the hair is brushed up and back, if possible, or cut so that the top hair may be arranged to cover the ear when you are ready to go home.

Will I have to have special care after the operation?

You will probably be on a fluid diet for the first few days because it may be painful to chew solid foods. You may be given antibiotics in large doses to control infection. Special attention will be paid to your mouth and to your teeth.

Does this kind of cancer usually recur?

Parotid tumors can recur. Sometimes they are treated with surgery again. The whole area may be treated with radiation. ✦

If the doctor removes one of the salivary glands, will I still have normal saliva production?

Yes. The remaining glands will take over for the gland that the doctor has removed.

CANCER OF THE THYROID

Questions to Ask Your Doctor About Thyroid Cancer

- How many thyroid operations have you performed in the last year? What are the usual results?
- Is there any indication that there is spread beyond the thyroid area?
- Is the nodule soft or hard?
- What tests are you planning for me?
- What type of cancer do you suspect?
- Will it be necessary to operate?
- Will it be possible for you to remove only the one nodule?
- If not, how extensive do you expect the operation to be?
- Do you think it will be necessary for you to remove both lobes?
- Will the diagnosis be made from the frozen section, or can we wait for a permanent section before proceeding with the removal of the thyroid?
- Are you planning to remove the regional lymph nodes?
- Will there be permanent hoarseness?
- Will I have trouble swallowing? For how long?

What is the thyroid?

This ductless gland, located in the front of the throat, below the Adam's apple and just above the breastbone, is roughly U-shaped and has two lobes—one on each side of the wind-pipe. The thyroid serves as the body's thermostat. It regulates the rate at which the body uses oxygen, the rate at which the body uses food, and the rate at which various organs function.

How is cancer of the thyroid usually discovered?

The patient may become aware of a growth in the neck, or the doctor may discover it during a regular examination. The lump usually is not painful or tender. A hard, irregular lump that does not seem to move is the most suspicious to the doctor's touch. Softness, mobility, the indication of more than one lump, and slow growth usually indicate a benign condition. There may also be enlargement of the nearby lymph nodes either above or below the level of the thyroid nodule. Any noticeable lump should be checked by a doctor, especially if it begins to increase in size. Sometimes there may be a history of persistent hoarseness or difficulty in swallowing.

Are all lumps in this area cancerous?

No. Only about 10 to 20 percent of patients with suspicious nodules actually prove to have cancer of the thyroid. Most of the tumors are cysts. However, removal is usually recommended because of the location.

Who is at a higher risk to get cancer of the thyroid?

Cancer of the thyroid is found twice as often in women as in men and more often in whites than in blacks. The majority of cases occur between the ages of 25 and 65. People who had radiation to the head and neck area when they were children are also at a higher risk for thyroid cancer. Cancer of the thyroid is not a common cancer—it accounts for less than 1 percent of all cancers. It is also one of the least frequent causes of death from cancer.

Why do people who had radiation treatment to the head and neck in childhood or adolescence get thyroid cancer?

X-ray treatment was used beginning in the 1920s and continued over 25 years to treat noncancerous conditions. Among the conditions which were treated with x-rays were ringworm of the scalp, enlargement of the thymus glands in infants, various types of ear inflammations, deafness due to overgrowth of the lymphoid tissue around the eustachian tubes, enlargement or inflammation of the tonsils and adenoids, inflammation of the sinuses, head and neck lumps, and acne. At the time the treatment was used, no one anticipated the aftereffects of the radiation.

Are x-rays to the head and neck still being used in treatment of children?

No. This kind of treatment is no longer prescribed for these childhood conditions.

Am I more likely to get thyroid cancer than the general population if I had x-ray treatment as a child?

You are at a higher risk, but only a small percentage of the people irradiated at an early age develop thyroid tumors. Most of the tumors are slow-growing. Most of the tumors are benign. Even those which are cancerous usually remain limited to the neck for many years and can be successfully removed by surgery.

What should I do if I was exposed to x-ray treatment when I was a child?

You should tell your doctor as much as you can about the kind of treatment which you had. It is important to find out, if you can, the kind of treatment you were given, what form it took, how many doses you were given, and any other details. This information should become a permanent part of your medical record. People with a history of radiation should be reexamined every 1 or 2 years. The most important part of the examination is careful inspection of the neck to detect the possible presence of nodules in the thyroid. Remember, the risk is for people who had x-ray *treatments* during childhood, not for people who had x-rays for diagnosing an illness.

Is a goiter cancerous?

Goiter is a term which means overgrowth of the thyroid. There are two kinds of goiters: colloid goiter, which comes from insufficient iodine in the drinking water and food, which is now rarely seen, and nodular goiter, which in some 10 percent of the cases may develop into cancer.

Is it unusual for a child to have cancer of the thyroid?

Cancer of the thyroid does occur in children and young adults. In contrast to cancers of some other organs, however, the statistics show that 90 percent continue to live normal lives with fairly normal life expectancies. Even when the disease is locally advanced with extensive involvement of the lymph nodes in the neck, this still holds true.

What kinds of tests are used to detect thyroid cancer?

The doctor will probably do several things. First he will look at the thyroid area for abnormalities. He will feel the thyroid gland and nearby areas for any lumps or swellings. If he suspects a tumor he will examine the inside of the throat with a small instrument called a laryngoscope, which lets him look with a mirror into the vocal cords. He might give you a thyroid scan or do a fine-needle biopsy. Depending on the size and extent of the growth, the doctor might do a barium swallow to examine the neck or chest films and a skeletal survey to determine if there are distant metastases. However, as in most kinds of cancer, the only true test is through biopsy, which is usually performed as part of an operation to remove the tumor.

How is a thyroid scan performed?

You will swallow a tiny dose of radioactive material. An instrument is moved back and forth over your neck to determine how actively your thyroid tissue is absorbing this substance. If it is quite active, the lump is called "hot." If it is not absorbing the substance, the lump is called "cold." Cold lumps may be cancerous, slow-growing, and slow to spread. Hot spots usually indicate a benign growth. Even if your scan shows that you have a cold spot, you should not worry, because about 80 percent of the time, cold spots, upon biopsy, prove *not* to be cancer. Sometimes two thyroid scan readings are taken—usually at 2 and 24 hours after administration of the radioactive material.

The Stages of Thyroid Cancer

CLASSIFICATION	EXPLANATION
Papillary, Stage I	Localized to thyroid gland. Stage IA means that only one lobe is affected. Stage IB indicates that both lobes are affected or that there are several sites within the gland.
Papillary, Stage II	Indicates spread to lymph nodes. Stages IIA and IIB are used to indicate whether lymph nodes in one or both lobes are affected as in Stage I.
Papillary, Stage III	Spread to the neck area, with or without lymph-node involvement.
Papillary, Stage IV	Spread to other organs—usually lungs and bone.
Follicular, Stage I	Localized to the thyroid gland. Stage IA means that only one lobe is affected. Stage IB indicates that both lobes are affected or that there are several sites within the gland.
Follicular, Stage II	Indicates spread to lymph nodes. Stages IIA and IIB are used to indicate whether lymph nodes in one or both lobes are affected as in Stage I.
Follicular, Stage III	Spread to head and neck area, with or without lymph-node involvement. May also have spread to blood vessels.
Follicular, Stage IV	Spread to other organs such as lung and bone—usually through blood vessels.
Medullary	No staging. Occurs in two forms: sporadic and familial.
Anaplastic	No staging. Classified as small cell or large cell. Both are rapid-growing and usually occur in older age group.

How long will the radioactive substance from the scan remain in my body?

The radioactive substance is quickly absorbed by the bloodstream and taken directly to the thyroid gland. It stays in the gland about 1 to 3 days—and then is excreted in the urine.

Are needle biopsies usually performed in the thyroid area?

Fine-needle biopsies are another method used to get a small specimen of thyroid tissue to study under the microscope. Using only skin anesthesia, the doctor can painlessly insert a narrow needle into the nodule and withdraw cells for microscopic study. This method, which was considered experimental five years ago, is today the method of choice for many doctors.

What are the cell types of thyroid cancer?

The major different cell types include papillary, follicular, medullary and undifferentiated (anaplastic). It is important for the doctor to determine the cell type because the treatment can differ depending on the type.

If a tumor is found in the thyroid gland, does the doctor usually operate?

It depends. An operation is usually necessary if there is an indication that the tumor is causing pressure, if there is a single nodule which shows rapid growth, if there are any signs of new growth, or if the patient is a child or young male. Sometimes the doctor will give you a thyroid hormone which cancels the need for the thyroid to produce its own hormones and causes the gland to shrink. The doctor may also use this technique in unclear cases, to let him feel for nodules which may lie hidden deep in the gland. He will probably watch the results for several months. If the tumor gets bigger or additional nodules appear, he will then operate. If there is a past history of x-ray treatment during childhood or adolescence, many doctors feel it is wiser to operate.

Treatment Choices for Thyroid Cancer

STAGE	POSSIBLE TREATMENTS
Papillary, Stage I	Surgery, followed by hormone treatment. I-131 sometimes used in addition to hormones. If lymph nodes involved, neck dissection may be required.
Papillary, Stage II	Surgery, followed by hormone treatment. I-131 sometime used in addition to hormones. If lymph nodes are definitely involved, neck dissection may be required.
Follicular, Stages I & II	Surgery, biopsy of regional lymph nodes. If involved, neck dissection. Hormone Treatment following surgery. I-131 sometimes used in addition to hormones.
Papillary and Follicular, Stage III	Total removal of thyroid by surgery. I-131 possible. Radiation if tumor is not responsive to I-131.
Papillary and Follicular, Stage IV	Following surgery, I-131 or radiation or hormones if not responsive to I-131. Chemotherapy if metastasized to lung, bone, or other distant sites. Investigational trials are available for extensive disease.
Medullary	Total removal of thyroid. Radical neck dissection if regional lymph nodes involved. Chemotherapy may be used for metastized disease.
Anaplastic	Total removal of thyroid. Radiation may be used to reduce tumor if surgery is not possible. Chemotherapy for distant metastasis or if tumor is unresponsive to radiation.
Recurrent	Radiation or chemotherapy. Investigational trials available.

Is surgery the main treatment for thyroid cancer?

Once diagnosed, surgery is usually the treatment of choice for thyroid cancer. In some cases the doctor will remove the entire thyroid gland. This procedure is called a thyroidectomy—either partial or total. Sometimes suspicious nearby lymph glands are also removed.

What is the difference between a lobectomy and a thyroidectomy?

Lobectomy (or hemithyroidectomy) indicates that one lobe of the thyroid (and sometimes the isthmus, or tissue connecting the two lobes) has been removed. Sometimes this is called a partial thyroidectomy. The total thyroidectomy includes removal of both lobes.

What is involved in a thyroidectomy?

There are several kinds. Subtotal thyroidectomy means the removal of parts of both lobes and of the isthmus of thyroid tissue over the windpipe or removal of a whole lobe and part of another. Total thyroidectomy means removal of all thyroid tissue.

How long will the thyroid surgery take?

Though not a dangerous procedure, thyroidectomy is a fairly complicated operation. If the entire thyroid is removed, it will take from 2 to 4 hours. The thyroid operation is complex, as it can involve nerves, veins, windpipe, and esophagus as well as parathyroid glands which lie directly under the thyroid. Most times the parathyroid glands are allowed to remain.

Is a neck dissection performed for cancer of the thyroid?

If lymph nodes are involved, a modified radical neck dissection may be necessary.

What kind of anesthesia is given?

A general anesthetic is usually used.

When can I expect to return to work after thyroid surgery?

Usually recovery is swift, and the patient can return to work within a few weeks. Hospital stay is usually 1 week. Because of the location of the operation, it is less painful than abdominal or chest surgery. The throat will probably be extremely sore, and hoarseness can be expected. A drain is usually left in place for 2 to 4 days and is removed with little or no discomfort.

What does the incision look like?

Generally a 3½-to-4-inch incision is made in the neck above the collarbone, usually in one of the creases of the neck. When the scar is healed it is barely noticeable, though the thin-line scar will never fully disappear.

Is there other treatment following surgery?

Yes. You will normally take hormones and/or a course of radioactive iodine (I-131) following surgery.

How does radioiodine work?

The thyroid gland gathers the radioactive iodine. The radiation given off by the iodine makes it difficult for the thyroid cells to work and to grow. Most of the radioactive iodine will be collected in your thyroid but some will go to other tissues in your body.

How long does the radioiodine stay in my body?

It stays in your body only temporarily and most of it that is not collected by your thyroid will leave your body within the first two days of treatment, primarily through your urine. Small amounts may also leave in your saliva, sweat and bowel movements.

Is there any possibility of radiation exposure to me or to others?

The small amount of radiation has not been shown to produce any harmful effects, and at the end of treatment, no radioiodine remains in your body. However, you need to take some steps to insure safety for yourself and others:

- Sleep alone for the first few days after your treatment. During this period, do not kiss anyone or have sexual intercourse.
- Keep your physical contact with others short, especially with children and pregnant women. The thyroid glands of children and unborn babies are more sensitive to the effects of radioiodine than those of adults. If you have a baby or are taking care of one, talk to your doctor about what you can and cannot do. It is probably better not to have the baby too close, such as sitting in your lap, for long periods of time during the first couple days of treatment.
- Do not breast feed. Talk with your doctor about when you can go back to breastfeeding.
- Wash your hands with soap and water when you go to the bathroom. Most of the radioactive iodine leaves your body in your urine.
- Keep the bathroom clean, especially the toilet (flush it two or three times after each use), the sink and tub (rinse thoroughly after you use them). Your sweat and saliva can also excrete radioactive iodine.
- Drink plenty of water and juices to help you go to the bathroom more often, helping the radioiodine leave your body faster.
- When you eat, especially for the first few days, use disposable dishes and utensils. If you do not, make sure you wash your dishes and utensils separately to lower the risk of exposure to others.
- Have separate towels and washcloths and wash them separately along with your bed linens and underclothes.

It is important for you to discuss with your doctor which of these precautions are important for you and how long to follow them.

Is thyroid cancer ever treated with radiation or chemotherapy?

Sometimes, if all the abnormal tissue cannot be removed by surgery or if the cancer has metastasized to other parts of the body, radiation therapy or chemotherapy may be used.

Can I continue to smoke after I have had a thyroid operation?

It certainly would be better if you stopped smoking. However, your doctor will probably tell you to stop for at least 2 weeks after the operation. This is because coughing can cause pain and stress on the muscles and skin close to the incision.

Will removal of the thyroid gland affect my sex life?

No. Removal of the thyroid gland should have no effect upon your sex life.

What are the parathyroid glands?

The parathyroids are four small glands which are attached to the thyroid gland. They secrete a hormone, parathormone, which is involved with the balance of the body and the excretion of calcium and phosphorus necessary for bone growth and maintenance. They are part of the endocrine system.

What are other parts of the endocrine system?

Other parts of the endocrine system include the adrenal glands and the pituitary glands.

Can one get cancer of any of the parts of the endocrine system?

Yes, it is possible to have cancer of the parathyroid glands, the adrenal glands, or the pituitary glands. Cancer of the endocrine system is relatively rare and is complex to diagnose.

Is cancer of the endocrine system difficult to treat?

Cancer of the endocrine system is difficult to treat because of hormonally produced changes in the patient. It is important, since a general practitioner rarely sees these cancers, to have endocrine cancer treated by a specialist.

Is surgery performed on the parathyroids?

Yes, surgery is the usual treatment. If a tumor is located in only one gland, it can be removed. The incision is similar to that for the thyroid operation: A 3½-to-4-inch incision is made in the neck above the collarbone. The doctor will take out as much tissue as necessary to remove the tumor. Recovery is quick from this operation. If the tumor reappears, surgery is usually performed again.

What is malignant thymoma?

This is a tumor of the thymus gland, highly curable with surgery. Thymomas are slow-growing tumors with a tendency to occur again locally. They seldom metastasize. Surgery is the usual treatment, with radiation sometimes given after the operation. In some selected patients, radiation therapy alone is used if surgery is not possible.

CANCER OF THE LARYNX

What is the larynx?

The larynx is the voice box. It is the upper part of the windpipe above the trachea. The larynx forms the Adam's apple in the neck. Air coming in passes through the larynx to the lungs. In front of the larynx are the vocal cords. Muscles move the vocal cords, which are made to vibrate by air exhaled from the lungs.

Who is at high risk to get cancer of the larynx?

Men are almost nine times more likely to get it than women, although the incidence in females is now rising. Most people who get it are in their fifties, although there are some cases in people in their twenties and thirties. People at high risk are those who smoke, drink to excess, and have frequent irritation to the larynx such as coughing frequently.

What the symptoms of cancer of the larynx?

The symptoms of cancer of the larynx occur early. They are noticeable hoarseness, a lump in the throat, difficult or painful swallowing, pain in the ear, shortness of breath, and harsh, noisy breathing. Some of the symptoms of more advanced cases are badly swollen neck glands, weight loss, and sometimes bleeding. If you have constant hoarseness

The Stages of Supraglottic Larynx Cancer

STAGE	OTHER CLASSIFICATIONS	EXPLANATION
Stage I	T1, N0, M0	Tumor is confined to region of origin with normal mobility of vocal cords.
Stage II	T2, N0, M0	Tumor involves adjacent supraglottic sites or glottis, without fixation of vocal cords.
Stage III	T3, N0, M0 T1–3, N1, M0	Tumor is confined to larynx but vocal cord(s) are fixed and/or tumor extends to postcricoid area, medial wall, or pre-epiglottic space. Or, tumor of any size that has spread to a lymph node on the same side as the tumor.
Stage IV	T4, N0 or N1, M0 Any T, N2–3, M0 Any T, any N, M1	Massive tumor extends beyond larynx to involve oropharynx, soft tissues of neck, or thyroid cartilage or there is one abnormal lymph node larger than 3 cm or there are many abnormal lymph nodes on both sides of the neck or one or more on the opposite side of the neck.

Treatment Choices for Supraglottic Larynx Cancer

STAGE	POSSIBLE TREATMENT
Stages I & II	Radiation therapy alone or supraglottic laryngectomy with voice preservation.
Stage III	Small tumors: radiation therapy alone or supraglottic laryngectomy with voice preservation. Large tumors: total laryngectomy with pre- or postoperative radiation therapy. Or, radiation therapy alone with plans to consider surgery if response is not satisfactory after radiation.
Stage IV	Total laryngectomy with pre- or postoperative radiation. Or, radiation alone with plans to consider surgery if response is not satisfactory. Investigational: chemotherapy.

that lasts for more than 3 weeks, it should be checked by a doctor.

Can cancer of the larynx be cured if treated early?

Yes. Hoarseness is an early symptom, and many of the cases of cancer of the larynx can be cured if seen at an early stage. It is estimated that 85 percent of larynx tumors could be cured, and the patient left with a fairly good speaking voice and a natural air passage, if diagnosed early and treated before there is spread to surrounding tissue.

Are all growths on the larynx cancerous?

No. Most tumors of the larynx are benign. Cancer of the larynx can be removed by surgery when found early, and the voice may be saved. Nonmalignant growths can also be removed and the voice restored to normal.

The Stages of Glottic Larynx Cancer

STAGE	OTHER CLASSIFICATIONS	EXPLANATION
Stage I	T1, N0, M0	Tumor is confined to the vocal cord or cords with normal mobility.
Stage II	T2, N0, M0	Tumor extends to the supraglottic or subglottic regions with normal or impaired vocal-cord mobility.
Stage III	T3, N0, M0 T1–3 N1, M0	Tumor confined to larynx with one or both vocal cords immobilized.
Stage IV	T4, N0–N1, M0 Any T, N2–3, M0 Any T, any N, M1	Large tumor with thyroid cartilage destruction and/or growth beyond larynx, or both.

Treatment Choices for Glottic Larynx Cancer

STAGE	POSSIBLE TREATMENT
Stage I	Removal of vocal cord, partial laryngectomy, radiation therapy with limited high-dose lymph-node radiation.
Stage II	Small tumors: partial laryngectomy or radiation therapy with limited high-dose lymph-node radiation. Advanced tumors: total laryngectomy with postoperative radiation. Nodes may be surgically removed or treated with radiation. Radiation therapy with limited high-dose lymph-node radiation.
Stage III	Small tumors: partial laryngectomy or radiation therapy with limited high-dose lymph-node radiation. Advanced tumors: total laryngectomy with possible postoperative radiation. Radiation therapy if medically inoperable or where tumor volume is minimal, followed by surgery. Investigational: chemotherapy in addition to other treatment.
Stage IV	Total laryngectomy with postoperative radiation. Surgery or radiation for nodes. Or radiation therapy for patients with advanced lesions where tumor volume is minimal, followed by surgery. Investigational: chemotherapy in addition to other treatment.
Recurrent	Surgery or radiation treatment depending on previous treatment. Investigational: chemotherapy.

What causes nonmalignant growth?

Noncancerous growths may be caused by allergy, irritation, infection, or overuse of the voice. Singers, teachers, and politicians often have nonmalignant growths or papillomas.

How is the nonmalignant growth treated? '

Usually, a hospital stay is required. Using a general anesthesia or local anesthetic, the doctor puts a tubular instrument (laryngoscope) through your mouth to the throat. He uses special instruments to cut away the tumor. You will feel some discomfort—similar to a very sore throat. You

will be on a liquid diet and will go home in 2 or 3 days.
The doctor will not let you use your throat for a week or
more. It is important to heed the doctor's advice in not using
the voice in order to have this area heal properly. You can
do permanent injury to your vocal cords if they do not heal
properly.

Do nonmalignant growths ever recur?

Yes, certain nonmalignant growths—those that are wart-
like—have a tendency to recur and are operated on again.

Where does cancer of the larynx occur?

Most cancer of the larynx occurs on the vocal cords. It can
also occur in the cartilage, muscles, passage from the throat,
or passage to the windpipe. For purposes of staging this
cancer the larynx is divided into three regions: the suprag-
lottis, the glottis (true vocal cords) and the subglottis.

How does the doctor diagnose cancer of the larynx?

The doctor may do an indirect laryngoscopy: He looks down
your throat with a long-handled mirror to see whether or
not the voice box shows signs of cancer of the larynx. This
can be done in the doctor's office and is painless. If he
needs to examine your throat more carefully, he may do a
direct laryngoscopy. For this examination your throat is
numbed and the doctor inserts a tube through which he
can inspect the area and take samples of the tissue if he
wishes. This examination takes only about 15 minutes but
must usually be done either in an outpatient clinic or in a
hospital. Diagnostic x-rays are also sometimes used, including a laryngeal tomograph (laryngogram) and chest
x-rays. As with other types of cancer, a biopsy is needed
for a final diagnosis. The biopsy is essential before any
treatment is planned.

How is cancer of the larynx treated?

It depends upon the exact location and site of the cancer.
Radiation therapy or surgery alone or in combination are
the usual treatments. Usually if the tumor is small, radiotherapy is used to shrink it enough so that your normal voice
returns. Since it is less disfiguring and equally effective,

The Stages of Subglottic Larynx Cancer

STAGE	EXPLANATION
Stage I	Confined to subglottic area.
Stage II	Tumor extends to vocal cords with normal or impaired cord mobility.
Stage III	Tumor confined to larynx with cord fixation.
Stage IV	Large tumor with cartilage destruction or extension beyond larynx, or both.

Treatment Choices for Subglottic Larynx Cancer

STAGE	POSSIBLE TREATMENT
Stage I	Radiation therapy, with preservation of normal voice. Surgery, if radiation not successful.
Stage II	Radiation therapy, with preservation of normal voice. Surgery, if radiation not successful.
Stages III and IV	Laryngectomy, followed by radiation therapy or radiation therapy alone, if inoperable. Investigational treatments also available.

radiation is more commonly used for small tumors. If the tumor is large, all or part of the voice box may be removed by surgery. Chemotherapy may be used in more advanced cancers as an investigational treatment.

Will I have a change in my voice if I am treated with radiation?

No, you will in all probability be able to continue talking in much the same way as before the treatment. If you are going to be treated with radiation, be sure to read the information in Chapter 7 on radiation.

What is a laryngectomy?

A laryngectomy is the complete removal of the voice box. In a partial laryngectomy, only part of the voice box is removed and the voice is preserved; just one vocal cord, half of both vocal cords, or the epiglottis (the lidlike structure that covers the entrance to the larynx) is removed.

How is a partial laryngectomy done?

This operation is performed under either general anesthesia or local anesthesia. An incision is made in the neck, starting at the top of the Adam's apple and extending about 2½ inches. The doctor will split the cartilage of the larynx and then cut away the growth on the vocal cord.

Will I have an opening in my throat from a partial laryngectomy?

An opening in the windpipe (tracheostomy) may be performed as part of the partial laryngectomy if a considerable amount of tissue is removed. This is to make sure that there is an adequate airway. A metal tube will be inserted and taken out a few days later. The opening will then close normally without any stitches being taken.

Will I be in pain after having a partial laryngectomy?

You will probably have a very sore throat. You will probably be told to sit halfway up in bed for the first few days to help you swallow. Your stitches will be taken out within a week, and you usually can go home in 10 days to 2 weeks.

Does a partial laryngectomy ever involve radical neck dissection?

It depends upon the extent of the cancer. The partial laryngectomy can involve different things. If the tumor is widespread, a radical neck dissection may be involved. If the cancer is in the leaflike flap of cartilage between the back of the tongue and the entrance to the larynx and windpipe (epiglottis), all of the larynx above the vocal cords may be taken out. In that case, the voice is preserved but you might have trouble swallowing. The doctor may put in a temporary feeding tube through the nose to the stomach for a week or longer until the swallowing becomes easier.

Will my voice change as a result of a partial laryngectomy?

Sometimes some change in voice occurs, such as a slight hoarseness. However, you will probably be able to continue talking in much the same way as before the operation.

How is a total laryngectomy performed?

The total laryngectomy is done under general anesthesia. It is a much more extensive operation than the partial laryngectomy. The incision is along the center of the neck, but is longer than for the partial laryngectomy. The windpipe is cut above the collarbone and a tube is inserted so that the anesthetic gas goes to the windpipe. The whole larynx is taken out.

Will I be in much pain after the total laryngectomy?

You will have a very sore throat. Sometimes the doctor will put in a plastic feeding tube through the nose to the stomach so that the area can heal more easily. This is not always necessary, and you may be able to swallow soft food within a few days. Your neck may feel weak, and it may be uncomfortable for you to move. You may need help to raise your head. You may have to have a special nurse or be in intensive care for a day or two.

Will I have a hole in my throat after a total laryngectomy?

Yes, you will. After a total laryngectomy you must breathe through a permanent opening in the neck. This opening is called a stoma.

I am afraid to have my voice box taken out. Is there any alternative?

If you have a large tumor there is probably no alternative, although you should talk to your doctor about it. It is only natural to be afraid, for you will be losing a part of your body which you use constantly. You should know, however, that many people who have had this operation have been able to resume their normal living. Most people have learned how to talk again. Many are people for whom talking is a livelihood, and they are able to talk fluently and understandably with their new voices.

What will I do while I am in the hospital and can't talk?

Some hospitals use simple charts with pictures of what you need, and in the early stage you can point to what you want. Some people find it easier to write a note for what they want. The nurses usually place a marker over your signal at their desks so that they can tell your calls from those of patients who can speak. If you wish, you can ask the nurse for a spoon and a water glass to signal with, or you can bring a bell to the hospital with you. One patient and his wife worked out a code which he could tap on the speaker of the telephone so she could call him in the morning and find out how he was. A magic slate or small blackboard can also be useful.

Will my lips and tongue be the same as before the laryngectomy?

Ordinarily, your lips, teeth, tongue, and nasal passages remain the same as before surgery.

What is a person who has lost his voice box called?

A person who has had his voice box removed is called a laryngectomee. Most of these people are men, and they have lost their ability to speak normally because they have had cancer of the larynx.

How soon will I be able to talk again?

That depends upon many factors. Mainly it depends on you. You need to have determination and the willingness to practice a new way of speaking. Some people say some words within 3 or 4 weeks after the operation. Others take several months. It will take time for you to be able to talk fluently so that everyone can understand you.

How can I breathe and speak if I am going to have my voice box removed?

Because your operation to remove the voice box removes the connection between the lungs and the nose and mouth, air from the lungs is no longer used to speak. You will breathe through an opening, called a stoma, in the front part of your neck. You will have to learn how to speak again.

Who will teach me to speak again?

If you are going to have this operation performed, it is important to talk with the doctor and the speech pathologist before the operation. That will be a big help in understanding what changes can be expected after surgery. Laryngectomees usually learn to talk again with the help of a speech pathologist. Occasionally some laryngectomees teach themselves. Talk to your doctor and to the local unit of the American Cancer Society to find out the names of speech clinicians or trained laryngectomees available. After you have learned basic speech you may wish to take advantage of group therapy available through such organizations as the International Association of Laryngectomees (see Chapter 23).

Is there more than one way to speak if you have had a voice box removed?

Basically there are three new ways to talk. One is by using esophageal speech, in which the tongue is used to force air into the very top part of the food pipe and that same air is forced back out through the mouth. By doing this, a sound is made deep in the throat that is used to form words in much the same way as in normal speech. The second method is pharyngeal speech, which uses the limited amount of air that goes into the nose and mouth when you breathe through the tracheostomy tube. You block this air with your tongue, making it vibrate against the roof of the pharynx at the back of the mouth. You can practice and make this speech sound almost normal—your voice will sound ordinary, but slightly hoarse. The third way uses a battery-operated device called an electro-larynx for speaking. The electro-larynx is held in the hand against the neck. When a button is pushed, the sound travels from the vibrating surface of this device through the neck and into the mouth, where the sound is formed into words. (This device is available from the telephone company's special-equipment service.)

Are there any other devices to help persons who have had a laryngectomy speak again?

There are two other devices for persons who cannot learn esophageal speech:

- The Blom-Singer device (named for its developers, Eric Blom, Ph.D., and Mark Singer, M.D., of Indianapolis) is a silicon tube, just over an inch long and rounded at one end into a one-way duckbill valve. It stays in place in a surgically made opening (tracheoesophageal puncture) in the neck. When the speaker blocks the opening in the neck with a finger, air is diverted from the lungs to the esophagus and from there to the mouth, where words are formed.
- Voice-button fistula procedure uses a small rubber device which is inserted into the back of the throat and allows one to expel air into the esophagus and thus make a sound. Surgery is required to insert the voice-button prosthesis.

All the ways seem very difficult. How will I be able to do it?

You will need a lot of practice and it will be quite a challenge for you. But most people want to learn to talk again so they can go back to the things they did before surgery as soon as they can. And many people have learned to talk in these ways.

When can I begin speech therapy?

You can start learning the new method of speaking as soon as your operation has healed. Your doctor will tell you when you can do this, but it is usually shortly after you can safely swallow liquids and solid foods.

Why is the opening in the neck necessary for a laryngectomy?

Before the operation, breathing and food passages had a common passage in the throat. Farther down, they divided into the windpipe for breathing and the esophagus for carrying food to the stomach. The voice box controlled the entry of air and guarded against food particles. The voice box has been taken out. It is necessary to relocate the end of the air passage as an opening at the front of the neck. This is called the stoma.

Will I always have to breathe through this opening?

Yes, you will always have to breathe through this opening, and once you learn how, you will do it without thinking about it. At first, you may have much mucus and coughing, but later you will cough no more frequently than someone who has not had the operation.

Will I always have to wear a tube in my stoma?

Probably for some time. A tube shaped to fit the tracheal opening (laryngectomy tube) is necessary to keep the breathing passage wide open until the tissues are healed. The doctor will tell you when it can be removed safely and how long you should wear it. Some people wear it all the time. You will get instructions on how to take it out and put it back in.

What is a stoma button?

A stoma button is a short, soft plastic tube put into the opening in your neck. Some people use a button instead of the laryngectomy tube. Some people do not need either the stoma button or the tube.

Do I keep the opening in my neck covered?

Yes. The opening in the neck needs to be covered all the time so you get warm, clean, moistened air. Air that is dusty, dry, or cold can dry your windpipe and cause coughing and make it harder for you to breathe.

Will material collect around my stoma?

Mucus, which is the liquid which is secreted normally by the lining of the respiratory tract, will be present in your stoma and sometimes will dry on the rim of it. If the mucus thickens, dries out, or collects at the edge of the stoma, it is called crustation.

How often do I have to clean my stoma?

It depends upon you. Some patients tell us they clean the stoma twice a day, once when they get up and again in the evening.

How do I clean my stoma?

You use plain water and soap and a soft cloth. It's usually easier if you are sitting down facing the mirror and leaning slightly forward. Do not use synthetic detergents or oil-based soaps.

Why is it important to have extra moisture in the air I breathe?

Before your operation, your nose helped to warm the air you were breathing and your respiratory tract helped to moisten it. Now there is no way to warm or moisten the air that comes into your lungs. It is a good idea to have a small vaporizer or a humidifier in your home so that the air you breathe is warm and moist. Some people keep a pot of water on the stove to moisten the air.

What do I do about blowing my nose?

You must remove the mucus manually. You can use a damp cloth to clean your nostrils but you cannot blow your nose. You also cannot suck on a straw, sip soup, gargle, or whistle because you cannot force air from your lungs out through your nose or mouth or force air through your mouth to your lungs.

How can I get rid of my secretions when I am wearing a shirt and tie?

Some patients tell us that they take off the second button on the shirt and sew it onto the buttonhole. That leaves an opening in which a handkerchief can be put to remove mucus. The shirt still looks as if it were buttoned.

Does my shirt have to be a bigger size than before?

Shirts usually need to be one to one and a half sizes larger than those worn before the surgery.

As a laryngectomee, can I take a shower?

You will have to be careful not to suck water into your lungs when you are bathing or showering. But baths and showers can provide moisture which you need. If you are taking a tub bath, pull the curtain around so that you keep the moisture in the air. Keep the drain partly open to keep the water from coming in high enough to get into the stoma. Keep a towel around your neck, and when you wash your face use a mirror so that you are sure water will not get into the stoma. If you are showering, adjust the stream so that it is chest-high. A special shower cover can be used to cover the stoma when you are in the shower.

Will I be able to swim?

No, you will no longer be able to swim when you are a laryngectomee. You should be careful when you are around water and you should not go boating.

Can I shave?

You must be careful if you are using a regular nonelectric razor. The area will be numb until the nerve endings return to normal, and that might take 6 months. You could cut yourself without knowing it. Don't let the shaving lather or toilet water get into the stoma. You could have severe coughing if they get into the trachea.

Is a laryngectomee a physically handicapped person?

Absolutely not. A laryngectomee can do most jobs that most others can do. You can farm, do plumbing, do officework, work in a factory, and so on. You can also participate in most sports, such as golfing, hunting, and gardening.

Can I go back to my regular job after I have my voice box removed?

Most people find they can return to their regular jobs. Talk to your doctor about when you can go back to work. It is essential that you get back to normal routines as soon as you can and take every opportunity to try out your new speech patterns.

Where can I get help for all this adjustment?

The American Cancer Society sponsors Lost Cord Clubs (sometimes called New Voice Clubs), which are groups of laryngectomees and their families dedicated to helping new members get used to the same physical and emotional changes they have been through. Many of the clubs offer group speech therapy as part of scheduled meetings. Members also visit new patients on the request of doctors, to show them how they speak and to answer questions. Some clubs also teach laryngectomees and their families special first aid. Don't hesitate to call on them if you need a helping hand. Since all these changes are sometimes difficult to deal with by yourself, it is important that you let family and friends help you through this period. The more you go out with friends and practice the new way of speaking, the more confident you will feel. Let your family and friends help, but try to get back to doing everything for yourself just as you did before.

Where can I find out about these clubs and other information about laryngectomies?

You can call the nearest office of the American Cancer Society, or the Cancer Information Service in your area.

Does a laryngectomee need a special kind of first aid if he becomes ill or is hurt in an accident?

A laryngectomee does need special first aid. First expose the neck. Give mouth-to-neck breathing only. Keep the person's head straight with the chin up. Keep the neck opening clear with cloth; don't use tissue. A laryngectomee should wear a special medic-alert identification bracelet or carry an emergency instruction card.

CANCER OF THE ESOPHAGUS

What is the esophagus?

The esophagus is the foodpipe. It is a long, hollow muscular tube which goes from the back of the throat down to the stomach. It carries food and liquid to the stomach.

Are most tumors of the esophagus cancerous?

Yes. Most tumors of the esophagus are malignant. More men than women have esophageal cancer, and it occurs most often between the ages of 50 and 70.

Is difficulty in swallowing one of the symptoms of cancer of the esophagus?

Difficulty in swallowing could be due to a number of conditions. If the problem lasts for more than 2 weeks, you should see a doctor, because cancer of the esophagus is one possibility. Because the tumors start in the lining of the membrane, the sensation may be that food, especially soft bread and meat, sticks behind the breastbone. Other warning signs of cancer of the esophagus include sensations of pressure and burning or pain in the upper middle part of the chest, hoarseness, cough, fever or choking. However, the main symptom is difficulty in swallowing (dysphagia). The food doesn't feel as if it is going down properly—but the feeling is different from the one you get from a sore throat. Because of the difficulty in swallowing, weight loss is sometimes a symptom.

Does the difficulty in swallowing continue as a symptom?

Sometimes the sensation seems to get worse and then to get better. Sometimes it comes and goes.

What tests are used to detect cancer of the esophagus?

Usually the first test will be a barium swallow. This is an x-ray procedure. You swallow a liquid containing barium, which outlines the esophagus. X-rays are taken. If a tumor is present, the lining of the esophagus will appear abnormal or narrowed. The doctor will be able to tell whether or not a tumor is there, the size of the tumor, and the extent of its growth.

What is an esophagoscopy?

This is the way a doctor usually confirms his diagnosis of esophageal cancer. A long, thin tube with a light and lens at the end of it (esophagoscope) is slid down the throat and into the esophagus. The doctor can see the inside of the esophagus and can tell whether or not a tumor is present. Sometimes he can also tell the size of the tumor with this instrument. The doctor also uses a biopsy forceps with the esophagoscope to take a tiny bit of tissue from the areas which look suspicious during the esophagoscopy. Or he might gather loose cells from the esophagus with a brush. Either the tissue or the cells are studied under the microscope to determine whether or not the tumor is cancer. Radioisotopes are also used sometimes in scanning to find tumors of the esophagus.

How is cancer of the esophagus treated?

Cancer of the esophagus is usually treated either by radiation or by surgery either alone or in combination. The radiation may be used either before or after the operation. The surgical operation is called an esophagectomy. It is performed under general anesthesia. The doctor makes a

The Stages of Cancer of the Esophagus

STAGE	OTHER CLASSIFICATIONS	EXPLANATION
Stage 0	T1S, N0, M0	A very early cancer that has not spread below lining of first layer of tissue.
Stage I	T1, N0, M0	Cancer involves a small portion of the esophagus (less than 5 cm) and shows no regional lymph-node involvement or spread to other organs.
Stage II	T1, N1–2, M0 T2, N0–2, M0	Cancer involves a large portion of the esophagus, produces symptoms of blockage, and involves entire circumference of esophagus but has not spread to nearby structures or to distant organs.
Stage III	T3, any N, M0 any T, N3, M0	Cancer has spread to nearby structures or there is extensive lymph-node involvement, but it has not spread to other organs.
Stave IV	Any T, any N, M1	Cancer had spread to other organs.

Treatment Choices for Cancer of the Esophagus

STAGE	POSSIBLE TREATMENTS
Stage 0	Surgery
Stage I, II	Surgery Radiation therapy Investigational: combinations of anticancer drugs and radiosensitizers in addition to surgery and radiation therapy (pre- and post-operative).
Stage III	Radiation therapy Investigational: Radiosensitizers and/or combination chemotherapy along with or instead of radiation therapy
Stage IV	Dependent on individual case Investigational: combination chemotherapy

10-inch incision between the ribs on the side of the chest and removes the whole cancerous area, if possible. The passage must again be connected to the stomach, either by replacement with a plastic tube, by using the remaining healthy tissue, or by using a portion of the intestine. The earlier the disease is detected, of course, the more successful the operation will be.

How long must I stay in the hospital with cancer of the esophagus?

After the operation, you will usually stay in for 2 to 4 weeks or longer. You will be in bed from 1 to 3 days.

Will I be able to eat?

After the operation you will be fed with intravenous fluids and/or by a rubber tube passed through the esophagus into the stomach. A rubber tube is also placed in the chest for a few days after surgery to drain the chest. Within 3 to 5 days you will probably be able to take fluids and soft food by mouth.

Is this major surgery?

Yes, surgery for cancer of the esophagus is major surgery. You will probably be uncomfortable for many days afterward.

chapter 19

Cancer of the Brain and Spinal Cord

The thought that a mass of abnormal tissue can grow in the brain, our center of thought, emotion, and feeling, terrifies us. Yet some brain tumors can be removed completely with surgery, leaving no trace of ever having been there. Even advanced cancers of the brain are being treated by new methods, making the diagnosis of brain cancer less ominous than it was even a few years ago. Many factors determine the outcome of brain cancer: the type and grade of tumor and, of course, the location of the tumor and whether it invades the tissues that surround it.

Persons Most Likely to Get Cancer of the Brain and Spinal Cord

- Young children and young adults to age 20
- People over 40; peak ages 50–60
- More men than women

Symptoms of Cancer of the Brain and Spinal Cord

The symptoms of cancer of the brain and spinal cord vary depending on where the tumor is located in the brain. Symptoms include:

- An unusual kind of headache, more painful than normal. A constant ache or soreness, located in the back, front, or side of the head or behind the eyes, often present upon waking in the morning
- Vomiting, usually in the morning
- Impaired speech
- Hearing loss or ringing and buzzing in ears
- Loss of ability to smell
- Muscle weakness of the face
- Abnormality in functioning of the eye
- Balance problems, or lack of coordination in walking or movement
- Changes in personality
- Convulsions or epileptic seizure
- Inability to sleep for long periods
- Drowsiness

Tests for Cancer of the Brain and Spinal Cord

- Complete medical history and physical
- Skull x-rays
- CT scan
- Electroencephalogram
- Brain scan
- Angiogram
- Pneumoencephalogram
- Echoencephalogram

Questions You Should Ask Your Doctor Before Agreeing to Treatment for Cancer of the Brain and Spinal Cord

- Where is the tumor located?
- What kind of tumor do you suspect?
- Where will the operation be?
- Will you shave my hair off?
- Will it be painful?
- What kind of diagnostic tests will I still need? How painful or dangerous are they?

- Will you have to drill a hole in my skull? Will it be painful?
- How long will I have to stay in the hospital?
- Will there be any side effects?
- Will there be any additional treatments?
- When will I be able to go back to work?

What kind of doctor should I see if I have symptoms of brain or spinal-cord cancer?

This is a specialized field, and you should be sure you have a skilled, competent diagnostician and surgeon. The physician who specializes in diseases of the nervous system—brain, spinal cord, and nerves—is called a neurosurgeon.

Is the National Cancer Institute supporting any studies on cancer of the brain and spinal cord?

Yes, many clinical cooperative group studies are being conducted by the National Cancer Institute on brain and other spinal-cord tumors. Numerous different drugs and radiation therapies are being used. For information on this subject, see Chapter 23.

What is meant by tumors of the central nervous system?

The central nervous system is made up of the brain and the spinal cord. Tumors can be found either in the brain or in the spinal cord. Sometimes brain tumors extend downward into the spinal cord. Usually, however, tumors of the central nervous system do not spread to any other part of the body. Cancer which starts in other parts of the body can, on the other hand, metastasize to the brain. About 80 percent of the central nervous system tumors involve the brain, and about 20 percent involve the spinal cord.

What is the brain?

The brain is a soft grayish-white structure enclosed by the skull. It weighs about 3 pounds and has some 15 million nerve units which permit it to store memory images and learning. Its connections control more than 600 muscles in the body. The brain is the seat of consciousness, sensation,

Cancer of the Brain and Spinal Cord

TYPE	CHARACTERISTICS
Glioma	Family of tumors which starts within brain substance itself.
Astrocytoma	Slow-growing, usually in shell-like capsule. May be malignant or benign. Found in both adults and children.
Glioblastoma multiforme	Most malignant type. Grows quickly. Term commonly used to describe a highly malignant astrocytoma.
Ependymoma	Begins in lining cells. Often benign. Usually occurs in children.
Medulloblastoma	Usually found in children. Usually malignant.
Oligodendroglioma	Adult central nervous system tumor.
Congenital tumors	Include dermoids, teratomas, cholesteatomas, and craniopharyngiomas. More common in children.
Meningioma	Starts in membranous tissue. Can grow to large size and destroy bone. Mostly benign. Occurs mostly in adults.
Neuroma (neurofibroma)	Arises in nerves. Usually occurs in adults over 40. Most common is acoustic neuroma (schwannoma), occurring in ear nerve. Benign, slow-growing.
Pituitary adenoma	Occurs in young or middle-aged adults. Almost always benign.
Metastatic	Starts somewhere else and spreads to brain. Usually comes from breast, lung, or melanoma.

and emotion. It directs all voluntary acts and controls all higher mental processes.

What are the parts of the brain?

The brain has four main structures: cerebrum (the largest area, which is divided into four lobes and controls movement, speech, and visual functions), cerebellum (second-largest area, involving muscular coordination), pons (which receives and sends impulses from the cerebrum and cerebellum to the spinal cord), and medulla oblongata (which regulates breathing, heartbeat, and vomiting). The brain also has many nerve structures, including twelve cranial nerves.

Is there any research on what causes brain tumors?

Little is known about the causes of brain cancers, although studies have linked them with occupational, environmental, viral, and genetic factors. Some cancers appear to be more frequent among workers in particular industries. Those who are exposed to vinyl chloride—chemists, pharmaceutical workers, embalmers, and workers in rubber manufacturing plants—appear to have a higher incidence of brain cancer than the general population. Cattle and sheep ranchers, dairy farmers, and grain millers, as well as those who are subjected to long-term pesticide exposure, have been shown in some studies to have a higher incidence of brain cancer. Other factors, such as high-dose x-rays, consumption of sodium nitrate (the meat preservative), and head injuries have also been suspected.

Who gets tumors in the brain?

About 85 percent of brain tumors occur in adults, with a peak age of 50 to 60. The remaining affect infants or children, with a peak age of 10 years. More men have brain cancer than women.

Are brain tumors common?

No. Brain tumors are relatively uncommon. They account for only 2 percent of all cancer deaths.

What are the symptoms of brain tumors?

The symptoms vary depending on where the tumor is located in the brain. They are caused by increasing pressure inside the skull as the tumor grows. Most common is a headache, more painful than usual, which results in a constant ache or soreness. It may be in the back, front, or side of the head or behind the eyes. Patients report that the headache will be there when they wake up in the morning,

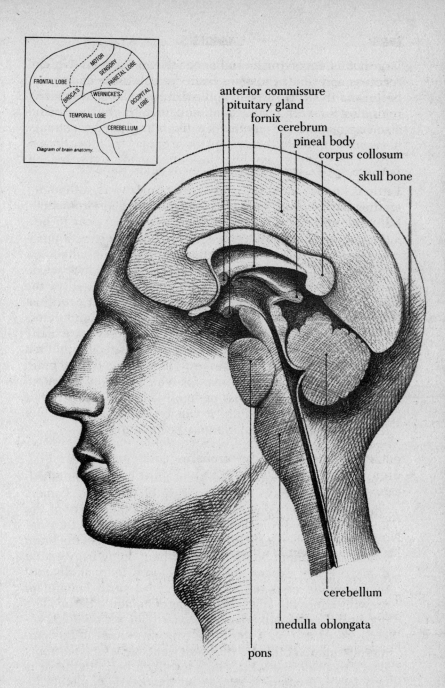

FRONTAL LOBE
BROCA'S
MOTOR
SENSORY
PARIETAL LOBE
WERNICKE'S
OCCIPITAL LOBE
TEMPORAL LOBE
CEREBELLUM

Diagram of brain anatomy.

anterior commissure
pituitary gland
fornix
cerebrum
pineal body
corpus collosum
skull bone

cerebellum

medulla oblongata

pons

Brain

or that it begins to ache right after they arise. Vomiting may accompany the headache. Some people note changes in personality or are more irritable than usual. Epilepsy is also a symptom, with convulsions, seizures, or short periods of unconsciousness. Sometimes patients say they hear strange sounds and smells that are not there or may fall into a dream-like state. There may be a loss of hearing, sight, speech, taste, smell, and balance.

Do some symptoms relate directly to the part of the brain the tumor is in?

Sometimes the symptoms are produced by the tumor push-ing into a particular area of the brain. Tumors which are located in the area controlling motion can produce weak-ness in the arm, the leg, or both. A tumor located in the cerebellum, for instance, might produce loss of coordina-tion, balance, or the ability to walk. However, brain tumors are very hard to diagnose, since the symptoms are usually difficult to pinpoint, may appear only occasionally, and are similar to those of other diseases. There is one type of brain tumor, olfactory meningioma, for which the key symptom is loss of smell. Since loss of smell is considered a minor problem by many people, it can be overlooked and not diagnosed until other symptoms become evident.

Are all brain tumors cancerous?

No. However, tumors in the brain must be thought of dif-ferently than tumors in other parts of the body. Tumors which would be considered benign in other parts of the body are more serious in the brain—not because they are cancerous but because they are located in a part of the brain where they cannot be taken out without doing irreversible damage. They expand inside the closed bony skull until they strangle essential centers. Even a small amount of growth occupying space can damage the nerve tissue. The doctor will often talk about a brain tumor which is encap-sulated—that is, in a shell-like capsule—and can be com-pletely removed. That is different from one which has roots like a plant or one which invades much brain tissue or is in a location where it cannot be removed completely by surgery.

Are those tumors which are in a capsule curable?

It depends upon the tumor. If it is discovered and removed when it is still in its capsule, the chances of cure are very good. If it goes untreated, it will eventually break through the capsule and spread cells into surrounding areas of the brain. When this happens, it is more difficult to treat. As with other cancers, the earlier it is discovered, the greater the possibility of successful treatment.

What causes the swelling in the brain?

Most tumors result in swelling (edema) of normal brain tissues. The swelling puts additional pressure on the brain and may cause a great deal of significant damage before the tumor grows to a large size. Sometimes steroid drugs are used to reduce the swelling in the brain. Steroid drugs are also sometimes used for pain of brain tumors, either alone or in addition to surgery or radiation.

How are brain tumors diagnosed?

There are several procedures which can help diagnose brain tumors. A complete medical history and physical, with the doctor looking for changes, watching movements, and looking at ear and eye nerves, and plain x-rays of the skull may sometimes give enough information. More specialized tests include:

- *Skull x-ray:* Reveals the effects that a tumor might have on the bone of the skull. It can show tiny deposits of calcium that may indicate the presence of a tumor.
- *CT scan:* Also called a CAT (computerized axial tomography) scan, a painless diagnostic technique. A computer, connected to a rotating x-ray machine prints out a pattern showing the concentration in the brain tumor of a radioactive substance. The CT scan causes the patient no discomfort. Where equipment is available, this test has largely replaced the vetriculogram and pneumoencephalogram.
- *Electroencephalogram:* Wires are taped to the skull to record brain waves from that area. Can show abnormal brain functioning but does not show the tumor itself. Causes patient no discomfort. Also called EEG.

- *Angiogram:* A small amount of contrast material is injected into arteries of the neck leading to the brain. X-rays are taken. Some patients have a painful, burning sensation as the contrast material is injected. A high-risk procedure. Anesthesia is used before the test is performed.
- *Pneumoencephalogram:* A needle is placed into the spinal canal, fluid is taken out, and air is injected. X-rays are taken. Following this procedure, many patients have headaches, nausea, vomiting, and fever which may last for several hours or days. A high-risk procedure.
- *Ventriculogram:* A burr hole is made in the skull and a needle is placed in one of the brain's ventricles (small cavities). A small amount of fluid is taken out and replaced by air, and x-rays are taken. A high-risk procedure.
- *Echoencephalography:* A picture of the brain is produced on a television screen by "echoes" of ultrasound. A technician passes an instrument that looks like a small microphone back and forth over the head. The instrument emits sound waves that strike the brain and bounce back against the instrument.
- *MRI:* Magnetic resonance imaging produces pictures of the body's internal tissues similar to CT scans. A new device, it uses electromagnets instead of x-ray tubes and is considered a safer procedure that produces sharper pictures. Nothing is injected into the body, and the body is not exposed to radiation. MRI equipment is usually available only at major medical centers.

What are the different kinds of brain tumors called?

There are several kinds of brain tumors, which are usually broken down into the following types: gliomas, meningiomas, neuromas, pituitary adenomas, congenital tumors, and metastatic tumors. Gliomas and meningiomas can also occur in the spinal cord.

How do doctors classify tumors of the brain and spinal cord?

Classifying brain and spinal-cord tumors is extremely difficult because of the nature of the tumors and the location.

Numerous methods are used, and most physicians and hospitals feel that the most critical features are the type of tumor, the extent of growth, and the location of the tumor. A "G" designation is sometimes used to indicate the biological activity of the tumor: G1, well differentiated; G2, moderately well differentiated with no mitoses; G3, poorly differentiated with occasional mitoses; G4, very poorly differentiated with frequent mitoses. "T" classifications are as follows:

- *T1:* Tumor less than 3 or 5 centimeters (size dependent on location), confined to one side
- *T2:* Tumor more than 3 or 5 centimeters (size dependent on location), confined to one side
- *T3:* Tumor invades or encroaches upon ventricular system. Greatest diameter may be less than 3 or 5 centimeters (depending on location in brain)
- *T4:* Tumor crosses the midline, invades opposite hemisphere, or extends into other sections of brain

What are the gliomas?

About half of the tumors inside the cranium originate within the brain substance itself and are called gliomas. There are a number of different types of gliomas.

- *Astrocytomas:* May be malignant or benign and are found in both adults and children. They grow slowly but penetrate into large areas. Sometimes astrocytomas are in a shell-like capsule and can be completely removed by surgery. Radiation and chemotherapy are sometimes used.
- *Glioblastoma multiforme:* The most malignant type of brain tumor. Accounts for more than half of all gliomas. It grows very quickly. It is treated by surgery but many times cannot be completely removed. Radiation and/or chemotherapy are used as secondary treatments.
- *Ependymomas:* Begin in the lining cells. Many of these are benign, but many cannot be removed because of location. Radiation and chemotherapy are sometimes used.
- *Medulloblastomas:* Most often found in children. Radiation and chemotherapy are often used.

What are congenital tumors?

The congenital tumors include dermoids (sometimes called dermoid cysts or cystic teratoma), cholesteatomas, and craniopharyngiomas. Craniopharyngiomas occur more commonly in children; they are benign but are sometimes difficult to remove because of their location.

What are meningiomas?

The meningiomas start in the meninges—the membranous tissue which surrounds, covers, and protects the brain. Some of these grow to a very large size and cause destruction of the bone. Most of them are benign. They vary in size from that of a small pea to that of a large grapefruit. They are usually distinct lumps. Meningiomas account for 10 to 15 percent of all tumors inside the brain and occur mostly in adults of middle age. They are more common in women than in men. They grow slowly and are usually treated by surgery. They can recur, usually in the same location.

What are schwannomas?

Schwannomas are tumors that arise from the Schwann cells, which form the fatty sheath that covers nerve fibers in the body. *Schwannoma* is a general term that includes neuromas.

What are neuromas?

Neuromas, or neurofibromas, as they are sometimes called, arise in the nerves of the brain. They rarely occur in persons under 40. They may develop at any nerve site, but the most common type is in the nerve of the ear, called acoustic neuroma. If left untreated, it can cause deafness. Neuromas are benign, grow slowly, and produce limited symptoms for a long period of time. Many of the acoustic neuromas are discovered early, because an early sign is difficulty in hearing, often accompanied by noises in the head. When discovered early, neuromas can be completely removed through the ear or through an opening in the back part of the skull. If they can be completely removed, they usually do not recur. Sometimes the patient's hearing can be saved.

Treatment Choices for Brain Cancer

STAGE OR TYPE	POSSIBLE TREATMENT
Adult Astrocytoma, Grade I and Grade II	Surgical removal of as much of tumor as possible Radiation Investigational: chemotherapy in addition to radiation
Adult Astrocytoma, Grade III	Surgical removal of as much of tumor as possible Radiation and chemotherapy Investigational: newer chemotherapy drugs, radiation sensitizers, new radiation therapy
Glioblastoma Multiforme	Surgery plus radiation treatment or surgery plus radiation and chemotherapy Investigational: newer chemotherapy drugs, radiation sensitizers, new forms of radiation therapy
Brainstem Glioma	Radiation therapy
Ependymoma	Surgery alone or followed by radiation if needed for known or suspected tumor not removed by surgery
Craniopharyngioma	Surgery alone or followed by radiation if needed for known or suspected tumor not removed by surgery
Medulloblastoma	Surgery plus radiation to brain and spinal cord Surgery plus radiation therapy plus chemotherapy
Meningioma	Surgery Surgery plus radiation if needed for known or suspected tumor not removed by surgery
Oligodendroglioma	Surgical removal plus radiation therapy
Recurrence	Investigational: newer chemotherapy to reduce or treat recurrence

What are metastatic brain tumors?

Metastatic brain tumors are different from other brain tumors because they are cancerous tumors which start somewhere else in the body and spread to the brain. Metastatic tumors make up about 10 to 15 percent of all brain tumors. They usually come from primary tumors of the breast or lung or from a melanoma. Radiation or hormone therapy is most often used.

Do tumors occur in the spinal cord?

Sometimes. Much that is true of brain tumors is also true of spinal-cord tumors, because the spinal cord and the brain together form the central nervous system. Sometimes tumors of the brain may extend down into the spinal cord. There are also separate spinal-cord tumors, but they are seen less often than brain tumors. Spinal-cord tumors may stop the flow of messages between the body and the brain in either one or both directions, similar to spinal-cord injuries which occur as a result of accidents.

Are most spinal-cord tumors cancerous?

Most of the spinal-cord tumors which start outside the cord itself (in the membrane around the cord or in a spinal nerve) are not cancerous. They cause pressure on the cord and the nerves. They can usually be removed completely by surgery.

Do tumors which are growing within the cord tend to be malignant?

Yes, tumors which are growing within the spinal cord are more often cancerous than those which start outside the cord itself. But they usually grow slowly. They are hard to remove without destroying a section of the spinal cord. However, they can be treated by radiation therapy, which stops the growth. Proton-beam radiation, available only in a few major centers, seems to be able to destroy spinal-cord tumors without damaging surrounding tissue. Cancer in other parts of the body sometimes spreads and involves the spinal cord. Radiation treatment is usually used in these cases.

How are spinal-cord tumors diagnosed?

Two tests can be done to diagnose spinal tumors:
* *Spinal puncture:* This will usually show an obstruction to the free flow of the spinal fluid. Chemical analysis of the fluid often provides additional useful information.
* *Myelogram:* The doctor injects a radioactive substance into the spinal fluid and then takes x-rays.

How are brain tumors treated?

Surgery is almost always the first step in treating brain tumors—and, if the tumor is completely removed, may be all the treatment needed. If additional treatment is needed, radiation therapy is usually the treatment used. Sometimes chemotherapy is added. The type, location, and extent of the tumor are very important in deciding the kind of treatment which will be used.

Are radiation implants ever used in treating brain tumors?

Yes, and with the advent of computers, it is now possible for implants to be placed with great accuracy. Some hospitals are presently experimenting with computer-assisted radiation implants.

Are lasers used to treat brain cancer?

Yes. In some major medical centers, computerized systems are used in conjunction with laser surgery as an investigational treatment.

What is a craniotomy?

A craniotomy is the operation for exposing the brain. It is usually performed under general anesthesia, although sometimes local anesthesia is used.

What preparations will be necessary before the operation?

Your head will be shaved and your scalp will be cleaned with water and soap. An antiseptic will be put on the area, and all but that portion to be operated on will be covered with sterile drapes.

How will the operation be done?

The doctor will make an incision in the shape of a semicircle facing downward in the skin on the affected part of the scalp. He will flap the skin down and drill holes in the skull. He will then connect the hole by sawing with a wire, air, or electric saw so that a block of bone (called a bone flap) can be taken out from the skull. In simple terms he has made a window into the skull through which to work. Directly underneath are the membranes which cover the brain. These will be cut so that the doctor can see the brain.

Will the block of bone be put back after the operation?

After the operation, the doctor will put the block of bone or flap back, or he will use a metal or fabric mesh to cover the opening. The doctor will fix it securely and then sew the skin back in place.

Can the exact location of the tumor usually be determined before the operation?

Yes, with the many tests available the exact location can usually be pinpointed.

Can the doctor always tell before the operation whether a brain tumor is malignant or benign?

No, that is not always possible.

Do brain operations take a long time to perform?

It depends upon the location of the tumor, the procedure which will be used, and the surgeon himself. Some operations are done within an hour or two. Others may take 3 or 4 hours. Because of improvements in giving anesthesia, even the lengthy operations are safe.

Will I have intravenous feedings after my brain surgery?

Sometimes feedings are done with a tube in the stomach or into the vein. Often you can be fed by mouth.

Will I need special nurses after brain surgery?

Yes, you will usually either be in intensive care or need special nurses for several days.

Will there be any aftereffects of the brain surgery?

It depends upon your condition before your surgery and what the outcome of the surgery is. Many people who have had brain surgery live normal lives. Usually the doctor will be able to tell you before the operation if you will have any defects after the operation—such as poor vision, hearing loss, difficulty in speaking, or problems with arms or legs. The operation itself usually does not cause the problems; usually the problems are there before the operation. Many times, physical therapy will be recommended by the doctor, especially to strengthen your arms and legs if they have been affected by your tumor. Many patients have learned to speak again if their speaking had been affected by the tumor.

Is radiation used in treating brain tumors?

Usually the surgeon will take out only as much of the tumor as is possible without damaging normal nerve tissue. The remaining tumor cells are often treated by radiation therapy. In many cases, radiation can stop the tumor from growing any further. Radiation is also used before surgery to reduce the size of the tumor.

Will my head hurt as a result of the radiation treatments?

Your head itself probably won't hurt, but the skin may become sensitive, and it might be a good idea for you to plan on clothes and pajamas which button down the front or back so you won't have to worry about pulling things over your head.

Is chemotherapy ever used in treating brain tumors?

Chemotherapy in treating brain tumors is still in the experimental stages. However, since brain cells do not multiply, they are less susceptible to some of the chemotherapeutic drugs than are the fast-growing tumor cells.

What is meant by the blood-brain barrier?

The brain has a special mechanism, called the blood-brain barrier, which keeps substances which might be harmful to it from getting from the blood into the tissues of the central nervous system. Consequently, some chemotherapeutic drugs are not effective in treating brain tumors because they cannot penetrate the blood-brain barrier. Several institutions are testing different types of drugs which have been able to get from the blood to the brain. Also under study are methods of delivering drugs directly to the tumors by implanting capsules into the brain.

What is pituitary adenoma?

Pituitary adenoma is a tumor of the pituitary gland. It occurs in young or middle-aged adults.

What is the pituitary gland?

The pituitary gland is a small gland about the size of a pea which is at the base of the brain just above the back of the nose. It secretes several hormones and influences many distant parts of the body. This gland is sometimes called the master gland because it influences body growth, metabolism, and other functions.

Is the pituitary gland ever removed?

The pituitary gland can be removed, and treatment for a tumor of this site is usually surgery and radiation. The pituitary gland is normally related to brain cancer, and its removal in that instance involves a craniotomy, which means opening the skull and pushing the brain aside to reach the gland.

Is the pituitary gland connected with breast and prostate cancer?

Some doctors are taking out the pituitary gland in breast-cancer patients and patients with prostate cancer because they believe that this eliminates various hormones that tend to support the growth of breast and prostate cancer. There is a new process in doing the operation for this purpose. Instead of a craniotomy, the surgeon goes through the upper gum and the nasal passage into the pituitary chamber below the brain. This operation is called a transsphenoidal hypophysectomy.

chapter 20

Childhood Cancer

Only a decade ago, the chances of surviving childhood cancer were very slim. Today, nearly 60 percent of children with cancer can be expected to be cured, about double the rate of three decades ago. It is estimated that by the late 1990s, 1 out of each 1,000 20-year-olds in the United States will be a cured cancer patient.

Leukemia, a blood cancer, is the most common childhood cancer. There are a number of different varieties. The most common is acute lymphocytic leukemia (ALL). It is called acute because without treatment the disease usually progresses rapidly. It is, however, the most treatable of all the leukemias. The second most common type of leukemia in childhood is acute nonlymphocytic leukemia (ANLL), a treatable and sometimes curable cancer. It also requires prompt treatment.

Childhood non-Hodgkin's lymphomas, which include lymphoblastic lymphoma and nonlymphoblastic lymphoma (undifferentiated lymphoma, Burkitt's and non-Burkitt's types, and large-cell lymphoma), are different from some of the lymphomas that occur in adults. The selection of treatment depends on cell type, stage of disease, and sites of involvement.

Brain tumors in children are treatable and often curable with modern therapy. How curable depends on how malignant a tumor is, whether or not it is sensitive to radiation and chemotherapy, and how completely it can be removed by surgery.

Osteogenic sarcoma, also called Ewing's sarcoma, usually occurs in teenagers. It is a bone sarcoma which may extend into the soft tissue around the bones. The two most important factors are the location and whether there has been any spread to other locations, such as to the lung, bone, or bone marrow.

Retinoblastoma may occur at any age, though it is usually seen in younger children. The goals of therapy are to cure the disease and to preserve as much vision as possible.

Childhood rhabdomyosarcoma is highly treatable and, in many patients, curable. It is a soft-tissue tumor that bears a resemblance to primitive muscle tissue. It usually involves the head and neck, the genital and urinary region, the arms or legs, or the trunk.

The evolution of treatment for *Wilms' tumor*, a childhood kidney tumor, is one of the remarkable efforts in cancer therapy. In 1938 the cure rate was less than 6 percent. Today, more than 80 percent of children with Wilms' tumor are cured.

Neuroblastoma, a cancer of the central nervous system, is one of the most common cancers found in children, usually occurring in children under 5 years of age. Patients with localized or regional disease are highly treatable and very curable.

Tests for Childhood Cancer

Acute lymphocytic leukemia (ALL) and Acute nonlymphocytic leukemia (ANLL)

* Complete blood count
* Bone marrow aspiration
* Cell marker studies
* Biopsy

Childhood non-Hodgkin's lymphoma

- Complete blood tests
- X-rays
- Bone marrow aspiration
- CT scans
- Ultrasound

Osteogenic sarcoma (osteosarcoma, bone tumor, or Ewing's sarcoma)

- X-rays
- Lung tomograms
- CT scans
- Bone scans
- Biopsy

Brain tumors

- Complete neurologic examination
- Electroencephalography
- Brain scan
- CT scans
- X-rays of skull and chest

Retinoblastoma

- Eye examinations
- X-rays
- CT scans
- Bone marrow examination
- Spinal fluid examination

Wilms' tumor

- Chest x-ray
- Complete blood count
- Urinalysis
- Intravenous pyelogram (IVP)
- Bone marrow tests
- CT scan
- Ultrasound
- Liver and bone scans
- Renal arteriogram

Neuroblastoma

- Intravenous pyelogram (IVP)
- Blood tests
- Ultrasound
- Urine tests
- Biopsy

Rhabdomyosarcoma

- X-rays
- Tomogram
- Gallium scan
- Intravenous pyelogram (IVP)
- Brain scan
- Bone and liver scans
- Bone marrow examination
- Biopsy

What kind of doctor should be treating my child?

Ideally, an oncological pediatrician should be responsible for the primary treatment of your child. Pediatricians who do not specialize in childhood cancer may see fewer than half a dozen cases in their careers. Therefore, your own pediatrician or surgeon will usually refer you to an oncologist, who may suggest that you take your child to one of the major medical centers for treatment. If you decide to use one of these, you could find total patient care; all the disciplines, including medical and other subspecialities, nursing, and social service, are orchestrated and individualized for the patient. However, the twenty comprehensive cancer centers now supply extensive information services to the local medical community, and specialists from many of the centers work with local physicians in planning followup treatment. New treatment methods require teamwork among radiologists, surgeons, medical oncologists, pediatric oncologists, physiotherapists, nurses, and social workers.

Questions to Ask the Doctor

- What kind of cancer does my child have?
- Has the diagnosis been checked with another pathologist?
- What kind of treatment are you advising?
- Will I be able to get these treatments locally?
- Will my child be receiving treatment following one of the new protocols?
- Will my child be part of a clinical study?
- Is it advisable to go to an out-of-town cancer center or specialized hospital for treatment?
- If no, why not?
- Does the hospital have provisions for living facilities for the parents while the child is undergoing his hospital treatment?
- How long do you think the child will be hospitalized?
- Have you treated other children with this type of cancer?
- How many?

Is the National Cancer Institute supporting studies on childhood cancer?

The National Cancer Institute's clinical cooperative groups have a great many studies under way, with oncologists, sur-

Childhood Cancer

Type	Age	Symptoms	Treatment
Acute lymphocytic leukemia (ALL)	Most between 2 to 8 years; boys more often than girls	Tired, pale, listless, swollen glands, easily bruised, infections that persist despite antibiotics, bleeding gums, nose bleeds, bone or joint pain	Chemotherapy with or without radiotherapy. New drugs and combined treatments have extended lives. Bone marrow transplants are sometimes used after chemotherapy and radiation.
Acute nonlymphocytic leukemia (ANLL)	All ages	Poor skin color, fever, infection, easy bruising, bleeding	Combination chemotherapy, radiation to skull, injection of drugs into spinal fluid. Bone marrow transplants may be used.
Osteogenic sarcoma (bone tumors or Ewing's sarcoma)	Peaks in late adolescence, usually occurs between 10 and 25 years; more in males than females	Swelling or pain in lower leg or forearm	Surgery combined with radiation and chemotherapy are bringing good results in 60% of all cases. Implants and limb preservation.
Neuroblastoma	May be present at birth; more than half before 2 years old	Swelling in abdomen, chest or eye	Surgery followed by chemotherapy and radiation.

Brain tumors	Tend to occur in first 10 years of life	Blurred or double vision, dizziness, difficulty in walking, unexplained nausea	Surgery, or radiation, or chemotherapy. Many are curable if diagnosed early. See Chapter 19.
Lymphomas (Hodgkin's and non-Hodgkin's)	11 up	Swelling of lymph nodes in neck, armpit, groin; weakness, fever	Chemotherapy. Radiation and surgery for local treatment. Picture improving every year. See Chapter 14.
Retinoblastoma (eye tumors)	Under 4	Squint, widening of pupil of eye, cat's-eye reflex	Surgery, radiation therapy, photocoagulation, cryotherapy, radiation implants.
Wilms' tumor (cancer of kidney or nephroblastoma)	From infancy to 15, most under 7	Swelling or lump in abdomen, blood in urine, fever, loss of appetite, paleness, lethargy	Surgery combined with radiation and/or chemotherapy.
Rhabdomyosarcoma	2–6, teens	Swelling, bleeding, unusual mass—found in head, neck, eyes, genitourinary system, extremities, chest, and abdomen see below	Surgery, followed by chemotherapy and radiotherapy.

geons, pathologists, and radiologists participating. Among the diseases being studied are leukemia, Wilms' tumor, neuroblastoma, rhabdomyosarcoma, Ewing's sarcoma, and other pediatric solid tumors. In Chapter 23 you will find the name of the chairman of each clinical cooperative group and the phone number for contact. The address listed is not an indication of where these groups are located. It is simply the information center for the specific type of study group. Your doctor or you may contact that person for information on what clinical trials are available in your area. You can get further information by calling the Cancer Information Service at 1-800-4-CANCER.

How common is childhood cancer?

Cancer is actually quite rare in children. Only 1 percent of all cancers appear in children. However, it is second only to accidents as a cause of death in children aged 3 to 14. Nearly half of the children with cancer are under the age of 5.

Are most tumors found in children cancerous?

No. Most tumors found in children are benign.

Is leukemia the most common childhood cancer?

Yes. Leukemia is the type of cancer most frequently found in children. Among the leukemias, acute lymphocytic leukemia, known by the abbreviation ALL, is the most common. For a disease that was once fatal in 99 percent of cases, the outlook is now bright, thanks to research in the last decade.

Is cancer fatal to most children?

No. Many adults—and many physicians in practice today— were taught that most cancers in children were incurable. In the last twenty years medical researchers have completely reversed this formerly hopeless prognosis. The enlightening news is that in some of the centers which specialize in childhood cancers, more than half of the children treated since the late 1960s have apparently been cured—and the cure rates are even higher among those presently being treated with the new drugs and combined treatments.

Are children ever born with cancer?

Yes. Wilms' tumor is a form of congenital kidney cancer. If detected early during infancy, Wilms' tumor can be removed and the child can grow to be a healthy adult. Scientists also believe that neuroblastoma may be present at birth. It appears to arise during fetal life and may be linked with inborn defects of nerve tissues.

Is leukemia contagious?

Leukemia is not contagious. Other children cannot "catch" leukemia from an affected child. Therefore, children with leukemia can continue to live at home, attend school, and play with their friends.

What causes leukemia?

At the present time, the cause of leukemia is unknown. It does not seem to be related to a child's past health, dietary history, or any of the other factors which appear to affect the onset and course of some other diseases. It is known that persons exposed to near-lethal doses of radiation at the atomic blasts at Hiroshima and Nagasaki developed leukemia. Researchers have also proved that some types of leukemia in animals are caused by virus. However, there is as yet no proven association with viruses in humans. ALL occurs more frequently among children with Down's syndrome (mongolism). It has been found that if an identical (not fraternal) twin is diagnosed with ALL, in 20 percent of cases, the other twin will also develop the disease.

What types of leukemia are usually found in children?

The most common type, accounting for 45 percent of all childhood leukemia, is acute lymphocytic leukemia, known as ALL for the initials of its name. It is most likely to occur in children below the age of 6. Acute nonlymphocytic leukemia (ANLL) is the second most common form of childhood leukemia.

The Stages of Childhood Acute Lymphocytic Leukemia (ALL) and Childhood Acute Nonlymphocytic Leukemia (ANLL)

STAGE	EXPLANATION
Untreated	Newly diagnosed with no previous treatment. Abnormal blood counts, abnormal bone marrow with more than 5% blasts, and signs and symptoms of disease.
In remission	Normal blood counts, bone marrow with less than 5% blasts, and no signs or symptoms of disease.
Relapsed	Disease has progressed, recurred, or relapsed.

Treatment Choices for Childhood Acute Lymphocytic Leukemia (ALL)

STAGE	POSSIBLE TREATMENTS
Untreated	Combination chemotherapy Central nervous system treatment, including combination chemotherapy with or without radiation treatment to the skull Investigational treatments, including combination chemotherapy with or without radiation treatment to the skull
In remission	Maintenance therapy can include: Combination chemotherapy Central nervous system treatment, including combination chemotherapy with or without radiation treatment to the skull Investigational treatments available
Relapsed	Investigational treatments, including bone marrow transplants

Treatment Choices for Childhood Acute Nonlymphocytic Leukemia (ANLL)

STAGE	POSSIBLE TREATMENTS
Untreated	Combination chemotherapy
	Radiation treatments to the skull and injection of medication into the spinal fluid
	Investigational treatments, including combination chemotherapy and bone marrow transplants
In remission	Maintenance chemotherapy
	Intensive chemotherapy followed by maintenance chemotherapy
	Bone marrow transplants
	Nervous system treatments with radiation, with or without chemotherapy
	Investigational treatments, including bone marrow transplants and chemotherapy combinations with or without radiation
Recurrent	Investigational treatments, including bone marrow transplants

What are the symptoms of childhood leukemia (ALL)?

Early symptoms often appear gradually and include fatigue; weakness; pallor; low-grade temperature; bleeding gums; frequent nosebleeds; bone or joint pain; enlargement of lymph nodes, liver, or spleen; pinpoint-sized red or deep-purple spots on the skin; and/or infection that does not respond well to antibiotics and persists.

What is childhood acute lymphocytic leukemia (ALL)?

This is the most common type of childhood leukemia. Leukemia begins when the bone marrow manufactures an overabundance of abnormal lymphocytic cells that are unable to mature or to function. These abnormal blood cells, called lymphoblasts (commonly referred to as "blasts"), crowd out normal bone marrow cells. These blasts may leave the marrow, circulate in the bloodstream, and end up in the liver, spleen, lymph nodes, and around the brain. The leukemic cells crowd the bone marrow so that it can no longer produce enough normal cells.

What is the usual treatment for childhood ALL?

The child must first be hospitalized. Intensive chemotherapy with a combination of drugs is usually the preferred treatment. Treatment to the central nervous system is also given including drugs put directly into the spinal fluid and in some cases radiation to the brain.

What is childhood acute nonlymphocytic leukemia (ANLL)?

This is the second most common type of leukemia in childhood and is referred to by the initials ANLL. Children with ANLL frequently have a high white-blood-cell count along with a low red-blood-cell count and a low platelet count. The usual symptoms include poor skin color, fever, infection, and easy bruising and bleeding.

What is the usual treatment for childhood ANLL?

Combination chemotherapy is usually the primary treatment. Radiation to the skull and the injection of medication into the spinal fluid by lumbar puncture is often prescribed. Because the treatment for childhood ANLL differs from the treatment for childhood ALL, it is essential that careful diagnosis be made before treatment begins. Special laboratory tests may be needed to distinguish between the types of leukemia. Since treatment is very specialized, it is important that it be given in a hospital with facilities that can deliver the optimum care.

Is acute nonlymphocytic leukemia in children different from the adult variety?

ANLL in children is essentially the same disease biologically as ANLL in adults. (See Chapter 14.)

Are there different types of childhood acute nonlymphocytic leukemia (ANLL)?

Childhood ANLL is categorized into the following major subtypes:

M1:   acute myelogenous leukemia (AML) without differentiation

M2:   acute myelogenous leukemia (AML) with differentiation

M3:   acute promyelocytic leukemia

M4:   acute myelomonocytic leukemia (AMML)

M5a: acute monoblastic leukemia without differentiation

M5b: acute monocytic leukemia with differentiation

M6:   acute erythroleukemia

Other types include:
acute eosinophilic leukemia
acute basophilic leukemia
acute megakaryocytic leukemia

Why are the first 6 months of treatment considered to be the most difficult?

The first 6 months following diagnosis are a time of intense medical treatment. At the same time, the patient and the family are faced with the emotional crisis of learning to live with leukemia. The outcome is unknown, and the whole family must accept and adjust to the many things that must be learned about the disease and its treatment.

What can I expect to happen during the initial treatment period?

This is a very critical time. Treatment, of course, varies with the severity of the symptoms, the treatment plan, the doctor, and the hospital. Generally, however, the child is anemic, susceptible to infections, and often at risk of bleeding. Various supportive measures may be necessary, including the use of blood transfusions to correct the anemia, platelet transfusions to prevent or treat bleeding, antibiotics, and sometimes white blood cell transfusions to cope with infections. Once the disease is in remission, these supportive measures will no longer be required.

What happens once remission takes place?

Though there is no single way to treat leukemia, once remission takes place, routine therapy makes life easier for the patient and his family. Combination chemotherapy is usually given as a maintenance treatment. Radiation treatments are sometimes given daily for several weeks after the child is released from the hospital. Sometimes brain and spinal-cord therapy—in the form of radiation and drugs given through a lumbar puncture—are prescribed as a preventive measure, because leukemia can affect the brain and spinal cord. The lumbar puncture, though it sounds traumatic, is similar to a routine blood or bone marrow test. Routine treatment, with blood tests and chemotherapy on a routine basis, bone marrow tests every few months, and lumbar punctures every 4 or 5 months will then continue.

What is a complete remission?

A complete remission means that the bone marrow, blood count, physical examination, and general well-being of the child are all within normal limits. In acute lymphocytic leukemia, complete remission usually takes about 4 weeks and is achieved in about 90 percent of all cases.

How long does a remission last?

Times vary. At least 50 percent of all children with acute lymphocytic leukemia should be in remission for at least 5 years. Many have had remissions that have lasted 10 years or more. The chances of a relapse after 10 years are considered rare. However, some remissions last a much shorter period of time. When a patient is no longer in remission, he is said to have had a relapse.

What is a relapse?

Relapse occurs when leukemic cells reappear in the bone marrow, blood, central nervous system, or any other site. The symptoms of relapse are usually similar to those at the time the disease was first diagnosed.

Can the same treatment be used to achieve another remission?

With the currently available therapy, children who relapse can usually be reinduced into remission. However, third and subsequent relapses are more difficult to control, because the cells become resistant to the chemotherapy.

Is it true that the faster the response to remission-inducing therapy, the more favorable the chances of a long remission?

In children with ALL and ANLL, it appears that those whose remission is more rapid have a better chance of having a long-term disease-free remission.

What kind of reactions can I expect my child to have from the various drugs he will be taking?

It depends on the drugs; the side effects will all be carefully outlined for you by the doctor and nurse when they review the treatment your child will be receiving. However, you should be sure to check Chapter 8 to refresh your memory.

How long does the usual leukemia treatment last?

The chemotherapy treatments usually last for about 3 years. Usually, the child misses a month or more of school at the start, during which time the disease is brought under control.

Do all cases of leukemia progress in the same way?

No two cases are alike—and exact predictions are impossible to make. Much depends on the type of leukemia, the treatment given, and the way in which the individual body reacts to treatment.

How can I be assured that the latest treatment methods are being used on my child?

To maximize the chance of cure, the first treatment your child receives must be the best available to totally eradicate his leukemia. The cancer centers and major medical institutions have teams that specialize in treating cancer in children.

Are bone marrow transplants being done for children with leukemia?

Yes. Bone marrow transplants are being used for over fifteen different diseases, including treatment of childhood leukemia and lymphoma. Since standard treatments for leukemia usually limit the dosages of chemotherapy drugs so they will not be too poisonous to the bone marrow, doctors have found that they can administer very large doses of drugs and then restore the patient's bone marrow to permanent production of all the normal components of the blood through the bone marrow transplant. The bone marrow transplant material is injected intravenously after chemotherapy, radiation, and other treatments have destroyed the leukemic cells from the patient's system and suppressed the patient's immunity to the donor's bone marrow. The transplanted bone marrow seeks out its place within the bone and begins to produce a whole new population of blood cells. If the bone marrow transplant is successful and the leukemic cells do not recur, the patient has a chance for therapy-free survival from leukemia. (More information about bone marrow transplants can be found in Chapter 14.)

What does it mean when the doctor talks about "lymphoma presenting as leukemia"?

Sometimes, even if the diagnosis is leukemia, the child responds poorly to the standard leukemia therapy and the doctor finds that using the treatment usually prescribed for lymphoma patients is more successful than treatment with the less intensive leukemia regimens.

Is it dangerous to a child with leukemia to be exposed to chicken pox?

Yes, it is. The doctor should be informed immediately if the child has been exposed. ZIG (zoster immune globulin) or ZIP (zoster immune plasma) are anti-chicken pox vaccines which can be used to reduce the chances of catching chicken pox. In order to be effective, ZIG or ZIP must be administered within 72 hours after your child has been exposed to chicken pox.

Is it dangerous for my leukemic child to be vaccinated?

Your child should not receive live-virus medicine—such as that used in smallpox and measles vaccinations. Always check with the doctor before allowing any such procedures on your leukemic child.

I've heard a lot about St. Jude Hospital in connection with leukemia. Can you tell me something about it?

St. Jude Hospital was founded by entertainer Danny Thomas. It is a research center to which patients are admitted only by physician referral, and only if their disease is under study. Research studies are under way in the various forms of childhood cancers as well as in severe infectious diseases and malnutrition.

Where can I turn for information about leukemia and how to handle telling my child, dealing with his siblings, and dealing with his disease?

Fortunately, there is a great deal of help available, on many different levels. An unusual amount of helpful, well-written literature is available from the National Cancer Institute, the American Cancer Society, and the U.S. Department of Health, Education and Welfare. In some states, the local crippled children associations also offer information and assistance. You can call 1-800-4-CANCER, the Cancer Information Service, and ask any questions you may have and request that they send a supply of all the literature they have available. The Candlelighters is an organization formed to help families cope with living with the disease. For information on the local chapter nearest you, write Candlelighters at 2025 I Street N.W., Washington D.C. 20006.

How do non-Hodgkin's lymphomas in children differ from those in adults?

These lymphomas in children, even though they come from cells that are part of the lymphatic system, usually cause masses *outside* of the lymph glands, such as in the abdomen, bone marrow, or chest. Treatment, therefore, usually calls for aggressive chemotherapy, sometimes combined with radiation or surgery.

The Stages of Childhood Non-Hodgkin's Lymphoma*

STAGE	EXPLANATION
Stage I	Single tumor or nodal area outside the abdomen or mediastinum
Stage II	Single tumor with involvement of regional nodes, two or more tumors or nodal areas on one side of the diaphragm, or a tumor of the primary gastrointestinal tract with or without involvement of regional nodes
Stage III	Tumors or lymph-node areas on both sides of the diaphragm and affecting the chest, abdomen, spine, or brain
Stage IV	Bone marrow or central nervous system disease regardless of other sites

Non-Hodgkin's lymphoma is also divided into lymphoblastic and nonlymphoblastic disease.

Treatment Choices for Childhood Non-Hodgkin's Lymphoma

STAGE	TREATMENT
Stages I, II, III, IV Lymphoblastic lymphoma	Chemotherapy Chemotherapy and radiation therapy Central nervous system treatment Investigational treatments available
Recurrent lymphoblastic	Investigational treatments available
Stages I, II Nonlymphoblastic lymphoma	Chemotherapy Chemotherapy plus either radiation therapy or surgery as local treatment Investigational treatments available
Stage III Nonlymphoblastic lymphoma	Chemotherapy Chemotherapy plus either radiation therapy or surgery or both as local treatment Central nervous system treatment Investigational treatments available

Treatment Choices for Childhood Non-Hodgkin's Lymphoma

STAGE	TREATMENT
Stage IV Nonlymphoblastic lymphoma	Chemotherapy
	Chemotherapy plus radiation therapy as local treatment
	Central nervous system treatment
	Investigational treatments available
Recurrent nonlymphoblastic	Investigational treatments available

Types of Childhood Non-Hodgkin's Lymphoma

- Lymphoblastic lymphoma
   thymic
   non-thymic
- Nonlymphoblastic lymphoma
   large cell
      immunoblastic
      diffuse histiocytic
   undifferentiated
      Burkitt's
      non-Burkitt's

What is Burkitt's lymphoma?

Burkitt's lymphoma, one of the fastest-growing human cancers, is rare in the United States, though it is a common childhood cancer in Africa. High doses of chemotherapeutic drugs have been found to be highly effective in treating Burkitt's lymphoma. In Americans, the usual site for this type of lymphoma is in the neck and digestive system. In African children, Burkitt's lymphoma most often starts in the jaw, ovaries, or kidneys. Because the cancer is fast-growing, surgery is sometimes needed to remove intestinal obstruction, either before or after chemotherapy begins. If surgery is not possible, radiation is used to reduce the size of the tumor.

What is Ewing's sarcoma?

This tumor occurs in children and young adults and may involve almost any part of the skeleton. It differs from other bone tumors in that it often attacks the shafts, rather than the ends, of the long bones. It is known to metastasize to the lungs and apparently to other bones. Pain, and later swelling, are the initial symptoms.

How is Ewing's sarcoma diagnosed?

X-rays are helpful, but diagnosis must be confirmed by biopsy.

Treatment Choices for Ewing's Sarcoma

LOCATION	POSSIBLE TREATMENTS
Localized in lower jaw, skull, face, shoulder blade, clavicle, or vertebra	Combination chemotherapy and radiation. Investigational treatments include surgery and presurgical chemotherapy.
Localized in rib	Radiation plus chemotherapy. Surgery may be used to control local disease. Investigational treatments are available, including bone marrow transplants.
Localized in upper arm or thigh bone	Chemotherapy plus radiation. Investigational treatments are available, including bone marrow transplants.
Localized in pelvis and sacrum (lower spine)	Radiation therapy plus chemotherapy. Investigational treatments are available, including bone marrow transplants.
Metastatic	When spread beyond the primary site to lung, bone, bone marrow, lymph nodes, or central nervous system, radiation therapy plus chemotherapy is used. Surgery may be used to remove individual tumors. Investigational treatments are available.
Recurrent	Dependent upon location and prior treatment. Investigational treatments are available.

What treatment is used for patients with Ewing's sarcoma?

The treatments use a combination of chemotherapy and radiation. (Surgery is sometimes used in addition.) This treatment has changed the statistics in the survival rate of children diagnosed with this disease. It was formerly fatal in more than 90 percent of cases, but today more than half of the children with localized Ewing's sarcoma are being saved.

What is osteogenic sarcoma?

This is one of the most common malignant bone tumors. It occurs most often in young persons, many only in their teens. It can occur in the long bones, flat bones, pelvis, and spine. The normal bone is destroyed and replaced by tumor cells. Metastases occur by way of the veins and usually first involve the lungs. The first symptom of osteogenic sarcoma is usually pain, followed by swelling.

How is osteogenic sarcoma diagnosed?

X-rays usually are taken, but final diagnosis is dependent upon biopsy.

How is osteogenic sarcoma staged?

There are only two stages: localized (when the sarcoma is confined to the bone area where the cancer is found) and metastatic (when the tumor has spread to other parts of the body, such as the lung or another bone).

What treatment is usually used for localized osteogenic sarcoma?

Surgery is the method of treatment used to eliminate the tumor, with chemotherapy given either before or after the operation. Before chemotherapy was available, amputation of the affected limb was necessary because lesser surgery usually resulted in return of the cancer at its original site. Now scientists are finding that when anticancer drugs are given before and/or immediately after the operation, limb-sparing surgery can be performed without increasing the risk of local recurrence in about half the cases. In the other half, amputation is necessary because of the size or location of the tumor, its involvement with major blood vessels or nerves, the presence of infection or for other reasons.

What is used to replace the diseased bone if the limb is being preserved?

In research programs where treatment to preserve the bone is being used, the doctors often use a prosthesis made of a metal called vitallium to replace the diseased bone. In some cases, bone from another part of the person's body is used. This procedure is called allografting. When only small pieces of bones that do not bear weight are removed, replacement is often not needed.

What treatment is prescribed for metastatic osteogenic sarcoma?

Metastatic osteogenic sarcoma is a treatable, sometimes curable cancer when a combination of therapies is used. The treatments may be as follows:

- Surgical removal of the primary tumor and metastases, where possible, followed by chemotherapy. Sometimes it is necessary to perform multiple operations on the chest to remove lung metastases.
- Chemotherapy before operation, followed by surgical removal of primary tumor and removal of lung metastases. Chemotherapy is given again postoperatively. If lung metasteses cannot be removed surgically, radiation may be helpful if chemotherapy is not successful.

What treatment is prescribed for recurrent osteogenic sarcoma?

If the metastases are confined to the lungs, the tumors may be removed, and chemotherapy may be prescribed. Further treatment depends on many factors, including the site of recurrence and prior treatment, as well as the wishes and needs of the patient.

What is parosteal sarcoma?

This is a less malignant form of bone cancer which involves the surface but not the interior of the bone. This type can often be cured by removing the affected section of bone, or by amputation. In children who have reached puberty, alternatives to amputation (such as bone-replacement grafts) are being investigated in major cancer centers.

What should a child with bone cancer who requires an amputation be told?

It is important to prepare the child ahead of time—and to be very honest. Usually, the surgeon will get to know the child during the workup and will explain exactly what will be done. It is possible, often, for the prosthesis to be applied in the operating room, allowing the surgeon to be able to assure the child that he will be able to use the limb within 2 or 3 days.

Are some tumors of the bone not really bone tumors at all?

That is correct. Malignant tumors in other parts of the body sometimes metastasize to the bone. In some cases, the metastases are discovered before the primary tumor is discovered. A biopsy can often give a clue as to the source of the metastasis.

What is neuroblastoma?

This is a cancer of the central nervous system, which is the second most common children's cancer—after leukemia. It is usually found in certain nerve fibers of the body—most commonly in the adrenal gland, abdomen, chest, or eye. It is a disease of infants and young children. More than 75 percent of all cases are diagnosed in children under 3 years of age. More males than females are found to have neuroblastoma. The older the child, the more difficult the disease is to treat. Neuroblastomas sometimes regress spontaneously and sometimes will revert to a benign state.

What treatment is usually used in neuroblastoma?

If the entire tumor can be removed, surgery is recommended. Chemotherapy or radiation therapy or both may also be used as treatments.

Treatment Choices for Neuroblastoma

STAGE	OTHER CLASSIFICATIONS	POSSIBLE TREATMENTS
Localized (located only in tissue where first began)	CCSG: Stage I St. Jude: Stages I & IIA POG: Stage A	Complete surgical removal of tumor
Regional (spread beyond original tissue to nearby tissue or to lymph nodes on both sides of body)	CCSG: Stages II & III St. Jude: Stage IIB POG: Stages B & C	Surgery only if complete removal of tumor is possible and no positive lymph nodes Surgery followed by chemotherapy or radiation or both Second surgery sometimes necessary
Disseminated (spread to other parts, such as bones, organs, or lymph nodes)	CCSG: Stage IV St. Jude: Stage III POG: Stage D	Aggressive chemotherapy Surgery and radiation therapy Investigational treatments available
Special Neuroblastoma (small tumor but spread to liver, skin, or bone marrow)	Stage: IVS	Treatment should be under observation of multidisciplinary team of physicians. May require little or no therapy.
Recurrent		Dependent on prior treatment, site, and individual circumstances. Investigational treatments available.

Are brain tumors often found in children?

Brain tumors account for 12 to 15 percent of childhood cancers. There is a great variety of brain tumors, affecting many different parts of the brain.

What symptoms signal a brain tumor?

Brain tumors are difficult to diagnose in young children. Symptoms vary a great deal, depending on the location of the tumor. If the tumor is located in a part of the brain that is not near a vital nerve center, it may grow quite large without producing any signs. However, disturbances such

Treatment Choices for Childhood Brain Tumors

Type	Possible Treatments
Medulloblastoma	Surgery followed by radiation Investigational: chemotherapy in addition to radiation
Cerebellar astrocytoma	Surgery Radiation if entire tumor cannot be removed surgically
Infratentorial ependymoma	Surgery followed by radiation Investigational: chemotherapy in addition to radiation.
Brainstem glioma	Radiation without surgery Investigational: chemotherapy before or after radiation, or both
Cerebral astrocytoma	Grade I: may be treated by surgery alone Other grades: surgery followed by radiation Investigational: chemotherapy prior to radiation
Supratentorial ependymoma	Surgery followed by radiation therapy Investigational: chemotherapy
Craniopharyngioma	Surgery Radiation if tumor not completely removed or if it recurs
Germ cell	Surgery followed by radiation Investigational: chemotherapy
Optic nerve glioma	Surgery or radiation or both Investigational: surgery, radiation, and chemotherapy
Recurrent	Investigational treatments may be considered.

as blurred vision, complaints of "seeing double," periph-
eral-vision problems, changes in muscular coordination,
unexplained vomiting, changes in personality, sudden
drowsiness, momentary loss of consciousness, convulsions,
and persistent headaches are all signs that should not be
ignored. Though these signs can be caused by many conditions totally unrelated to brain tumors, the appearance of
many of them suggests the need for investigation.

What kinds of tests can be done to detect brain tumors?

Careful studies must be made before any steps are taken.
Complete neurologic examination, testing of vision and
hearing, electroencephalography, brain scans, and x-rays of
skull and chest (to rule out involvement in other parts of
the body) must all be completed before any conclusions are
reached.

How are brain tumors treated?

Once the tumor has been pinpointed, a decision will be
made about whether it can be removed safely with surgery.
Surgery is the usual treatment followed by radiation therapy. Many brain tumors are responsive to treatment and
when discovered early are quite curable. Because brain
tumors are relatively rare in children, treatment should be
planned by a multidisciplinary team at cancer specialists
experienced in this pediatric field. (More information on
brain tumors can be found in Chapter 19.)

What is retinoblastoma?

This is an eye cancer which affects children under the age
of 4. Usually, a change in the appearance of the pupil of
one eye will be noticed, making the size of the two pupils
look uneven. The widening of the pupil allows a peculiar
white reflection to shine through the pupil of the eye, which
is actually the tumor itself. There may also be pain, redness,
and vision loss. If allowed to advance, swelling will occur,
closing the eye. In one out of every four or five cases,
retinoblastoma can affect both eyes.

Does retinoblastoma run in families?

Because so little is known of the genetics of most types of
cancer, precisely how the disease is transmitted is still un-

known, but retinoblastoma seems to have a hereditary factor. The fact that multiple cases are found in some families suggests that some cases are due to a dominant gene. It is now estimated that about 40 percent of cases are inherited. Young children in families where the disease has occurred should be watched carefully and examined frequently for early signs.

Is there any way that retinoblastoma can be detected in the fetus?

A new diagnostic test makes it possible to predict the possibility of retinoblastoma in pregnant women where there is a history of this cancer. The infant's eyesight can be saved by prompt use of radiation on tumors that would not ordinarily be detected at an early stage. The diagnostic tests are based mainly on studies of chromosome 13 and on the use of genetic markers that indicate variations in the chemistry of the DNA.

Treatment Choices for Retinoblastoma

STAGE	POSSIBLE TREATMENTS
Intraocular: one eye (unilateral)	If no useful vision can be preserved, no radiation. Surgery if potential for preservation of sight. Radiation, cryosurgery, photocoagulation, implant.
Intraocular: both eyes (bilateral)	Radiation, only if potential for vision in both eyes. If vision cannot be preserved, surgery on eye with most advanced disease. Radiation and/or other types of treatment listed above. Investigational chemotherapy treatments available.
Extraocular	Radiation and chemotherapy. Investigational treatments available.
Recurrent	If small, confined to eye, local therapy. Investigational treatments available.

Is vision usually lost in patients with retinoblastoma?

No. Even in patients where the disease is quite advanced, partial vision can often be saved. Where discovered early, vision is preserved in 95 percent of cases.

How is retinoblastoma treated?

Radiation therapy, surgery, photocoagulation, cryotherapy and radiation implant are all treatments for retinoblastoma. Treatment is planned after the extent of the tumor within and outside the eye is known. When both eyes are affected, surgery is usually performed on the most severely involved eye and radiation is used on the other in an effort to preserve the greatest amount of sight.

What is Wilms' tumor?

Wilms' tumor, which is a cancerous tumor, is usually found in children 1 year of age and older. Peak incidence occurs at about 3 years of age. The tumor is uncommon after 8 years of age. More boys than girls are found to have Wilms' tumor. Wilms' tumor is sometimes referred to as nephroblastoma or cancer of the kidney.

What are the symptoms of Wilms' tumor?

In the majority of children, an abdominal mass is discovered by the parents. Symptoms can also include abdominal pain, nausea, vomiting, diarrhea, fever, and blood in the urine.

Do these young children have to undergo all the same testing an adult would before surgery is performed?

Yes. It is important that the disease be properly evaluated before surgery. Therefore, diagnosis for Wilms' tumor would probably include a chest x-ray, intravenous pyelogram, liver and bone scans, complete blood count, urinalysis, and bone marrow examination. These tests are usually done in the hospital prior to surgery.

What is the treatment for Wilms' tumor?

Usually surgery is followed by radiotherapy and chemotherapy. Radiotherapy is sometimes used prior to surgery to reduce the size of the tumor if it is very large.

The Stages of Wilms' Tumor

STAGE	EXPLANATION
Stage I	Tumor limited to kidney; completely removed. Tumor did not rupture before or during removal. No apparent tumor remains.
Stage II	Tumor extends beyond outer surface into soft tissues. Or areas outside kidney are affected. Or tumor was biopsied and spillage is confined to flank. Or, though tumor extended to outer surface, tumor was completely removed by surgery.
Stage III	Lymph nodes are affected. Or growth has penetrated through peritoneal surface. Or tumor extends beyond surgery. Or tumor cannot be completely removed because of growth into other organs.
Stage IV	The tumor has spread to lung, liver, bone, brain, etc.
Stage V	Tumor affects both kidneys.

*Each tumor is designated as favorable histology (FH) or unfavorable histology (UH).

Treatment Choices for Wilms' Tumor

STAGE	POSSIBLE TREATMENTS
Stage I	Surgery plus chemotherapy or surgery plus radiation plus chemotherapy, depending on cell type.
Stage II	Surgery plus chemotherapy. Radiation may or may not be used. Investigational: surgery plus chemotherapy without radiation.
Stage III	Surgery plus radiation plus chemotherapy.
Stage IV	Surgery plus radiation plus chemotherapy
Stage V	Surgery plus chemotherapy or surgery plus chemotherapy plus radiation. Investigational treatments are available.
Recurrent	Aggressive multimodal treatment.

Is there a good chance a child with Wilms' tumor can live a normal life?

The outlook for Wilms' tumor has changed completely in the last 40 years. Whereas Wilms' tumor was previously considered a fatal disease, today between 80 and 90 percent of children suffering from it can be cured. If the child remains disease-free for two years following surgery and treatments, he will be considered cured.

What is rhabdomyosarcoma?

This is the most common soft-tissue cancer among children—usually found in the head, neck, eyes, genitourinary area, extremities, chest, and abdominal cavity. It occurs most frequently between the ages of 2 and 6 and in the teens. Symptoms depend upon where the tumor is located: a swelling in the eye, a bloody nasal discharge, a mass in an extremity, grapelike clusters protruding from the vagina, vaginal bleeding, or obstruction of the urinary outlet.

How is rhabdomyosarcoma treated?

Treatment depends upon where the tumor is located and the cell type. The usual treatment is surgery followed by chemotherapy and sometimes radiation therapy. Since this cancer may spread to other sites, the stage at which it is found is an important factor. Metastase occur early and often spread to distant organs, generally the lung. Biopsy is usually performed to establish the diagnosis.

Are there any new studies being done on rhabdomyosarcoma?

Yes—and they are encouraging, especially for patients with localized nonmetastatic rhabdomyosarcoma. Children with localized rhabdomyosarcoma are potentially curable with intensive chemotherapy and radiotherapy following surgery. The results are much less encouraging if the disease has spread. For information on National Cancer Institute studies, see Chapter 23.

Treatment Choices for Rhabdomyosarcoma

STAGE	POSSIBLE TREATMENTS
Group I	Surgery followed by chemotherapy. Radiation may be used.
Group II	Surgery followed by radiation and chemotherapy. Investigational treatments available.
Group III	Surgical biopsy followed by chemotherapy and radiation. Investigational treatments include bone marrow transplant following surgery, chemotherapy and radiation.
Group IV	Surgery limited to biopsy unless primary tumor can be removed. Radiation and chemotherapy. Investigational treatments available.
Recurrent	Treatment depends on site of recurrence and prior treatment as well as individual considerations. Investigational treatments available.

Should I tell my child he has cancer?

Openness and honesty are usually the best depending, naturally, upon the age and understanding of the child. The toddler can be told that he is sick and needs to take his medicine to get better. Older children need to know that cancer is a serious but treatable illness. Many of them have the impression from watching television that everyone who has cancer or leukemia dies. They need reassurance that there are successful treatments and that new treatments are being used with very hopeful results. Try not to avoid the subject because you are afraid of saying something wrong. Painful and awkward though you may feel, it is better to deal with the question honestly and to keep communication open between you and the child.

My child gets angry over the inconveniences that the treatments impose. How do I handle this anger?

Anger is a very normal reaction—and you should allow the child to vent some of it. Let him know you share his concerns but that the treatment is necessary for him to be able to lead a normal life.

Should the other children in the family be told when a brother or sister has cancer?

It really is best to do this right at the start. Children are concerned and worried and need to be included and re-assured. The age of the child dictates how much needs to be told. A three- or four-year-old can be told that his brother is sick and needs to go to the hospital and will be taking medicine for a long time. Young children often feel guilty when another member of the family becomes sick and need to be reassured that they are not responsible. Children also worry that they might come down with the same illness. Being aware of these fears and understanding that the special attention the sibling is receiving does not detract from their own specialness will help keep them from becoming resentful about the time you must spend with the sick child. Let them know that anger and guilt feelings are normal and that you understand.

Where can I get more information about childhood cancers?

The Cancer Information Service 1-800-4-CANCER phone service will be able to give you information about the specific disease which has been diagnosed. Their trained counselors can tell you what hospitals in your local area are participating in the latest treatments. They can also send you a supply of the most recent booklets that are available. Some wonderfully helpful and sensitive material has been written by parents who have cared for their children at home to the end. One of the most informative and most poignant, *Coping at Home with Cancer, for Parents, by a Parent*, by Nina Cottrell, may be purchased from Children's Hospital of St. Paul, 311 Pleasant Ave., St. Paul, Minn. 55102.

Is financial help available for children with cancer?

Some help is available through the American Cancer Society, the Leukemia Society of America, and, in some states, through the local associations for crippled children. The Leukemia Society will often help in paying costs of anti-leukemic drugs, transportation to and from treatment centers, and costs of typing and cross-matching of blood, and in some states provides aid to families whose medical costs in the course of a year have gone beyond $20,000.

What is the Ronald McDonald House?

This is a "home away from home" for families with children under treatment for serious illnesses. The program was started with the help of McDonald's restaurants to provide comfortable, accessible quarters for families of children undergoing treatment which required long stays in hospitals away from the family's home. Food supplies are usually available, and most Ronald McDonald facilities ask for a donation of $10 a night, which can be waived if the family is without financial means. To find out if there is a Ronald McDonald House close to the treatment center you are using, call the Cancer Information Service (1-800-4-CANCER) or the American Cancer Society.

How do I get in touch with the organization that makes wishes come true for children with cancer?

There are a number of these organizations across the country (see listing in Chapter 23)—and additional information is available through your Cancer Information Service or local American Cancer Society office. When the committee receives a request from a parent, members check with the child's doctor. If the trip is approved, the doctor notifies a physician in the area the child will visit and gives the parents a letter detailing all necessary medical information in case the child needs help while away. Many children have had their wishes to take trips to Disneyland or Disney World, to meet a movie star or professional athlete, to fly a plane, or to ride with a fireman come true thanks to volunteers who staff these organizations.

Are there summer camps for children with cancer?

There are a growing number of summer camps for children with cancer. The camps are medically staffed, and many of the programs are free. They give children with cancer a normal camping experience, shared with others who have the same problems. A listing of camps is included in Chapter 23. You can get additional information about summer camps in your area from the Cancer Information Service, Candlelighters, or the American Cancer Society.

What is Children's Hospice International?

Children's Hospice International is a nonprofit agency that promotes the hospice concept through pediatric care facilities, encouraging the use of hospices and home-care programs for children. Most of the present hospice programs focus on adults. This program hopes to give the same attention to the needs of dying children and their families. The organization's address is 501 Slater's Lane, N. 207, Alexandria, Virginia 22314.

chapter 21

Coping When Cancer Spreads or Comes Back

The greatest fear of any cancer patient is that the cancer will spread or recur. And, unfortunately, sometimes, despite all efforts to take the recommended treatments, to eat properly, to act positively, we are faced with the fact that the cancer which we thought we'd beaten, has returned. It's a time of difficult challenges. And after you get over being angry with the unfairness of life, the feelings of fear, the agony of thinking about submitting yourself to more treatment, you are able to face what is happening at this turning point in your life with greater knowledge and understanding. By learning all you can about your illness and treatment, you make it possible to be a part of what happens to you. Through your own understanding of your case and type of cancer, you gain positive reinforcement that will help you control and deal with some of your emotional and physical reactions—and the reactions of those around you. The most important thing to remember is not to "run scared." Remember that there still are many appropriate treatments available. And, though cancer may have taken away the feeling that your tomorrows would go on forever, you can pride yourself in having gained the vision and wisdom of recognizing the preciousness of each and every day.

For most patients, the fear of pain is one of the most significant and difficult aspects they feel they must face. Pain, if it occurs, usually happens in the later stages of cancer, and though it is a commonly held belief that all cancer patients experience unbearable pain, in actual fact, this is not so. It is estimated that about one-third of all patients with advanced cancer have pain which requires the use of a prescribed drug. With new advances in understanding pain and pain management, many causes of cancer pain are being managed without narcotics. Where narcotics are required, pain control can be achieved in 90 to 95 percent of patients.

Pain centers—designed to study and deal with people in pain—have opened in many hospitals across the country, including one at the National Institutes of Health (NIH). Some health professionals are now dealing in pain management as a specialty. Patients are usually accepted to pain centers by referral only, so it is necessary to check with your doctor for a referral for assistance in controlling pain. Most pain clinics are affiliated with university medical schools or teaching hospitals. Their staffs represent the full spectrum of methods of pain relief therapy: surgery, neurology, psychiatry, psychology, and pharmacology. Both inpatient and outpatient services are usually available for relief of both acute and chronic pain.

Why does cancer recur?

Recurrent cancer gets its start from cells that break away from the original tumor and travel through the lymph system or bloodstream to start new cancer growths. The original treatment is always designed to destroy the original cancer and any of the cells that may have become detached from it. Sometimes, however, microscopic cells too small to be detected may survive and eventually start to grow in another location.

What does it mean when the cancer has metastasized?

It means that the cancer has spread from its original location to other parts of the body. The cancer in its original location is called the primary cancer. A second cancer growth in another part of the body is called a metastasis. (The plural of *metastasis* is *metastases*.) It is important to know where the primary cancer is located, because cancer that metastasizes usually has the same properties as the original cancer. For example, a doctor can tell if a cancer that grows in the bone of a breast cancer patient is a metastasis when he examines the cancerous tissue under a microscope, for it will resemble the tissue from the breast site.

Can you have a metastasis without having primary cancer?

No. A metastasis is a cancer growth that starts from a cancer cell or cells from another site. Sometimes the metastasis is discovered first, such as when pain is experienced from a metastatic cancer of the bone before any symptoms are noticed from a primary lung cancer.

My doctor says I have a metastasis, but he cannot find the primary tumor. Does this mean he doesn't know what he's doing?

No. A small number of cancer patients have tumors which clinically and pathologically can be proven to be cancer metastases, yet tests and examinations do not reveal where the first cancer is located. Even after extensive diagnostic studies, some of these cancers are impossible to detect. There are a number of ways in which such cases are managed, depending on the history, the site of the metastatic cancer, and where the doctor suspects the primary cancer is located. In such cases, it is especially important that your pathology be completely reviewed by the doctor who knows your case best and the pathologist. Be sure to report to your doctor any previous problems with what were thought to be harmless symptoms: skin tumors, removal of benign polyps of the colon, D & C or conization procedures, biopsies of the prostate, etc. The tissue that was removed may have been considered benign, but could be the location of the original tumor. Think carefully about your past medical history, any pains, change in bowel habits or voiding pattern, vaginal or other bleeding, or pelvic discomfort to give the doctor any clues that may help determine where the original cancer might be located. Usually, the tumors, when finally detected, are smaller than the tumor in the metastatic site. It is sometimes necessary to start treatment before the original cancer is found—and many times the original site is never pinpointed.

What is the difference between local, regional, and metastatic recurrence?

Local recurrence means that the cancer has come back in the same place as the original cancer. The term *local* also means that there is no sign of cancer in nearby lymph nodes or other tissues. For instance, a woman who has had a mastectomy could later have a local recurrence of breast cancer in or around the area of the original surgery. The same is true of colon or bowel cancer, where sometimes recurrences occur in the scar area or nearby. A *regional* recurrence involves growth of a new tumor in lymph nodes or tissues near the original site, but with no evidence of growth at distant sites. A woman treated for breast cancer, for instance, might have a regional recurrence in the lymph nodes under her arm. The third type of recurrence is a *metastatic* recurrence, where the cancer has spread to organs or other tissues at some distance from the original site—such as in the bone, lung, or brain.

How is a metastasis found?

When any cancer is discovered, careful testing is usually done to determine if there are any signs that the cancer has spread. This is part of the staging process. The most common places for cancers to spread are to the lungs, bones, liver, or brain. Unfortunately, although x-rays, CT scans, ultrasound, and radioisotope scans are helpful in detecting metastases, no test yet devised is able to pinpoint a very small number of cancer cells as soon as they have been shed from a primary tumor.

How can a doctor tell if a cancer is a primary or a secondary tumor?

The cell structure of a metastasis resembles that of the primary cancer. When cancer is discovered elsewhere in a patient already known to have cancer, it most often is a metastasis rather than another primary tumor. These secondary cancers may appear at about the same time as the primary tumor, or they may not become evident until months or years later.

Where do metastases occur most frequently?

The most common locations are the lungs, bones, liver and brain. In the brain, metastases are most often in the front lobe. The symptoms include headache, loss of motor function, vision problems, seizures or loss of feeling. CT scans are now able to pinpoint a brain metastasis. Radiation therapy is usually used to treat a metastasis in the brain. Some metastatic tumors, though malignant, are totally separated from normal brain tissue and can be completely removed. Chemotherapy may also be used.

Metastases to the lung are found by using chest x-rays, tomograms or CT scans. Some doctors recommend CT scans at regularly scheduled intervals for patients with testicular, kidney, breast, or colon cancer or for those with osteogenic and soft-tissue sarcomas, so that any metastases can be detected in their earliest, most curable stages. The use of chemotherapy as a treatment for the primary tumor has reduced, though it has not eliminated, the number of patients who later have metastatic lung cancer. Chemotherapy is often the treatment of choice for metastases to the lung.

Cancers of the lung, breast, and gastrointestinal system sometimes spread to the liver. Depending on the size of the tumor, surgery may be recommended. Since the recuperative powers of the liver are amazing, many people live with only 20 to 25 percent of their livers. Chemotherapy and radiation therapy are also used. Infusion pumps are sometimes used to deliver chemotherapy drugs directly to the liver.

Metastases to the bone are seen most often in patients with breast, lung, or prostate cancer. Metastatic bone cancer rarely is life-threatening, and many patients live for years after the discovery of bone metastases. Fractures and forced immobility are the two most difficult side effects of bone metastases. Treatment usually centers on relieving pain, which may develop gradually over weeks or months. Chemotherapy and hormonal treatment can delay the progression of bone metastases. Radiation is sometimes used to provide pain relief.

What is ascites?

Ascites is a medical term for severe swelling of the abdomen. Ascites results when fluid accumulates because stray cancer cells plug small lymphatic vessels, thus blocking the normal draining of fluids. It is most often seen in cancers of the ovary, uterus, breast, colon, stomach and pancreas. The patient may feel a painful tightness as a result of this condition. Sometimes, the fluids also begin to accumulate in the legs. It is important to get medical and nursing treatment for this condition.

How is ascites treated?

Usually, a procedure called paracentesis is performed to determine what is causing the problem. Fluid is withdrawn with a needle and looked at under the microscope to see if it contains cancer cells. If it does, chemotherapy is usually given.

What if the patient cannot be given chemotherapy?

If the patient cannot be given chemotherapy for some reason, a LeVeen shunt may be used. A small plastic valve is inserted to drain the fluid into the large vein. This is usually done under local anesthesia.

What special care is needed for patients with ascites?

Patients usually need to be propped up at an angle to help them breathe more easily. They may need help in moving, even in turning over in bed. Because there is pressure on the stomach, they may have a poor appetite. Help from the visiting nurse or a dietitian may be needed if the patient is at home.

Why do I feel as though the whole idea of going through treatments again is more than I can face?

This is a normal reaction. It is certainly easy to understand your reluctance to undergo further discomfort and disability. Ask the doctor to give you a frank assessment of the possible outcome of the treatment, arranging for a second opinion with another doctor if you feel it would be helpful.

In many cases, the second treatment regimen will be successful. Your attitude toward the treatment is an important factor in a return to health, and if it is possible for you to think of your cancer as a chronic disease, much as you would if you had diabetes, it is easier to deal with facing the necessary treatment. Unfortunately, too many of us continue to have the mistaken idea that cancers are not curable—making further treatment and positive attitudes difficult.

I find myself blaming myself, the doctor, the hospital, the whole world for what's happening to me. Is this usual?

Absolutely. You probably feel that you have been betrayed by your body and by the medical profession—and may have serious doubts about the value of future treatment since the initial attempt was, in your mind, unsuccessful. Cancer is a life-threatening physical disease. Yet anyone who has fought the battle of cancer knows that it is as much a psychological battle as a physical one. Anyone who has dealt with cancer patients has seen patients who, through a tremendous amount of positive energy, have successfully dealt with treatments and forced their bodies back to health. Anger at your present fate is a normal reaction—and a healthy one. But, be sure your anger is directed in a nondestructive direction. The doctors and nurses you have dealt with are trying to help you. Your family, friends, doctors, nurses and others around you are not to blame for your setbacks, so try to turn your anger into constructive directions. Try to set goals for yourself—even small goals—on a daily basis. The attainment of goals gives you emotional strength and helps you stay in control of your problems.

I just feel as though I want to give up. What can I do about that feeling?

Many people experience this emotion. Generally, the best cure for it seems to be to find meaningful things to do. We all need responsibilities as well as diversions, regardless of whether or not we have cancer. Many times people try to do too much for the patient. If you are physically able, you should insist on participating in your normal range of activities and responsibilities. Helplessness is one of the worst feelings—because it makes us lose our sense of self-worth. Though it hasn't been scientifically proven, cancer patients who feel they are in control and have a goal in life seem to live longer—or at least the lives they live are fuller. Doing as much as you can, while recognizing your limitations, is important. So, plan for rest, but keep yourself busy with things that make you feel good. We recommend that you read three excellent publications, available free by calling your local Cancer Information Service: *Taking Time: Support for People with Cancer and the People Who Care About Them*; *When Cancer Recurs: Meeting the Challenge Again*; and *Advanced Cancer: Living Each Day*. Published by the National Cancer Institute, they offer wonderful insights and help for the patient and his family.

What can I do to help myself feel more like a normal person?

One approach is to try to live as normally as possible. Surround yourself with familiar things. Even in the hospital, you can wear your own clothes, have your own blanket and pillows, keep pictures of your loved ones close by. Try to keep up with local and national news through newspapers and television. Call and invite friends to visit. Many people may not contact you because they don't know how to react to your problems. But there's no reason why you can't call them and talk to them naturally about what is happening to you. As you get stronger, start doing more of your normal tasks and keeping up with things that interested you before you got sick. Seek out new interests and new challenges.

Why is it that when you have a life-threatening disease like cancer, you're treated as though you don't exist?

There sometimes does seem to be an unconscious conspiracy between the medical profession and the family of the patient to "protect" the patient from what is happening. It is important to continue to be assertive. Even if you are bedridden, you are still able to discuss treatment options, financial arrangements, and family problems. It is important for families to make every effort to preserve the patient's usual role within the family as much as possible.

I recognize that my cancer is advanced and I worry about how my life will end. Who can I talk with about this?

Family, friends, clergymen, your doctor, and other health professionals can all help you if you express your concerns to them. For most of us, it is usually not death we fear, but the days, weeks, or months that precede it. It is perfectly normal to be afraid of the pain you may have to bear and to be concerned that you may become a burden to others. Those around you want to help. Try to talk with them. Or, if it is easier for you, try to write out some of your thoughts, feelings and desires. Be honest and open about your feelings and desires. It may be a good idea to include those closest to you in talks with your doctor about your own and your family's concerns to give everyone a better understanding. You will be relieved to learn, as the next pages explain, that there are many ways of dealing with pain that have been perfected in the last several years so that most cancer patients no longer have to suffer as they once did.

Treatments for Pain

TREATMENT	WHAT IS DONE	COMMENTS
Drugs: non-prescription and prescription	Pain medication is given either orally or by injection.	Doctor usually starts with mild drug and moves to stronger medication (tranquilizers, anti-depressants, and narcotics), depending upon severity of pain. Continuous medication is better than medication given only when need arises. Medication can sometimes be placed directly where pain is.
Non-medical methods	Relaxation techniques, imagery, distraction, skin stimulation, acupressure	Pain sensation is lessened or blocked through the use of a variety of methods.
Acupuncture	Thin needles are put into body at key points	Opinion of effectiveness varies.

Treatments for Pain

TREATMENT	WHAT IS DONE	COMMENTS
Hypnosis	Person is put in state of intense concentration.	No one knows how hypnosis works to control real pain. Opinion of treatment varies.
Biofeedback	Patient learns how to control inner functions of body through mind control and electronic survey.	Usually used in combination with another method. Opinion of effectiveness varies.
Transcutaneous nerve stimulation	Electrical impulses are sent through pads applied to the skin in the affected area.	Pain is relieved for period longer than application time.
Epidural dorsal column stimulator	Electrodes are surgically implanted over spinal cord. Patient controls electrical impulses.	Surgery required to implant electrodes.
TENS or TNS	Electric nerve stimulation	Small electric impulses are used to interfere with pain sensations.
Infusion pump	A self-contained ambulatory device is used to deliver a constant flow of medication to relieve pain.	For patients who do not respond to conventional treatment.
Nerve blocks	Anesthesia or alcohol is injected at a point in the nerve to deaden the nerve fibers.	Local nerve blocks give temporary relief. Sometimes used in combination with steroids. Nerve blocks with alcohol injected into or around spinal cord deaden nerves for longer period of time.
Cordotomy	Precise area in the spinal cord where bundles of nerves are located is cut.	Surgeon must be careful not to destroy nerve fibers that control muscle movement.
Percutaneous cordotomy	Electric current is used to destroy nerve fiber.	Can be performed on awake patient; can be repeated as required.

Treatments for Pain (continued)

TREATMENT	WHAT IS DONE	COMMENTS
Nerve-root clipping	Nerve roots are clipped high in neck.	Used for pain problems in upper part of body.
Rhizotomy	Pain nerve is cut where it enters spinal cord.	Dangerous because it can leave organs or limbs useless.

Is it true that most cancer patients do not experience any pain?

This is true. Most people think of cancer as a painful disease. The truth is that most cancers cause no pain in their early stages. Therefore, the people whose cancers are treated early usually have only the pain or discomfort which is part of any operation or treatment. This pain is temporary. It can be easily tolerated and can be controlled with medicine, if necessary.

Is pain more of a problem with advanced cancers?

Yes, pain occurs more often in people with advanced cancers. But even among people with advanced disease, more than half have little or no pain or discomfort. Some of the advanced patients require some light medication. For those who experience severe pain, there are several modern methods of pain relief which can be prescribed.

Is cancer pain different from pain of other illnesses?

Some recent studies seem to indicate that when cancer pain occurs, it has different characteristics, since it may be both severe and of long duration. And since it is a reminder of the disease, the pain of cancer patients is also believed to have psychological consequences.

Do some people feel more pain than others?

Some people's nervous systems are naturally more sensitive to pain than others'. A person's response to pain depends upon his general makeup and how much pain he can endure (called tolerance or threshold). The pain also depends upon the type of cancer and whether or not it is located in a place in the body where the nerves are especially sensitive.

Can worry, unhappiness, or fear cause pain?

Studies have shown that fear, worry, or unhappiness can make pain more intense. This does not mean that pain is not there physically; it means that if you can take some positive steps to keep yourself from worrying about it, it can be lessened and more easily tolerated.

Are there any cancer patients who do not suffer pain in their terminal illness?

Yes, a large percentage of cancer patients have little or no pain even in later stages.

Can pulse and blood pressure indicate how much pain a person has?

No. Pulse and blood pressure are not reliable measures of the amount of pain a person is experiencing.

What are the main causes of pain for patients with advanced cancer?

In patients with advanced cancer, pain that lasts a few days or longer may result from any of the following causes:
- Pressure placed on a nerve by the tumor
- Infection or inflammation
- Poor blood circulation because of blocked blood vessels
- Blockage of an organ or tube in the body
- Bone fractures caused by cancer cells that have spread to the bone
- Aftereffects of surgery, stiffness from inactivity, or side effects from medications
- Non-physical responses to illness—such as tension, depression, or anxiety

What kinds of things should I tell my doctor about my pain?

Pain is very difficult to describe, so you must try to be as specific as you can when discussing pain with your doctor. Try to answer each of the following questions in the course of your description:

- Where do you feel your pain?
- When did it begin?
- What does it feel like? (Sharp, dull, throbbing, steady, pinching, stabbing, intense, fiery, etc.)
- Where does the pain start?
- Do you feel pain in more than one spot?
- Does the pain move, or is it constantly in one spot?
- What relieves your pain?
- What makes the pain worse?
- What have you tried for pain relief? What helped? What did not help?
- What have you done in the past to relieve other kinds of pain?
- Is the pain constant? If not, how many times a day or week does it occur?
- How long does it last each time?
- Is the pain related to an event? Does it come after treatment? After eating? When you are overtired?

How can I remember all the details of my pain?

It is helpful to keep a diary of your pain and what you have done to try to relieve it. Note the time the pain started and disappeared. Assign a number from 0 to 5 for your pain level. Zero would be the absence of pain; 1 would indicate discomfort; 2, mild pain; 3, distress; 4, severe pain; and 5, excruciating pain. Also note any activity that seems to be affected by the pain or that increases or decreases the pain, the time pain medicine is taken (as well as the kind and amount). Any pain-relief methods other than medication— such as rest, relaxation techniques, distraction, skin stimulation, or imagery—should also be noted. Such a chart or diary will be helpful to you, to your family, and to your doctor in helping to determine how best to deal with the pain.

Who decides on which method of pain management should be used?

The doctors (oncologist, radiologist, neurosurgeon, chemotherapist) and the patient are the main decision-makers, although sometimes social workers, nurses, the clergy, and the family are also involved. In deciding which method is best, health professionals will look at the site and type of the cancer, the general health of the patient, where the pain is, the type of pain and how severe it is, the life expectancy of the patient, the temperament and psychological state of the patient, the background of the patient (occupational, domestic, and economic), and the availability and practicality of the various methods of pain relief. The management of pain is a complex problem.

Is it best to wait to take medication until the pain really is severe?

Sometimes people think they should wait as long as they can before taking medicine. Pain professionals have found that pain medication is more effective if taken on a scheduled basis to prevent pain from starting or getting worse. A mild pain reliever taken three or four times a day on a regular schedule, rather than when the pain returns, may be all the medication needed.

What is the benefit of prescribing pain medicine regularly rather than only when the need arises? Won't that lead to addiction?

If the medicine is taken regularly, the patient does not have to worry about when he will feel the pain next and how long it will take the medicine to work again. It has been found that fear and anxiety help to intensify pain. The medication is not given as needed (PRN), but instead is given before it is needed to prevent pain and fear of pain as well as to prevent feelings of dependency in patients who have to ask for relief. Some doctors using this method have found that less medication is required when medicine is given in this manner than if the patient has to ask for it.

Is it true that it takes longer for a drug to work if the pain is very severe?

Generally, that is true. If you wait too long to seek relief from pain, the pain may become more severe and more difficult to relieve. It might take twice as much medicine to control the pain adequately. That is why it is important to seek help before the pain becomes too severe.

Do drugs taken orally or drugs given by needle take longer to take effect?

Drugs taken orally generally take longer to work than those that are injected. Most injected drugs reach their peak in about an hour. The peak effect of oral drugs takes longer to achieve. On the other hand, oral drugs are effective for a longer time than injected drugs. It usually takes a smaller amount of an injected drug than an oral drug to give relief.

Does the same amount of drug give the same results for each patient?

Different people react differently to drugs. That is why it is important to tell the doctor and/or the nurse about your experience with the pain medication being given to you. They can give you a greater dose if the original dosage does not work for you, or cut the dosage if it is too strong. It is important not to change the dose yourself without telling the doctor and not to stop taking the drug without talking to someone on the medical team.

What methods are used to relieve the pain of cancer patients?

There are many ways in which the pain of cancer can be relieved.
* Non-prescription pain relievers
* Prescription pain relievers
* Relaxation techniques
* Imagery
* Distraction
* Skin stimulation
* Surgical procedures

What are non-prescription pain relievers?

Non-prescription pain relievers are analgesics that can be bought without a doctor's prescription. The most common are aspirin and acetaminophen (such as Tylenol and Datril). Equal doses of these two types of non-prescription pain relievers give about equal pain relief, and both reduce fever. However, aspirin reduces swelling from inflammation, which acetaminophen does not. Aspirin, on the other hand, can cause stomach upset or stomach bleeding, while acetaminophen does not have these side effects.

Which is better—aspirin or acetaminophen?

It depends upon your condition. Aspirin should be avoided by people who are on any of the cancer chemotherapeutic drugs that may cause bleeding, or are on steroid medication such as prednisone. Aspirin should be avoided within a week of scheduled surgery. It should be avoided if you are on blood-thinning medicine or have stomach ulcers, gout, or bleeding disorders. You should be aware that many nonprescription drugs contain aspirin. Aspirin is in Excedrin (a pain reliever), Coricidin (a cold or allergy medicine), and Alka Seltzer (an antacid), as well as in some prescription drugs such as Percodan and Empirin with codeine.

Aren't there stronger pain relievers that I can take?

In many cases, aspirin or acetaminophen are all you will need to relieve pain—especially if you take them on a regular, preventive basis. Aspirin and acetaminophen are stronger than many people realize. Certain doses of prescription pain relievers given by mouth are no more effective than two or three regular tablets (650 mg) of plain aspirin or acetaminophen. Two aspirin or acetaminophen tablets provide as much pain relief as the following prescription medications taken by mouth:

32 mg	codeine
50 mg	Demerol
30 mg	Talwin
65 mg	Darvon
100 mg	Darvon-N
1.25 mg	Dilaudid

What can be done if my narcotic pain medicine doesn't work as well as it used to?

After taking narcotic pain relievers for a time, you may develop a drug tolerance, which means that your body does not respond to the drugs as well as it once did. You are the best judge of how well your pain is relieved. Some doctors are reluctant to prescribe large enough doses or stronger narcotics for pain control. Until recently it was thought that increasing the dose of strong narcotics such as morphine and methadone would increase serious side effects without adding to pain relief. However, with careful medical observation, the doses of strong narcotics, by mouth or injection, can be raised to high levels safely so that severe pain can be eased. If you still have pain and your doctor does not seem to be aware of other alternatives, it would be helpful to ask for a consultation with a pain specialist.

How many aspirin or acetaminophen tablets can I safely take each day?

Naturally, dosage varies among individuals according to size, condition, and other factors, and only the doctor who is treating you and knows you can give you a complete answer. However, as a rule of thumb, eight aspirin or acetaminophen per day is considered a moderate dose, and many adults can safely take a total of twelve tablets per day (two or three tablets, three or four times a day). Extra-strength forms (such as Extra-Strength Tylenol) equal about one and a half regular tablets, so a maximum of eight per day would be considered the safe dose for this type. Higher dosages should be taken only with regular medical supervision.

Can I still take aspirin or acetaminophen if my doctor has also prescribed stronger medication?

It is wise to discuss this question with your doctor or nurse. Many persons who need prescription drugs can also take regular doses of aspirin or acetaminophen, since different drugs relieve pain in different ways. However, since some prescription pain tablets contain a small amount of aspirin or acetaminophen, it is important to check with your doctor or pharmacist to see how much aspirin or acetaminophen you can safely add. The total daily dose of either aspirin or acetaminophen should not be greater than 2600 to 3900 mg unless your doctor specifically recommends more.

Will I become addicted if I use narcotic pain killers?

Fear of addiction is very common among those taking narcotics for pain relief. Narcotic addiction usually is defined as dependence on the regular use of narcotics to satisfy physical, emotional, and psychological needs rather than for medical reasons. Pain relief is a medical reason for taking narcotics. Although drug addiction in patients with cancer pain can occur, it is not a major problem. As long as narcotics are used under proper medical supervision, the chance of becoming addicted is small. Most patients who take narcotics for pain relief can stop taking these drugs if their pain can be controlled by other means. Your doctor will try to prescribe the amount of narcotic that will be both safe for you and effective for your pain. The dose may have to be changed to a smaller or larger amount, depending upon how it affects you and how well it relieves your pain. You should be certain to tell the doctor at once if your pain is not controlled or if you have severe side effects, such as extreme drowsiness or difficulty in breathing.

What are the usual narcotic pain relievers?

Frequently used narcotic pain relievers include codeine, hydromorphone (Dilaudid), levorphanol (Levo-Dromoran), meperidine (Demerol), methadone (Dolophine), morphine, oxycodone (in Percodan), and oxymorphone (Numorphan). These are available only with a doctor's written prescription.

Are there any prescription pain relievers that are not narcotics?

A group of prescription pain relievers has been developed for the treatment of mild to severe pain. This group, known as nonsteroidal anti-inflammatory agents, includes products such as Zomax, Anaprox, and Motrin. These drugs relieve pain more effectively than aspirin or codeine. Your doctor or nurse can tell you if these drugs might be helpful in treating your pain.

If the pain really is severe, will narcotic injections for pain relief help?

Most severe pain can usually be relieved by narcotics taken orally. Narcotic rectal suppositories also can be effective. Sometimes injections are used usually for a few days at a time.

Is it true that heroin is the most effective drug for really severe pain?

It is believed that the reported success with heroin was due more to how the drug was given (in a preventive way) than to the effects of the drug itself. In the United States, heroin is classified as a controlled substance and is not available for medical purposes except for research. Strong narcotics such as morphine and Dilaudid are used to relieve very severe pain. The body, in fact, converts heroin to morphine. Even in England, where heroin is available for treatment of cancer patients, morphine is now being used routinely because it has been shown to be just as effective as heroin.

What is Brompton cocktail or Hospice mix?

Brompton cocktail or Hospice mix is a mixture of drugs in liquid form (varying doses of morphine, heroin, cocaine, alcohol, syrup, and chloroform water) which was first used at St. Christopher's Hospice in England in the 1970s to treat pain in cancer patients. The physicians at this hospital used the medication regularly, increased the doses of the narcotic as necessary to overcome the body's tolerance to it, and carefully adjusted the dose to the needs of the patient. Many of the new methods being used in pain management are based on procedures originally developed at St. Christopher's, as is much of the ongoing research in that field.

Are antidepressants helpful in relieving pain?

Doctors sometimes prescribe antidepressants such as Sinequan, Elavil, and Tofranil to help relieve depression associated with pain. Antidepressants can work with other medicine for more effective pain relief. Usually, it takes about 14 to 21 days before action is noted. Many of the beneficial effects are not noticeable immediately. Dizziness and nausea sometimes are reported as side effects, as well as dry mouth, bad dreams, and a "spaced-out" feeling. Most side effects, except for dry mouth, usually end within 2 weeks.

Can alcohol help relieve pain?

Alcohol can sometimes provide pain relief, increase appetite, reduce anxiety, and help induce sleep. Drinking small amounts of alcoholic beverages with meals or in the evening can be beneficial. However, you should check with your doctor before using alcohol, because it can be very dangerous when combined with some drugs.

Is marijuana used to relieve pain?

Current research has shown that marijuana is not the wonder drug as some thought in the 1970s. The active substance in marijuana, tetrahydrocannabinol, known as THC, has been found to have mild analgesic effects, but it also is known to cause hallucinations and extreme drowsiness. Some cancer patients have reported that smoking marijuana actually increased their pain. Marijuana has been available to physicians on an investigational basis for the treatment of nausea and vomiting in cancer patients who are receiving chemotherapy. It is now being manufactured commercially and is available by prescription.

What kinds of procedures on nerves are used to control pain?

There are several procedures—surgical or injections of substances—which interrupt the nerve pathways and may be used to control pain in patients. The objective of all these procedures is the same: to interrupt the nerves that carry pain messages to the brain. The nerves can be interrupted anywhere between the brain and the cancer: along the nerve to the cancerous organ, in the nerve roots of the spinal cord, and within the spinal cord proper.

What relaxation techniques can I use to relieve pain?

There are many methods. Here are some you can try:

Visual concentration and rhythmic massage: Open your eyes and stare at an object, or close your eyes and think of a peaceful, calm scene. With the palm of your hand, massage near the area of pain in a circular, firm manner, avoiding red, raw, swollen, or tender areas. You may wish to ask someone to do the massage for you.

Inhale/tense, exhale/relax: Breathe in deeply. At the same time, tense a muscle or group of muscles of your choice. (Squeeze your eyes shut, frown, clench your teeth, make a fist, stiffen your arms and legs, or draw up your arms and legs as tightly as you can.) Then, hold your breath and keep your muscles tense for a second or two. Now, let your body go limp as you breathe out. Relax.

Slow rhythmic breathing: Stare at an object, or close your eyes and concentrate on your breathing or on a peaceful scene. Take a slow, deep breath; as you breathe in, tense your muscles, such as your arms. As you breathe out, relax and feel the tension draining. Remain relaxed and begin breathing slowly and comfortably, concentrating on your breathing, taking about six to nine breaths a minute. It may help to say to yourself, "In, one two; out, one two." Each time you breathe out, feel yourself relaxing and going limp. Continue slow, rhythmic breathing for a few seconds or up to 10 minutes, depending on your need.

Relaxation tapes: Ask your doctor or nurse about obtaining relaxation tapes. These are commercially available tape recordings that provide step-by-step instructions in relaxation techniques.

Are there any other non-medical methods that can be tried to relieve pain?

Some success has been reported with techniques such as imagery, distraction, and skin stimulation. *Imagery* is used to create mental pictures or situations that concentrate the mind and distract it away from the pain. One often-used exercise is to imagine a ball of energy that forms in your lungs or on your chest. As you breathe in, imagine the ball blowing to the area of your pain, where the ball heals and relaxes you. When you breathe out, imagine the air blowing the ball away and taking with it the discomfort and tension. *Distraction* is another method that many people use without realizing it when they watch television, listen to the radio, read, knit, or work on crafts such as model building to take their minds away from the pain. *Skin stimulation* is the use of pressure, friction, temperature changes, chemical substances, or mild electrical current to excite the nerve endings in the skin. It is done either on or near the area of pain, on the same or opposite side of the body as the pain. Massage is also very effective, especially if slow, steady circular motions are used. Vibration devices can also be helpful in bringing relief of pain through skin stimulation.

What is acupuncture, and how is it done?

Acupuncture has been used in China and elsewhere to treat pain for thousands of years. Special needles are inserted into the body at certain points and at various depths and angles. Particular groups of acupuncture points are believed to control specific areas of pain sensation. The patient is given no painkiller and usually feels no pain from the insertion of the needles. Treatments are generally given in a series—sometimes every day for a week or more. Most doctors believe acupuncture is not harmful so long as the needles are sterile. Acupuncturists are often listed in the yellow pages of the telephone directory.

What is acupressure?

Acupressure is based on principles similar to those of acupuncture, but it can be performed by anyone without using anything except fingertip pressure. The method concentrates on stimulating trigger points in the body, in the area of pain. The technique is simple and involves deeply probing with the tip of the thumb or forefinger until a sharp twinge is felt, and then stimulating as deeply as possible for from a few seconds to 4 minutes. The same spot on the opposite side of the body is then given the same treatment for the same amount of time. Trigger points are believed to be caused by injury to the muscle. The original injury heals, leaving behind a sensitive spot, a sort of muscular memory. Physical or mental stress activates the spot, causing pain. Holding steady pressure while counting to twenty, and repeating on the opposite side of the body, appears to relax the tenseness and relieve the pain. It is worth trying, since it is free of any harm and can be done at any time, at any place.

What is hypnosis?

Hypnosis is usually defined as intensive concentration, a state in which the person is open to suggestions on which he will then or later act, often without realizing why. It is total concentration on a thought or object so that the hypnotized person is out of touch with the world. There is little agreement on what hypnosis is or why or how it accomplishes what it does.

Has hypnosis ever been used to manage cancer pain?

Yes, in several places in the country, hypnosis is being used in an attempt to relieve cancer pain.

Are there any benefits to hypnosis over other kinds of pain management?

Hypnosis seems to offer many benefits and few drawbacks, mainly because hypnosis does not usually have any unpleasant side effects. Some doctors have found that hypnosis is so effective that some patients are able to give up painkilling drugs.

How does hypnosis work on cancer pain?

It depends upon the techniques being used. Hypnosis has been used to block awareness of pain, to substitute another feeling for the pain, to move the pain to a smaller or less significant area of the body, to change the sensation to one that is not painful, and in extreme cases to dissociate the body from the awareness of the patient. Although no one knows exactly how hypnosis works to control real physical pain, there are cancer patients who feel they have been helped by this treatment.

Is hypnosis dangerous?

Hypnosis can be dangerous if it is not being done by a trained professional. A trained hypnotist will not usually attempt to remove pain unless the cause has been fully probed and definitely known, because hypnosis can also succeed in concealing real pain and thus concealing the underlying condition.

Can hypnosis be used with other remedies?

Sometimes it is used alone. In other cases it can be used in combination with other techniques—painkilling drugs, blocks, and biofeedback, for instance.

How many hypnosis sessions are necessary to achieve results in pain control?

Hypnotists maintain that it takes only a few sessions to teach a person to become hypnotized. Thereafter, the person can hypnotize himself when necessary. It is this self-hypnosis that is found to be most useful in pain control.

What is biofeedback?

Biofeedback is a system by which you can monitor the signals coming from the various organs of your body—heart, brain, muscles, stomach, etc. Using electronics, biofeedback tunes in on body functions and transposes them into a visible or audible signal that an individual can actually hear or see so he can be aware of what is going on in his own body. Biofeedback has been shown to be useful in slowing or speeding up heart rates, and in relaxing tense muscles. In learning how to relax muscles which produce tension headaches, for example, patients are hooked up to a machine which picks up the electrical current produced by a muscle when it contracts. The machine converts this signal to a tone which the patient can hear. The person can reduce the tone by relaxing the muscle. With practice he learns to relax his muscles and keep them relaxed and thus eliminates his headaches.

Is biofeedback being used for cancer patients?

Sometimes it is used if the patient cannot take medications or use other pain-reducing techniques. Biofeedback has usually been used in combination with other methods. Certainly if the pain being suffered by the cancer patient is due to causes other than the cancer itself—such as tension headaches or hypertension—then biofeedback can be used to control this kind of pain. It can also be used to lessen tension which might be increasing the patient's pain.

I am a cancer patient and my doctor told me not to take aspirin for any reason, including pain. Why is this?

Aspirin is known to cause bleeding, particularly in patients with gastrointestinal problems. Therefore doctors usually prescribe an acetaminophen such as Tylenol or Datril, instead of aspirin.

I had radiation as part of my treatment. Can I use a heating pad for relieving pain?

No. Patients who have received radiotherapy should not apply heat (whether with a warm cloth or a heating pad) directly on the part of the body that was treated. Radiotherapy can lessen nerve activities and so the body becomes less sensitive to heat and the patient is more susceptible to burns.

When I get a pain, I worry about how long it is going to last. Am I unusual?

No, you certainly are not. It is common for people in pain to worry about whether or not the pain will last. They also are concerned about what is causing it, whether or not it will get worse, and whether or not they will be able to stand it, all of which seems to help intensify the pain.

Are there any ordinary things which can be done to help a person in pain?

Since some people's pain is caused by anxiety, talking can be useful. Good mouth care, a back rub or massage, putting on clean bed linen, offering special foods, giving the person something else to think about such as watching television, doing a crossword puzzle, needlework, model construction, reading a book, listening to music, or talking to friends and relatives on the phone, applying compresses of warm heat to the affected areas can be helpful.

When a person is in bed, little things like changing the angle of the bed, or sometimes just adding an extra pillow, can make a lot of difference. If the person is not in bed, keeping busy is important.

How are electrical signals used to relieve pain?

There are two devices which use painless electrical impulses to control pain: the transcutaneous nerve stimulator and the epidural dorsal-column stimulator. Both work on the theory that nerves can transmit only one sensation at a

time and that there is a gate in the spinal cord through which
messages are sent to the brain. If the nerves are stimulated
artificially, pain impulses apparently cannot get through the
gate.

What is TENS or TNS?

These initials stand for transcutaneous electric nerve stimulation, a technique in which mild electric currents are
applied to selected areas of the skin by a small power pack
connected to two electrodes. The sensation is a buzzing,
tingling, or tapping feeling. It does not feel like a shock.
The small electrical impulses seem to interfere with pain
sensations. The current can be adjusted so that the sensation
is pleasant and relieves the pain. Pain relief lasts after the
current has been turned off.

What is an epidural dorsal-column stimulator?

This is another device for controlling pain by using electrical signals. In the epidural dorsal-column stimulator,
electrodes are implanted surgically over the spinal cord.
They are connected to receivers usually put on the patient's
left side under his arm. When the person feels a small pain,
he connects the antenna to a small transmitting box. This
box is placed over the receiver and the patient turns on the
transmitter. Electrical impulses are sent to the electrodes,
which stimulate the nerves to relieve pain.

Are there any new techniques being used to give pain kill-ers directly to the affected nerves?

Several centers have been experimenting with different
methods of directing pain control medications. They can
be infused directly into the spinal fluid, through a catheter
inserted into the lower spine or into the brain. Because the
drugs go directly to the pain control center, they can be
given in smaller doses than would be necessary if it were
taken intravenously or by mouth. Other centers are implanting catheters to bring the pain medication directly to
the affected areas.

What kind of surgery can be performed for pain control?

There are several surgical procedures which can be used for pain control. They include cordotomy, percutaneous cordotomy, nerve-root clipping, and rhizotomy. However, these operations are performed only after the many other techniques for relieving pain have been tried.

How are these operations usually performed?

The doctor first determines the location of the painful tumor. He then figures out which nerve carries the pain sensations from the area of the tumor to the spinal cord and from there to the brain. When he has found the correct nerve, he performs a delicate neurosurgical operation to destroy the pain-carrying nerve at some point along the path—either before or after it enters the spinal cord. Because the nerve has been cut, it cannot carry sensations to the brain. Therefore, the patient will not feel the pain.

What is a cordotomy?

A cordotomy cuts the precise areas in the spinal cord where bundles of nerves are located. The surgeon removes bone from the spinal column, making a hole in the bony back wall of the spinal-cord tunnel. The operation is performed either under local anesthesia (there will be some pain if it is done in this manner) or under general anesthesia. The surgeon must be careful to clip the pain-nerve bundles without destroying those nerve fibers that control muscle movements.

What is percutaneous cordotomy?

It is a technique for selectively destroying the nerve fibers. The doctor uses an x-ray for guidance. He inserts the tip of a hollow needle directly through the skin into the pain-nerve bundle along the front and side of the spinal cord. The nerve bundle is destroyed by an electric current passed through the needle. The operation is usually performed high in the back of the neck. Local anesthesia is used. Some of the advantages of the percutaneous cordotomy are that it can be performed while the patient is conscious, it has low mortality, and it can be repeated as required.

Does a person sometimes have to have more than one percutaneous cordotomy?

Sometimes, yes. It is not uncommon if the cordotomy was performed on one side to have the pain or the awareness of the pain move to the originally pain-free side. Apparently, the pain on the side where the cordotomy was performed was intense enough to mask pain on the original pain-free side. If this happens, a second cordotomy may be necessary.

Do I have to take any special precautions after having a cordotomy?

You will usually be up and around and able to eat anything you wish after 1 or 2 days. Some patients complain of headaches, but these are usually easily treated with mild medication. Because you will not feel pain or temperature on the side where the cordotomy has been done, you should avoid doing things that might cause burns, scratches, and bruises.

What is rhizotomy?

In performing a rhizotomy the surgeon cuts the pain nerve where it enters the spinal cord. This procedure can eliminate pain—for example, in the arm or leg—but it also leaves the area treated (the arm or leg) without sensation so that it is not usable. A rhizotomy can also be used to relieve abdominal and chest pain, but there may be loss of bladder and bowel control. Chemical rhizotomies are now being performed with alcohol or phenobarbital injected into the spaces around the spinal cord. This type of rhizotomy may relieve pain for a period of time without many of the unpleasant aftereffects of the surgical rhizotomy.

Under what circumstances would a physician use a nerve-root clipping operation?

Nerve-root clipping is usually done for pain problems in the upper part of the body. Nerve roots are clipped high in the neck. Individual head nerves—cranial nerves which lead out from openings in the skull bones—also can be clipped.

What is an ambulatory infusion pump?

This is a device that makes it possible for a patient to have medication, such as continuous morphine infusions, away from the hospital. The pump operates on a 7-day rechargeable power pack. It fits into a pocket so that the patient can receive continuous medicine and ongoing pain relief, while continuing usual activity.

What options do I have if my pain is not relieved and my doctor says nothing more can be done for me?

You can ask for a consultation with a pain specialist. This new field is attracting many qualified professionals—oncologists, anesthesiologists, physicians in other specialties, nurses, and pharmacists. New developments and research in this field have proceeded rapidly in the last few years. An excellent booklet called *Questions and Answers About Pain Control* is available from the Cancer Information Service or the American Cancer Society near you. Many of the larger hospitals now have pain clinics, devoted to helping patients cope with pain. There are many different techniques being used to relieve pain, and many professionals feel that much suffering can be eliminated through the use of proper pain-control techniques. Chapter 23 includes a listing of programs funded by the National Cancer Institute to study pain control.

chapter 22

Living with Cancer

This chapter deals with the many practical aspects as well as with the whole range of emotions which are encountered in living with cancer on a day-to-day basis. It covers a wide range of subjects. Consequently, some of the questions apply to all patients, while some are relevant to only a few, and some are directed to members of the patient's family. You'll find helpful information on nutrition, talking about cancer, and on sexual problems. Since dying is part of living, this chapter deals frankly with that subject and includes information on caring for the patient at home, euthanasia, the hospice movement, dying, death, and autopsies. The information on health insurance and wills should be of interest to the healthy as well as to those who are ill, since they are subjects best considered before the need arises.

What do I do if I feel that the treatment is worse than the disease?

In the midst of treatments, many patients feel this way, and you would be wise to talk through your feelings with your doctor or nurse. Don't discontinue taking your treatments without discussion with your doctor—it is unfair to yourself to do this. He can explain the alternatives to you, and you can then make the decision about how you will proceed.

Why is it important to eat well when a person has cancer?

There are several reasons:

- A balanced diet can help maintain strength, prevent body tissues from breaking down, and rebuild normal tissues which have been affected by the treatments.
- Patients who eat well during treatment periods—especially foods high in protein and calories—are better able to stand the side effects of treatments, whether the treatment is chemotherapy, radiation therapy, immunotherapy, or surgery. It may even be possible for the patient to withstand a higher dose of certain treatments.
- Patients with good eating habits tend to have fewer infections and are often able to be up and about more.
- When a person eats less, for whatever reason, the body uses its own stored-up fat, protein, and other nutrients, such as iron.

What exactly is meant by "eating well"?

"Eating well" means using a variety of foods to provide the vitamins, minerals, protein, and other elements necessary to keep the body working normally. It means

- Having a diet that is high enough in calories to keep up a normal weight.
- Eating foods which are high in protein needed to build and repair the skin, hair, muscles, and organs in the body. People who have had surgery or are ill need extra protein and other nutrients for repair of body tissues. Protein can be used for repair only if the body is also getting enough calories. If it is not, the body will use the protein for energy instead of for repair.
- Eating a mixed diet, including the basic four groups of food: salads, cooked vegetables, raw or cooked fruits; meats, fish, poultry, eggs, or cheese; grains and cereals; milk or other dairy products.

While I am having my treatments, is it a good idea for me to go on the higher-fiber, lower-fat diet recommended by the National Cancer Institute to help prevent cancer?

No. For individuals under treatment for cancer, the highest priority is a diet adequate in calories, protein, and vitamins.

After completing treatment, you may wish to consider modifying your diet in order to lower fat and raise fiber levels. However, there is no evidence at this time that changes in your diet will prevent a *recurrence* of your cancer (for information on cancer prevention, call the Cancer Information Service 1-800-4-CANCER or the American Cancer Society).

Are there any general hints for cancer patients who are having difficulty in eating?

There are a few, including the following:
- Remember that what sounds unappealing today may sound good tomorrow.
- When feeling well, take advantage of it by eating well and by preparing meals which you can freeze for the "down" days. On good days, eat when you feel hungry, even if it is not mealtime. Eat food with good nutritional value, for many nutrients can be stored in your body for later use.
- Talk to your doctors and your health team about your eating problems. Many hospitals and Visiting Nurse Associations have dietitians and nutritionists on their staffs who can help you with these problems. Before you try home remedies, be sure that your problems are not symptoms needing medical attention.
- Take advantage of time-saving foods, such as those which can be prepared as a meal-in-a-dish, with little preparing and cooking. Blenders, food processors, microwave ovens, and toaster ovens save time and effort.
- Make your eating atmosphere pleasant, with an attractively set table, varying the place in your home where you eat, or eating with friends. A glass of wine or beer before meals (with your doctor's approval) helps to relax you and can help to make you hungry.

I am not hungry. Is that a common problem among cancer patients?

This seems to be a common complaint. Loss of appetite (*anorexia*, in medical terms) sometimes is caused by treatments, such as radiation or chemotherapy. But it also happens to people who are not having treatments. No one really knows whether the loss of appetite is due to illness, fatigue, pain, stress, or depression—or to a combination of all of these. Some people's appetites come and go. Others rarely feel hungry. Among patients' complaints are that food doesn't taste right (especially meat), that they have a bitter metal taste in their mouths or on their tongues, and that they simply get full too soon.

My loss of appetite has caused conflict with my family. Is this unusual?

This is a common problem. When attention becomes focused on your diet, other areas of your relationship seem to be affected, too. In our society, food is used to express care and love, so when you are unable to eat, especially food that has been prepared for you by a loved one, the reaction is likely to be disappointment and rejection. In turn, you may feel guilty because you aren't hungry. It's important for everyone to understand the many emotions behind food preparation and eating, and try to work together to help resolve them.

Are there any hints for increasing one's appetite?

Here are several things you can try:
- Eat small meals more often. Keep snacks handy for nibbling. Try eating a good snack before going to bed in addition to your regular meals.
- Mix ice cream with ginger ale or a favorite carbonated beverage. Drink milk shakes. Eat frozen yogurt.
- Tart food may enhance flavors (for people who have no problems with their mouths and throats). Pickles, lemonade, and orange juice may help. Use vinegar and lemon juice for flavorings.
- Add bacon bits, sliced almonds, ham strips, or pieces of onion to vegetables for added flavor and nourishment. Chicken and fish can be added to cream soups for flavor and protein.
- Wine, beer, or mayonnaise added to soups and sauces makes them taste better.
- Marinate meat, chicken, or fish in sweet fruit juices, sweet wines, Italian or French dressing, or sweet-sour sauce for more taste. Use more and stronger seasonings

in your cooking, such as basil, oregano, rosemary, tarragon, lemon juice, or mint.

- If meat doesn't taste right, cook chicken, turkey, or fish instead (choose fish that does not have a strong flavor and cook it on a barbecue, if possible). Use eggs and dairy products as substitutes.
- If you have a strange taste in your mouth, try taking it away by drinking more liquids (water, tea, or ginger ale) or by eating foods which leave their own taste in your mouth (fresh fruit or sugar-free hard candy).
- If you feel you are full when you've only eaten a little, chew your food more slowly to prevent your stomach from becoming too full too quickly, don't drink liquids with your meals (take them 30 to 60 minutes before meals to reduce the volume of material in your stomach), and make sure that the liquids have nutritional content (such as juices, milkshakes, or milk).
- Try to add protein to your foods without increasing the amount of food you eat.

How can I add protein to my food without increasing the amount of food I eat?

- Skim-milk powder adds protein. Try adding 2 tablespoons of dry skim-milk powder to the regular amount of milk in recipes. Add milk powder to hot or cold cereals, scrambled eggs, soups, gravies, ground meat (for patties, meatballs, meatloaf), casserole dishes, desserts, and in baking.
- Use milk or half-and-half instead of water when making soup, cereals, instant cocoa, puddings, and canned soups. Soy formulas may also be used.
- Add diced or ground meat to soups and to casseroles.
- Add grated cheese or chunks of cheese to sauces, vegetables, soups, and casseroles.
- Add peanut butter to butter on hot bread.
- Choose dessert recipes which contain eggs such as sponge cake, angel-food cake, egg custard, bread pudding, or rice pudding.
- Add peanut butter to sauces and use it on crackers, waffles, or celery sticks.

I have trouble eating enough food to keep up my weight. What should I do?

If you are having trouble eating enough food to keep up your weight, you could add some high-fat or high-carbo-hydrate foods to your diet. For instance:

- Spread peanut butter on fruit (such as an apple, banana, or pear) or stuff celery with it. Add it to a sandwich with mayonnaise or cream cheese. Peanut butter is high in both calories and protein.
- Spread honey on toast, use it as a sweetener in coffee or tea, or add it to cereal in the morning.
- Mix butter or margarine into hot foods such as soups, vegetables, mashed potatoes, cooked cereal, and rice. Serve butter on hot bread (more butter is used when it melts into hot bread).
- Use mayonnaise (it has 100 calories per tablespoon, which is about twice as much as salad dressing) in salads, in eggs, or with lettuce on sandwiches.
- Add sour cream and yogurt to vegetables (potatoes, beans, carrots, squash), to gravies, or as a salad dressing for fruit.
- Use sour cream as a dip for fresh vegetables. Scoop it on fresh fruit and add brown sugar for a quick dessert.
- Add whipped cream to pies, fruit, puddings, hot choc-olate, Jell-O, and other desserts (it has 60 calories in a tablespoon).
- Snack with foods such as nuts, dried fruits, candy, pop-corn, crackers and cheese, granola, ice cream, and pop-sicles. Add marshmallows to fruit and to hot chocolate.
- Add powdered coffee creamers to gravy, soup, milk-shakes, and hot cereals. Creamers add calories without volume.
- Bread meat, chicken, or fish before cooking.
- Add raisins, dates or chopped nuts, and brown sugar to hot or cold cereals for a snack.

I am bothered by nausea and vomiting because of my treat-ment. What can I eat to help this problem?

There are several things you can try. You will need to ex-periment to see which ones will work for you. New antinausea drugs are available from your doctor. In addition, relaxation methods such as tension reduction, rhythm, imagery, distraction, biofeedback, and hypnosis are being used to help cope with the discomfort of nausea and vomiting. You may also wish to incorporate some of the following suggestions into your daily eating habits:

- Eat smaller portions of food that is low in fat (be sure to eat more often to make up for your calorie and protein needs if you are eating foods low in fat).
- Take whatever liquids you feel you can handle, such as clear soups, flavored gelatin, carbonated beverages (ginger ale), popsicles, and ice cubes made of any favorite kind of liquid. Sip liquids slowly through a straw.
- Eat dry foods such as toast and crackers, especially soon after getting up in the morning.
- Avoid liquids at mealtimes. Take them 30 to 60 minutes before eating.
- If you have been vomiting, eat salty foods. Don't eat overly sweet ones.
- If the smell of food makes you feel nauseated, let someone else do the cooking while you sit in another room or take a walk. Use prepared foods from the freezer that can be warmed at a low temperature, or eat a meal of food that does not need to be cooked.
- Do not lie down flat for at least 2 hours after eating. You might want to rest after eating, since activity can slow down digestion and increase your discomfort. If you wish to rest, sit down. If you do lie down, make sure your head is at least 4 inches higher than your feet.
- If your problems with nausea or vomiting are severe, talk with your doctor or nurse about it. If you are bloated, have pain, or have a swollen stomach before nausea and vomiting occur (and if these problems are relieved by vomiting), call the doctor.

What are some of the foods which are low in fat?

Foods which are low in fat include:
- Crab, white fish, shrimp, light tuna (packed in water)
- Veal, chicken and turkey breast, and lean cuts of other meats which are braised, roasted, or cooked without adding fats

- Broth-type soups
- Spaghetti with plain sauces
- Fruits and fruit juices, vegetables and vegetable juices
- Hot and cold cereals except granola-type cereals
- Low-fat yogurt, low-fat cottage cheese, 1-percent buttermilk, 1-percent low-fat milk
- Plain bread, soda crackers, pretzels, toast with jelly or honey (no butter)
- Popsicles, sherbet, gelatin ices
- Angel-food cake, Danish pudding and fruit-pie fillings, sauces, junket, pudding, or shakes made with skim milk
- Hard and jelly candies

My mouth and throat are sore, which makes it very hard for me to eat. Do you have any suggestions?

Yes. The linings of the mouth and throat are among the most sensitive areas of the body. Cancer patients, especially those receiving chemotherapy or radiation treatments, often complain of soreness in these areas. There are a few important things to remember:

- If you have sores under your dentures, do not wear dentures when you do not need them for eating.
- Drink lots of fluids and eat well, because part of the healing in these sensitive areas depends upon your having good food and liquids for your body.
- If you have mouth or throat problems, be sure your doctor examines the area to see whether or not you need special medication.
- Make sure you see your dentist for special care of your teeth during this period.
- If your mouth is dry, ask the doctor whether the medicines you are taking are causing the dryness.
- Cold foods can sometimes be soothing. Add ice to milk and milkshakes for extra coldness. Eat ice cream or yogurt and make popsicles with milk or milk substitutes.
- Use gravies and sauces on meats and vegetables. Cook stews and casseroles, adding more liquids to make them softer.
- Cut your meats up in small pieces. Use a blender (cook your food first and then put it in the blender to make it easy to eat).

- Choose soft foods such as mashed potatoes, yogurt, scrambled or poached eggs, egg custards, ricotta cheese, milkshakes, puddings, gelatins, creamy cereals, and macaroni and cheese.
- Stay away from foods that sting or burn such as citrus-fruit juices and tomatoes. Fruits low in acid (bananas, canned pears) and nectars (peach, pear, apricot) are easier to swallow. Use a little sugar to tone down acid or salty foods.
- Soak foods in coffee, tea, milk, cocoa, or warm beverages. Try taking a swallow of liquid with each bite of food.
- Eat food lukewarm or cold rather than hot. Do not use hot spices such as pepper, chili powder, nutmeg, and cloves. Avoid rough or coarse foods such as raw vegetables and bran. Don't eat dry foods like toast or hard bread unless you soak them (they can scratch delicate tissues).
- If you smoke or drink, talk to your doctor about it. Certain alcoholic beverages can irritate your mouth and throat, as does any smoking.
- If your house is heated with dry heat, a humidifier or a steam kettle in the bedroom may help.
- Rinse your mouth whenever you feel you need it—to remove debris, to stimulate your gums, to lubricate your mouth, or to put a fresh taste in your mouth. You can make a mouthwash from 1 teaspoon of salt to 1 quart of water (or 1 teaspoon of baking soda to 1 quart of water). A mixture of equal parts of glycerine and warm water is also effective. Do not use a commercial mouthwash without your doctor's permission. Do not use hot water; let it cool before using. Rinsing with club soda can relieve dry mouth or thick saliva. Oragel, available at the pharmacy, can help deaden the pain.
- Stay away from strong fumes such as cleaning solutions and paints.
- If your problem is severe, talk to your doctor about medicine to numb your gums and tongue. If you need it, artificial saliva is also available.

I feel too tired to eat. What should I do?

Try resting first and then eating later on. Many times you will feel more like eating after you have napped or rested. In addition:

- Rely on meals you have frozen when you felt well or on convenience foods that are easy to prepare.
- If your tired feeling is related to your recovery from surgery or from other treatments and you are gradually building up your strength, start by eating smaller portions of easily digested foods and slowly work back to normal.
- Accept the offers of friends to help you. Tell them what you need. People like to do things for others. Do not be embarrassed to ask for help and to accept and direct your friends' aid.
- If you live alone, you might wish to arrange for "Meals on Wheels" to prepare your meals. Many communities offer this service. Contact your doctor, Visiting Nurse Association, or American Cancer Society for information on this service.
- If you feel tired when you wake up or if you are not sleeping at night, talk with your doctor. Do not take sleeping pills without the doctor's permission.

I have diarrhea. Is this a common problem with cancer patients?

Some patients with some kinds of cancers (such as tumors in the pancreas) and on some kinds of treatment (radiation and chemotherapy) may have problems with diarrhea, excessive gas, or a bloated feeling.

What can I do about these problems?

Here are several suggestions:

- Drink liquids between meals instead of with them. Make sure you drink plenty of liquids, since diarrhea causes you to lose fluids and salts which you must replace.
- Eat smaller amounts of food more often. Eat foods which help control diarrhea, such as applesauce, bananas,

boiled white rice, tapioca, and plain tea. Stay away from fatty foods and foods which are highly spiced.

- Use less fiber (roughage) in your diet. If your intestines are irritated, the normal amount of fiber may be too much for them. Use only cooked fruits and vegetables, omitting those with seeds and tough skins, beans, broccoli, corn, onions, and garlic.
- Potassium, an important element to your body, is lost in great quantities when you have diarrhea. If you are lacking potassium, you can feel very weak. Make sure you eat some foods that are high in potassium but won't worsen the diarrhea, such as bananas, apricot or peach nectar, fish, potatoes, and meat. If you cannot eat these foods, talk to your doctor about taking potassium supplements.
- If you have cramps, stay away from foods that may encourage gas or cramping such as carbonated drinks, beer, beans, cabbage, broccoli, cauliflower, highly spiced foods, too many sweets, and chewing gum.
- Do not skip meals. Try to chew with your mouth closed. Talking while you chew may cause you to swallow too much air, which can cause gassiness or cramps.
- If your diarrhea is persistent or has blood in it or if you start to lose weight, be sure to tell the doctor.

What can I do about constipation?

Constipation can be a problem for people with cancer. It may result from treatment with some drugs. Try the following suggestions one at a time to see what works best for you:

- Make sure your regular diet includes whatever has helped you move your bowels before, such as a variety of fruits and vegetables, breads, cereals, bran, dried fruits (raisins, prunes, or apricots), and nuts to add more fiber. If you cannot chew or swallow these, try grating them or putting them in a blender.
- Drink plenty of liquids (eight or ten glasses each day are needed). You can drink prune juice to stimulate bowel activity.
- Add 1 or 2 tablespoons of bran to your foods to keep you

regular. Try it in cooked cereals, casseroles, eggs, or baked goods, or eat it as a raw cereal.

- Eat high-fiber snack foods such as sesame sticks, date-nut bread, oatmeal cookies, fig newtons, date or raisin bars, granola, prune bread, or corn chips.
- Do some light exercise. Set aside 10 to 20 minutes a day to sit quietly on the commode.
- If you are undergoing treatment, check with the doctor or nurse before taking a laxative or stool softener.

What suggestions do you have if I need to eat soft foods?

- Use tender cuts and ground meat. Use moist-heat cookery such as braising, simmering, and poaching.
- Use only cooked eggs. Make omelets or scrambled, poached, or soft-boiled eggs.
- Choose soft breads, hot or soaked cereals, and cooked grains such as rice or macaroni.
- Use cooked vegetables, removing seeds and tough skins.
- Choose fruits which are well ripened, canned, or cooked. Remove seeds and tough skins.
- Warm meats, vegetables, or potatoes before putting in the blender.
- Cut meat finely. Blend with liquids such as broth or gravy.
- Strain liquid meals if you want to avoid particles.
- Include pancakes, pudding, gelatin, custard, and similar foods which can be served without blending.
- If you need tube or gastrostomy feeding, ask for a consultation with the nutritionist or dietitian at the hospital to determine the contents, method of preparation, and feeding techniques.

How much protein and how many calories do I need?

The needs will differ for each person. However, the following basic facts can help you:

- Protein and calorie needs are greater during illness, treatment, and recovery than in normal times.
- Maintaining your weight is a good indication that you are getting enough calories each day.
- Protein needs are more rigid than calorie needs. There-

fore, your diet should emphasize such protein-rich foods as meat, fish, poultry, milk, cheese, eggs, nuts, and seeds.

- Daily needs for calories and protein for healthy adults (U.S. Recommended Dietary Allowances) are 2,700 calories and 56 grams of protein for men; 2,000 calories and 45 grams of protein for women. During illness, treatment, and recovery, 90 grams of protein for men and 80 grams of protein for women plus an additional 200 to 300 calories are usually recommended.
- You can get simple calorie guides in most department or discount stores, or you can ask the dietary staff at your own hospital for help.
- A copy of a booklet published by the National Cancer Institute, titled *Eating Hints: Recipes and Tips for Better Nutrition During Cancer Treatment*, may be helpful to you. You can get a free copy by calling the Cancer Information Service 1-800-4-CANCER.

Can physical therapy really help to make me feel better?

Whether your disabilities are permanent or only temporary, and whether they are caused by the cancer or its treatment, there is therapy available which can help you to cope with your daily tasks. One of the most common problems is loss of strength or paralysis. It is amazing what simple exercises designed to strengthen muscles or improve balance and coordination can do to help make normal movement return.

What is a physical therapist, and where can I find one to help me?

The role of the physical therapist is to help maintain and increase normal body function, to prevent loss of function where possible, to help teach a patient to substitute when loss occurs, and to help the patient become as independent as possible. Special exercises needed by the patient are determined by testing. Then a plan of activity is prescribed to suit the needs and limitations of the patient. This kind of help can mean the difference between a helpless invalid and someone who is able to care for himself. Physical therapists can be recommended by your doctor or are available through cancer rehabilitation hospital services and visiting nurse associations. There is a listing in the phone book, usually under "Physical Therapists."

I've heard of homemaker services. What do they do?

Homemaker services provide well-trained, adaptable, mature women to help keep the household running. Homemaker service may be available in your area through a community health or welfare agency, a church, a club, or some other organization.

What can visiting nurses do to help?

Visiting nurse associations or city health departments provide part-time nursing help to patients at home and offer advice and guidance to help the family and others in the care of the patient. A visiting nurse will give health instructions and referrals to other agencies that may be of help. You can contact the visiting nurse either directly or through the doctor. If you have health insurance which covers nursing care, the charges (which are adjusted to the patient's ability to pay) may be payable under the policy. Medicare covers some part-time public health nursing in the home. Many public-health nursing organizations use practical nurses, who attend to all general health needs of the patient and work under the direction of the professional nurse.

How can I possibly deal with the idea that I might be dying?

There are no simple answers to that question except to try to put into perspective the whole idea of death and dying. Simplistic as it may sound, everyone is one day closer to dying every day of his life. If at all possible, try to talk about your fears and the possibility of dying. As Orville Kelly, founder of Make Today Count, says: "We don't have to like death, but we don't have to be terrified of it, either." He learned to "live with cancer, not die from it."

What is Make Today Count?

Make Today Count was founded by Orville Kelly, a cancer patient who felt the need for patients and their families to have group support of their problems. An organization was formed and there are now over 100 chapters across the coun-

try. Meetings and workshops are conducted, and a news-
letter is published. The organization's address is MTC, Box
222, Osage Beach, Missouri 65065.

Does the fear that cancer will recur ever disappear?

Usually the fear remains in the back of the mind. This is a
normal reaction—one that is shared by every patient who
has ever had cancer. However, if you learn to face the fact
that you have cancer and know as much as you can about
your own case, you can lay to rest many of these fears in
the knowledge that you have been treated with the best
methods known to date.

What can I do about job discrimination against me as a cancer patient?

If cancer treatment meant leaving your old job, discrimination may be a problem when you are ready to return to
work. From the experiences of cancer patients, we know
that even those who are completely recovered may find it
difficult to become employed. For your own information,
the Rehabilitation Act of 1973, a federal statute, includes
persons who have been treated for cancer among the handicapped, and thus are covered by the Act. You may not think
of yourself as handicapped, but fortunately, the Act does
cover those who have had cancer and need protection in
finding a job. The Act requires firms with contracts or sub-
contracts to the federal government of $50,000 or more, and
with fifty or more employees, to prepare and maintain an
affirmative action program for the handicapped. The Act
makes it illegal to discriminate against a handicapped individual by any entity, regardless of size, if it receives money,
regardless of amount, from the Department of Health and
Human Services. If you apply to a company with government contracts and believe you did not get the job because
of your cancer history, you can file a complaint under Section 503 of the Rehabilitation Act with the Office of Federal
Contract Compliance Programs of the U.S. Department of
Labor. If your complaint is against an agency receiving
money from the Department of Health and Human Services, your complaint falls under the regulations in Section
504 of the Act and should be filed with the Department of

Health and Human Services, Office of Civil Rights. In addition, your local State Department of Labor or Office of Civil Rights can advise you of state statutes prohibiting discrimination against those with a cancer history.

What should I tell relatives, friends, neighbors, and others?

Knowing what to tell others, and how much, is something that each patient or family must come to grips with. Experience indicates that it is better to discuss the subject than to try to hide it. However, the way in which this is done depends upon your own lifestyle—whether you prefer to share your problems with those around you fully or whether you prefer to keep discussions of problems at a low level. In the case of schoolchildren with cancer, it is wise to inform schoolteachers, administrators, and nurses, as they can be most helpful when they understand the situation.

I want to talk about my feelings about my having cancer, but I can't because I'm trying to protect other people's feelings. What can I do?

Cancer is a very stressful disease, and even the most well-adjusted people sometimes need help in dealing with all the complicated feelings that go with it. You might try discussing your problem with your doctor or with the nurses where you are getting treatment. If you would like to become involved in group discussion, the hospital where you are receiving treatment or the American Cancer Society may help by bringing people together and can tell you where support groups are meeting. These groups, offered in many areas to cancer patients and their families, give reassurance that there are many others who are going through what you are going through, others who share your concerns, your anger, and your problems. Some patients and family members have found seeing a psychologist or a social worker helpful.

I notice my friends don't discuss the nature of my illness with me. Should I bring up the subject?

You can help communication with your friends if you initiate the discussion and use the word *cancer* in discussing your illness. Many people are afraid and inhibited at the thought of cancer—and this is misinterpreted by the patient as a lack of empathy and concern at a time when it is most needed. Often a patient wonders if the lack of conversation about his illness means that his family knows something they aren't telling him. It's up to the patient to lead the way in discussing his illness.

Shouldn't children be protected from knowing that a parent has cancer?

It really is best not to try to protect children. You'll find that they intuitively know what is going on anyway. It is frightening and confusing to them not to understand what is happening. Children need support and reassurance that whatever happens, they will continue to live, to be loved, and to grow. Better to tell them as much as they are able to understand and give them a chance to share and help. It is also sometimes helpful to tell a child's teacher when there is serious illness in the family.

Is it normal to feel depressed following cancer surgery?

Yes. It is the most normal reaction in the world. Fear and anger are very normal reactions, and you should allow yourself to express them. Once expressed and understood by those around you, your depression will be easier to deal with. If you can acknowledge and come to terms with your own fear and anger, you should be better able to face your daily life.

I am convinced that my surgery—that is, losing a part of my body—is more difficult for me to accept than having cancer. Am I unusual in feeling this way?

Any loss of a part of the body—even loss of a tooth—is likely to bring about such feelings. Therefore, it's not surprising that the loss of a body part or function may be more devastating than the fear of cancer. It will take time for these feelings to lessen. Awareness of them can be the first step in developing acceptance.

Why do I feel such anger at having cancer that it affects all my relationships?

It's not unusual for deep feelings of anger to surface after cancer diagnosis and treatment. Most people feel some form of anger at having a disease over which they feel they have no control. The feeling of helplessness about the situation, the endless indignities of hospitalization, and the difficulty of treatments all combine to bring about feelings of anger. Your partner as well as others who are close to you often also have feelings of anger. Because there seems to be a close connection between anger and sexual feelings, problems in sexual expression may result. Though anger reactions may be different for each partner and each couple, they often exist and are often repressed. An important part of the healing process is to allow these feelings to be expressed. Once the anger has been confronted, steps can be taken toward understanding and accepting it and the other emotions that are triggered by a cancer diagnosis.

My partner and I have never had any sexual problems before. Why is it that we are suddenly having problems now, when we should be most supportive of each other?

Since 50 percent of the healthy population has sexual problems caused by stress, it's certainly understandable why cancer and cancer treatments may put stress on sexual relationships. In addition, as people age, changes take place in enjoyment and performance as well as in attitudes toward sexuality. These changes may not be noticed until a crisis occurs. Open, honest communication with your partner is essential. Try to be honest about your feelings and concerns.

Why is it that since I've had cancer I find I have little or no sex drive?

The way you feel is quite normal and can be expected to change as stress decreases. Lessening of sex drive can occur during many different stages of the disease: at diagnosis, at various times during treatment, when new treatments need to be undertaken, or when you feel ill. At these times, there is a great need for physical contact, though not necessarily for sexual intercourse. Partners should be aware that the special warmth of a loving touch conveys feelings in a very direct way. Sitting or lying together holding each other, cuddling, a warm hug, a hand squeeze, a kiss on the cheek, gentle stroking of the hair, or a relaxing back rub are all ways of being sexual and fulfilling the need to be physically close. You need to tell your partner how important it is to you to be touched and held even if you do not want to have intercourse. Try not to make your partner guess at your feelings.

My partner is not as creative sexually with me now as before I had cancer. I think my partner fears that cancer may be contagious. Is that true?

There is a great deal of anxiety about sexual transmission of disease, due largely to publicity about herpes and AIDS. However, there is no evidence to show that cancer is contagious. Sexual contact will not cause your partner to "catch" your cancer or to develop cancer of the sexual organs, mouth, hands, or any other body part. Nor will you develop a recurrence or spread of your cancer as a result of having sexual intercourse.

I feel very alone with a body that doesn't respond as it used to. It's as though I'm the only person who ever had this problem, and it's very lonely. Will it ever get better?

The realization that body responses are not the same as before, is a very frightening and lonely feeling. By accepting the lonely and fearful feelings, acknowledging them to someone else, and having your feelings accepted, you begin an important process. Try giving yourself the freedom to explore and perhaps to define what gives you sexual pleasure. You can help bring new closeness by talking about the changes with the people you love. It takes flexibility and deep concern to change attitudes. Examining alternatives is, in itself, an important step.

Why is it so hard to talk to my doctor about intimacy and sexual feelings?

In their book *Sexual Turning Points*, Lorna and Philip Sarrel explain that we tend to be afraid that others will be shocked or embarrassed if we bring up *that* subject when we "should" be concentrating on our health and well-being, as though sex weren't a natural part of well-being. Fortunately, an increasing number of people will respond to direct questions about sexual function without embarrassment or shock. And if you make it a habit to try to have a continuing dialogue with your partner and those who love you, you will be keeping communication lines open so that you can continue to express yourself and your needs.

I tried to talk about my sexuality problems with my doctor, but he avoided answering my questions. To whom can I talk about this?

It's reasonable for you to say to your doctor, "I have concerns about sex. Is this a problem you can help me with, or can you refer me to someone else?" Some doctors are uncomfortable with questions that pertain to personal relationships. It may be tempting to give up when you've been rebuffed, but remember that your concerns are legitimate and that support and information are available.

How do I find a professional sex therapist or counselor?

The professionals most qualified to deal with your sexuality problems include psychiatrists (medical doctors who specialize in mental health), psychologists (people with a Ph.D. or master's degree in psychology), licensed marriage and family therapists, and social workers. Those who specialize in marriage or family counseling usually are best qualified to deal with the kinds of problems you may be experiencing. Those who are most highly trained usually belong to one or more of the following organizations:

- American Association of Sex Educators, Counselors and Therapists
  11 Dupont Circle, Suite 220
  Washington, D.C. 20036
- American Association for Marriage and Family Therapy
  1727 K Street, N.W.
  Washington, D.C. 20006
- American Family Therapy Association
  15 Bond Street
  Great Neck, New York 11021

- National Association of Social Workers
  1425 H Street, N.W.
  Washington, D.C. 20005

If your physician or other health professional or minister cannot make a referral, you can locate members of these organizations by looking in the yellow pages under "Marriage and Family Counseling" or by consulting the American Cancer Society, Cancer Information Service, local Family Service, or United Way agencies, or you may contact the organizations listed above for referrals.

What kinds of questions should I ask the therapist before starting therapy?

You can ask the therapist a number of questions to find out about his or her professional training and counseling techniques. Some questions you might want answered include:

- What is your professional training and degree?
- Have you had training and experience in dealing with sexual problems relating to cancer?
- Do you usually see partners together or as individuals? (It is advisable in dealing with sexual problems if both partners are together when advice is given.)
- How frequently do we meet?
- How long are the sessions?
- What does each session cost?
- Does insurance cover the cost?

What does a sex therapist do?

Usually, a sex therapist wants to hear from both partners about problems and how each partner views them. Just bringing problems into the open and discussing them with a professional can be a big help.

I'm single and interested in socializing with potential partners. How do I deal with telling them about my cancer history?

This is a difficult question with different answers for different people. Much, of course, depends upon your own medical situation. To help you with your perspective, try to think about how you would tell someone about yourself if you had heart disease or diabetes rather than cancer. Usually, dealing honestly and openly is the best policy—which does not mean that you need to discuss your problems with everyone you meet in a casual way. If the subject should naturally arise in the course of conversation, then you can contribute insights from your own personal experience. This is a subject that is often discussed in support groups, and it might be possible for you to find a group in your area with others who have the same concerns as you do.

Being single and having cancer makes me feel more alone than ever. What can I do to fulfill my needs to be touched and held?

It is difficult to be alone during times of stress, and the need to have real contact with others is one that needs to be recognized and fulfilled.

- Reach out to friends, letting them know your needs. Greet them with a warm embrace; encourage friendly warmth.
- Massage can give real relief from depression, anxiety, and pain. Perhaps a friend can give you a simple back rub. Or you might treat yourself to the services of a massage therapist. Check with local YMCAs, health clubs, or beauty salons for names of qualified massage therapists.
- Giving pleasure to yourself, through masturbation, is a possible avenue for some to explore.

It is important, especially in time of crisis, to have the support of friends, neighbors, family, religious or social groups—in short, to rely on others. Cancer support groups can also be helpful to those who are single and feeling the loneliness of illness.

My doctor told me to find "other means of sexual expression," but I am not sure I know what he means. What other means are there besides sexual intercourse?

Genital intercourse is only one way of expressing physical love. People find that using hands, thumbs, fingers, tongues, lips, and mouths can provide exciting and pleasurable alternatives to "normal" intercourse. A visit with a sex therapist may be helpful to both you and your partner to help you understand your particular situation better. There are also helpful books which you can read.

Is masturbation a solution?

If your religious, social, and cultural background permits it, masturbation is a form of sexual activity that can be a satisfactory alternative form of gratification when sexual intercourse is not possible or not desired. Some women have found that mechanical vibrators can be used, either alone by themselves or along with other sexual activities with their partners.

I am in pain most of the time. What can I do to be more comfortable when I wish to have sex?

- Make sure you take your pain medicine before you have intercourse or time your sexual activity to take place during the hours you feel best. (Don't forget that too much pain medication may decrease desire and interfere with ability to achieve an erection.)
- Use relaxation techniques both before and after you have sex; some of these techniques are explained in the booklet *Questions and Answers about Pain Control,* which is available through the Cancer Information Service (1-800-4-CANCER) or the American Cancer Society.
- Try different positions and use pillows to make yourself more comfortable during intercourse.
- Try different, less energetic types of sexual activity, such as massage, or stimulating sex organs by hand or by mouth.

Are there some suggestions that might be helpful to me in understanding the intimate needs of my partner who has cancer?

- Most people who were comfortable with and enjoyed their sexuality before illness can be helped to adjust to sexual problems caused by the illness. Encourage talk about feelings and needs.
- Many patients feel a need for more physical closeness than before. Cuddling, holding hands, sitting very close,

hugging, kissing, feeling loved and being loved, and being comforted and reassured become as important as sexual intercourse.

- Massage can be a satisfying extension of sexuality.
- Try to be aware of what is comfortable for the patient in lovemaking. Remember that you cannot develop any type of cancer through intercourse.
- Careful planning may be necessary for your intimate moments. Take into consideration the patient's emotional as well as physical state. Choose a quiet time when the ill partner is rested and free from symptoms and discomfort.
- People who have been through illness, particularly serious operations and treatments, may need help deciding when and how they can resume sexual activity. If doctors, nurses, or social workers don't bring up the subject, be sure the patient or you ask for help in regaining one of the most important parts of your personal life. There are also good books which can help you.

My partner has told me that he doesn't want to resume intimacy because he knows he is going to die and doesn't want to make it more difficult for me. What can I do?

In dealing with this type of rejection, you should understand that your partner may be trying to shield you and himself from the fear of his illness as well as the fear of being unacceptable, abandoned, or left alone. He needs reassurance. Let him know that you realize he is in a difficult situation and that you understand his feeings, but that you want to continue to be intimate and loving. Help him to realize that there are many ways to be close and maintain the special bond and relationship you have, that you want to be with him as long as you can. Continue to treat him as a functioning, useful, and responsible person and as a partner in your decisions, be they for his emotional needs, health needs, or business or family needs. In this way, you may be able to help lift his despair and make life more meaningful for him.

Is it right for me even to be thinking about sex when my partner has such a serious illness?

Yes, it's perfectly natural and understandable for you to be thinking about sex even though your partner is ill. Serious illness may directly change your partner's sexuality, but the illness does not erase your own sexual needs. Hospitalization and illness may make it very difficult to spend time alone together. You need to seek ways for you and your partner to express sexuality and meet your varying needs, preferences, and desires. Talk together about ways of maintaining sexual intimacy even if sexual intercourse is not possible at times. Don't hesitate to discuss with the doctor when sexual intercourse can be resumed.

I've come to the conclusion that my partner is so ill and in such pain most of the time that sexual intercourse is just not a possibility for us anymore. Is that a reasonable conclusion?

No, it is not. It is important that you do not make such a decision without discussing it with your partner and the doctor. If you have, and it is agreed that this is the outlook, then it is important for you and your partner to talk about using touch and words to continue your relationship. Some people with cancer fear intimacy and sex and are afraid of being engaged in these life-affirming activities. Rather than risking the feelings these changes arouse, some ill people, and those around them, simply withdraw. Contact with other people is a human need. Being close and being held can help allay fears, provide encouragement to endure treatments, and help erase some of the dehumanizing effects of the disease.

I think the doctor is avoiding me because he thinks I'm dying. What do I do about the situation?

You may not be dying at all. You should talk to your doctor quite frankly. Difficult as it may sound, your best bet is to confront your doctor with your feelings. Many physicians, because their training has been in "curing" patients, find it difficult to accept long-term disease. The fact is, however, that there are many treatment alternatives available to you

as a patient, and you should be sure that the doctor understands that you expect to continue to have his support or,
if he is unwilling to give you that kind of care, the support
and care of some other health professional. As a consumer,
you are entitled to personalized care. You are entitled to be
informed about what is happening to you. You have a right
to be included in the decisions affecting your treatment.
You should feel free to be able to talk about your situation
fully and frankly with your doctor. The question is still
"How does one go about confronting a doctor with so basic
a problem?" Perhaps you do not feel you can do this alone.
You could ask someone in your family, someone you trust,
to talk with the doctor alone or in your presence about the
situation. If at all possible, you should try to voice your own
feelings to the doctor. It will help him in understanding
you and will make it easier for him to deliver the kind of
care you expect and deserve.

**As a patient who has a visitor but just doesn't feel like
talking, what can I say?**

Just clue your visitor in on how you're feeling, emotionally
as well as physically. You might say, "It's nice just to have
you sitting there, even though I don't feel much like talking."

**Is it unusual for friends to stop coming to visit when they
think someone is dying of cancer?**

The fact that a person may be dying of cancer seems to have
a profound effect on his relationship with others. The fault
lies with society's uncomfortableness with the whole area
of dying—which has been a taboo subject for so long. Cou-
pled with what has always been thought of as the dread
disease, "cancer," makes it difficult for people to handle
the situation comfortably—and so they just withdraw. Even
doctors and nurses have a difficult time, and this leaves the
patient without the emotional support so desperately
needed. The patient and his family can help the situation
by encouraging people to visit, by letting friends know when
is the best time for a visit, by discussing the illness, and by
letting others share the concern and the needs.

Is it possible for me to choose not to prolong dying?

There is a document called the Living Will which may help. Issued by an organization called Concern for Dying, it reads: "To my family, my physician, my lawyer and all others whom it may concern: Death is as much a reality as birth, growth, maturity and old age—it is the one certainty of life. If the time comes when I can no longer take part in decisions for my own future, let this statement stand as an expression of my wishes and directions, while I am still of sound mind. If at such a time the situation should arise in which there is no reasonable expectation of my recovery from extreme physical or mental disability, I direct that I be allowed to die and not be kept alive by medications, artificial means or 'heroic measures.' I do, however, ask that medication be mercifully administered to me to alleviate suffering even though this may shorten my remaining life. This statement is made after careful consideration and is in accordance with my strong convictions and beliefs. I want the wishes and directions here expressed carried out to the extent permitted by law. Insofar as they are not legally enforceable, I hope that those to whom this Will is addressed will regard themselves as morally bound by these provisions." (The will should be signed, dated, and witnessed by two persons.)

If this reflects your feelings, your family, your close friends, and your regular physician should be informed of this will and be given a copy of it. If the physician is unwilling to comply, another more sympathetic physician should probably be sought. A copy should also be submitted to the hospital to be entered with your charts. Material, including copies of the Living Will, is available from Concern for Dying, 250 West 57th St., New York, N.Y. 10019, telephone, 212-246-6962.

Will I be allowed to make a decision about whether I plan to die at home or in the hospital?

It is important for you to let your feelings be known to your doctor so that he can do everything possible to see that your wishes are followed. For those who prefer to spend their last days at home, some forward-looking hospitals, and the program known as Hospice, have instituted home-care programs, with medical supervision in the home under trained medical staff. Hospice emphasizes the management of pain and other symptoms, providing help for the family as well as the patient. Hospice makes the family the unit of care, centering much of the caring process in the home, and seeks to enable the patient to carry on an alert and pain-free existence. The decision of how your illness will be managed depends on many different factors—but if you feel strongly about your desire to die at home, be certain that you tell your doctor and discuss it with your family so that when the time comes, your wishes can be carried out.

What is the hospice program?

There has been a growing interest in the hospice concept of care in the past decade, as we have come to realize that dying people and their families have needs that differ from those of people with curable disease. Hospices offer care for terminally ill patients and provide supportive services for family members. In a hospice, the primary concern is quality of life, not cure. Hospices stress controlling pain and other symptoms so that the patient can remain as alert and comfortable as possible. There are many kinds of hospice programs. Some offer home care, some provide services in a hospice center, others are located within a hospital or skilled nursing facility—and many offer a combination of these services.

What services do hospices offer?

A key element of hospices is encouraging families to care for a dying person at home whenever possible. Some hospices have buildings where patients may be admitted for short periods of treatment, but home care is the heart of the program. The concept is the management of terminal disease to make it possible for the patient to live at home as long as possible, with the family being involved to the end. Some provide help for the family for a year after the patient dies. Home-care teams, involving doctors, nurses, and social workers as well as volunteers, help in practical ways to make it possible for the whole family to help the dying person really "live" his last days.

What is the National Hospice Organization?

The National Hospice Organization is a specialized home health-care program. The goals of Hospice are to help the terminally ill patient to live as fully as possible, to support the family as the unit of care, to keep the patient at home for as long as appropriate, to educate health professionals and lay people, to supplement rather than duplicate existing services, and to keep costs down. Following the precept that pain is nearly always manageable, its goal is to enable patients to carry on an alert and pain-free existence through the administration of drugs and other types of therapy. Care of the family continues through the period of bereavement. Members of Hospice make regular visits and are on call 24 hours a day, 7 days a week to make house calls on patients.

How can I find out about hospices in my area?

For information on hospices, contact the National Hospice Organization (see Chapter 23). The Cancer Information Service and the American Cancer Society may also be able to guide you to hospices in your area.

Where can I get more information on questions of death and dying?

The whole subject has been covered most beautifully and practically by Elisabeth Kubler-Ross in her books *On Death and Dying, Questions and Answers on Death and Dying,* and *On Children and Death,* all published by Macmillan. The first two are presently available in paperback. We especially recommend *Questions and Answers on Death and Dying,* which consists of the questions most frequently asked of Dr. Kubler-Ross.

As a friend I want to be able to talk freely about cancer. What kinds of needs do cancer patients have that I should understand?

Most people feel first and foremost that they want to maintain control over their situation. In some cases this is difficult—but it is important for family and friends to allow it as much as possible. Further, they need to be able to share with friends and family the feeling of being robbed of the ability to function and of life itself by something which they are unable to control. Try to be sensitive to how your friend is feeling. Try to plan simple outings—visiting a friend, going for a ride, going out to lunch or for an ice cream soda, doing an errand—on those days when your friend feels up to doing these things. Keep in close touch by telephone. Just a quick call at a set time every day, every other day, or once a week lets your friend know you're thinking of him or her.

When someone close to me who has cancer starts to talk about the disease, should I change the subject?

Please try not to. If the person feels he can talk with you about this difficult subject, help to keep that communication going. Be honest about how difficult it is for you to talk about it. But try to give realistic support and reassurance. Help to maintain hope. Don't brush off conversation with a comment like "Don't worry about it" or "Don't be silly, you're not going to die." Help bolster hope by reminding the person that he's not a statistic, that every case is different, that he's responding to this drug and there are others that can be tried in the future—but discuss it. A reminder that hope survives in the thought of being able to go home, get outdoors, or resume old interests and hobbies can be helpful.

Isn't it better if everyone just pretends that the patient isn't dying?

When death is imminent and inevitable, pretending that a patient isn't dying is very difficult both for the patient and for his family and friends. It puts a tremendous burden on the patient, often plunging him into depression. Accepting the fact that the patient is going to die opens the way for the patient to dissipate his loneliness and depression by allowing him to verbalize some of his feelings. Naturally, if stoicism is the family's way of life, they can deal with this in their accustomed ways. But stoicism is not denial, and pretense really does not make it easier for the patient.

Is it normal for me to feel angry that my husband/wife/child has had such a long illness?

This is a perfectly natural response that has nothing to do with your feelings about the person—so don't punish yourself by feeling guilty.

How can I respond or find out if my friend wants to talk about cancer?

Many comments will lead you to an opening where you can ask a question which leads into whatever that friend wants to tell you. Just say, "Do you feel like talking about it?"

Where can I look for information on the different kinds of health services available in my community?

Many communities, even quite small ones, have a directory of health agencies available in the community. Ask at the public library—you'll be amazed to find agencies you never knew existed. Look also in the yellow pages, ask your doctor, call the social services department at your hospital, the Cancer Information Service, the American Cancer Society, or the local visiting nurse association.

What kinds of help are available in the community which might make it possible for me to care for a patient at home?

The American Cancer Society is a good place to turn for information, counseling, transportation help, nursing care, medications, blood, loans of such items as wheelchairs, beds, walkers, bedpans, etc. The United States Department of Health, Education and Welfare and state, city, and county health departments as well as family service agencies can be contacted for advice and guidance. The important thing to remember is that you must let others know you need help—and you must not be shy about asking for it. There are many skilled professionals and volunteers out there who want to be of help, but you have to let them know your needs.

What kind of outside services are needed to care for a patient at home?

Naturally, much depends on the condition of the patient. Often a patient can be cared for at home with little more professional assistance than a periodic visit by a nurse. If the patient is more seriously ill, part- or full-time nursing care may be necessary. If round-the-clock nursing care is performed by registered nurses, the cost can be almost as much as hospital care. Often, a nurse can be retained for a few hours a day or several days a week to give enough care to avoid hospitalization. Many nursing tasks can be performed by licensed practical nurses (LPNs) or nurse's aides. If family members are willing and able to perform bedside duties, an agency-supplied part-time homemaker may be able to relieve the family of domestic duties so that their time can be spent caring for the patient.

What happens if the health-care services don't work out?

No patient or family should feel obligated to continue receiving home health-care services which prove unsatisfactory for any reason. When you hire professional health services, you retain the right to discharge employees whose performance is unsatisfactory. Complaints about services obtained through hospital home-care programs or public agencies should be brought to the sponsoring agency. Complaints about the performance of a private company should be directed to that company's director of consumer affairs.

Where can I get some information about caring for a patient at home?

The American Red Cross offers a course which teaches home-nursing skills as well as first aid. Learning the basics and following the guidance of available health personnel can make it possible for you to care for the patient at home— bringing comfort and peace to convalescence. There is a great deal of helpful written material on the subject of home nursing available either through your library or other resources. One of the most comprehensive is *Home Care*, by Jane Henry Stolten, R.N. (New York: Little, Brown). Inexpensive pamphlets are available through the U.S. Department of Health, Education and Welfare, Washington, D.C. or from your local state, county, and city health departments.

How can I create a restful atmosphere for convalescence?

The best way is to be aware. To someone who is ill, little things can be disturbing—a noisy TV, loud music, heavy footsteps, a rattling window, incessant telephone ringing, constant chattering. Being alert to such patience-triers and resolving them before they become problems can help to make convalescence easier. Turning down the bell sound on the telephone, wearing rubber-soled shoes, and in other small ways giving consideration to the patient's needs can make life easier for everyone.

What suggestions do you have for setting up the sickroom?

- Make sure the room is near a bathroom.
- Give the patient a handbell so you can be called when needed. A small transistorized walkie-talkie set might also be used for this purpose.
- A hospital bed is helpful if the patient will spend much time in bed. A low bed is best for a patient who is able to move from bed. Be sure such a bed is firmly anchored and will not slip when the patient uses it to support himself.
- Mattresses can be protected with a waterproof pad. Placing a drawsheet on the bed under the patient's hips provides added protection. Disposable waterproof bed pads are a great innovation.
- A visitor's chair encourages relaxed visiting.
- A bedside table with space for tissues, drinking water, a radio, extension telephone, and reading and writing material should be provided.
- A good light, firmly attached and within easy reach, is a must.
- A pull-up device can be made to help some patients in rising from bed or in changing position. A strong rope, tied to the end of the bed, knotted at intervals, is very useful.

- Other special items such as bathtub handrails, a commode or a raised seat in the bathroom, bed tables, and such items available at surgical supply houses should be considered.
- Whenever possible, help the patient to enjoy a change of scenery by making it possible for him—through the use of a wheelchair or walker if necessary—to spend part of the day sitting up or resting in the family living room or kitchen, where he can join the rest of the family and not feel so isolated.

What is a normal temperature?

Depending on where the temperature is taken—mouth, rectum, or under the armpit—the temperature varies slightly. When the thermometer is placed under the tongue and held there for 3 minutes with the mouth firmly closed, the normal oral temperature is 98.6° Fahrenheit or 37° Celsius. When taken rectally—and this method is usually used when the patient is having difficulty breathing, is confused, or is a small child—the normal temperature is 99.6° Fahrenheit or 37.5° Celsius. A rectal thermometer has a fat, bulb-like silver tip and should be lubricated before being inserted. An oral thermometer has a long, slender silver tip. Either an oral or a rectal thermometer may be used to take the armpit (axillary) temperature. The silver tip should be placed well inside the armpit and the arm held tight against the body. The thermometer is left in place for ten minutes. Normal armpit (axillary) temperature is 97.6° Fahrenheit or 36° Celsius.

How is a sterile dressing applied?

A sterile dressing is one which is free of germs, and it is used to protect a wound from infection or to absorb a discharge. Usually the doctor or nurse will instruct you in how a dressing should be applied. If medication is to be used, the object which will be used to apply the medication must be sterilized. You can use a spoon, a round-edged silver knife, or a wooden tongue depressor. Sterilize by placing in a pan, completely covered with water, and boiling for 10 minutes. Holding cover in place, drain off water, leaving articles in the covered pan. After removing the soiled dressing, carefully unwrap the sterile dressing, apply medication to the inside of the dressing with the sterile knife, spoon, or wooden blade, and apply dressing to the wound. Be careful not to touch anything but the edges of the dressing (or, better yet, wear sterilized gloves). If you touch any part being placed on the patient's wound, you will contaminate the dressing and it will no longer be sterile.

Is it a good idea to get a hospital bed for use at home?

Hospital beds are a wonderful help and may be purchased or rented (the monthly fee may be covered by your medical insurance or Medicare), or they may be borrowed from the American Cancer Society, visiting nurses, or various voluntary health agencies.

How can I help prevent bedsores?

It is important to change the position of the patient frequently. Pillows of various sizes, both hard and soft, are a help, and it is a good idea to have a variety of them on hand to help make the patient comfortable. Rolled-up pillows can also be used to help keep the weight of bedclothes off the toes, knees, or other parts of the body. Covered cardboard cartons placed under the upper sheet at the foot of the bed to protect the toes or next to the thigh or abdomen will help keep the weight of bedclothes away from the body. Also available are bedpads of real or synthetic sheepskin which form a soft, comfortable surface for the frail patient. Eggcrate mattresses, made of foam with indentations to keep the patient comfortable, may also be used.

What can I do about leg cramps when I'm in bed?

Leg cramps can be a problem when a person must lie in bed for long periods of time. One simple exercise which is effective in relieving leg cramps is pumping the toes. This can be done with the legs extended or with the knees bent. All that is needed is to flex the toes toward the sole of the foot, then straighten them out flat. Doing this regularly, several times a day, can help prevent leg cramps.

What can be done to treat dry mouth?

There are a number of reasons for the dry mouth syndrome. Dry mouth is listed as a side effect of more than 200 medications—including antihistamines and decongestants as well as chemotherapy drugs and radiation. A fluoride-containing mouthwash, preferably one that does not contain alcohol, can be helpful. A homemade sodium borate mouthwash may also be helpful. There are several artificial saliva products, including Saliv-Aid, Moi-Stir, Salivart, and Xero-Lube which are sold in pharmacies. They help with lubrication, though they lack infection-fighting substances and digestive enzymes. If the problem persists, talk to the nurse about it.

How do you give a back rub?

Warm body lotion or alcohol by placing the bottle in a pan of warm water. Then, starting at the patient's neck, move gently with long, firm strokes down to the lower spine and buttocks and up again to the neck. Repeat several times. Circular motions can also be used. Back rubs are a wonderful way to help the patient to relax, and they help to stimulate circulation.

Can I learn how to give a bed bath?

This is one of the techniques which the visiting nurse can teach. Briefly, these are the things to remember:

- Always follow the same order, starting with the eyes, face, neck, and ears. Then proceed to the chest and abdomen, far arm, near arm, hands, far leg, near leg, feet, back, buttocks, genitals. You'll notice that this order is designed to use the cleanest water on the most sensitive areas. Another method used recommends face, arms, and trunk to hips, back, and buttocks, legs, feet, and genitals. Bath water can be changed before the back, buttocks, and genitals are washed. Hands and feet can be washed in the basin. Allow the patient to wash the genitals if he or she is able to do so.
- Prepare washbasin, warm water, washcloths, towels, soap, and toilet articles beforehand. An extra cotton blan-

ket or large bathtowel will be needed to cover the patient
when you remove the gown or pajamas. Expose only the
part of the body to be washed. Place a towel under each
part as you wash it, dry thoroughly, and cover. Remember to support the patient's arms and legs directly under
the joints during the bath.

- Allow the patient to do as much for himself or herself
  as is safely possible.

How do you give a patient a shower?

A shower is less strain on a patient than a tub bath and is
often recommended by the doctor. A shower chair—a small
straight chair on locking wheels—is most useful. Some have
a cut-out seat for easier bathing of genitals. Soap on a string
around the patient's neck is another convenience. A ramp
so that the shower chair can be wheeled into the shower
will help simplify the procedure. Be sure to test the strength,
direction, and temperature of the water before the patient
enters. Aim the spray to reach below shoulder level. Lock
brakes on the shower chair. Never leave the patient alone
in the shower.

What is the best way to help clean the teeth and mouth and to shave a patient?

If the patient needs help in doing these tasks, place a towel
under his or her chin and across the chest and clean the
teeth and gums gently with toothpaste and toothbrush or
large cotton swabs and mouthwash. Have the patient turn
the head to the side and hold the basin snugly under the
chin so he or she can rinse when you have finished. If the
patient wears dentures, they should be put on before attempting to shave. Soften the whiskers by leaving a towel
wrung out in hot water on the face for a few minutes. Stretch
the patient's skin tight at all times to prevent cutting skin.
Shave by stroking upward and returning downward over
the same area.

How can I cope with home-care problems like incontinence and bedsores?

There are numerous ways of dealing with these problems,
which often loom as barriers to providing home care for a

patient. The doctor and visiting nurse will be most helpful in the decision as to how the patient can be handled best. Incontinence is an embarrassment to the patient—and comes often as such a shock that the patient becomes depressed, cries, and even may insist he or she wants to die rather than be a bother. Organizing the changing process so that it is done quickly and simply helps to alleviate guilt feelings. The use of adult toss-away diapers, sanitary napkins, and bed pads can be helpful. In the case of the male patient, a plastic bag, filled with absorbent toweling or tissues, secured to the patient with masking tape can sometimes help solve much of the problem. The visiting nurse can be most helpful in teaching you specific techniques for handling this difficult job.

How can I keep track of the medicines that need to be taken?

It is a good idea to keep a daily written record of the type and amount of medicine and the time it was given, along with a record of the patient's temperature and pulse, etc., as recommended by the doctor—especially when more than one person is helping care for the patient. Remember that you must give only the medicines prescribed by the physician at the times and in the amounts specified. One helpful idea for pills is to set out the amount needed for the day when the first pill is taken. This makes it easy to check to see that all medications are taken each day. There are also compartmentalized plastic containers available at pharmacies and by mail order for this purpose.

What do the abbreviations mean on prescriptions?

The typical prescription gives the dosage strength in milligrams (mg), usually notes the type of medicine such as capsule or tablet, how many times a day it should be taken, and how much of the medicine you can get from the prescription. How many times the prescription can be refilled is also noted on the prescription blank. Some of the terms commonly used include:
- a.c. (ante cibos): before meals
- ad lib. (ad libitum): at pleasure, at discretion; take drug freely as needed

- d. (die): day
- dur. dolor (durante dolor): while the pain lasts
- g: gram
- h. (hora): hour
- h.d. or h.s. (hora somni): at bedtime
- mg: milligrams
- omn. hor. *or* omn. noct.: every hour or every night
- p.c. (post cibos): after meals
- p.o. (per os): by mouth
- p.r.n. (pro re note): whenever necessary
- q. (quaque): every
- q.2h. (quaque 2 hora): every 2 hours (number in middle changes)
- q.d. (quaque die): every day

What is parenteral feeding?

This form of feeding is used for patients who, as a consequence of surgical or radiation treatment, are unable to eat normally or patients who need to build up their bodies nutritionally before surgery, chemotherapy, or radiation treatments. A hollow plastic tube is inserted surgically into a central vein. The parenteral fluids—a mixture of amino acids, fat, sugar, vitamins, and other essential nutrients—are slowly infused into the tube by means of a small pump which the patient operates. It takes 10 to 14 hours to infuse a full day's nourishment, but the patient can usually rest or sleep while the food is being injected. Any patient who requires long-term parenteral feeding and who does not otherwise require being in a hospital can be cared for at home.

Is it possible to arrange for intravenous therapy at home?

Many visiting nurse associations and other nursing services across the country now have programs which provide intravenous therapy to patients at home. The home intravenous treatment, which covers the nursing charge plus the cost of medication and equipment, which is usually provided by the hospital, costs an average of $50 to $80 a day, compared with $200 to $400 a day for a hospital stay. The nurses' association will train patients and their families to administer the medication themselves, but nurses are available for visits as needed on a 24-hour-a-day basis.

What should I tell the doctor when I call him to report a change in the patient's condition?

Always start by giving your name and the patient's name, address, and telephone number. Explain that you are calling because of changes in the patient's condition. Before calling, write down all the pertinent information, such as:

- What has happened to prompt you to call the doctor—heavy breathing, weak pulse, rise in temperature, etc.
- The time when the changes took place and how the patient's condition has changed

If you want the doctor to visit the patient, be sure to say so. Listen carefully and write down any instructions you are given.

Should I feel guilty about not being able to care for my child/parent/spouse at the end?

Many people who have been able to take part in care during the course of the illness find it impossible to cope with the final stages of the illness. This is a very painful time, and each family must find its own answers. If the patient is hospitalized, arrangements can usually be made for some member of the family to stay at the hospital, helping as much or as little as he or she chooses.

How can the patient be helped to die in comfort?

When it is determined that the patient is dying and there is no reasonable hope that he will recover, the family and his doctor can make plans to help the patient die comfortably. Either at home or in the hospital, all testing and transfusions, etc., can cease. This means that temperature no longer needs to be taken at the usual intervals, and the measuring of intake and output and the obtaining of blood samples can all be curtailed so that the patient will not be disturbed. Glucose and water can be given intravenously if the patient cannot eat or drink and complains of thirst. Morphine, or whatever drugs are most effective, should be prescribed to be given continuously to relieve pain. Oxygen may be used if there is shortness of breath. A catheter can be inserted in the bladder for comfort. The important thing for everyone to keep in mind is that any measures that are taken should be only for the purpose of maintaining the patient's comfort.

What kind of care must be given to the dying patient?

Being with the patient as much as possible is the most important consideration. Remember that even if the patient does not seem to be able to hear what is happening, his awareness may be very acute. The patient may want to talk about dying, and those close to the patient can help him to do so. He may be in physical distress and frightened, restless, gasping for breath, and disoriented. Keep the patient warm. Most important, keep the mouth moist. Special oiled swabs which can be used to remove mucus from inside the mouth and which help keep the mouth and lips moist are most helpful. Placing the patient on his side helps drain mucus from mouth and nose. Every effort must be made to reduce irritating conditions, and provide an atmosphere that is peaceful and comfortable.

What can the family do when the hospital wants to continue to prolong life but the patient and his family do not want heroic measures used?

This is not an uncommon situation—and it is a difficult one for the patient, family, doctor, and hospital. The hospital is geared to prolonging life, and health-care personnel often find it difficult to deal with death. Ideally, the question should be discussed with the doctor early in the illness so that he understands the family's viewpoint from the outset. But ideal conditions do not always prevail and the doctor's views may not always coincide with the feelings of the family and his patient. Several avenues can be considered. Asking for a consultation with another doctor is a possibility. The patient can be transferred to another facility—or, better still, brought home. Though it may be frightening to think of caring for the patient at home, most families are able to handle the patient very well in the home with the support of some outside help—such as the visiting nurses and an understanding physician.

What is the final stage in the life of most cancer patients?

Every case is different, so there is no certainty regarding the pattern the disease will follow. Most cancer patients die of something other than cancer itself. If there is extensive involvement of cancer with various body systems, a great strain is placed on the heart and respiratory system. The patient often lapses into a coma or intermittent unconsciousness. It is at this time that decisions regarding life-prolonging measures must be made—and they should be made in accordance with the patient's wishes if they have been made known. When it is no longer possible to communicate with the patient, it is the patient's known feelings and the family's wishes that will help to guide the physician to what course must be taken: whether to continue to keep the patient alive (and this can be done, these days, almost indefinitely, if that is desired) or to allow the patient to die naturally.

What are the specific signs of impending death?

People in the health-care field who see death almost every day tell us that although many people think of death as being a traumatic time for the patient, in reality, most people die very peacefully, in their sleep or while at rest. The signs of death will vary from patient to patient. It is very important to note changes in the patient's normal status. Some of the significant changes to be aware of include:

- Marked changes in breathing: labored, spasmodic heavy breathing, followed by quiet or shallow breathing or a decreased number of breaths per minute (sometimes referred to as Cheyne-Stokes respiration)
- Heartbeat rate either faster or slower than usual
- Change in skin texture and temperature; though the patient feels cold to the touch, he may perspire profusely
- Lapsing in and out of consciousness, being confused, or going into a coma
- Loss of sensation, power of motion, and/or reflexes first in legs, then in arms
- A tendency to turn the head toward the light as a result of failing sight and hearing

When the patient dies, be sure the body is laid flat on the back with one pillow under the head. Close the eyes and mouth. If necessary, clean the patient. Put any dentures or artificial parts in place. Fold the hands on the chest.

Why are autopsies necessary after someone has suffered so much?

This final examination, made so the physician may see the effects of the disease and gather new information for use in the future, is sometimes requested. By comparing clinical findings, treatment for others with the same disease may be improved in the future.

The medical profession treats an autopsy as a surgical procedure with full respect of the individual.

My husband's/child's/parent's illness was so prolonged that I felt only relief when the end came, and this makes me feel so guilty.

When the illness is prolonged, often the grieving process is completed before the actual death. It is not uncommon for the family to feel relief that the pain, suffering, and uncertainty have ended. Some people may misinterpret this acceptance and think that you are hard-hearted and unfeeling. You must not feel guilty, for this has been found to be a perfectly normal reaction. People experience grief in different ways, and often the deepest grief is felt by those who do not show grief outwardly.

I'd like to make a contribution in memory of a friend who died of cancer. How can I do this?

There are several ways. The American Cancer Society, listed in the white pages of the telephone directory, accepts contributions to their programs. You can send contributions to the oncology department of your local hospital or to one of the cancer centers listed in Chapter 23. Hospice, St. Jude's, and other such organizations accept contributions in the name of someone who has died of cancer. Be certain that you include with your contribution the name of the deceased, the name and address of the person to whom you wish the acknowledgment sent, and your own name and address.

Do you have suggestions on ways I can express my sympathy?

Most of us say, "If there's anything I can do, let me know"—and feel terribly helpless and disappointed if our friends do not ask for help. Better to look for an immediate need and try to fill it—helping with baby sitting, or providing food, being there when needed, taking charge of some routine task such as telephoning those who need to be notified, quietly returning the rented hospital bed or wheelchair, meeting an incoming train or plane, offering a spare room to an overnight visitor, or providing transportation for necessary errands. When bringing food, it is wisest to use a container that can be discarded. If you bring food in your own dish, be sure to mark your name on the bottom, and stop by to pick up the dish so the family won't have to think about returning it. A little note with a personal reference, recalling some special quality you will remember about the deceased, or referring to some event that was shared, makes it easier to write something meaningful and comforting. The important time to be aware is after the funeral is over and all the relatives have departed. Stay in touch, suggest an outing, include your friend in your family plans, and help your friend to get involved in outside activities.

Types of Health Insurance

KIND OF POLICY	COVERAGE
Hospital	Covers costs during hospital stays as a result of illness or accident. Policies usually include payment in whole or part for room, drugs, general nursing, operating and recovery room, laboratory tests.
Surgical	Covers whole or partial cost of operation. Preset schedule of allowable fees.
Medical	Covers doctor's services other than surgery, such as home, office, and hospital visits. Check to see if this covers diagnostic examination and checkups.

Types of Health Insurance

KIND OF POLICY	COVERAGE
Major medical	Covers major illness and accidents. Usually a deductible amount before payment starts. Covers hospital, surgical, drug, and medical. Usually there is a maximum amount. Some pay 75 to 80 percent of covered expenses.
Medicare, Plan A	Covers inpatient hospital care, skilled-nursing-facility care, part-time skilled nursing care at home. Not covered: prescription drugs.
Medicare, Plan B	Covers x-ray treatments, lab services, services of physician, emergency-room and clinic services, physical therapy, lab and diagnostic tests, x-ray, radiology, rental or purchase of medical equipment, ambulance services. Not covered: prescription drugs.
HMO	Health Maintenance Organization. Covers almost all costs of doctors, hospitals, lab services, tests and treatments. Patient is limited to use of those physicians and facilities involved in the particular HMO.

Items to Check on Your Policy

ITEM OR FEATURE	COMMENTS
Number of days of hospitalization	The very least should be 30 days. Many have special provisions for over 90 days.
Outpatient services	Check carefully, since vital cancer treatments such as chemotherapy and radiation are usually given on an outpatient basis.
In-hospital services	Check to see if nursing care, anesthesia, x-rays, laboratory tests, drugs, CT scans, etc., are covered.
Home health benefits	Check to see if your plan offers some payment for services of homemakers and visiting nurses.

Items to Check on Your Policy

ITEM OR FEATURE	COMMENTS
Deductibles	Often the first $100, $500, or $1,000 may not be covered. *Often policies with the higher deductible figures give better long-range coverage.* For long illnesses, such as some cancer illnesses, this type gives better protection, since it gives long-range help.
Who is covered	Check especially if you have stepchildren or foster children, or expect more children.
Retirement benefits	Check limitations relating to age or place of employment. Can benefits be converted from group to individual policy upon termination or retirement?
Cancellation	Under what terms can the policy be canceled? Check to be sure you will be covered even if health deteriorates or you have severe or repeated need for treatment.
Maximums or benefit limits	Check to see what the maximum figure refers to. Is it paid in full for each illness or all illnesses in the course of a year? Is it paid only once in the life of the policy?
Preexisting conditions	If there is an exclusion against coverage of preexisting conditions, it should never go back longer than 1 year.
Waiting period	In buying a new policy, check to see if there is a waiting period longer than 30 or 60 days during which new illnesses will not be covered. You should know this in making your plans. The shorter the waiting period, the better.
Guaranteed renewable	This means that the policy stays in effect up to a specified age as long as the premium is paid promptly. The premium rate cannot be raised for any one individual but only for all policyholders with the same type of benefits.
Noncancellable—guaranteed renewable	This is the safest type. It cannot be canceled, and the premium rate cannot be changed.

Questions to Ask About Your Heath/Surgical/Medical Insurance

- What kind of hospital room will my insurance allow?
- What percentage of daily rate is paid?
- How many days are covered? (It can vary from 30 days to a year.)
- What is the current cost of a hospital room in my locality?
- What is the current cost of a nurse for one shift?
- What is the current cost of a doctor's visit—office, hospital, home?
- What in-hospital procedures are covered? General nursing care? Anesthesia? Operating room? X-rays? Laboratory tests? Drugs? Surgical supplies? Doctors' fees? Radiation therapy? Chemotherapy?
- Is there a limitation on the amount paid for these hospital services?
- Is there a deductible toward hospital expenses before benefits start?
- What provisions exist for renewing the policy?
- What exclusions or limitations are contained in the policy?
- Are surgical fees paid by the insurance in line with surgeons' fees in my community?
- What kind of limitations are placed on surgical fees?
- Is hospitalization for diagnostic purposes covered?
- How much does the policy pay for each time my doctor visits me in the hospital?
- How many visits are allowed per confinement?
- How much is allowed for a house call or office visit?
- Is there a deductible, either a dollar amount or number of visits not covered before benefits start?
- Is there a waiting period before any conditions are covered?
- What is the maximum lifetime amount my policy will pay?
- What maximum yearly amount per family member will the policy pay?
- How much must I pay before insurance benefits start (deductible amount)?

- Is there a deductible for each claim for a different illness or injury?
- Is the deductible on a calendar-year basis with one deductible in a given year charged against total bills? Or is it on a per-illness basis?
- What percent of the total cost above the deductible does the policy pay?
- Is the policy renewable?
- What top benefit limits, if any, exist for such expenses as hospital room and board, surgery, consultations, treatments?

Questions to Ask About Your Disability Insurance

- Is there a waiting period before benefits begin?
- Does the waiting period vary depending on whether sickness or an accident is involved?
- How is total disability defined?
- Are there any benefits for partial disability?
- What is the amount of weekly or monthly benefits? (Between 50 and 75 percent of gross income should be covered.)
- How long do regular payments continue?
- Are lifetime payments available?
- What provisions exist for renewing the policy?

General Questions to Ask About Insurance?

- Can benefits be converted from group to individual policy?
- What benefits will be continued after retirement?
- Can the policy be changed or canceled?

What types of health insurance are available?

Sometimes several types are combined in one policy, such as hospital/surgical and medical. *Hospital insurance* pays certain costs during hospital stays. *Surgical insurance* covers whole or partial cost of operations within a schedule of allowable fees. *Medical insurance* covers the doctors' services such as home, office, and hospital visits. *Major-medical insurance* usually covers expenses above an established deductible amount with a maximum limit. *Disability or loss-of-income insurance* pays monthly income benefits to offset the loss of income because of total disability resulting from an accident or sickness.

Medicare, Part A, covers most of the hospital costs for those 65 and over. *Medicare, Part B,* is similar to a major-medical plan, paying 80 percent of doctors' bills, plus extras such as outpatient hospital services, home health services, and medical supplies.

Where can I get information about the types of health policies available?

The Health Insurance Institute (277 Park Avenue, New York, N.Y. 10017) has information available to help guide you in purchasing your health-insurance policies. Your place of business has information on the group insurances available to you. If you are not eligible for group insurance or wish to seek insurance in addition to the group plan, you should contact an insurance agent for information about the various policies available. Be sure that he is a licensed representative of the company issuing the policy or a reputable insurance broker in the community. You might also check out your library for a copy of *Best's Insurance Reports* or *Timesaver for Health Insurance*, published by the National Underwriter Co.·

Is there some way I can check out my health insurance company?

Yes. The leading authority on the financial strength of insurance companies is the rating it receives in *Best's Insurance Reports*. Copies of this report are sometimes available in the reference room of the public library.

Is there some way I can compare health insurances?

Since there is no standard of comparison, comparing health insurances is not an easy job. However, one comparison that can be made is by looking at the loss ratios of different companies. This can be tricky, because different policies within the same company may have different loss ratios. However, it is a starting point. The loss ratio is the percentage of premiums which a company pays back to its policyholders in benefits. A high loss ratio means a good value for the buyer. For instance, a company which returns 60 percent of its premiums to its policyholders gives a better value than one which returns only 30 percent. Some companies return as much as 95 percent. Some Blue Cross/Blue Shield groups return better than 100 percent. Others return as low as 30 percent. Steer clear of any company which returns less than 50 percent. Check *Best's Insurance Reports* for ratings. *Timesaver for Health Insurance*, available through the National Underwriter Co. (420 East Fourth Street, Cincinnati, Ohio 45202), lists descriptions of various policies.

If I have the opportunity to get group insurance, should I take it?

Group insurance is usually offered by employers, labor unions, professional organizations or other groupings of people (such as those offered by AAA's or other organizations). These policies, because of the large number of persons covered and the subsequent pooling of risks, will usually have lower premiums than individual policies. In addition, the employer or group policyholder often pays part or all of the premium. Individuals are eligible for protection regardless of physical condition. For these reasons group insurance is usually desirable.

Are individual policies better than group policies?

Health policies written individually represent the poorest form of health-care financing. They should be considered only as carefully planned supplements to group coverage or as last-resort attempts to gain some security when nothing else is available. Most individual and family hospital and surgical policies available are totally inadequate in terms of modern price tags. If you are not eligible for a group policy, your best bet is probably the Blue Cross and Blue Shield policies, which are recognized by most hospitals and generally offer better benefits than individual policies.

Do all health policies cost the same for the same kind of protection?

No, they do not. Nor are the benefits for all policies the same. If you're not in a group and must buy an individual policy, the coverage, value, and claims practices vary widely from company to company. First, consider Blue Cross and Blue Shield. Almost every state has a Blue Cross and Blue Shield plan, and most provide comprehensive benefits at a fair value. Since they are nonprofit companies, normally more of the dollars they receive in premiums are returned to the policyholder in benefits. The cost of the total package, however, is high. If you can't afford Blue Cross and Blue Shield premiums, then look at other health policies. The premiums charged will usually be lower, but so will the benefits. Check them carefully against the questions list so that you know exactly what is being provided.

I always get Medicare and Medicaid mixed up. What is the difference.

Medicare is the federally sponsored program for people who are 62 and over. Medicaid is a public assistance program for people of all ages; it is run by the state and pays hospital bills and doctors' fees and covers additional services as well. Benefits for Medicare are the same in all states. Those for Medicaid vary from state to state.

What is Medicare?

Medicare is the health-insurance program of the federal government provided through Social Security or Railroad Retirement for people 62 and older and some people under 65 who are disabled. The program is available in two parts— A and B. Benefits automatically go into effect when you reach age 65, though it is wise to apply to your Social Security office for your Medicare card a few months before you reach 65 to be sure you are covered.

What does regular Medicare cover?

Medicare Hospital Insurance, Part A, covers room and board in a semiprivate room, nursing care, supplies and equipment, x-ray, radiology, operating room, drugs, medical supplies, and lab tests. The patient assumes a portion of the bill as a deductible. In addition, the patient may be eligible for limited care in a skilled nursing facility or convalescent home which is a participant of Medicare. Medicare may also cover care at home and visits of part-time public-health skilled nursing caregivers—including physical, occupational, or speech therapists or skilled home health aides. It is important to know that further coverage, known as Medical Insurance, Part B, is available.

What do Medicare Supplementary Benefits (Part B) cover?

This part of Medicare insurance, known as Medical Insurance, Part B, is available to all those age 65 and over and to some people under 65 who are disabled. However, you must apply for these benefits and agree to pay part of the premium cost, which is deducted from your Social Security payments. Under this plan, a portion of the medical bills must be paid by the patient. Thereafter, Medicare will assume 80 percent of the allowable charge. Covered items include medical and surgical services of physician, in hospital, nursing home, office, clinic, or patient's home. They include radiology and pathology costs as well as services prescribed by the physician in connection with his diagnosis or treatment. X-ray treatments, lab services, and physician's services in a convalescent home are also covered. Additionally, emergency-room and clinic services, physical therapy, lab tests, diagnostic tests, x-rays, radiology services, surgical dressings and casts, and rental or purchase of medical equipment such as oxygen, wheelchairs, prosthetic devices to replace internal organs, and colostomy equipment are covered. Medicare will also help pay for transportation by an approved ambulance service to a hospital or skilled nursing facility if used to avoid endangering the patient's health.

What is Medicaid?

Medicaid is a federally sponsored plan which is administered by the states—and therefore each state sets its own rules for eligibility and coverage. Contact your city or county government Social Services office for information on eligibility. Medicaid in some states helps with hospital bills and bills for inpatient physician services when those costs exceed 25 percent of annual net income. Medicaid also may cover the following: recipients of old-age assistance, persons with income or resources sufficient to meet general living expenses but not enough to meet the cost of medical care, those receiving Medicare but whose medical needs are not fully met under that program, recipients of aid to the disabled and blind, and persons under 21 whose resources are insufficient to meet the cost of medical care. Those receiving Medicare benefits can check with their local Medicaid or Social Security offices to see if they are eligible.

Is insurance to supplement the Medicare A and B plans available?

Yes. Some companies offer plans with an annual premium based on age, sex, and number in the family. Most of these are guaranteed renewable and offer hospital payments. These are in addition to the Medicare benefits.

If I have Medicare do I need any other insurance?

As good as Medicare is, it was never meant to cover all the health-care expenses of older people. Medicare, Plan B, helps to cover major-medical expenses. However, with Medicare, as with most health insurance, there are deductible amounts and percentages of charges for various services which you must pay before you become eligible for payment. Whatever type of basic health insurance you have—Medicare or other—adding some supplemental protection can be a wise idea. Some companies offer a special Medicare supplement insurance. Some Blue Cross/Blue Shield companies have a "65-Special" which will fill most of the gaps in Medicare A and Medicare B.

What Social Security disability benefits are available?

Workers who become disabled before they are 65 as well as certain family members may be eligible for income benefits under Social Security starting with the seventh full month of disability. Persons disabled in childhood who continue disabled are covered, as are disabled widows, dependent widowers, and disabled surviving divorced wives. Claims for benefits are made by contacting the local Social Security office.

Is cancer insurance available?

Cancer insurance, as a supplement to existing health insurance, is available in most states. Many of the benefits offered are similar to those available through a hospital, surgical, or major-medical plan which also covers the family in other medical emergencies and usually gives more economical coverage. The prospective buyer is asked to sign a pledge that he does not have cancer and never had it before being accepted. Payments are made in addition to claims paid by basic health insurance. Some of the policies specifically state that they do not cover diagnostic x-ray and laboratory examinations. Most insurance experts feel that good general medical and surgical policies are a better investment than specialized cancer insurance.

How can I be sure I'm getting all the benefits to which I am entitled?

Take the time to read through your insurance policies. Check to see that you have the necessary insurance forms. Keep all your medical bills and information together in one spot. Accept the help of a friend who has some knowledge of insurance or hire a tax accountant to go over your bills with you to be certain you are getting all the benefits available to you. The social service department of your hospital can also be helpful.

Are mail-order policies a good buy?

As with every other type of product, there are good and poor buys in mail-order policies, but in every case you should check the company and the policy carefully before buying. The buyer should bear in mind that any omission of pertinent health information will be held against him when he tries to collect. At claim time, some companies have been known to find some preexisting condition to justify nonpayment of claims. Furthermore, the benefits in many of the mail-order health-insurance policies are based on the number of days you spend hospitalized. Usually they are advertised as having a maximum payment of $400, $800, or $1,000 a month. The payment is usually a cash payment made directly to you. $1,000 a month breaks down to $33.33 a day—far less than daily hospital costs and far less coverage than most people need. The average hospital stay is usually 8 days, and 14 days for people over 65. As you can well understand, this type of policy is a very inadequate one as a basic protection plan, but might be a useful supplement.

What is an HMO (Health Maintenance Organization)?

HMOs are medical supermarkets in which a group of doctors join together to provide almost all your health-care needs. Instead of operating on a fee-for-service basis, the way most doctors and hospitals do, they work on a prepaid basis, much as an insurance company does. You pay one premium, and your coverage includes most of your medical expenses. Since the doctors' incomes are fixed in advance, their incentive is to keep you healthy and out of the hospital to keep costs down. They emphasize preventive medicine—keeping you well rather than treating you after you are sick. You are limited in using the doctors and institutions covered by the HMO you have joined. More and more doctors are joining HMO groups. It is important for you to research the HMO you are considering before you join. Be sure you understand which physicians will be involved in your care, the policy on second opinions and any restrictions before you make your decision.

Do health-insurance companies ever turn down claims?

Indeed they do. The most standardized policy provisions are subject to widely different interpretations from company to company. If you have a complaint or feel you have been treated unfairly by your insurance company, agent, or broker, be sure to report it to your state insurance department. Send a copy of your letter to your state representative or senator.

Do I have to pay state sales taxes for medical devices?

In some states, sales tax is not charged on such items as ostomy equipment, mastectomy prosthesis and bra, braces, supports, artificial electrolarynx and batteries, crutches, wheelchairs, oxygen, etc. Be sure to check your local laws so that you will know whether or not you are eligible for these deductions.

How can I possibly keep track of all the bills?

Bills and insurance forms are part of all our lives—but they are especially important when they involve hospitalization and medications. It is helpful from the start to keep all of your medical records in one spot, so that they are available to you or to your accountant when tax time rolls around. Keep a running record—just a sheet of paper will do—with date, check number, who the bill is from, total charge, and any other information such as how much was reimbursed by the insurance company. Records of mileage driven (or cab fares paid) to appointments, treatments, hospitals, and pharmacies should all be kept.

Whom can I turn to for help in solving my financial problems due to prolonged cancer treatment?

The social service department of your hospital should be able to give you advice about financial help which is available in your locality. The American Cancer Society also offers financial counseling in many parts of the country as well as information about local programs.

The drugs I am taking for cancer are so expensive. Is there any program that can help me pay for them?

Check your insurance coverage carefully. If you have a major-medical policy, check to see if it pays for chemotherapy drugs and medicines dispensed by a licensed pharmacist or given in a doctor's office.

Can the American Cancer Society or the Leukemia Society provide financial help?

The ability of these organizations to provide financial help in any great amount is limited—and such aid may be determined by a means test. However, these organizations may be able to help provide transportation to and from treatment centers, baby-sitting services, and special equipment and dressings for home care. If you get in touch with them early in your illness, they can sometimes intervene in your behalf in the area of doctor and medical bills. Don't wait to call them for help. Have someone talk with them while you are still in the hospital so they can help investigate financial help possibilities before the bills begin to come in. Do not expect these organizations to call you; privacy laws do not allow them to initiate calls to people who have been diagnosed.

What other local organizations can I contact for help?

Services are sometimes available from the Red Cross, Salvation Army, labor unions to which any family member belongs, churches, and fraternal or social organizations. In time of need, do not hesitate to reach out for help. These organizations exist to perform many services. Be sure to contact them and let them know you need help.

What help is available through the Veterans Administration hospital or state veteran's hospitals?

Bonafide veterans of the United States services are eligible to receive full benefits from the various veterans hospitals across the country. Hospital care may be authorized for the veteran if Veterans Administration or state veterans hospital facilities are unavailable or if conditions warrant admission to another hospital.

Are there any special places to turn for help in rehabilitation?

Yes. Many states have a department of vocational rehabilitation or department of health which provides assistance for the rehabilitation of cancer patients, including prostheses and ambulatory training. It may even help pay for college education of recovering cancer patients.

What sorts of specialized organizations are available?

Reach to Recovery programs are available in most states for mastectomy patients. Candlelighters organizations have been formed to help families of children stricken with cancer. Ostomy patients can turn to the Ostomy Association, and laryngectomees have the support of New Voice Clubs. Many American Cancer Society units are also running self-help groups for cancer patients and their families. The American Cancer Society or the Cancer Information Office in your locality can give you the names and phone numbers of local chapters for these organizations (see Chapter 23).

Should I be thinking about writing a will?

Everyone should have a will, and this is probably as good a time as any to think about it. You would be wise to consider having a lawyer draw one up for you. A lawyer can help you with all the intricacies of your own special situation. If you do not have a lawyer, you can find one by checking the yellow pages for "Attorneys" or "Lawyer Referral Services." Lawyer Referral Services is run by bar associations in many cities and counties and allows lawyers to register, often indicating whether they specialize in wills, divorce, criminal law, etc. For a small set fee, you may have an initial office consultation to review your problem, discuss fees, and determine whether you will choose him as your lawyer. If Lawyer Referral Services is not listed in your phone book, you can write to the American Bar Association (1155 East 60th Street, Chicago, Ill. 60637) for a free copy of the *Directory of Lawyer Referral Services*. If your will is a simple one, it can be drawn up for between $50 and $100—sometimes less. If you wish, you can call the lawyer, outline the sort of will you feel you need, explaining your property worth, and ask about the charge for such a will. Of course, the more complicated your situation, the higher the cost.

Can I write my own will?

If there are any complicated trust or tax situations, this can be risky. However, in every state, you can buy a standard will form from a stationery store.

Many people have a legally drawn up will and a handwritten will for their personal possessions. Some states will accept an unwitnessed will in the form of a letter or note written entirely in your own handwriting. However, most states require at least two witnesses, while some require three.

How can I make arrangements to donate my body?

A uniform anatomical gift act or similar law has been passed in all fifty states. Persons can become donors by signing a card in the presence of two witnesses. The card allows the person to specify what donation is desired. He may contribute any needed organs or parts, restrict donation to certain organs or parts, or give the entire body for anatomical study. More information can be obtained by writing to Living Bank, P.O. Box 6725, Houston, Texas 77005 or by calling 713-528-2971.

chapter 23

Where to Get Help

Although the information given in this chapter is as up to date as possible, the fields of cancer research and treatment are dynamic and constantly changing. You should expect to find that some of your inquiries will be routed to different organizations or individuals, and you should not limit your investigations to the organizations listed here.

Where is the best place to start to get help?

There are two major sources of information: the Cancer Information Service, which is supported by the National Cancer Institute, and the American Cancer Society.

What is the Cancer Information Service?

The Cancer Information Service (CIS) is a nationwide telephone service with funding in some areas by the National Cancer Institute. A trained staff answers (or will find answers) to questions for the general public (in layman's language) and for health professionals. The staff can give you information on causes of cancer, how to help prevent it, methods of detection, how cancer is diagnosed, ways of treatment, rehabilitation assistance, medical facilities, home-care assistance programs, financial aids, emotional counseling services, and patient referrals. It can provide support, understanding, and rapid access to the latest information on cancer and local resources. It can tell you where in the country investigational treatment is being conducted, and what hospitals and doctors in your area are involved in which kinds of investigational treatment. If, for instance, your relative lives in a different part of the country, the staff can get information on treatment available for you. In many places, the Cancer Information offices are affiliated with comprehensive cancer centers (specialized research and treatment centers recognized by the National Cancer Institute) and the American Cancer Society.

What kind of questions should I ask when I call the Cancer Information Service?

The more specific you can be with your questions, the better the information you will receive. It is wise to think through what you want to know and to write down the questions you want to have answered before you call. You can call as many times as you wish. You do not have to give your name if you do not want to. All calls are kept confidential.

Can the Cancer Information Service send me written information about cancer?

The Cancer Information Offices are supplied with a wealth of printed information about cancer. All of them have brochures which are supplied by the National Cancer Institute. Some also have available brochures from the American Cancer Society. The material will be sent to you free of charge.

How can I call the Cancer Information Service?

By dialing an easy-to-remember number: 1-800-4-CANCER (1-800-422-6237). The Cancer Information Service covers the entire United States. Based on the area code from which you are dialing, you will be connected to the regional center which covers your area. There are three areas of the country which do not share the 1-800-4-CANCER number. They are Hawaii, 808-524-1234; Washington, D.C., 202-636-5700; and Alaska, 1-800-638-6070.

Can I call the Cancer Information Service at any time?

In the majority of offices, service is on a 9:00 A.M. to 4:30 P.M. basis. After regular hours, until 9:00 P.M. Eastern

Time, and on Saturdays, callers are routed to the central office at the National Cancer Institute.

Can the Cancer Information Service tell me where different kinds of investigational treatments are available in the United States? Overseas?

Yes, the Cancer Information Service has information on the investigational treatments being conducted in the cancer centers and community hospitals around the country and overseas.

What is PDQ?

PDQ, Physician Data Query, is a computerized service of the National Cancer Institute which informs doctors of the latest and best treatments for cancer patients. It provides the latest information on the state-of-the-art treatment for each type and stage of cancer. It also gives information on more than 1,000 active treatment studies under way in the country, as well as access to a directory of 10,000 doctors who devote a major portion of their practices to treating cancer and 2,000 institutions which have organized programs for cancer. The doctor can "look up" the latest information by simply dialing up the database from a home, hospital, or office computer.

How can a cancer patient get the same kind of information that is available to doctors through PDQ?

Because the information available from PDQ is written in medical language and needs interpretation, the database itself is not available to the public. However, by calling the Cancer Information Service's 1-800-4-CANCER number, you can get the latest information on cancer treatment. Trained counselors use many information resources, including PDQ, to help patients and have many different kinds of materials which can be sent to callers, including information on the latest treatments, investigational studies, and physicians who are caring for cancer patients.

What is the American Cancer Society?

The American Cancer Society (ACS), a voluntary organization of some 2.5 million Americans, is a national organization fighting cancer through research, education, and patient service and rehabilitation programs. It is composed of a national society with 58 chartered divisions and nearly 3,000 local units. The national society administers programs of research, medical grants, and clinical fellowships and is charged with carrying out public and professional education at the national level. The divisions are in all states, in addition to six metropolitan areas, the District of Columbia, and Puerto Rico. The units are organized to cover the counties in the United States. Some units have branches which cover smaller geographic areas.

What kind of help can I get through the American Cancer Society?

The units of the American Cancer Society conduct basic service programs, including information and counseling service for the cancer patient and the patient's family (information and guidance concerning ACS services, community health services, and other resources), equipment loans (sickroom supplies and special comfort items to assist in caring for the homebound patient, such as hospital beds, walkers, aspirators, blenders, bedpans, urinals, pressure pillows, incontinence pads, and wheelchairs, etc.), surgical dressings prepared by volunteers, and transportation to and from a doctor's office, clinic, or hospital for treatment. Some units also provide home health care, blood programs, assistance with employment problems, social-work assistance, and medications. Rehabilitation programs, primarily directed toward laryngectomy, mastectomy, and ostomy patients, are an important part of the service offered. These include Lost Cord clubs, Reach to Recovery volunteers, ostomy clubs, and Candlelighters, as well as support groups for patients and their families.

How can I reach the American Cancer Society?

You can reach local units in most areas of the country by telephone. Look in the white pages under "American Cancer Society." Ask for the person in charge of patient services. The American Cancer Society can also answer many questions by telephone and offers printed material on cancer free of charge.

Will I have to visit the offices of the American Cancer Society in order to get help?

It depends upon what you are looking for. If you want counseling help or are looking for guidance in finding resources for financial aid, you will probably need to visit the office to discuss your problems. If you are looking for loan equipment, you will have to make arrangements to pick it up. If you have a simple question, it will probably be answered immediately on the phone. Your first step in all cases, however, is to make a telephone call.

What is the mailing address for the American Cancer Society?

The address for the national office is American Cancer Society, 90 Park Avenue, New York, New York 10016. The addresses for the divisions are as follows:

Alabama Division, Inc.
402 Office Park Drive
Suite 300
Birmingham, Alabama 35223
(205) 879-2242

Alaska Division, Inc.
1343 G Street
Anchorage, Alaska 99501
(907) 277-8696

Arizona Division, Inc.
634 West Indian School Road
P.O. Box 33187
Phoenix, Arizona 85067
(602) 234-3266

Arkansas Division, Inc.
5520 West Markham Street
P.O. Box 3822
Little Rock, Arkansas 72203
(501) 664-3480-1-2

California Division, Inc.
1710 Webster Street
P.O. Box 2061
Oakland, California 94604
(415) 893-7900

Colorado Division, Inc.
2255 South Oneida
P.O. Box 24669
Denver, Colorado 80224
(303) 758-2030

Connecticut Division, Inc.
Barnes Park South
14 Village Lane
P.O. Box 410
Wallingford, Connecticut 06492
(203) 265-7161

Delaware Division, Inc.
1708 Lovering Avenue
Suite 202
Wilmington, Delaware 19806
(302) 654-6267

District of Columbia Division, Inc.
Universal Building, South
1825 Connecticut Avenue, N.W.
Washington, D.C. 20009
(202) 483-2600

Florida Division, Inc.
1001 South MacDill Avenue
Tampa, Florida 33609
(813) 253-0541

Georgia Division, Inc.
1422 W. Peachtree Street, N.W.
Atlanta, Georgia 30309
(404) 892-0026

Hawaii Pacific Division, Inc.
Community Services Center
Bldg.
200 North Vineyard Boulevard
Honolulu, Hawaii 96817
(808) 531-1662-3-4-5

Idaho Division, Inc.
1609 Abbs Street
P.O. Box 5386
Boise, Idaho 83705
(208) 343-4609

Illinois Division, Inc.
37 South Wabash Avenue
Chicago, Illinois 60603
(312) 372-0472

Indiana Division, Inc.
9575 N. Valparaiso
Indianapolis, Indiana 46268
(317) 872-4432

Iowa Division, Inc.
Highway #18 West
P.O. Box 980
Mason City, Iowa 50401
(515) 423-0712

Kansas Division, Inc.
3003 Van Buren Street
Topeka, Kansas 66611
(913) 267-0131

Kentucky Division, Inc.
Medical Arts Bldg.
1169 Eastern Parkway
Louisville, Kentucky 40217
(502) 459-1867

Louisiana Division, Inc.
Masonic Temple Bldg.
7th Floor
333 St. Charles Avenue
New Orleans, Louisiana 70130
(504) 523-2029

Maine Division, Inc.
Federal and Green Streets
Brunswick, Maine 04011
(207) 729-3339

Maryland Division, Inc.
1840 York Rd., Suite K-M
P.O. Box 544
Timonium, Maryland 21093
(301) 561-4790

Massachusetts Division, Inc.
247 Commonwealth Avenue
Boston, Massachusetts 02116
(617) 267-2650

Michigan Division, Inc.
1205 East Saginaw Street
Lansing, Michigan 48906
(517) 371-2920

Minnesota Division, Inc.
3316 West 66th Street
Minneapolis, Minnesota 55435
(612) 925-2772

Mississippi Division, Inc.
345 North Mart Plaza
Jackson, Mississippi 39206
(601) 362-8874

Missouri Division, Inc.
3322 American Avenue
P.O. Box 1066
Jefferson City, Missouri 65102
(314) 893-4800

Montana Division, Inc.
313 N. 32nd Street
Suite #1
Billings, Montana 59101
(406) 252-7111

Nebraska Division, Inc.
8502 West Center Road
Omaha, Nebraska 68124
(402) 393-5800

Nevada Division, Inc.
1325 East Harmon
Las Vegas, Nevada 89109
(702) 798-6877

New Hampshire Division, Inc.
686 Mast Road
Manchester, New Hampshire
03102
(603) 669-3270

New Jersey Division, Inc.
CN2201, 2600 Route 1
North Brunswick, New Jersey
08902
(201) 297-8000

New Mexico Division, Inc.
5800 Lomas Blvd., N.E.
Albuquerque, New Mexico
87110
(505) 262-2336

New York State Division, Inc.
6725 Lyons Street, P.O. Box 7
East Syracuse, New York 13057
(315) 437-7025

☐ **Long Island Division, Inc.**
145 Pidgeon Hill Road
Huntington Station, New York
11746
(516) 385-9100

☐ **New York City Division, Inc.**
19 West 56th Street
New York, New York 10019
(212) 586-8700

☐ **Queens Division, Inc.**
112-25 Queens Boulevard
Forest Hills, New York 11375
(718) 263-2224

☐ **Westchester Division, Inc.**
901 North Broadway
White Plains, New York 10603
(914) 949-4800

North Carolina Division, Inc.
11 South Boylan Avenue
Suite 221
Raleigh, North Carolina 27603
(919) 834-8463

North Dakota Division, Inc.
Hotel Graver Annex Bldg.
115 Roberts Street
P.O. Box 426
Fargo, North Dakota 58102
(701) 232-1385

Ohio Division, Inc.
1375 Euclid Avenue
Suite 312
Cleveland, Ohio 44115
(216) 771-6700

Oklahoma Division, Inc.
3800 North Cromwell
Oklahoma City, Oklahoma
73112
(405) 946-5000

Oregon Division, Inc.
0330 S.W. Curry
Portland, Oregon 97201
(503) 295-6422

Pennsylvania Division, Inc.
Route 422 & Sipe Avenue
P.O. Box 416
Hershey, Pennsylvania 17033
(717) 533-6144

☐ **Philadelphia Division, Inc.**
1422 Chestnut Street
Philadelphia, Pennsylvania
19102
(215) 665-2900

Puerto Rico Division, Inc.
(Avenue Domenech 273
Hato Rey, P.R.)
GPO Box 6004
San Juan, Puerto Rico 00936
(809) 764-2295

Rhode Island Division, Inc.
400 Main Street
Pawtucket, Rhode Island 02860
(401) 722-8480

South Carolina Division, Inc.
2214 Devine Street
Columbia, South Carolina 29205
(803) 256-0245

South Dakota Division, Inc.
1025 North Minnesota Avenue
Hillcrest Plaza
Sioux Falls, South Dakota 57104
(605) 336-0897

Tennessee Division, Inc.
713 Melpark Drive
Nashville, Tennessee 37204
(615) 383-1710

Texas Division, Inc.
2433 Ridgepoint Drive A
Austin, Texas 78754
(512) 928-2262

Utah Division, Inc.
610 East South Temple
Salt Lake City, Utah 84102
(801) 322-0431

Vermont Division, Inc.
13 Loomis Street, Drawer C
Montpelier, Vermont 05602
(802) 223-2348

Virginia Division, Inc.
4240 Park Place Court
P.O. Box 1547
Glen Allen, Virginia 23060
(804) 270-0142

Washington Division, Inc.
2120 First Avenue North
Seattle, Washington 98109
(206) 283-1152

West Virginia Division, Inc.
Suite 100
240 Capitol Street
Charleston, West Virginia 25301
(304) 344-3611

Wisconsin Division, Inc.
615 North Sherman Avenue
P.O. Box 8370
Madison, Wisconsin 53708
(608) 249-0487

□ **Milwaukee Division, Inc.**
 11401 West Watertown Plank
 Road
 Wauwatosa, Wisconsin 53226
 (414) 453-4500

Wyoming Division, Inc.
Indian Hills Center
506 Shoshoni
Cheyenne, Wyoming 82009
(307) 638-3331

What are other organizations which give direct help to cancer patients and their families?

There are several.

ASSOCIATION FOR BRAIN TUMOR RESEARCH
6232 North Pulaski Road, Suite 200
Chicago, IL 60646
312-286-5571

A voluntary organization which supports research, promotes the understanding of brain tumors and offers printed materials that deal with research and treatment of brain tumors.

CANDLELIGHTERS
2025 I Street, N.W., Suite 1101
Washington, DC 20006
202-659-5136

Organization of parents of young cancer patients. Helps other families of cancer patients cope with living with disease. Regular meetings held to discuss problems and exchange ideas. Nationally, supports programs for cancer research with 225 groups throughout the world. Call the American Cancer Society or the Cancer Information Service to get information about groups in your area.

CANSURMOUNT
90 Park Avenue
New York, NY 10016
212-736-3030

A group that offers patient and family education and support. It tries to match a volunteer who has had cancer with a patient for hospital visits. Local information is available through the American Cancer Society.

CHILDREN'S HOSPICE INTERNATIONAL
501 Slater's Lane, N 207
Alexandria, VA 22314

Non-profit agency that encourages use of hospices and home care programs for children.

CORPORATE ANGEL NETWORK, INC.
Westchester County Airport, Building 1
White Plains, NY 10604
914-328-1313

A service which fills available space on corporate airplanes with cancer patients in need of transportation to treatment centers.

ENCORE
Young Women's Christian Association (YWCA)
Encore Supervisor—National Board
126 Broadway
New York, NY 10003

For postoperative breast-cancer patients. Exercise plan (usually includes some swimming) plus discussion group. Call your local YWCA branch.

HOSPICE
NATIONAL HOSPICE ORGANIZATION
1901 North Fort Meyer Drive, Suite 902
Arlington, VA 22209
703-243-5900

Hospice concept is modeled after St. Christopher's Hospice in England. Can include both home care and inpatient services. Focuses on quality of life, not cure. To be admitted in most cases, patient must be referred by physician, and live in area served by hospice. For

home care, must have a family member, friend, or other helper available on around-the-clock basis. The national organization, established in 1978 to promote and maintain quality hospice care and to
encourage support for patients and family members, can provide information about hospice services in your area.

I CAN COPE
90 Park Avenue
New York, NY 10016
212-736-3030

A course designed to address the educational and psychological needs
of people with cancer. Patterned after a program which was begun
by two nurses in Minnesota, I Can Cope is run locally, usually by
nurses and social workers. Information about local courses is available
through local American Cancer Society units.

INTERNATIONAL ASSOCIATION OF LARYNGECTOMEES (IAL)
90 Park Avenue
New York, NY 10016
212-736-3030

Voluntary organization composed of 190 member clubs. Also called
Lost Cord, Anamilo, or New Voice clubs. Assists people who have
lost their voices as a result of cancer, provides education in skills
needed by laryngectomees, and works toward total rehabilitation of
patient. Maintains registry of postlaryngectomy speech instructors,
publishes educational materials, sponsors meetings and other activities. Sponsored by American Cancer Society. Look in phone book
for local chapter or call local ACS office.

INTERNATIONAL UNION AGAINST CANCER
(UNION INTERNATIONALE CONTRE LE CANCER—UICC)
3 rue du Conseil-General
1205 Geneva
Switzerland
Tel: (41-22) 20 18 11

Nongovernmental, voluntary organization devoted solely to promot-
ing throughout the world the campaign against cancer in its research,
therapeutic, and preventive aspects. Worldwide association with
member organizations in 78 countries. Facilitates exchange of information between national cancer organizations. Publishes, with NCI
support, *International Directory of Specialized Cancer Research and
Treatment Establishments.*

LEUKEMIA SOCIETY OF AMERICA, INC.
733 Third Avenue
New York, NY 10017
212-573-8484

National voluntary health agency which provides supplementary financial assistance to patients with leukemia, the lymphomas, and Hodgkin's disease as well as referral services to other sources of help in the community. Program is administered through society chapters located throughout the United States. Payment can be made for drugs used in care, treatment, and/or control of disease; transfusing of blood; transportation to and from a doctor's office, hospital, or treatment center; and x-ray treatment. There are chapters in Alabama, Arizona, California, Colorado, Connecticut, Delaware, District of Columbia, Florida, Georgia, Illinois, Indiana, Kansas, Kentucky, Louisiana, Maryland, Massachusetts, Minnesota, Missouri, New Jersey, New York, North Carolina, Ohio, Oklahoma, Pennsylvania, Rhode Island, South Carolina, Tennessee, Texas, Virginia, Washington, and Wisconsin. Look in your local directory or write to the address above.

MAKE TODAY COUNT, INC.
P.O. Box 222
Osage Beach, MO 65065
314-348-1619

Provides psychological assistance to patients with advanced cancer and to their families. Helps people live each day as fully and happily as possible. Group meetings, home visit programs, newsletters, and material distribution. Founded by Orville E. Kelly, a cancer patient. About 300 chapters throughout the United States and in several foreign countries. Look in local directory or write to address above.

REACH TO RECOVERY
American Cancer Society
90 Park Avenue
New York, NY 10016
212-736-3030

Offers assistance to breast-cancer patients. Trained volunteers who have had breast cancer lend emotional support and furnish information. In most places, must have physician referral. Look in phone book for number of local American Cancer Society office.

RONALD McDONALD HOUSE
National Coordinator
500 N. Michigan Avenue
Chicago, IL 60614
312-836-7129

Non-profit organizations that offer a home away from home for parents and families of children being treated for a serious illness. Can be found in over 60 cities in the United States and Canada and in Sydney, Australia. Each Ronald McDonald House is different, created by a team of concerned local citizens to meet the needs of their own community. Each House is owned and operated by a local not-for-profit organization comprised of volunteers and is primarily funded by local contributions.

UNITED CANCER COUNCIL, INC.
650 East Carmel Drive, Suite 340
Carmel, IN 46032
317-844-6627

Federation of voluntary agencies that offer service, education and research programs. Composed of 37 affiliated member agencies in 12 states that receive partial support through the United Way. Mastectomy groups, health promotion, loan closets, assistance with services. Some give direct financial assistance.

UNITED OSTOMY ASSOCIATION (UAC)
2001 West Beverly Boulevard
Los Angeles, CA 90057
213-413-5510

Organized and administered by ostomates. Helps ostomy patients return to normal life through mutual aid and moral support. Has over 600 local chapters. Provides information to patients and public and contributes to improvement of ostomy and supplies. Publishes *Ostomy Quarterly* and other educational materials. American Cancer Society also furnishes services to ostomates through its ostomy rehabilitation program. Helps ostomates adjust to everyday experiences of work, travel, and recreation. Offers ostomy therapy training. Call the American Cancer Society for information about local chapters.

Where are camps located which serve children with cancer or their brothers or sisters?

There are many around the country. Among them are:

ARIZONA

CAMP SUNRISE
Contact: Division Director of Medical Affairs, American Cancer Society, PO Box 33187, Phoenix AZ 85067. One week medically staffed program for children 7–15. Funded by the American Cancer Society; transportation provided.

CALIFORNIA

CAMP GOOD TIMES
Contact: Pepper Abrams, 201 N. Carmelina Ave., Los Angeles CA 90049. Two six day sessions for children and young adults 8 and up who are being or have been treated for cancer. Teenagers 15–18 are junior counselors and young adults 19 and older are counselors. Medically staffed.

CAMP OKIZU
Contact: Coral Cotten, Director of Camping, Alameda-Contra Costa Council of Camp Fire, 1201 E. 14th St., Oakland CA 94606.

One week oncology camp for children with cancer, leukemia, or other life-threatening illnesses. Medical supervision; oral medications given.

CAMP REACH FOR THE SKY
Contact: Ann Buckley, S.W., American Cancer Society, 2251 San Diego Ave., Suite B 150, San Diego CA 92110. (619) 299-4200. Five day overnight camp.

CAMP SUMMERSAULT
Contact: John Altman, Long Beach Cancer League of the American Cancer Society, 936 Pine Ave., Long Beach CA 90813 (213) 437-0791. Free day camp for children with cancer.

CAMP SUNBURST
Contact: Geri Brooks, Executive Camp Director, Columbia Pacific Univ. Foundation, 150 Shoreline, Mill Valley CA 94941. (415) 459-1650. Two week summer residential program for chronically ill children 6–16.

COLORADO

SKY HIGH HOPE CAMP
Contact: Nancy King, R.N., Camp Director, 2430 E. Arkansas Ave., Denver CO 80210. One week camp for children 8–17 who have or have had leukemia or cancer.

CONNECTICUT

CAMP RISING SUN (Hemlocks Outdoor Education Center)
Contact: Jane Bemis, American Cancer Society Connecticut Division, Inc., PO Box 410, Wallingford CT 06492 (203) 265-7161. Overnight program for children 6–18. Physician and nurse available.

FLORIDA

R.O.C.K. CAMP (Lake Wales Camp)
Contact: Beverly Deason, Director of Service & Rehabilitation, American Cancer Society Florida Division, 1001 S. MacDill Ave., Tampa FL 33709. (813) 253-0541. Two week overnight camp for children 7–17.

GEORGIA

CAMP SUNSHINE
Contact: CURE, PO Box 1321, Lawrenceville GA 30246. (404) 493-8966. One week

medically staffed camp for Georgia children and adolescents who have or have had leukemia or other forms of cancer.

IDAHO

CAMP BETCHACAN
Contact: Pam Smith, American Cancer Society Idaho Division, Inc., PO Box 5386, Boise ID 83705. (208) 343-4609. Medically staffed camp for children with cancer and siblings.

ILLINOIS

ONE STEP AT A TIME CAMP
Contact: Children's Oncology Services of Illinois, 120 S. Lasalle St., Chicago IL 60603. Two one week sessions for children with cancer from Illinois and Wisconsin.

THE DREAM FACTORY CAMP
Contact: Arthur A.H. Nehring, Director, RR 2, Box 277, Pinckneyville IL 62274. (618) 684-2240. One week overnight camp.

SUMMER SUNRISE (Parkview School, Morton Grove IL)
Contact: Deb Wetherbee, Maine Niles Assoc. of Special Recreation, 7640 Main St., Niles IL 60648. (312) 966-5522. Day camp for children with cancer and siblings 4–10. Oncology nurse on duty.

TLC (Together Through Love and Caring) CAMP
Contact: Nancy Kohl, Lombard Junior Women's Club, Lombard IL 60148. One week day camp for children 5–12 with cancer or leukemia. Staffed by oncology nurses.

INDIANA

THE LITTLE RED DOOR
Contact: Marion County Cancer Society, Inc., c/o United Cancer Council, Inc., 1803 N. Meridian St., Indianapolis IN 46202. One week summer camp for cancer patients 8–18.

IOWA

CAMP AMANDA
Contact: JoAnn Zimmerman, c/o Catholic Council for Social Concern, 700 3rd St., Des

Moines IA 50309. Weekend program for children who lost family member to cancer, other diseases or accidents.

KANSAS

CAMP HOPE
Contact: Norma Meddendorf, MSW, VP for Medical Affairs, American Cancer Society Kansas Division, Inc., 3003 Van Buren, Topeka KS 66611. One week free camp for 50 children. Medically staffed.

KENTUCKY

INDIAN SUMMER CAMP
Contact: Darlo Tanner, 469 Longbranch Rd., Union KY 41091. One week summer program for children 7–17 with leukemia and other forms of cancer. Medical personnel available to administer routine chemotherapy, perform blood counts and handle emergencies.

MICHIGAN

SPECIAL DAYS SUMMER CAMP
Contact: Steve Farris, 1340 Wines Dr., Ann Arbor MI 48103. One week summer camp for children 8–18 with cancer. Winter weekend camp is also held.

MINNESOTA

CAMP COURAGE
Contact: Sandy Miller, 3801 Yates North, Crystal MN 55422. Six day session for pediatric oncology patients 7–13.

MISSOURI

KIWANIS CAMP WYMAN
Contact: Paige S. Vemer, (314) 938-5245. Eleven day summer program for children with cancer. Financial assistance available.

NEW JERSEY

CAMP HAPPY TIMES
Contact: Sy Frankel, Valerie Fund, 40 Somerset St., Plainfield NJ 07060. One week medically staffed camp for children from New York and New Jersey treatment centers.

HAPPINESS IS CAMPING
Contact: Murray Struver, Gramercy Boy's Club, 2169 Grand Concourse, Bronx NY 10453. One week session for children with cancer and leukemia. Medical staff for chemotherapy and blood counts.

NEW MEXICO

CAMP WORLD COLLEGE
Contact: World College, Las Vegas NM 87701.

NEW YORK

BEST (Brothers and Sisters Together)
Contact: Polly Schwensen, S.W., University of Rochester Medical Center, PO Box 650, Rochester NY 14642. Weekend program for siblings 7–17 of children with cancer.

CAMP GOOD DAYS AND SPECIAL TIMES
Contact: Gary Mervis, Director, PO Box 245, Pittsford NY 14534. (716) 427-2650. For children with cancer whose illness is either in remission or under control with oral chemotherapy.

HAPPINESS IS CAMPING
See **NEW JERSEY.**

CAMP OPEN ARMS
Contact: United Cancer Council, 1441 East Ave., Rochester NY 14610. Two week day camp for children with cancer and blood diseases and their siblings or friends.

NORTH CAROLINA

CAMP RAINBOW
Contact: Brenda Martin, Medical Social Worker, East Carolina School of Medicine, Greenville NC 27834. (919) 757-2892. One week medically staffed camp cosponsored by East Carolina School of Medicine Dept. of Pediatrics and Pitt Memorial Hospital Therapeutic Recreation Dept. Free to eastern North Carolina pediatric cancer patients 5–18.

OHIO

CHILDREN'S HOSPITAL HEMATOLOGY CAMP
Contact: Jim Miser, M.D., Children's Hospital, 700 Children's Dr., Columbus OH 43205. One weekend program.

CAMP FRIENDSHIP–CAMP KERN
Contact: Powell R. Zeit, M.D., Director American Cancer Society, Ohio Division, Inc., 1375 Euclid Ave., Rm. 312, Cleveland OH 44115. (216) 771-6700. One week camp.

INDIAN SUMMER CAMP
See **KENTUCKY.**

OKLAHOMA

FUN IN THE SUN & FUN IN THE FALL
Contact: Marianne B. Jost, Ped. Oncology
Social Worker, Oklahoma Children's Memorial Hospital, 940 NE 13th, Oklahoma
City OK 73104. (405) 271-4412. No charge
Friday-Sunday program, limited to children in therapy. Medically staffed.

CAMP WALUHILI
Contact: Peggy Jacks, Camp Director, Camp
Fire, Inc., 5305 E. 41st, Tulsa OK 74135.
Special one week oncology session for children 7 and older. Medically staffed.

OREGON

CAMP GOODTIME
Contact: Oregon Candlelighters, c/o American Cancer Society, Oregon Division, Inc.,
0330 SW Currey St., Portland OR 97201.
Camp on Vashon Island, Washington for
children with cancer 7–15 and their siblings.

PENNSYLVANIA

CAMP CAN-DO
Contact: Kathy Nelson, RN, Children's
Hospital of Pittsburgh, 125 DeSoto St.,
Pittsburgh PA 15213. Co-sponsored by the
American Cancer Society and the Pennsylvania Federation of Women's Clubs for
children 8–14 who have been treated or
who are currently being treated for cancer.
Medically staffed.

CAMP DOST
Contact: Paul Kettlewell, M.D., Geisinger
Medical Center, Danville PA 17822. One
week summer program for cancer patients
8–18. Medically staffed.

**SOUTH
CAROLINA**

CAMP KEMO
Contact: Frances Friedman, Director, Richland Memorial Hospital, 3301 Harden St.,
Columbia SC 29203. (803) 765-7011. One
week overnight camp.

CAMP HAPPY DAYS
Contact: Debby Stephenson, 7821 Dorchester Rd., Charleston SC 29418. (803) 552-2905.

TENNESSEE

CAMP
Contact: East Tennessee Children's Hospital, Knoxville TN. Camp cosponsored by Xerox for children 6–18 from the East Tennessee Children's Hospital Oncology/ Hematology Clinic.

CAMP REMISSION
Contact: Leila Rust, Director of Service, American Cancer Society Tennessee Division, Inc., 713 Melpark Drive, Nashville TN 37204. (615) 383-1710. One week overnight camp.

TEXAS

CANDLELIGHTERS CAMP COURAGEOUS
Contact: PO Box 31146, El Paso TX 79931. Medically staffed camp for children with cancer 7–18. Some financial aid available.

CAMP ESPERANZA
Contact: Sally Francis, Child Life Dept., Children's Medical Center, 1935 Amelia, Dallas TX 75235. Free one week program for children 6–16 who have or have had cancer. Medically staffed.

CAMP PERIWINKLE
Contact: Judy Packler or Elsie McDermott, c/o Research Hematology, Texas Children's Hospital, Houston, TX 77030. Free one week medically staffed camp for children 6–16 currently being treated at Texas Children's Hospital. Transportation provided.

CAMP SANGUINITY
Contact: Ellen North, Camp Director, c/o Cook Children's Hospital, 1212 W. Lancaster Ave., Fort Worth TX 76102.

CAMP STAR TRAILS
Contact: Jan Johnson, University of Texas
M.D. Anderson Hospital and Tumor Institute, 6723 Bertner, Houston TX 77030. (713)
792-2465.

CAMP DISCOVERY
Contact: American Cancer Society, Professional Pediatric Committee, 8214
Wurzbach Rd., San Antonio TX 78229. (512)
696-4211.

UTAH

CAMP KOSTOPULOS
Contact: Miles Shepherd (801) 486-1267 or
Ellen Eckels (801) 322-0431, American
Cancer Society Utah Division, 610 E. South
Temple, Salt Lake City UT 84102. Medi-
cally staffed camp for children with cancer
and their siblings.

VIRGINIA

CAMP FANTASTIC
Contact: Tom Baker, Special Love, Inc., PO
Box 3243, Winchester VA 22601. One week
overnight camp for children with cancer
8–16 from the National Cancer Institute
Pediatric Branch. Counselor in training
program for teenagers over 16. Staffed by
NCI medical personnel.

CAMP HOLIDAY TRAILS
Contact: PO Box 5806, Charlottesville VA
22903. Therapeutic camp for children with
special health needs provides camping experience for children with cancer.

WASHINGTON

CAMP BET 'U CAN
Contact: PO Box 1362, Richland WA 99352
or Jan Oser, Clark County Chairman American Cancer Society (509) 256-8970 or Margaret Graham (509) 423-3230. Medically
staffed camp sponsored by the American
Cancer Society.

CANADA

CAMP MAGIC MOMENTS
Contact: Judy Steen, McDonald's Restaurants of Canada, 20 Eglinton Ave. West,
Toronto, Ontario, Canada, M4R 2E6 (416)
486-4392.

Where in the country are there organizations which grant wishes to chronically or terminally ill children?

The following is a list of those organizations which try to make the wishes of children who are chronically or terminally ill come true:

BRASS RING
SOCIETY, INC.
7020 South Yale Ave.
Suite 103
Tulsa, OK 74103
(918) 496-2838

Helps terminally ill children to see their "impossible dream" come true. Has groups forming across the country.

CAROLINA
SUNSHINE FOR
CHILDREN
PO Box 1803
Columbia, SC 29202

Grants wishes to children with life-threatening illnesses at a time in their lives that it is critical for them and their families.

CHILDREN'S HOPES
& DREAMS FOUNDA-
TION
284 Rt. 46
Dover, NJ 07801
(201) 361-7348

Fulfills dreams of children with life-threatening illnesses. Families included. No boundaries.

A CHILD'S WISH
COME TRUE
PO Box 377
Western Springs, IL
60558
(312) 366-3315 Lori Anthony
(312) 349-7967 Debbie
DeRuntz

Fulfills dreams of terminally ill children.

DREAMS COME
TRUE, INC.
Emory University Clinic
Pediatric Hematology/On-
cology
1365 Clifton Rd., NE
Atlanta, GA 30322
(404) 329-4451

Any child with cancer or a chronic blood disease treated at Emory University Pediatric Clinic. Family included. Dreams submitted by children.

THE DREAM
FACTORY, INC.
PO Box 188
Hopkinsville, KY 42240
(502) 443-2143

Makes wishes come true for children twelve or under who are seriously or terminally ill. Chapters in other states.

FULFILL A DREAM
3653 Presley
Ft. Smith, AR 72903
(501) 783-7559

GRANT A WISH
FOUNDATION
c/o Brian Morrison
Office of Community
Relations
University of MD Baltimore
County
Catonsville, MD 21228

GRANT A WISH
FOUNDATION OF
MASSACHUSETTS, INC.
756 Washington St.
Canton, MA 02021
(617) 828-8248

Grants wishes of terminally ill child, family included.

HIGHHOPES
FOUNDATION
Box 172
North Salem, NH 03073
(603) 898-5333

Helps the families and friends of seriously ill children by funding and facilitating the fulfillment of the last or fondest wishes.

LOLLIPOP
FOUNDATION
PO Box 12453
Overland Park, KS 66212
(816) 421-4980

Provide chronically and terminally ill children in the Greater Kansas City area with gifts which will make their illnesses easier to live with.

MAKE-A-WISH-
FOUNDATION
(National Office)
4601 N. 16th St.,
Suite 206
Phoenix, AZ 85016
(602) 234-0960

Grants wishes to terminally ill children, up to age eighteen. Affiliates in other states. No boundaries.

OPERATION
LIFTOFF
c/o Ernest Bischoff
1171 Kings Ave.
Bensalem, PA 19020
(215) 639-1586

Takes children with terminal illnesses to Disneyworld.

PROJECT TAKE
HEART
Michelle Caropenuto
American Cancer
Society
120 Washington St.
PO Box 2325 R
Morristown, NJ 07960
(201) 538-5336

ROTARY WISHING
WELL
PO Box 43
Redmond, WA 98052
(206) 883-1933

Provides "significant life experiences" for children with life-threatening or chronic illness. Recipients
selected from hospitals serving WA,
OR, ID, MT, AK.

STARLIGHT
FOUNDATION
9021 Melrose Ave.
Suite 206
Los Angeles, CA 90069
(213) 276-6331

Grants wishes to chronically and terminally ill children.

STATE SERTOMA
CLUB
Capitol Station
PO Box 11476
Columbia, SC 29211

Grants wishes to chronically and terminally ill children.

SUNSHINE
FOUNDATION
2842 Normandy Dr.
Philadelphia, PA 19154
(215) 743-2660

Grants wishes to chronically and terminally ill children. Affiliates in other
states.

TEDDI PROJECT
c/o Camp Good Days
PO Box 245
Pittsford, NY 14534
(716) 288-1950

Accepts wishes of terminally or seriously ill children through age eighteen.

A WISH COME TRUE, INC.
PO Box 1067
Webster, MA 01570
(617) 943-1509

Aids terminally and chronically ill children's dreams come true. Has chapters in other states. Has also helped parents who are terminally ill to have their children's wishes fulfilled.

WISH UPON A STAR FOUNDATION
1681 N. Laurel #129
Boise, ID 83706
(208) 322-5141

Deals with smaller wishes (dinner, movies, fair passes, food, etc.) and includes families.

A WISH WITH WINGS, INC.
Pat Skaggs
PO Box 110418
Arlington, TX 76007
(817) 261-8752

Enables catastrophically and terminally ill children to live out a wish they have which would be otherwise financially impossible. No geographic boundaries. Also consultant to help others start groups for wish fulfillment. Will send out information. No obligation and no charge.

What is the National Cancer Institute?

The National Cancer Institute (NCI) is the federal government's principal agency for research on cancer prevention, diagnosis, treatment, and rehabilitation and for dissemination of information for the control of cancer. The Institute is one of eleven research institutes and four divisions that form the National Institutes of Health, located in Bethesda, Maryland. As an agency of the Department of Health and Human Services, the NCI receives annual appropriations from Congress. These funds support cancer research in the Institute's Bethesda headquarters and in about 1,000 laboratories and medical centers throughout the United States. Director of the NCI is Vincent DeVita, M.D. The address is National Cancer Institute, National Institutes of Health, Bethesda, Maryland 20205.

Where are the comprehensive cancer centers located?

There are twenty comprehensive cancer centers designated by the National Cancer Institute. These medical research centers investigate new methods of diagnosis and treatment of cancer patients and provide new scientific knowledge to doctors who are treating cancer patients. They must meet ten specific criteria, which include basic and clinical research and patient care. Comprehensive cancer centers have teams of experts working together on problems of research, teaching, and patient care. They are knowledgeable about the latest developments in cancer treatment.

ALABAMA

Dr. Albert F. LoBuglio
Director, Comprehensive Cancer
  Center
University of Alabama in
  Birmingham
University Station
1824 Sixth Avenue, S., Room 214
Birmingham, AL 35294
205-934-5077

CALIFORNIA

Dr. Brian E. Henderson
Director, Kenneth Norris, Jr.
  Cancer Research Institute
University of Southern California
Comprehensive Cancer Center
P.O. Box 33804
1441 Eastlake Avenue
Los Angeles, CA 90033-0804
213-224-6416

Dr. Richard J. Steckel
Director, Jonsson Comprehensive
  Cancer Center
UCLA Medical Center, Room 10/
  247
Louis Factor Health Sciences
  Building
10833 Le Conte Avenue
Los Angeles, CA 90024
213-825-1532/5268

CONNECTICUT

Dr. Alan C. Sartorelli, Director
Yale University Comprehensive
  Cancer Center, School of
  Medicine
333 Cedar Street, Room WWW
  205
New Haven, CT 06510
203-785-4095

DISTRICT OF COLUMBIA

Georgetown Univ./Howard Univ.
  Comprehensive Cancer Center

Dr. John F. Potter
Director, Vincent T. Lombardi
  Cancer Research Center
Georgetown University
  Medical Center
3800 Reservoir Road, N.W.
Washington, DC 20007
202-625-2042

Dr. Jack E. White, Director
Cancer Research Center
Howard University Hospital
2041 Georgia Avenue, N.W.
Washington, DC 20060
202-636-7697

FLORIDA

Dr. C. Gordon Zubrod, Director
Papanicolaou Comprehensive
  Cancer Center
University of Miami Medical
  School
1475 N.W. 12th Avenue
P.O. Box 016960 (D8-4)
Miami, FL 33101
305-548-4810

ILLINOIS

Illinois Cancer Council (Includes institutions listed and several other health organizations)

Dr. Shirley B. Lansky
Director
Illinois Cancer Council
36 S. Wabash Avenue, Suite 700
Chicago, IL 60603
312-346-9813

Dr. Nathaniel I. Berlin
Director
Northwestern University Cancer Center
Health Sciences Building
303 E. Chicago Avenue
Chicago, IL 60611
312-908-5250/5251/5400

Dr. John E. Ultmann
Director
University of Chicago Cancer Research Center
5841 S. Maryland Avenue
Box 444
Chicago, IL 60637
312-962-6180

MARYLAND

Dr. Albert H. Owens, Jr.
Center Director, Professor of Oncology & Medicine
Johns Hopkins Oncology Center
600 North Wolfe Street, Room 157
Baltimore, MD 21205
301-955-8822

MASSACHUSETTS

Dr. Baruj Benacerraf
President
Dana-Farber Cancer Institute
44 Binney Street
Boston, MA 02115
617-732-3555

MICHIGAN

Dr. Michael J. Brennan
Director, Comprehensive Cancer Center/Metropolitan Detroit
110 East Warren Street
Detroit, MI 48201
313-833-1088

MINNESOTA

Dr. John Kovach, M.D.
Director, Mayo Comprehensive Cancer Center
Mayo Clinic
200 First Street, S.W.
Rochester, MN 55905
507-284-2511

NEW YORK

Dr. Paul Marks
President
Memorial Sloan-Kettering Cancer Center
1275 York Avenue
New York, NY 10021
212-794-6561

Dr. Thomas B. Tomasi
Director
Roswell Park Memorial Institute
666 Elm Street
Buffalo, NY 14263
716-845-5770

Dr. I. Bernard Weinstein
Director
Columbia University Cancer Center
College of Physicians & Surgeons
701 West 168th Street, Room 1208
New York, NY 10032
212-694-3647

NORTH CAROLINA

Dr. William Shingleton
Director, Comprehensive Cancer
 Center
Duke University Medical Center
227 Jones Building, Research
 Drive
P.O. Box 3814
Durham, NC 27710
919-684-2282

OHIO

Dr. David S. Yohn
Director
Ohio State University
 Comprehensive Cancer Center
410 W. 12th Avenue, Suite 302
Columbus, OH 43210
614-422-5022

PENNSYLVANIA

Fox Chase/Univ. of Pennsylvania
 Comprehensive Cancer Center

Dr. John R. Durant
President
Fox Chase Cancer Center
7701 Burholme Avenue
Philadelphia, PA 19111
215-728-2781

Dr. Richard A. Cooper
Director
University of Pennsylvania
 Cancer Center
7 Silverstein Pavilion
3400 Spruce Street
Philadelphia, PA 19104
215-662-3910

TEXAS

Dr. Charles A. LeMaistre
President
University of Texas System Cancer
 Center
M.D. Anderson Hospital & Tumor
 Institute
6723 Bertner Avenue
Houston, TX 77030
713-792-6000

WASHINGTON

Dr. Robert W. Day
Director
Fred Hutchinson Cancer Research
 Center
1124 Columbia Street
Seattle, WA 98104
206-467-4302

WISCONSIN

Dr. Paul P. Carbone
Director
University of Wisconsin Clinical
 Cancer Center
600 Highland Avenue
Madison, WI 53792
608-263-8610

Where are clinical and laboratory cancer centers?

Clinical and laboratory cancer centers are medical
centers which have support from the National Cancer
Institute for programs to investigate promising new
methods of cancer treatment or for research programs.

ARIZONA

Dr. Sydney E. Salmon*
Director, Arizona Cancer Center
University of Arizona
College of Medicine
1501 N. Campbell Avenue, Room
 7925
Tucson, AZ 85724
602-626-6044/7925

CALIFORNIA

Dr. Saul A. Rosenberg*
Director
Northern California Cancer
 Program
1801 Page Mill Road
Building B, Suite 200
P.O. Box 10144
Palo Alto, CA 94303
415-497-7431

Dr. William H. Fishman**
Director, Cancer Research Center
Cancer Research Center
La Jolla Cancer Research
 Foundation
10901 North Torrey Pines Road
La Jolla, CA 92037
619-455-6480

Dr. John Mendelsohn*
Director, UCSD Cancer Center,
 T-010
University of California at San
 Diego
School of Medicine
La Jolla, CA 92093
619-294-6930

Dr. Charles Mittman*
Director, Cancer Research Center
Beckman Research Institute
City of Hope
1450 East Duarte Road
Duarte, CA 91010
818-357-9711, x 2705

*Clinical Cancer Center
**Laboratory Cancer Center

Dr. Walter Eckhart**
Professor and Director
Armand Hammer Center for
 Cancer Biology
Salk Institute
P.O. Box 85800
San Diego, CA 92138
619-453-4100, x 386

Dr. Leroy E. Hood**
Director, Cancer Center
California Institute of Technology
Biology Division 156-29
Pasadena, CA 91125
818-356-4951

HAWAII

Dr. Laurence N. Kolonel*
Acting Director, Cancer Research
 Center of Hawaii
University of Hawaii at Manoa
1236 Lauhala Street
Honolulu, HI 96813
808-548-8415/8416

INDIANA

Dr. D. James Morre**
Director, Cancer Research Center
Purdue University, Stadium Mall
Pharmacy Building, Room 506
West Lafayette, IN 47907
317-494-1388

MAINE

Dr. Barbara H. Sanford**
Director
The Jackson Laboratory
Bar Harbor, ME 04609
207-288-3371, x 206

MASSACHUSETTS

Dr. Thoru Pederson**
Director, Cancer Center
Worcester Foundation for
  Experimental Biology
222 Maple Avenue
Shrewsbury, MA 01545
617-842-8921

Dr. Phillip A. Sharp**
Director
Massachusetts Institute of
  Technology, Room E17-113
77 Massachusetts Avenue
Cambridge, MA 02139
617-253-6401/6421

NEBRASKA

Dr. Edward Bresnick**
Director and Eppley Professor of
  Oncology
Eppley Institute for Research in
  Cancer
University of Nebraska Medical
  Center
42nd and Dewey Avenue
Omaha, NE 68105
402-559-4238

NEW HAMPSHIRE

Dr. O. Ross McIntyre*
Director, Norris Cotton Cancer
  Center
Dartmouth-Hitchcock Medical
  Center
Hanover, NH 03755
603-646-5505

NEW YORK

Dr. James F. Holland*
Chairman, Department of
  Neoplastic Diseases
Mt. Sinai School of Medicine
Fifth Avenue at 100th Street
New York, NY 10029
212-650-6361

Dr. Enrico Mihich**
Director, Grace Cancer Drug
  Center
Roswell Park Memorial Institute
666 Elm Street
Buffalo, NY 14263
716-845-5759

Dr. Harry Eagle*
Director, Cancer Research Center
Albert Einstein College of
  Medicine
Chanin Building, Room 330
1300 Morris Park Avenue
Bronx, NY 10461
212-430-2302
212-792-2233

Dr. Vittorio Defendi*
Director, Cancer Center
New York University Medical
  Center
550 First Avenue
New York, NY 10016
212-340-5349

Dr. Robert A. Cooper, Jr.*
Director
University of Rochester Cancer
  Center
601 Elmwood Avenue, Box 704
Rochester, NY 14642
716-275-4865

Dr. Arthur C. Upton**
Professor and Chairman
Department of Environmental
  Medicine
Director, Institute of
  Environmental Medicine
New York University Medical
  Center
Medical Science Building, Room
  213
550 First Avenue
New York, NY 10016
212-340-5280

*Clinical Cancer Center
**Laboratory Cancer Center

Dr. Ernst L. Wynder**
President and Medical Director
American Health Foundation
320 E. 43rd Street
New York, NY 10017
212-953-1900

NORTH CAROLINA

Dr. Joseph S. Pagano*
Director, Lineberger Cancer
  Research Center
University of North Carolina
School of Medicine at Chapel Hill
  (237H)
Chapel Hill, NC 27514
919-966-3036

Dr. Robert L. Capizzi*
Director, Oncology Research
  Center
Bowman Gray School of Medicine
  of Wake Forest University
300 South Hawthorne Road
Winston-Salem, NC 27103
919-748-4464

OHIO

Dr. Ralph J. Alfidi**
Director of Specialized Cancer
  Research Center
Case Western Reserve University
University Hospitals
MacDonald House, Room
  B006
2074 Abington Road
Cleveland, OH 44106
216-844-3858/3539

PENNSYLVANIA

Dr. C. Max Lang**
Director, Cancer Research
  Center

Pennsylvania State
  University
College of Medicine
P.O. Box 850
Hershey, PA 17033
717-534-8462

Dr. Hilary Koprowski**
Director
Wistar Institute of Anatomy and
  Biology
36th Street at Spruce
Philadelphia, PA 19104
215-898-3703

Dr. Peter N. Magee**
Director
Fels Research Institute
Temple University School
  of Medicine
3420 N. Broad Street
Philadelphia, PA 19140
215-221-4312

RHODE ISLAND

Dr. Paul Calabresi*
Professor, Department of
  Medicine
Brown University
Roger Williams General Hospital
825 Chalkstone Avenue
Providence, RI 02908
401-456-2070

TENNESSEE

Dr. Joseph V. Simone*
Director
St. Jude Children's Research
  Hospital
332 North Lauderdale
Memphis, TN 38101
901-522-0301

*Clinical Cancer Center
**Laboratory Cancer Center

TEXAS

Dr. John J. Costanzi*
Director, UTMB Cancer Center
University of Texas Medical
  Branch
11th at Mechanic
Microbiology Building
Room G.104, Rt J20
Galveston, TX 77550
409-761-2981/1862

VERMONT

Dr. Roger S. Foster, Jr.*
Director, Vermont Regional
  Cancer Center
University of Vermont
1 South Prospect Street
Burlington, VT 05401
802-656-4414

VIRGINIA

Dr. Walter Lawrence, Jr.*
Director, Massey Cancer Center
Medical College of Virginia
Virginia Commonwealth
  University
MCV Station, Box 37
Richmond, VA 23298
804-786-9322/9323/0448

WISCONSIN

Dr. Henry C. Pitot**
Director
McArdle Laboratory for Cancer
  Research
University of Wisconsin
450 N. Randall Avenue
Madison, WI 53706
608-262-2177

*Clinical Cancer Center
**Laboratory Cancer Center

Where are clinical cooperative groups located?

Clinical cooperative groups, which are funded by the National Cancer Institute to investigate promising new methods of cancer treatment, are located in many of the medical institutions in the United States and abroad. Some 4,000 cancer-research physicians in the United States and abroad are involved. Following laboratory research, the treatment under study is evaluated in cancer patients. Clinical cooperative groups are working on anticancer drugs, radiotherapy, immunotherapy, and surgery, alone or in various combinations.

Listed below are the various clinical cooperative groups and institutional projects funded by the National Cancer Institute, with the names and institutions of the chairmen of the groups. Information on the kinds of cancers being studied by these groups is available through PDQ (Physician Data Query) for physicians who wish to enroll patients in a study. If you want to know whether a doctor or an institution in your area is participating in any of the groups, call the Cancer Information Service.

DETERMINANTS OF
RESPONSE IN ACUTE
MYELOCYTIC LEUKEMIA
(AML)
Harvey D. Preisler, M.D.
Roswell Park Memorial Institute
Buffalo, New York

BRAIN TUMOR COOPERATIVE
GROUP
William R. Shapiro, M.D.
Memorial Sloan-Kettering Cancer
Center
New York, New York 10021

CANCER AND LEUKEMIA
GROUP B (CALGB)
Emil Frei III, M.D.
Dana-Farber Cancer Institute
Boston, Massachusetts

CHILDREN'S CANCER STUDY
GROUP (CCSG)
Denman Hammond, M.D.
University of Southern
California
Los Angeles, California

EASTERN COOPERATIVE
ONCOLOGY GROUP (ECOG)
Paul Carbone, M.D.
University of Wisconsin Clinical
Center
Madison, Wisconsin

EUROPEAN ORGANIZATION
FOR RESEARCH ON
TREATMENT OF CANCER
(EORTC)
Maurice J. Staquet, M.D.
rue Heger, Bordet 1
1000 Brussels, Belgium

GYNECOLOGIC ONCOLOGY
GROUP (GOC)
George C. Lewis, Jr., M.D.
American College of Obstetricians
and Gynecologists
Philadelphia, Pennsylvania

LUNG CANCER STUDY
GROUP (LCSG)
E. Carmack Holmes, M.D.
UCLA School of Medicine
Los Angeles, California

PATHOLOGY CENTER FOR
LYMPHOMA CLINICAL
STUDIES
Henry Rappaport, M.D.
City of Hope National Medical
Center
Duarte, California

NATIONAL BLADDER
CANCER COLLABORATIVE
GROUP A (NBCCG)
George R. Prout, M.D.
Massachusetts General
Hospital
Boston, Massachusetts

NATIONAL SURGICAL
ADJUVANT PROJECT FOR
BREAST AND BOWEL
CANCERS (NSAPB)
Bernard Fisher, M.D.
University of Pittsburgh School of
Medicine
Pittsburgh, Pennsylvania

NATIONAL WILMS' TUMOR
STUDY GROUP (NWTSG)
Giulio D'Angio, M.D.
Children's Cancer Research
  Center
Children's Hospital of
  Philadelphia
Philadelphia, Pennsylvania

NORTH CENTRAL CANCER
TREATMENT GROUP
(NCCTG)
Charles Moertel, M.D.
Mayo Clinic Comprehensive
  Cancer Center
Rochester, Minnesota

PEDIATRIC ONCOLOGY
GROUP (POG)
Teresa J. Vietti, M.D.
Washington University
St. Louis, Missouri

RADITATION THERAPY
ONCOLOGY GROUP (RTOG)
Luther W. Brady, M.D.
Hehnemann University
Philadelphia, Pennsylvania

RADIOTHERAPY HODGKINS'
DISEASE GROUP
George B. Hutchinson, M.D.
Harvard University School of
  Public Health
Boston, Massachusetts

INTERGROUP
RHABDOMYOSARCOMA
STUDY
Harold M. Maurer, M.D.
Medical College of Virginia
Richmond, Virginia

SOUTHWEST ONCOLOGY
GROUP (SWOG)
Charles Coltman, Jr., M.D.
Cancer Therapy and Research
  Center
San Antonio, Texas

Are there clinical cooperative groups in Canada and Europe?

There are some groups, both in Canada and Europe, which are studying various treatments, some in collaboration with U.S. scientists, researchers, and doctors. You can get information by calling the Cancer Information Service.

What are community clinical oncology programs?

The National Cancer Institute has funded fifty-eight community clinical oncology programs, known as CCOPs, in thirty-three states across the country at community hospitals or groups of community cancer specialists. The program is designed to combine the expertise of community doctors with ongoing research projects and to introduce the newest clinical research findings into community settings. Qualified community physicians participate in clinical trials by affiliating with treatment study programs at major medical centers and national and regional clinical cooperative groups that conduct large treatment studies. Some CCOPs are located at individual community hospitals, single clinics, or with groups of practicing oncologists. Others are affiliated with consortia of physicians, clinics, and hospitals.

Where are the CCOPs located?

Following is a listing of CCOPs presently funded, along with the hospitals and physicians' offices affiliated with them:

ARIZONA

Phoenix

GREATER PHOENIX CCOP
1010 E. McDowell, Suite 201
Phoenix, AZ 85006
602-239-2413

Hospitals
Good Samaritan Medical Center
John C. Lincoln Hospital and
  Health Center
Maricopa Medical Center
Maryvale Samaritan Hospital
St. Joseph's Hospital and
  Medical Center
Phoenix Children's Hospital

Offices
Internists, Oncologists, Ltd.
Palo Verde Hematology,
  Oncology
Affiliated Medical Specialists, P.C.
Hematology Associates Ltd.
Baranko, Wood & McCallister

ARKANSAS

Little Rock

ARKANSAS ONCOLOGY CLINIC CCOP
500 South University, Suite 401
Little Rock, AR 72205
501-664-3008

Hospital
Arkansas Oncology Clinic

CALIFORNIA

Fresno

SAN JOAQUIN VALLEY CCOP
P.O. Box 1232
Fresno, CA 93715
209-442-6429

Hospitals
Fresno Community Hospital and
    Medical Center, Radiation
    Oncology Department
Veterans Administration
    Hospital
Clovis Community Hospital
Valley Medical Center
Sierra Hospital
Merced Community Hospital

Offices
Nagen Bellare, M.D.
Hematology-Medical Oncology
    Group of Fresno
B. Peck Lau, M.D.
Edward Felix, M.D.
Anthony Cheng, M.D.
Victor Capostagno, M.D.
Medrano & Reinsch, M.D.s
Morgan & Prather, M.D.s
Richard W. Wolk, M.D.
Paul Frye, M.D.
Thomas Glenchur, M.D.
Hoffmann and Hackette, M.D.s
Hanson & Kemp, M.D.s
Michael Maruyama, M.D.
James Sung, M.D.

Bakersfield

Greater Bakersfield Memorial
    Hospital
Kern Medical Center
Mercy Hospital
San Joaquin Community
    Hospital

Rodger Bick, M.D.
Edward P. Fischer, M.D.
Lloyd I. Gillan, M.D.
G. Gordon McCormack, M.D.
Madan Mukhopadhyay, M.D.
William Wilson, M.D.

Los Angeles

GREATER LOS
    ANGELES CCOP
616 South Witmer Street
Los Angeles, CA 90017
213-977-2427

Hospitals
Hospital of the Good
  Samaritan
Los Angeles Orthopedic
  Hospital

**CENTRAL LOS
  ANGELES CCOP**
2131 West Third Street
P.O. Box 57992
Los Angeles, CA 90057
213-484-7086

Hospitals
St. Vincent Medical
  Center

Pasadena

**SAN GABRIEL VALLEY
  CCOP**
100 Congress Street, P.O.
  Box 7013
Pasadena, CA 91105-
  7013
818-440-5186

Hospitals
Community Hospital of
  San Gabriel
Huntington Memorial
  Hospital
Methodist Hospital of
  Southern California
St. Luke's Hospital

Sacramento

KAISER FOUNDATION RESEARCH INSTITUTE
Department of Pediatrics, Station D
2025 Morse Avenue
Sacramento, CA 95825
916-486-6679

Hospitals
David Grant Medical Center
Sacramento Medical Center

Offices
Kaiser-Permanente
  Medical Group

COLORADO

Denver

COLORADO CANCER RESEARCH PROGRAM
1719 E. 19th Avenue
Denver, CO 80218
303-839-7788

Hospitals
Presbyterian/St. Luke's Medical
   Center
St. Joseph's Hospital

CONNECTICUT

Hartford

GREATER HARTFORD CCOP
114 Woodland Street
Hartford, CT 06105
203-548-5474

Hospitals
Hartford Hospital
Mount Sinai Hospital
St. Francis Hospital and
   Medical Center
New Britain General Hospital

New Haven

HOSPITAL OF ST.
   RAPHAEL CCOP
Main 238
1450 Chapel Street
New Haven, CT 06511
203-789-4347

Hospitals
Hospital of St. Raphael

Offices
Hematology-Oncology, P.C.
Medical Oncology and
   Hematology, P.C.
Martin E. Katz, M.D.

FLORIDA

Daytona Beach

HALIFAX HOSPITAL MEDICAL CENTER
P.O. Box 1990
Daytona Beach, FL 32015
904-254-4211, Ext. 3913

Hospitals
Regional Oncology Center
Halifax Hospital Medical Center

Gainesville

FLORIDA PEDIATRIC
CCOP
P.O. Box 13372,
University Station
Gainesville, FL 32604
904-375-6848

Hospitals
All Children's Hospital
Jacksonville Wolfson Children's
Hospital
Orlando Regional Medical
Center
Sacred Heart Children's
Hospital

GEORGIA

Augusta

UNIVERSITY HOSPITAL CCOP
1350 Walton Way
Augusta, GA 30910
404-722-9011

Hospitals
University Hospital
Medical College of Georgia

HAWAII

Honolulu

HAWAII CCOP
320 Ward Avenue, Suite 203
Honolulu, HI 96814
808-536-7702, Ext. 57

Hospitals
Kaiser Foundation
Straub Clinic and Hospital
Kapiolani/Children's Medical
  Center
Kauai Veterans Memorial
  Hospital
Kuakini Medical Center
St. Francis Hospital
The Queen's Medical Center
Tripler Hospital
Maui Memorial Hospital
G. N. Wilcox Memorial Hospital
Castle Memorial Hospital

Offices
Fronk Clinic

ILLINOIS

Chicago

SAINT MARY OF NAZARETH HOSPITAL CENTER
2233 West Division Street
Chicago, IL 60622
312-770-3205

Hospitals
St. Mary of Nazareth Hospital
  Center

Evanston

EVANSTON HOSPITAL
2650 Ridge Avenue
Evanston, IL 60201
312-492-3989

Hospitals
Evanston Hospital Corporation

Peoria

METHODIST MEDICAL CENTER OF ILLINOIS
221 N.E. Glen Oak Avenue
Peoria, IL 61636
309-672-5521

Hospitals
The Methodist Medical Center of
   Illinois

Offices
Oncology/Hematology Associates
Midwest Radiation Therapy
   consultants

Urbana

CARLE CANCER
   CENTER CCOP
602 West University
   Avenue
Urbana, IL 61801
217-337-3010

Hospitals
Carle Clinic Association

IOWA

Des Moines

IOWA ONCOLOGY RESEARCH ASSOCIATION
1048 4th Avenue
Des Moines, IA 50314
515-244-7586

Hospitals
Iowa Methodist Medical Center
Iowa Lutheran Hospital
Mercy Hospital Medical Center
Des Moines General Hospital
Charter Community Hospital

KANSAS

Wichita

WICHITA CCOP
929 N. St. Francis
Box 1358
Wichita, KS 67201
316-268-5784

Hospitals
St. Francis Regional Medical
    Center
St. Joseph Medical Center
Wesley Medical center

LOUISIANA

New Orleans

OCHSNER CLINIC
1514 Jefferson Highway
New Orleans, LA 70121
504-838-3758

Hospitals
Ochsner Clinic and Ochsner
    Foundation Hospital
Baton Rouge Clinic
Hattiesburg Clinic
South Louisiana Medical Center

MAINE

Bangor

EASTERN MAINE MEDICAL CENTER
489 State Street
Bangor, ME 04401
207-945-7481

Hospitals
Eastern Maine Medical Center

Portland

SOUTHERN MAINE
  CCOP
22 Bramhall Street
Portland, ME 04102
207-871-2213

Hospitals
Maine Medical Center
Mid-Maine Medical Center

Offices
Oncology/Hematology
  Associates
Marjorie Boyd, M.D.
Louis Bove, M.D.
Stephen Blattner, M.D.
Eugene Beaupre, M.D.
Joseph Hiebel, M.D.
Thomas Ervin, M.D.

MASSACHUSETTS

Boston

NEW ENGLAND COLLABORATIVE CCOP
185 Pilgrim Road
Boston, MA 02215
617-732-9237

Hospitals
New England Deaconess
  Hospital
St. Luke's Hospital
Wentworth-Douglass Hospital
Frisbie Hospital
Elliot Hospital
Portsmouth Hospital
Symmes Hospital
Choate Hospital
St. Anne's Hospital
Exeter Hospital

MICHIGAN

Grand Rapids

GRAND RAPIDS CCOP
100 Michigan N.E.
Grand Rapids, MI 49503
616-774-1230

Hospitals
Blodgett Memorial Medical Center
Butterworth Hospital
Ferguson Hospital
Grand Rapids Osteopathic
    Hospital
Saint Mary's Hospital

Kalamazoo

KALAMAZOO CCOP
1521 Gull Road
Kalamazoo, MI 49001
616-383-7007

Hospitals
Borgess Medical Center
Bronson Methodist Hospital

MINNESOTA

Duluth

DULUTH CLINIC, LTD
400 East Third Street
Duluth, MN 55805
218-722-8364

Hospitals
The Duluth Clinic, Ltd.
Miller-Dwan Hospital & Medical
    Center Radiation Unit
Adams Clinic

St. Louis Park

W. METRO-
MINNEAPOLIS
CCOP
5000 West 39th Street
St. Louis Park, MN
55416
612-927-3491

Hospitals
Abbott-Northwestern Hospital
Fairview-Southdale Hospital
Mercy Medical Center
Methodist Hospital
Metropolitan Medical Center
North Memorial Medical Center
Unity Medical Center

MISSISSIPPI

Tupelo

NORTH MISSISSIPPI CCOP
806 Garfield
Tupelo, MS 38801
601-844-9166

Hospitals
North Mississippi Medical
Center

Offices
North Mississippi Hematology and
Oncology Association, Ltd.

MISSOURI

Kansas City

ST. LUKE'S HOSPITAL
Wornall Road at Forty-fourth
Kansas City, MO 64111
816-932-2085

Hospitals
St. Luke's Hospital of Kansas City
Bethany Medical Center
The Children's Mercy Hospital

Offices
University of Health Sciences
Larry Rosen, M.D.
Richard Morrison, M.D.

KANSAS CITY CCOP
6601 Rockhill Road
Kansas City, MO 64131
816-361-5288

Hospitals
Baptist Memorial Hospital
Menorah Medical Center
Research Medical Center
Shawnee Mission Medical Center
St. Mary's Hospital
Trinity Lutheran Hospital

St. Louis

ST. LOUIS CCOP
Mercy Doctors Building
621 South New Ballas
    Road, Suite 3018
St. Louis, MO 63141
314-569-6573

Hospitals
Christian Hospitals
DePaul Health Center
Missouri Baptist
    Hospital
St. Anthony's Medical
    Center
St. John's Mercy Medical
    Center

MONTANA

Billings

BILLINGS INTERHOSPITAL ONCOLOGY PROJECT
1145 N. 29th Street, Suite 1B
Billings, MT 59101
406-259-2452

Hospitals
St. Vincent's Hospital
Billings Deaconess Hospital

Offices
Northern Rockies Cancer Treatment
    Center
Internal Medicine Association
Surgical Clinic

NEVADA

Las Vegas

SOUTHERN NEVADA RESEARCH FOUNDATION
2040 West Charleston Boulevard
Suite 204
Las Vegas, NV 89102
702-384-0013

Hospitals
Nevada Radiation Oncology Center
Southern Nevada Memorial
    Hospital
Valley Hospital Medical Center

Offices
Robert Belliveau, M.D.
B. Norman Brown, M.D.
Kirk Cammack, M.D.
Cancer Care Consultants
Stephen Kollins, M.D.
Dermot O'Rourke, M.D.
William Rydell, M.D.

NEW JERSEY

Hackensack

BERGEN-PASSAIC CCOP
30 Prospect Avenue
Hackensack, NJ 07601
201-441-2363

Hospitals
Beth Israel Hospital
Hackensack Medical Center
Holy Name Hospital

Livingston

ESSEX COUNTY CANCER CONSORTIUM
Old Short Hills Road
Livingston, NJ 07039
201-533-5917

Hospitals
St. Barnabas Medical Center
The Hospital Center at Orange
The Mountainside Hospital

Newark

MEDICAL CENTER CCOP
   CONSORTIUM
201 Lyons Avenue
Newark, NJ 07112
201-926-7230

Hospitals
Newark Beth Israel
   Medical Center
Christ Hospital
West Hudson Hospital
Memorial General
   Hospital

Summit

NORTHERN NEW
   JERSEY CCOP
193 Morris Avenue
Summit, NJ 07901
201-522-2043

Hospitals
Overlook Hospital
Morristown Memorial
   Hospital
Elizabeth General
   Medical Center

NEW YORK

Binghamton

TWIN TIERS CCOP
169 Riverside Drive
Binghamton, NY 13905
607-798-5431

Hospitals
Our Lady of Lourdes Hospital
Robert Packer Hospital

Brooklyn

LUTHERAN MEDICAL
   CENTER
150 55th Street
Brooklyn, NY 11220
718-630-7065

Hospitals
Lutheran Medical Center
Maimonides Medical Center
Methodist Hospital
New York Infirmary—Beekman
   Downtown Hospital

Cooperstown

MARY IMOGENE
   BASSETT HOSPITAL
   CCOP
Atwell Road
Cooperstown, NY 13326
607-547-3339

Hospitals
Mary Imogene Bassett Hospital

Manhassett

NORTH SHORE
   UNIVERSITY
   HOSPITAL
300 Community Drive
Manhasset, NY 11030
516-562-4161

Hospitals
North Shore University Hospital

Offices
Klaus Dittmar, M.D.
Frank Tomao, M.D.
Francis X. Moore, M.D.
Robert Levy, M.D.
Jakow Diener, M.D.
Jerome Appelbaum, M.D.
John Lovecchio, M.D.
Samuel Packer, M.D.
Jay Bosworth, M.D.

Mineola

NASSAU REGIONAL
   CANCER PROGRAM
222 Station Plaza North,
   Room 300
Mineola, NY 11501
516-663-2310

Hospitals
Lydia Hall Hospital
Nassau Hospital

Rochester

ST. MARY'S HOSPITAL
   CCOP
89 Genesee Street
Rochester, NY 14611
716-464-3521

Hospitals
St. Mary's Hospital

Syracuse

CCOP OF CENTRAL
   NEW YORK
101 Union Avenue, Suite
   817
Syracuse, NY 13203
315-424-1188

Hospitals
St. Joseph's Hospital
Crouse-Irving Memorial
Community General

Offices
Manuel G. Dalope, M.D.
Nabila A. Elbadawai, M.D.
Abdul G. Musa, M.D.
J. Robert Smith, M.D.
Richard W. Weiskopf, M.D.

NORTH DAKOTA

Fargo

ST. LUKE'S HOSPITAL CCOP
5th Street North at Mills Avenue
Fargo, ND 58122
701-237-2446

Hospitals
St. Luke's General Hospital
Fargo Clinic
The Neuropsychiatric Institute
St. John's Hospital
St. Ansgar Hospital

OHIO

Columbus

COLUMBUS CCOP
111 South Grant Avenue
Columbus, OH 43215
614-461-3049

Hospitals
Grant Hospital
St. Anthony Hospital
Doctors Hospital

Kettering

DAYTON CCOP
3525 Southern Boulevard
Kettering, OH 45429
513-299-7204, Ext. 322

Hospitals
Good Samaritan Hospital
Grandview Hospital
Kettering Medical Center
Miami Valley Hospital
St. Elizabeth Medical Center

Toledo

TOLEDO CCOP
5200 Harroum Road
Sylvania, OH 43560
419-885-1444, Ext. 2003

Hospitals
Flower Hospital
St. Charles Hospital
St. Joseph Mercy Hospital
The Toledo Hospital
The Toledo Clinic, Inc.

PENNSYLVANIA

Danville

GEISINGER CLINIC CCOP
North Academy Avenue
Danville, PA 17822
717-271-6413

Hospitals
Geisinger Clinic and Medical
  Center

Pittsburgh

ALLEGHENY CCOP
320 East North Avenue
Pittsburgh, PA 15212
412-359-4054

Hospitals
Allegheny General Hospital
Jameson Memorial Hospital

SOUTH CAROLINA

Spartanburg

SPARTANBURG CCOP
101 East Wood Street
Spartanburg, SC 29303
803-573-6921

Hospitals
Spartanburg General Hospital
Mary Black Memorial Hospital
Doctor's Memorial Hospital

SOUTH DAKOTA

Sioux Falls

SIOUX FALLS COMMUNITY CANCER CONSORTIUM
1301 South 9th Avenue, Suite 501
Sioux Falls, SD 57105
605-331-3160

Hospitals
McKennan Hospital
Central Plains Clinic
Sioux Valley Hospital
Veterans Administration
  Hospital

Offices
Medical Oncology Associates
L. Gilbert Thatcher, M.D.

TEXAS

Fort Worth

FORT WORTH/ARLINGTON CCOP
1401 S. Main
Fort Worth, TX 76104
817-336-9371, Ext. 7273

Hospitals
St. Joseph's Hospital

Offices
Radiation Therapy & Chemotherapy
  Associates, Fort Worth

VERMONT

Rutland

GREEN MOUNTAIN ONCOLOGY GROUP
Rutland Regional Medical Center
Rutland, VT 05701
802-775-7111, Ext. 184

Hospitals
Rutland Hospital, Inc.
Putnam Memorial Hospital

Offices
Mildred Reardon, M.D.
John Valentine, M.D.
Peter P. Bradley, M.D.
Mark Donavan, M.D.

VIRGINIA

Roanoke

CCOP OF ROANOKE
P.O. Box 13367
Roanoke, VA 24033
703-981-7009

Hospitals
Roanoke Memorial Hospitals
Community Hospital of
    Roanoke
Lewis-Gale Hospital
Veterans Administration
    Medical Center

WASHINGTON

Seattle

VIRGINIA MASON MEDICAL CENTER CCOP
1100 Ninth Avenue
Seattle, WA 98111
206-223-6742

Hospitals
Virginia Mason Medical Center
Valley General Hospital

Tacoma

SOUTHWEST CCOP
    WASHINGTON
314 South K Street
Suite 108
Tacoma, WA 98405
206-597-7461

Hospitals
Auburn General Hospital
Good Samaritan Hospital
St. Joseph Hospital
Allenmore Community Hospital
VA Medical Center
Mary Bridge Children's Health
    Center
St. Peter Hospital
Community Hospital
St. Joseph Hospital in Aberdeen
Tacoma General Hospital

WEST VIRGINIA

Charleston

WEST VIRGINIA COOPERATIVE CCOP
3200 MacCorkle Avenue, S.E.
Charleston, WV 25304
304-348-9541

Hospitals
West Virginia University
Hospital, Morgantown
United Hospital Center, Clarksburg
Charleston Area Medical Center
Veterans Administration Medical
Center, Huntington
Ohio Valley Medical Center,
Wheeling
Raleigh General Hospital,
Beckley
City Hospital of Martinsburg
Marshall University School of
Medicine, Huntington
St. Mary's Hospital, Huntington
Cabell-Huntington Hospital,
Huntington

WISCONSIN

Marshfield

MARSHFIELD CCOP
1000 North Oak Avenue
Marshfield, WI 54449
715-387-5241

Hospitals
Marshfield Clinic
St. Joseph's Hospital

What are the National Cancer Institute's clinical treatment programs?

The National Cancer Institute conducts research clinical programs at the Clinical Center of the National Institutes of Health in Bethesda, Maryland. Doctors who are engaged in studies of particular types of cancer will accept limited numbers of patients for treatment. Nursing and medical care are provided to study patients without charge. You must be referred by your doctor, who must furnish full medical reports. The telephone number of the Patient Referral Service is (301)-496-4891. The clinical director of the institute is Vincent T. DeVita, Jr., M.D. The various branches and kinds of cancer being treated are listed.

BIOLOGICAL THERAPEUTICS BRANCH

Chief, Clinical Investigations Section: Stephen A. Sherwin, M.D.
301-695-1520

The Biological Therapeutics Branch of the Biological Response Modifiers Program is solely devoted to the early clinical testing (Phase I, Phase II) of biological agents with potential in the treatment of cancer. The agents being examined in detail include immunoaugmenting and immunomodulatory agents, lymphokines, interferon, thymic factors, maturation and differentiation factors, anti-tumor monoclonal antibodies, and anti-tumor effector cells. The clinical research facilities of the Biological Therapeutics Branch are located in Frederick, Maryland, in conjunction with the National Cancer Institute's Frederick Cancer Research Facility. There is a small inpatient unit located in Frederick Memorial Hospital as well as a larger outpatient facility, including a cytapheresis unit, located near the hospital. Both units are staffed by NCI oncologists and research nurses.

Current studies are focused on early clinical testing of interferon and anti-tumor monoclonal antibodies. The interferon trials are generally open to patients with histologically proven recurrent cancer of any type and who are refractory to curative therapy. In addition, patients must be ambulatory and not have received chemotherapy, radiation, or corticosteroid therapy within 4 weeks of entering the trial. The anti-tumor monoclonal antibody trials are open to patients with chronic lymphocytic leukemia and cutaneous T-cell lymphoma, and in the future to patients with disseminated melanoma. Monoclonal antibody trials in other malignancies may also be available in the future. The eligibility requirements for patients on these latter trials are similar to those for the interferon trials.

Patients entering research trials of the Biological Therapeutics Branch will be referred back to their primary physician after the completion of the trial for ongoing care and follow-up. While patients are under the care of the Biological Therapeutics Branch, research funds will be made available to help defray hospitalization and travel expenses.

DERMATOLOGY BRANCH

Chief: Stephen I. Katz, M.D.
301-496-2481

Selected patients with the following diseases will be admitted for study:

Benign Mucosal Pemphigoid (ocular pemphigoid)

Bullous Pemphigoid

Cystic Acne

Dermatitis Herpetiformis

Epidermodysplasia Verruciformis (genetic predisposition for flat warts and squamous-cell carcinoma)

Erythema Elevatum Diutinum

Herpes Gestationis

Multiple Warts

Pemphigus Vulgaris

Sezary Syndrome

Tuberous Sclerosis Vasculitis

Skin Cancer—Selected patients with extensive cutaneous basal-cell carcinoma will be admitted for study and investigative therapy.

Xeroderma Pigmentosum—Selected patients will be admitted for treatment, study, and long-term follow-up.

EPIDEMIOLOGY BRANCHES

Environmental Epidemiology Branch

Chief: Joseph F. Fraumeni, Jr., M.D.
301-496-1611

Persons with cancer or at high risk of any type of cancer are sought for studies of the causes of cancer. On referral, patients are considered for inclusion in studies because of:

1. A strong family history of malignant or benign neoplasia of an unusual type, pattern, or frequency (e.g., three or more relatives with cancer); or

2. Known or suspected factor(s) that predispose to neoplasia: either environmental exposures (occupation, drugs, radiation, diet, viruses, etc.) or genetic and/or congenital factors (Mendelian traits associated with neoplasia, birth defects, and chromosomal anomalies); or

3. A tumor presenting with peculiar demographic or clinical features, such as unusual age of onset, bilaterality, unusual histopathology or response to therapy, or associated medical conditions, like autoimmune disease or immune deficiency; or

4. Documented history of T-cell malignant leukemia and/or lymphoma for study of human T-cell leukemia/lymphoma virus (HTLV).

Studies consist of 1) verifying the patient's personal and family history by means of questionnaire, interview, and review of records and histologic slides and, sometimes, 2) offering the opportunity for an in-depth clinical and laboratory evaluation to clarify the mechanism of carcinogenesis. Study may involve drawing blood, skin biopsy, and radiographic examinations, as well as use of clinically available tissue for laboratory assays. No therapy beyond counseling is offered, but referral to other clinical branches of the National Cancer Institute will be expedited.

IMMUNOLOGY BRANCH

Acting Chief: David H. Sachs, M.D.

Immunotherapy and Immunobiology of Neoplastic Diseases—The role of adjuvant immunotherapy is being evaluated in patients between the ages of 15 and 70 with malignant melanoma. Patients with Stage I (level IV or V) or Stage II disease who have been or can be surgically rendered free of clinical disease are candidates for this protocol. Initial evaluation includes clinical and laboratory staging as well as assessment of each patient's immune status. Patients are randomly assigned to treatment with adjuvant immunotherapy, chemotherapy, or no further treatment. During follow-up they are monitored for evidence of antibody and cell-mediated immune responses to melanoma cells, in parallel with clinical and laboratory monitoring for evidence of tumor recurrence. In addition, the nature of the immunologic response of patients to selected tumors other than melanoma is under investigation.

MEDICINE BRANCH

Chief: Robert C. Young, M.D.
301-496-4916

Patients with the following diseases are eligible for admission to the Medicine Branch for definitive treatment, provided they have not received prior chemotherapy or, where indicated, prior radiotherapy. A serious underlying illness in addition to the patient's neoplasm will disqualify the patient from eligibility for these studies.

Hodgkin's Disease and Non-Hodgkin's Lymphoma—Patients with biopsy-proven diagnosis of Hodgkin's disease or non-Hodgkin's lymphoma not previously treated are eligible for admission and treatment in collaboration with the Radiation Oncology Branch.

Ovarian Carcinoma—Patients who have epithelial tumors of the ovary are eligible for this program. All stages of disease are acceptable, provided patients have had no prior chemotherapy or radiotherapy.

Breast Carcinoma—Patients with disseminated breast cancer, and with evaluable metastatic lesions, are eligible for admission for chemotherapeutic trials. Patients are excluded if they have received prior chemotherapy with more than one agent. Patients will also be accepted for evaluation and treatment of primary breast masses. Primary treatment protocols consist of a comparison of breast irradiation and lymph node dissection vs. modified radical mastectomy.

Testicular Carcinoma—Patients with poor prognosis bulky non-seminomatous testicular cancer metastatic to abdominal lymph nodes or distant sites are eligible for this study if they have received no prior radiotherapy or chemotherapy. In addition, patients with bulky disseminated seminoma may be admitted for combined modality therapy.

Cervical Carcinoma—Patients who have had no prior radiation or chemotherapy are eligible provided they have invasive carcinoma of the cervix *and* para-aortic lymph-node involvement.

METABOLISM BRANCH

Chief: Thomas A. Waldmann, M.D.
301-496-6653

Agammaglobulinemia—Selected patients with X-linked agammaglobulinemia and thymoma and agammaglobulinemia are being studied.

Antibody Deficiency with Normal Immunoglobulins—Selected patients with recurrent infections, normal immunoglobulin levels, but the inability to produce specific antibodies are being studied.

Ataxia-Telangiectasia—Patients with ataxia-telangiectasia are admitted for thorough evaluation as well as intensive study of immunologic function. Selected patients with this syndrome and demonstrable T-cell deficiency will receive thymosin therapy.

DiGeorge Syndrome (Thymic-Parathyroid Aplasia)—Selected patients with the DiGeorge syndrome are being admitted for study and therapy.

Growth Hormone Deficiency—Selected patients 4 to 20 years of age with isolated growth hormone deficiency or growth hormone deficiency as part of panhypopituitarism are being studied.

Hyper IgE Syndrome—Selected patients with recurrent severe bouts of furunculosis and pneumonia secondary to *Staphylococcus aureus* from early infancy and markedly elevated serum IgE levels are being studied.

Hypogammaglobulinemia—Patients with common, variable hypogammaglobulinemia and with different forms of dysgammaglobulinemia are being studied.

Isolated IgA Deficiency—Selected patients with isolated IgA deficiency or IgA deficiency associated with autoimmune disorders are being studied.

Serum Protein Abnormalities—Protein metabolism is being studied in patients with congenital and acquired disorders of the serum proteins, including subjects with idiopathic hypoproteinemia, gastrointestinal protein loss, intestinal lymphangiectasia, allergic gastroenteropathy, and analbuminemia.

Severe Combined Immunodeficiency—Selected patients with the severe combined immunodeficiency syndrome are being admitted for study and therapy.

Cutaneous T-Cell Lymphomas (Sézary Syndrome) and Adult T-cell Leukemia—Selected patients with cutaneous T-cell lymphomas and high circulating neoplastic cell counts are being admitted for study, and when indicated, chemotherapy will be given in collaboration with the Division of Cancer Treatment.

Wiskott-Aldrich Syndrome—Patients are admitted for extensive evaluation of their immunodeficiency state. Selected patients are being evaluated in terms of their response to transfer factor therapy.

NCI-VA MEDICAL ONCOLOGY BRANCH

Chief: John D. Minna, M.D.

Veteran and non-veteran patients with various unresectable neoplastic diseases may be referred to this branch for primary treatment protocols. Various clinical and basic research programs are conducted. Combination chemotherapy, radiation therapy, and immunotherapy are under clinical investigation. In addition, basic research in tumor cell virology, genetics, cytogenetics, and immunology is conducted on clinically available material.

Non-military and military patients with small-cell lung cancer and mycosis fungoides/Sézary syndrome are of particular interest. Patients eligible for military care are entered onto therapeutic trials in a variety of malignant diseases.

Patients accepted for study and treatment in these programs will be admitted to the NCI-VA Medical Oncology Branch research ward at the National Naval Medical Center across the street from the main NIH campus.

PEDIATRIC ONCOLOGY BRANCH

Chief: Philip A. Pizzo, M.D.
  301-496-4256

The Pediatric Oncology Branch accepts patients with selected neoplasms who are between 1 and 25 years of age. In most situations, patients must be previously untreated to be eligible for active protocols. However, previously treated patients may be considered for Phase I or II studies. All patients accepted for admission to this branch may be enrolled in studies of optimal supportive care techniques. Selected patients are considered for autologous marrow rescue after high-dose chemotherapy. Clinically available materials are employed in basic studies of tumor virology, kinetics, biology, biochemistry, immunology, and genetics.

Acute Leukemia—Untreated patients, usually under 25 years of age, will be considered for admission. In patients with acute lymphocytic leukemia, the therapeutic emphasis is on the evaluation of drug combinations, new agents, and various methods for cranial prophylaxis.

Neuroblastoma—Previously untreated patients over 2 years old are being sought for treatment. Studies of cultured tumor cells and biological markers are carried out.

Ewing's Sarcoma—Previously untreated patients with a biopsy-proven diagnosis are eligible for admission and treatment with radiation and chemotherapy. Patients at high risk for relapse are offered high-dose chemotherapy, total-body irradiation, and maximum supportive care.

Non-Hodgkin's Malignant Lymphoma (especially Burkitt's Lymphoma)—Patients under 25 years of age with a suspected or proven diagnosis of non-Hodgkin's lymphoma are being sought. While untreated patients are preferred, selected treated patients may be accepted. The treatment emphasis is on combined modality therapy including surgery, radiation, and chemotherapy.

Osteogenic Sarcoma—Previously untreated patients with non-metastatic disease are offered surgery and adjuvant chemotherapy in conjunction with the Surgery Branch. Patients with metastatic disease, with or without previous treatment, are considered for admission at any age.

Rhabdomyosarcoma and Undifferentiated Sarcomas—Previously untreated patients with extensive disease are considered for admission. Combined modality therapy will be evaluated.

RADIATION ONCOLOGY BRANCH

Chief: Eli Glatstein, M.D.
    301-496-5457

Breast Cancer—Patients with Stage I or II breast cancer will receive either modified radical mastectomy or primary radiotherapy to the breast. This study is performed in collaboration with the Surgery and Medicine Branches.

Unresectable Chondrosarcoma or Osteogenic Sarcoma—Patients with locally unresectable tumors will receive radiation therapy and radiosensitizers.

Gliomas—Patients without prior radiation therapy are eligible for a variety of radiotherapy studies performed in conjunction with the Neurological Surgery Branch of NINCDS.

Hodgkin's Disease—Patients with previously untreated disease are eligible for full staging and therapy with radiation and/or combination chemotherapy. This study is performed in collaboration with the Medicine Branch.

Malignant Lymphoma of Non-Hodgkin's Type—Patients with a biopsy-proven diagnosis of lymphoma are eligible for admission and treatment if they have had no prior treatment.

Oat Cell Cancer—Patients with biopsy-proven oat cell carcinoma of the lung are eligible for admission and treatment. This study is performed in collaboration with the NCI-VA Medicine Branch.

Gastric Cancer and Pancreatic Cancer—Patients with these neoplasms who have no distant metastases are eligible for studies involving intraoperative irradiation in conjunction with radical surgery performed by the Surgery Branch.

Carcinoma of the Nasopharynx—Patients without distant hematogenous metastases are eligible for studies of radiotherapy in conjunction with experimental radioprotecting agents.

SURGERY BRANCH

Admitting Officer: David N. Danforth, M.D.
    301-496-1534

Sarcomas of Bone and Soft Tissues—Patients who have had biopsies and may or may not have had definitive surgical therapy are eligible for admission for treatment with new radiotherapeutic and chemotherapeutic adjuvant combined modality protocols.

Colorectal Neoplasms—All patients who are at high risk for recurrent colon or rectal cancer after standard surgical procedures have been completed are eligible for adjuvant chemotherapy trials. Patients at high risk are those with Dukes C lesions, perforating tumors, obstructing tumors, or those with adjacent organic involvement.

Also patients with solitary or multiple hepatic metastases will be considered for hepatic resection, adjuvant intraperitoneal chemotherapy, or chemotherapy by hepatic artery infusion.

Combined modality trials for primary rectal and primary squamous-cell cancer of the anus are currently in effect.

Breast Cancer—Patients with untreated, Stage I–II epithelial cancers of the breast diagnosed clinically or by biopsy and patients with breast masses which require biopsy to exclude malignancy will be considered.

Cancer of the Pancreas—Patients with suspected or documented nonmetastatic pancreatic carcinoma are eligible for consideration for treatment on protocols combining surgical resection and intraoperative radiotherapy.

Cancer of the Stomach—Patients with suspected, documented, or locally recurrent carcinoma of the stomach may be considered for treatment on combined modality surgery-radiation therapy protocols.

Testicular Tumors—Selected patients with testicular cancers are considered for treatment. Data derived from investigations of various immunologic factors in these patients are being used to develop improved methods of treatment of testicular malignancies.

Bladder Tumors—Protocols are being developed for patients with suspected or documented invasive bladder carcinoma. These patients may be considered for treatment on combined modality surgery-radiation therapy protocols.

Prostate Tumors—New protocols are being developed for patients with local or metastatic prostate carcinoma. Patients with local and metastatic malignancies will be considered for chemotherapeutic, radiation, and/or endocrinologic treatment.

What institutions are accepting patients for research studies in particle-beam therapy?

There are eight:

Cleveland Clinic
Lewis Research Center (NASA)
Cleveland Ohio
206-444-5570
Neutron therapy

Fermi National Accelerator Laboratory (Fermilab)
Batavia Illinois
312-840-3865
Neutron therapy

Fox Chase Cancer Center and
   University of
   Pennsylvania
Philadelphia, Pennsylvania
205-728-2582
Neutron therapy

Massachusetts General Hospi-
   tal
Harvard University
Cambridge, Massachusetts
617-726-8150
Proton therapy

M.D. Anderson Hospital and
   Tumor Institute
University of Texas
Houston, Texas
713-792-3410
Neutron therapy

University of California
Lawrence Berkeley
   Laboratory
Berkeley, California
415-486-6325
Helium and heavy ions

University of California
Wadsworth VA Medical Center
Los Angeles, California
213-825-9304
Neutron therapy

University of Washington
Seattle, Washington
206-543-3390
Neutron therapy

Can I get a list of pain clinics?

For a directory of pain clinics, write Committee on Pain Therapy and Acupuncture, American Society of Anesthesiologists, 515 Busse Highway, Park Ridge, Illinois 60068 or American Pain Society, 340 Kingsland Street, Nutley, New Jersey 07110.

Does the National Institutes of Health have a pain clinic?

Yes. The National Institutes of Health (NIH) has established a multidisciplinary pain clinic at the Clinical Center in Bethesda, Maryland, to improve the understanding of pain mechanisms and to develop better ways of assessing and treating pain. Scientists and research physicians in the pain clinic are available to the medical community for consultation regarding special difficulties in pain management.

What institutions are funded by the National Cancer Institute to study pain control?

The following institutions have been founded by the National Cancer Institute to do research in pain control:

A PILOT STUDY OF CANCER PAIN
Dr. Charles Cleeland
Principal Investigator
University of Wisconsin
Madison, WI 53706

CANCER PAIN: PHARMACO-
KINETIC CORRELATES OF AN-
ALGESIA
Dr. Kathleen M. Foley
Principal Investigator
Memorial Sloan-Kettering In-
stitute
New York, NY 10021

IMPROVING MANAGEMENT OF
CHEMOTHERAPY TOXICITY: A
MULTIDISCIPLINARY   AP-
PROACH (This grant has a ma-
jor component of cancer pain
research)
Dr. C. Richard Chapman
'Principal Investigator
Fred Hutchinson Cancer Re-
search Center
Seattle, WA 98104

CANCER PAIN: INTRASPINAL MS
VS. CONVENTIONAL NARCOT-
ICS
Dr. Dennis W. Coombs
Principal Investigator
Department of Surgery
Dartmouth Medical School
Hanover, NH 03756

Where can I find someone trained in hypnotism to help me?

For lists of trained personnel who use hypnotism, write Society for Clinical and Experimental Hypnosis, 129A Kings Park Drive, Liverpool, New York 13088 or The American Society of Clinical Hypnosis, 2400 East Devon Avenue, Suite 218, Des Plaines, Illinois 60018.

How can I find people working on biofeedback in my area?

To locate those in your area working on biofeedback, write Biofeedback Research Society, University of Colorado, Medical Center, Denver, Colorado 80262.

What are the cancer programs approved by the American College of Surgeons?

The American College of Surgeons maintains a certification program relating to the quality of cancer care in hospitals in the United States. Cancer programs are surveyed at the request of their administrators or their medical staffs or both. The approved status is based on the level of excellence in relation to standards established by the College of Surgeons. In order to be certified, the hospital must have a cancer committee, a cancer registry, a clinical education program, and means for evaluating the quality of care in the hospital. Hospitals listed in the directory, published annually and updated twice during the year, have been approved for cancer treatment by the College. The directory (*Cancer Programs Approved by the American College of Surgeons*) is available from the Cancer Department, American College of Surgeons, 55 East Erie Street, Chicago, Illinois 60611. Inquiries about current status of an institution's cancer program should be sent to the same address.

What is meant by a cancer program approved by the Commission on Cancer of the American College of Surgeons?

The Commission on Cancer of the American College of Surgeons sets forth basic criteria for approval of organized cancer programs. The criteria stress the importance of multidisciplinary cancer conferences and accurate recording of diagnostic and treatment data in a cancer registry for meaningful patient-care evaluation. The activities are primarily patient-oriented through emphasis on the education of physicians and allied-health professionals in new knowledge gained from basic clinical research.

The program is to assure that the proper atmosphere and organization exist in each approved cancer program. The approval of a program only assures that the necessary program elements are in place and are functioning at a satisfactory level.

Those cancer programs approved as of November, 1986 include:

ALABAMA
Birmingham
Baptist Medical Center
Brookwood Medical Center
Carraway Methodist Medical
  Center
Saint Vincent's Hospital
University of Alabama Hospitals
Veterans Administration Hospital

Mobile
Mobile Infirmary
University of South Alabama
  Medical Center

Selma
Selma Medical Center Hospital

Tuskegee
Veterans Administration Hospital

ALASKA
Fairbanks
Fairbanks Memorial Hospital

ARIZONA
Mesa
Desert Samaritan Hospital
Mesa Lutheran Hospital

Phoenix
Good Samaritan Hospital
Maricopa Medical Center
Memorial Hospital
Veterans Administration Medical
Center

Scottsdale
Scottsdale Memorial Hospital

Tucson
Tucson Medical Center
University Medical Center

ARKANSAS

Fayetteville
Washington Regional Medical
Center

Fort Smith
Sparks Regional Medical Center
St. Edward Mercy Medical Center

Little Rock
John McClellan Memorial
Veterans Hospital

Rogers
St. Mary-Rogers Memorial
Hospital

CALIFORNIA

Alhambra
Alhambra Community Hospital

Anaheim
Anaheim Memorial Hospital
Martin Luther Hospital
West Anaheim Humana Hospital

Apple Valley
St. Mary Desert Valley Hospital

Arcadia
Methodist Hospital of Southern
California

Bakersfield
Kern Medical Center
San Joaquin Community Hospital

Bellflower
Bellwood General Hospital
Kaiser Foundation Hospital

Berkeley
Alta Bates Hospital
Herrick Hospital and Health
Center

Buena Park
La Palma Intercommunity
Hospital

Burbank
St. Joseph Medical Center

Burlingame
Peninsula Hospital and Medical
Center

Castro Valley
Eden Hospital

Chico
N.T. Enloe Memorial Hospital

Concord
Mount Diablo Hospital Medical
Center

Covina
Inter-Community Medical Center

Daly City
Seton Medical Center

Downey
Downey Community Hospital

Duarte
City of Hope Medical Center
Santa Teresita Hospital

Encino
Encino Hospital

Escondito
Palomar Memorial Hospital

Fontana
Kaiser Foundation Hospital

Fountain Valley
Fountain Valley Regional
   Hospital

Fresno
Fresno Community Hospital
   Medical Center
Valley Children's Hospital
Veterans Administration Medical
   Center

Fullerton
St. Jude Hospital and
   Rehabilitation Center

Glendale
Glendale Adventist Medical
   Center
Memorial Hospital of Glendale

Glendora
Foothill Presbyterian Hospital
Glendora Community Hospital

Granada Hills
Granada Hills Community
   Hospital

Harbor City
Bay Harbor Hospital
Kaiser Foundation Hospital

Hawthorne
Robert F. Kennedy Medical
   Center

Huntington Beach
Pacifica Community Hospital

Imola
Napa State Hospital

Indio
John F. Kennedy Memorial
   Hospital

Inglewood
Centinela Hospital Medical
   Center
Daniel Freeman Memorial
   Hospital

La Jolla
Green Hospital of Scripps Clinic
Scripps Memorial Hospital

La Mesa
Grossmont District Hospital

Laguna Hills
Saddleback Community Hospital

Lakewood
Doctors Hospital of Lakewood

Livermore
Veterans Administration Medical
   Center

Loma Linda
Loma Linda University Medical
   Center

Long Beach
Long Beach Community Hospital
Los Altos Hospital
Memorial Hospital Medical
   Center
St. Mary Medical Center
Veterans Administration Medical
   Center

Los Alamitos
Los Alamitos Medical Center

Los Angeles
California Hospital Medical
   Center
Cedars-Sinai Medical Center
Children's Hospital of Los
   Angeles
Hollywood Presbyterian Medical
   Center
Hospital of the Good Samaritan
Kaiser Foundation Hospital—
   Cadillac
Kaiser Foundation Hospital—
   Sunset
Los Angeles County, USC Medical
   Center
Martin Luther King, Jr., General
   Hospital
Orthopaedic Hospital Medical
   Center

Queen of Angels Medical Center
St. Vincent's Medical Center
Santa Marta Hospital and Clinic
UCLA Hospital and Clinics
White Memorial Medical Center

Lynwood
St. Francis Medical Center

Martinez
Veterans Administration Medical
   Center

Mission Viejo
Mission Community Hospital

Modesto
Memorial Hospitals Association

Montebello
Beverly Hospital

Monterey Park
Garfield Medical Center
Monterey Park Hospital

Napa
Queen of Valley Hospital

Newport Beach
Hoag Memorial Hospital—
   Presbyterian

Northridge
Northridge Hospital Medical
   Center

Oakland
Naval Hospital
Samuel Merritt Hospital

Oceanside
Tri-City Hospital

Orange
Children's Hospital of Orange
   County
St. Joseph Hospital
University of California Irvine
   Medical Center

Oxnard
St. John's Hospital Regional
   Medical Center

Palm Springs
Desert Hospital

Palo Alto
Veterans Administration Medical
   Center

Panorama City
Kaiser Foundation Hospital
Panorama Community Hospital

Pasadena
Huntington Memorial Hospital
St. Luke Hospital of Pasadena

Pomona
Pomona Valley Community
   Hospital

Poway
Pomerado Hospital

Rancho Mirage
Eisenhower Medical Center

Redlands
Redlands Community Hospital

Redondo Beach
South Bay Hospital

Redwood City
Sequoia Hospital

Riverside
Parkview Community Hospital
Riverside Community Hospital

Sacramento
Mercy General Hospital
Sutter Community Hospital of
   Sacramento
University of California Davis
   Medical Center

San Bernardino
St. Bernadine Community
   Hospital
San Bernardino County Medical
   Center
St. Bernardine Hospital

San Clemente
San Clemente General Hospital

San Diego
Children's Hospital & Health
    Center
Sharp Memorial Hospital
Kaiser Foundation Hospital
Mercy Hospital and Medical
    Center
Naval Hospital
University Hospital

San Dimas
San Dimas Community Hospital

San Francisco
Children's Hospital of
    San Francisco
French Hospital/Medical Center
Letterman Army Medical Center
Marshal Hale Memorial Hospital
Mount Zion Hospital and Medical
    Center
Pacific Presbyterian Hospital
Ralph K. Davis Medical Center
San Francisco General Hospital
    Medical Center
St. Francis Memorial Hospital
St. Luke's Hospital
St. Mary's Hospital and Medical
    Center
University of California Hospitals
    and Clinics

San Gabriel
Community Hospital of San
    Gabriel

San Jose
Good Samaritan Hospital
O'Connor Hospital
San Jose Hospital
Santa Clara Valley Medical Center

San Pablo
Brookside Hospital

San Pedro
San Pedro Peninsula Hospital

San Rafael
Marin General Hospital

Santa Ana
Western Medical Center

Santa Barbara
Galeta Valley Community Hospital
Santa Barbara Cottage Hospital
St. Francis Hospital

Santa Cruz
Dominican Santa Cruz Hospital

Santa Monica
Santa Monica Hospital Medical
    Center
St. John's Hospital and Health
    Center

South Laguna
South Coast Medical Center

Stockton
Dameron Hospital Association
St. Joseph's Hospital

Tarzana
Medical Center of Tarzana
    Hospital

Thousand Oaks
Los Robles Regional Medical
    Center

Torrance
Little Company of Mary Hospital
Los Angeles County Harbor—
    UCLA Medical Center
Torrance Memorial Hospital
    Medical Center

Travis AFB
David Grant USAF Medical
    Center

Upland
San Antonio Community Hospital

Van Nuys
Valley Presbyterian Hospital

Victorville
Victor Valley Community Hospital

Visalia
Kaweah Delta District Hospital

Walnut Creek
John Muir Memorial Hospital

West Covina
Queen of the Valley Hospital
West Covina Hospital

Whittier
Presbyterian Intercommunity
 Hospital

COLORADO

Aurora
Fitzsimons Army Medical Center

Colorado Springs
Penrose Hospital

Denver
Porter Memorial Hospital
Presbyterian Denver Hospital
Rose Medical Center
St. Joseph Hospital
St. Luke's Hospital
St. Anthony Hospital Systems
University of Colorado Medical
 Center
Veterans Administration Medical
 Center

Englewood
Swedish Medical Center

Fort Carson
Evans Army Community Hospital

Fort Collins
Poudre Valley Hospital

Greeley
North Colorado Medical Center

Lakewood
AMC Cancer Research Center and
 Hospital

Longmont
Longmont United Hospital

Montrose
Montrose Memorial Hospital

Pueblo
St. Mary-Corwin Hospital

Wheat Ridge
Lutheran Medical Center

CONNECTICUT

Bridgeport
Bridgeport Hospital
Park City Hospital
St. Vincent's Medical Center

Bristol
Bristol Hospital

Danbury
Danbury Hospital

Derby
Griffin Hospital

Farmington
University of Connecticut Health
 Center—John Dempsey
 Hospital

Greenwich
Greenwich Hospital Association

Hartford
Hartford Hospital
Mount Sinai Hospital
St. Francis Hospital and Medical
 Center

Meriden
Meriden-Wallingford Hospital

Middletown
Middlesex Memorial Hospital

New Haven
Hospital of St. Raphael
Yale-New Haven Hospital

Norwalk
Norwalk Hospital

Sharon
Sharon Hospital

Stamford
St. Joseph Medical Center
Stamford Hospital

Torrington
Charlotte Hungerford Hospital

Waterbury
St. Mary's Hospital
Waterbury Hospital

DELAWARE

Dover
Kini General Hospital

Lewes
Beebe Hospital of Sussex County

Wilmington
St. Francis Hospital
The Medical Center of Delaware

DISTRICT OF COLUMBIA

Washington
Georgetown University Hospital
Greater Southeast Community
  Hospital
Howard University Hospital
Veterans Administration Hospital
Walter Reed Army Medical Center
Washington Hospital Center

FLORIDA

Boca Raton
Boca Raton Community Hospital

Bradenton
Manatee Memorial Hospital

Clearwater
Morton F. Plant Hospital

Daytona Beach
Halifax Hospital Medical Center

Dunedin
Mease Hospital

Fort Lauderdale
Broward General Medical Center

Gainesville
Shands Teaching Hospital at the
  University of Florida

Jacksonville
Jacksonville Wolfson Childrens
  Hospital
Naval Hospital
St. Vincent's Medical Center
University Hospital of
  Jacksonville

Largo
Medical Center Hospital

Miami
Baptist Hospital of Miami
Cedars Medical Center
Jackson Memorial Hospital
North Shore Medical Center
South Miami Hospital

Miami Beach
Mount Sinai Medical Center

Naples
Naples Community Hospital

Ocala
Marion Community Hospital
Munroe Regional Medical Center

Orlando
Orlando Regional Medical Center

Pensacola
Baptist Hospital
Naval Hospital
West Florida Hospital

Tallahassee
Tallahassee Memorial Regional
  Community Hospital

Tampa
St. Joseph's Hospital
Tampa General Hospital
University Community Hospital

GEORGIA

Americus
Sumter Regional Hospital

Atlanta
Crawford W. Long Memorial
  Hospital
Emory University Hospital
Georgia Baptist Medical Center
Grady Memorial Hospital
Northside Hospital
Piedmont Hospital
St. Joseph's Hospital
West Paces Ferry Hospital

Augusta
Eugene Talmedge Memorial
  Hospital
University Hospital

Austell
Cobb General Hospital

Columbus
Medical Center

Dalton
Hamilton Medical Center

Decatur
De Kalb General Hospital
Veterans Administration Medical
  Center, Atlanta

East Point
South Fulton Hospital

Fort Benning
Martin Army Community Hospital

Fort Gordon
Dwight D. Eisenhower Army
  Medical Center

Gainesville
Northeast Georgia Medical Center

La Grange
West Georgia Medical Center

Marietta
Kennestone Hospital

Rome
Floyd Medical Center

Savannah
Memorial Medical Center

Staleboro
Bulloch Memorial Hospital

Toccoa
Stephens County Hospital

Valdosta
South Georgia Medical Center

HAWAII
Honolulu
Kaiser Foundation Hospital
Kuakini Medical Center
Queen's Medical Center
St. Francis Hospital
Straub Clinic and Hospital
Tripler Army Medical Center

Lihue
G.N. Wilcox Memorial Hospital
  and Health Center

Wailuku
Maui Memorial Hospital

Waimea
Kauai Veterans Memorial Hospital

IDAHO
Blackfoot
Bingham Memorial Hospital

Boise
St. Alphonsus Regional Medical
  Center
St. Luke's Hospital & Mountain
  States Tumor Institute

Burley
Cassia Memorial Hospital and
  Medical Center

Lewiston
St. Joseph's Hospital

Nampa
Mercy Medical Center

Pocatello
Bannock Memorial Hospital
Pocatello Regional Medical
  Center

Twin Falls
Magic Valley Regional Medical
 Center

ILLINOIS

Arlington Heights
Northwest Community Hospital

Aurora
Copley Memorial Hospital
Mercy Center for Health Care
 Services

Barrington
Good Shepard Hospital

Belleville
St. Elizabeth Hospital

Berwyn
Macneal Memorial Hospital

Blue Island
St. Francis Hospital

Carbondale
Memorial Hospital of Carbondale

Centralia
St. Mary's Hospital

Champaign
Burnham Hospital

Chicago
Bethany Methodist Hospital
Central Community Hospital
Children's Memorial Hospital
Columbus Hospital
Cook County Hospital
Edgewater Hospital
Franklin Boulevard Community
 Hospital
Holy Cross Hospital
Illinois Masonic Medical Center
Jackson Park Hospital
Louis A. Weiss Memorial Hospital
Mary Thompson Hospital
Mercy Hospital and Medical
 Center
Michael Reese Hospital and
 Medical Center

Mount Sinai Hospital Medical
 Center
Northwest Hospital
Northwestern Memorial Hospital
Ravenswood Hospital Medical
 Center
Ressurection Hospital
Rush-Presbyterian Ressurection
 Hospital
 Medical Center
South Chicago Community
 Hospital
St. Anne's Hospital
St. Elizabeth's Hospital
St. Joseph Hospital
St. Mary of Nazareth Hospital
 Center
Swedish Covenant Hospital
University of Chicago Medical
 Center
University of Illinois Hospital
Veterans Administration West Side
 Hospital

Chicago Heights
St. James Hospital

Danville
Lake View Medical Center
St. Elizabeth Hospital

Dekalb
Kishwaukee Community Hospital

Decatur
Decatur Memorial Hospital
St. Mary's Hospital

Des Plaines
Holy Family Hospital

Dixon
Katherine Shaw Bethea Hospital

Downers Grove
Good Samaritan Hospital

Effingham
St. Anthony's Memorial Hospital

Elgin
St. Joseph Hospital
Sherman Hospital

Elk Grove Village
Alexian Brothers Medical Center

Elmhurst
Elmhurst Memorial Hospital

Evanston
Evanston Hospital
St. Francis Hospital

Evergreen Park
Little Company of Mary Hospital

Galesburg
St. Mary's Hospital

Granite City
St. Elizabeth Medical Center

Great Lakes
Naval Regional Medical Center

Harvey
Ingalls Memorial Hospital

Highland Park
Highland Park Memorial

Hinsdale
Hinsdale Hospital

Joliet
St. Joseph Hospital

Kankakee
St. Mary's Hospital

La Grange
La Grange Memorial Hospital

Lake Forest
Lake Forest Hospital

Libertyville
Condell Memorial Hospital

Macomb
McDonough District Hospital

Maywood
F.G. Mcgaw Hospital—Loyola
    University Medical Center

McHenry
McHenry Hospital

Moline
Lutheran Hospital

Naperville
Edward Hospital

Oak Lawn
Christ Hospital

Oak Park
West Suburban Hospital Medical
    Center

Olney
Richland Memorial Hospital

Park Ridge
Lutheran General Hospital

Peoria
Methodist Medical Center of
    Illinois
St. Francis Hospital and Medical
    Center

Pontiac
St. James Hospital

Quincy
Blessing Hospital
St. Mary Hospital

Rockford
Rockford Memorial Hospital
St. Anthony Hospital Medical
    Center
Swedish-American Hospital

Skokie
Skokie Valley Hospital

Springfield
Memorial Medical Center
St. John's Hospital

Sterling
Community General Hospital

Urbana
Carle Foundation Hospital
Mercy Hospital

Waukegan
St. Therese Hospital
Victory Memorial Hospital

Winfield
Central DuPage Hospital

INDIANA

Bluffton
Caylor-Nickel Hospital, Inc.

Columbus
Barholomew County Hospital

East Chicago
St. Catherine Hospital

Evansville
Deaconess Hospital
St. Mary's Medical Center
Welborn Baptist Hospital

Gary
Methodist Hospital of Gary

Hammond
St. Margaret Hospital

Indianapolis
Community Hospital of
    Indianapolis
Methodist Hospital of Indiana
St. Vincent Hospital and Health
    Care Center

Lafayette
St. Elizabeth Hospital Medical
    Center

New Albany
Floyd Memorial Hospital

South Bend
Memorial Hospital
St. Joseph's Medical Center

Terre Haute
Terre Haute Regional Hospital
Union Hospital

Vincennes
Good Samaritan Hospital

IOWA

Des Moines
Iowa Methodist Medical Center
Mercy Hospital Medical Center
Veterans Administration Medical
    Center

Iowa City
University of Iowa Hospitals and
    Clinics

Mason City
North Iowa Medical Center
St. Joseph Mercy Hospital

Sioux City
Marian Health Center
St. Luke's Regional Medical
    Center

KANSAS

Fort Riley
Irwin Army Hospital

Hays
Hadley Regional Medical Center
St. Anthony Hospital

Kansas City
Bethany Medical Center
Providence-St. Margaret Health
    Center
University of Kansas Medical
    Center

Shawnee Mission
Shawnee Mission Medical Center

Topeka
St. Francis Hospital and Medical
    Center

Wichita
St. Francis Regional Medical
    Center
St. Joseph Medical Center
HCA Wesley Medical Center

KENTUCKY

Fort Campbell
F.A. Blanchfield Army Community
   Hospital

Fort Thomas
St. Luke Hospital

Lexington
Central Baptist Hospital
Good Samaritan Hospital
University Hospital

Louisville
Highlands Baptist Hospital
Humana Hospital University
Kosair-Children's Hospital
Norton Hospital
Veterans Administration Medical
   Center

Madisonville
Regional Medical Center of
   Hopkins County

LOUISIANA

Alexandria
Rapides Regional Medical Center
St. Frances Cabrini Hospital

Lafayette
University Medical Center

Lake Charles
St. Patrick's Hospital

New Orleans
Charity Hospital of Louisiana
Touro Infirmary
Veterans Administration Medical
   Center

Shreveport
Louisiana State University
   Medical Center University
   Hospital
Veterans Administration Medical
   Center

MAINE

Augusta
Kennebec Valley Medical Center

Bangor
Eastern Maine Medical Center

Lewiston
Central Maine Medical Center
St. Mary's General Hospital

Portland
Maine Medical Center

Presque Isle
Aroostook Medical Center

Rockland
Penobscot Bay Medical Center

Rumford
Rumford Community Hospital

Skowhegan
Redington-Fairview General
   Hospital

Togus
Veterans Administration Medical
   Center

Waterville
Mid-Maine Medical Center

MARYLAND

Annapolis
Anne Arundel General Hospital

Baltimore
St. Agnes Hospital
Johns Hopkins Hospital
Sinai Hospital of Baltimore
University of Maryland Medical
   Center

Bethesda
Naval Hospital

Cumberland
Sacred Heart Hospital

Frederick
Frederick Memorial Hospital

Olney
Montgomery General Hospital

Salisbury
Penninsula General Hospital

Takoma Park
Washington Adventist Hospital

MASSACHUSETTS

Arlington
Choate-Symmes Health Services

Beverly
Beverly Hospital

Boston
Boston City Hospital
Brigham & Women's Hospital
Carney Hospital
Children's Hospital
Faulkner Hospital
Massachusetts General Hospital
New England Deaconess Hospital
St. Elizabeth's Hospital of Boston
University Hospital
Veterans Administration Medical
  Center, *Jamaica Plain*

Brockton
Brockton Hospital
Cardinal Cushing General Hospital

Burlington
Lahey Clinic Hospital

Cambridge
Mount Auburn Hospital

Chelsea
Lawrence F. Quigley Memorial
  Hospital

Concord
Emerson Hospital

Danvers
Hunt Memorial Hospital

Fall River
Charlton Memorial Hospital
St. Anne's Hospital

Framingham
Framingham Union Hospital

Gloucester
Addison Gilbert Hospital

Greenfield
Franklin Medical Center

Holyoke
Holyoke Hospital
Providence Hospital

Hyannis
Cape Cod Hospital

Lowell
Lowell General Hospital
St. John's Hospital
St. Joseph's Hospital

Lynn
Allanticare Medical Center

Malden
The Malden Hospital

Melrose
Melrose-Wakefield Hospital

Natick
Leonard Morse Hospital

Needham
Glover Memorial Hospital

Newton Lower Falls
Newton-Wellesley Hospital

Norfolk
Southwood Community Hospital

North Adams
North Adams Regional Hospital

Northampton
Cooley Dickenson Hospital

Norwood
Norwood Hospital

Palmer
Wing Memorial Hospital

Pittsfield
Berkshire Medical Center

Plymouth
Jordan Hospital

Salem
Salem Hospital

South Weymouth
South Shore Hospital

Springfield
Baystate Medical Center
Mercy Hospital

Stoneham
New England Memorial Hospital

Stoughton
Goddard Memorial Hospital

Turners Falls
Farren Memorial Hospital

Waltham
Waltham Weston Hospital and
    Medical Center

Winchester
Winchester Hospital

Worcester
St. Vincent Hospital
University of Massachsetts Medical
    Center
Worcester Memorial
    Hospital

MICHIGAN

Allen Park
Veterans Administration Medical
    Center

Ann Arbor
University Hospital

Battle Creek
Leila Hospital and Health Center

Bay City
Bay Medical Center

Dearborn
Oakwood Hospital

Detroit
Detroit-Macomb Hospital Corpo-
    ration
Harper Grace Hospital
Henry Ford Hospital

Flint
Hurley Medical Center
St. Joseph Hospital

Grand Rapids
Blodgett Memorial Medical Center
Butterworth Hospital
Ferguson Hospital
St. Mary's Hospital

Kalamazoo
Borgess Medical Center
Bronson Methodist Hospital

Lansing
Edward W. Sparrow Hospital

Marquette
Marquette General Hospital

Midland
Midland Hospital Center

Muskegon
Hackley Hospital and Medical Cen-
    ter

Petoskey
Northern Michigan Hospitals

Rochester
Crittenton Hospital

Royal Oak
William Beaumont Hospital

Saginaw
St. Mary's Hospital

Southfield
Providence Hospital

MINNESOTA

Fridley
Unity Medical Center

Grand Rapids
Itasca Memorial Hospital

Mankato
Immanuel-St. Joseph Hospital

Minneapolis
Abbot-Northwestern Hospital
Hennepin County Medical Center
Methodist Hospital
Metropolitan Medical Center
Minneapolis Children's Medical
  Center
St. Mary's Hospital
Veterans Administration Medical
  Center

Moorhead
St. Ansgar Hospital

Rochester
Mayo Clinic

St. Paul
St. Paul-Ramsey Medical Center

MISSISSIPPI

Biloxi
Biloxi Regional Medical Center
Veterans Administration Medical
  Center

Gulfport
Memorial Hospital at Gulfport

Hattiesburg
Forest County General Hospital
Methodist Hospital

Jackson
University of Mississippi Medical
  Center
Veterans Administration Medical
  Center

Keesler
USAF Medical Center

Oxford
Oxford-Lafayette Community Hospital

Pascagoula
Singing River Hospital

Tupelo
North Mississippi Medical Center

Vicksburg
Mercy Regional Medical Center

MISSOURI

Cape Girardeau
St. Francis Hospital
Southeast Missouri Hospital

Columbia
Boone Hospital Center
Columbia Regional Hospital
Ellis Fischel State Cancer Center
University of Missouri Hospital and
  Clinics

Fort Leonard Wood
General Leonard Wood Army Hospital

Jefferson City
Memorial Community Hospital

Joplin
St. John's Medical Center

Kansas City
Baptist Memorial Hospital
Children's Mercy Hospital
Menorah Medical Center
St. Luke's Hospital
St. Joseph Hospital of Kansas City
Truman Medical Center West

Poplar Bluff
Doctors Regional Medical Center

Sikeston
Missouri Delta Community Hospital

St. Joseph
Hartland Hospital West

St. Louis
Barnes Hospital
Christian Hospitals Northeast/
    Northwest
Deaconess Hospital
Jewish Hospital of St. Louis
St. Anthony's Medical Center
St. John's Mercy Medical Center
St. Mary's Health Center
Veteran's Administration Medical
    Center

MONTANA
Great Falls
Columbus Hospital

NEBRASKA
Hastings
Mary Lanning Memorial Hospital

Kearney
Good Samaritan Hospital

Lincoln
Bryan Memorial Hospital
Lincoln General Hospital
St. Elizabeth Community Health
    Center
Veterans Administration Medical
    Center

Omaha
Archbishop Bergan Mercy Hospital
Bishop Clarkson Memorial Hospi-
    tal
Immanuel Medical Center
Lutheran Medical Center
Nebraska Methodist Hospital
St. Joseph Hospital
University of Nebraska Hospital and
    Clinics

Scottsbluff
West Nebraska General Hospital

NEVADA
Las Vegas
Humana Hospital Sunrise
University Medical Center of
    Southern Nevada

Reno
Washoe Medical Center

NEW HAMPSHIRE
Concord
Concord Hospital

Dover
Wentworth-Douglass Hospital

Exeter
Exeter Hospital

Hanover
Mary Hitchcock Memorial Hospital

Keene
Cheshire Hospital

Lanconia
Lakes Region General Hospital

Littleton
Littleton Hospital

Manchester
Catholic Medical Center
Elliot Hospital
Veterans Administration Medical
    Center

Portsmouth
Portsmouth Hospital

Rochester
Frisbie Memorial Hospital

Woodsville
Cottage Hospital

NEW JERSEY
Atlantic City
Atlantic City Medical Center

Belleville
Clara Maass Memorial Hospital

Camden
West Jersey Hospital

Denville
St. Clare's Hospital

Dover
Dover General Hospital and Medical Center

East Orange
Veterans Administration Medical Center

Elizabeth
Elizabeth General Hospital
St. Elizabeth Hospital

Englewood
Englewood Hospital

Hackensack
Hackensack Medical Center

Hackettstown
Hackettstown Community Hospital

Livingston
St. Barnabas Medical Center

Long Branch
Monmouth Medical Center

Montclair
Mountainside Hospital

Morristown
Morristown Memorial Hospital

Mount Holly
Burlington County Memorial Hospital

Neptune
Jersey Shore Medical Center Fitkin Hospital

New Brunswick
Robert Wood Johnson University Hospital
St. Peter's Medical Center

Newark
Newark Beth Israel Medical Center
University Hospital

Newton
Newton Memorial Hospital

Orange
Hospital Center at Orange

Passaic
Beth Israel Hospital

Paterson
St. Joseph's Hospital and Medical Center

Phillipsburg
Warren Hospital

Princeton
Medical Center at Princeton

Red Bank
Riverview Hospital

Ridgewood
Valley Hospital

Somerville
Somerset Medical Center

Summit
Overlook Hospital

Sussex
Wallkill Valley Hospital

Teaneck
Holy Name Hospital

Trenton
Mercer Hospital
St. Francis Medical Center

Westwood
Pascack Valley Hospital

NEW MEXICO

Albuquerque
Lovelace Medical Center
St. Joseph Hospital
Presbyterian Hospital Center

University of New Mexico Hospital
Veterans Administration Medical
Center

NEW YORK

Albany
Albany Medical Center Hospital
Veterans Administration Medical
Center

Binghampton
Our Lady of Lourdes Memorial
Hospital

Brooklyn
Brookdale Hospital Medical Center
Brooklyn Hospital
Caledonia Hospital
Coney Island Hospital
Health Sciences Medical Center at
Brooklyn
Interfaith Medical Center
Kings County Hospital Center
Long Island College Hospital
Lutheran Medical Center
Maimonides Medical Center
Methodist Hospital
Wyckoff Heights Hospital

Bronx
Bronx-Lebanon Hospital Center
Our Lady of Mercy Medical Center
Veterans Administration Medical
Center

Bronxville
Lawrence Hospital

Buffalo
Roswell Park Memorial Institute
Veterans Administration Medical
Center

Cobleskill
Community Hospital of Schoharie
County

Cooperstown
Mary Imogene Bassett Hospital

East Meadow
Nassau County Medical Center

Elmhurst
City Hospital Center at Elmhurst
St. Johns Queens Hospital

Elmira
Arnot-Ogden Memorial Hospital
St. Joseph's Hospital

Flushing
Booth Memorial Medical Center
Flushing Hospital and Medical
Center

Forest Hills
La Guardia Hospital

Glen Cove
Community Hospital at Glen Cove

Jamaica
Jamaica Hospital
Mary Immaculate Hospital
Queens Hospital Center

Jamestown
Woman's Christian Association
Hospital

Johnson City
United Health Services

Manhasset
North Shore University Hospital

Mineola
Winthrop University Hospital

Mount Kisco
Northern Westchester Hospital
Center

Mount Vernon
Mount Vernon Hospital

New Hyde Park
Long Island Jewish Medical Center

New Rochelle
New Rochelle Hospital Medical
Center

New York City
Bellevue Hospital Center
Beth Israel Medical Center
Cabrini Medical Center
Harlem Hospital Center
Manhattan Eye, Ear and Throat Hospital
Memorial Sloan-Kettering Cancer Center
Montefiore Medical Center
New York Infirmary Beekman Downtown Hospital
New York University Medical Center
Presbyterian Hospital
St. Luke's Hospital Center
St. Vincent's Hospital and Medical Center
Veterans Administration Hospital Medical Center

Oceanside
South Nassau Communities Hospital

Patchogue
Brookhaven Memorial Hospital Medical Center

Plainview
Central General Hospital

Port Jefferson
John T. Mather Memorial Hospital
St. Charles Hospital

Port Jervis
Mercy Community Hospital

Poughkeepsie
Vassar Brothers Hospital

Rochester
Genessee Hospital
Highland Hospital of Rochester
Park Ridge Hospital
Rochester General Hospital
St. Mary's Hospital
Strong Memorial Hospital

Rockville Center
Mercy Hospital

Saratoga Springs
Saratoga Hospital

Schenectady
Ellis Hospital

Staten Island
Bayley Seton Hospital
Doctors' Hospital of Staten Island
St. Vincent's Medical Center of Richmond
Staten Island Hospital

Syracuse
St. Joseph's Hospital Health Center
University Hospital of Upstate Medical Center

Troy
Samaritan Hospital

Valley Stream
Franklin General Hospital

Valhalla
Westchester County Medical Center

Walton
Delaware Valley Hospital

NORTH CAROLINA
Asheville
Memorial Mission Hospital

Camp Le Jeune
Naval Regional Medical Center

Chapel Hill
North Carolina Memorial Hospital

Durham
Duke University Medical Center

Shelby
Cleveland Memorial Hospital

Valdese
Valdese General Hospital

Winston-Salem
North Carolina Baptist Hospital

NORTH DAKOTA

Bismarck
Medcenter One Hospital
St. Alexius Medical Center

Fargo
Dakota Hospital
St. John's Hospital
St. Luke's Hospitals
Veterans Administration Medical
Center

Grand Forks
The United Hospital

Mandan
Mandan Hospital

Minot
St. Joseph's Hospital

Rugby
Good Samaritan Hospital Association

Williston
Mercy Hospital

OHIO

Akron
Akron City Hospital
Akron General Medical Center

Barberton
Barberton Citizens Hospital
St. Thomas Hospital Medical Center

Canton
Timken Mercy Medical Center

Chardon
Geauga Community Hospital

Cincinnati
Bethesda Hospital
Children's Hospital Medical Center
Good Samaritan Hospital
Jewish Hospital of Cincinnati
St. Francis-St. George Hospital
The Christ Hospital
University of Cincinnati Hospital

Cleveland
Cleveland Clinic Foundation Hospital
Deaconess Hospital of Cleveland
Huron Road Hospital
Lutheran Medical Center
St. Alexis Hospital
St. Vincent Charity Hospital
University Hospitals of Cleveland

Columbus
Children's Hospital
Grant Hospital
Mt. Carmel Health Centers
Ohio State University Hospitals
Riverside Methodist Hospital

Dayton
Good Samaritan Hospitals and
Health Centers
Miami Valley Hospital
St. Elizabeth Medical Center

Dover
Union Hospital Association

Elyria
Elyria Memorial Hospital

Gallipolis
Holzer Medical Center

Kettering
Kettering Medical Center

Lima
St. Rita'sMedical Center

Lorain
St. Joseph's Hospital

Marion
Marion General Hospital

Mayfield Heights
Hillcrest Hospital

Medina
Medina Community Hospital

Middlebury Heights
Southwest General Hospital

Oregon
St. Charles Hospital

Parma
Parma Community General Hospital

Revenna
Robinson Memorial Hospital

Sandusky
Firelands Community Hospital
Providence Hospital

Springfield
Community Hospital of Springfield and Clark County
Mercy Medical Center

Sylvania
Flower Memorial Hospital

Steubenville
Ohio Valley Hospital

Toledo
Medical College of Ohio Hospital
St. Vincent's Medical Center

Urbana
Mercy Memorial Hospital

Warren
Trumbull Memorial Hospital

Wright-Patterson AFB
USAF Medical Center

Xenia
Greene Memorial Hospital

Youngstown
Northside Medical Center
St. Elizabeth Hospital Medical Center

OKLAHOMA

Ada
Valley View Hospital

Bartlesville
Jane Phillips Episcopal Memorial Medical Center

Chickasha
Grady Memorial Hospital

Muskogee
Muskogee General Hospital

Oklahoma City
Baptist Medical Center of Oklahoma
Mercy Health Center
Oklahoma Children's Memorial Hospital
Oklahoma Memorial Hospital
Presbyterian Hospital
South Community Hospital
St. Anthony's Hospital

Okmulgee
Okmulgee Memorial Hospital Authority

Shattuck
Newman Memorial Hospital

Shawnee
Shawnee Medical Center Hospital

Tulsa
Hillcrest Medical Center
St. Francis Hospital
St. John's Hospital Medical Center

OREGON

Albany
Albany General Hospital

Clackamus
Sunnyside Medical Center—Kaiser Foundation

Corvallis
Good Samaritan Hospital

Eugene
Sacred Heart General Hospital

Grants Pass
Josephine General Hospital

Klamath Falls
Merle West Medical Center

Medford
Providence Hospital
Rogue Valley Memorial Hospital

Oregon City
Williamette Falls Community Hospital

Pendleton
St. Anthony Hospital

Portland
Bess Kaiser Medical Center
Emanuel Hospital
Good Samaritan Hospital and Medical Center
Oregon Health Sciences University
Portland Adventist Medical Center
Providence Medical Center
St. Vincent Hospital and Medical Center
Veterans Administration Medical Center

Salem
Salem Hospital

Tualafin
Meridian Park Hospital

PENNSYLVANIA

Allentown
Allentown Hospital
Leigh Valley Hospital Center
Sacred Heart Hospital

Altoona
Altoona Hospital
Mercy Hospital

Bethlehem
St. Luke's Hospital

Bryn Mawr
Bryn Mawr Hospital

Danville
Geisinger Medical Center

Drexel Hill
Delaware County Memorial Hospital

Easton
Easton Hospital

Erie
Hamot Medical Center

Franklin
Franklin Regional Medical Center

Greensburg
Westmoreland Hospital

Greenville
Greenville Hospital

Hersey
Milton S. Hersey Medical Center

Johnstown
Conemaugh Valley Memorial Hospital

Lancaster
Lancaster General Hospital
St. Joseph Hospital

Lansdale
North Penn Hospital

Latrobe
Latrobe Area Hospital

Lewistown
Lewistown Hospital

Natrona Heights
Allegheny Valley Hospital

New Castle
Jameson Memorial Hospital

Norristown
Montgomery Hospital
Sacred Heart Hospital

Paoli
Paoli Memorial Hospital

Philadelphia
Albert Einstein Medical Center—
Northern Division
American Oncologic Hospital
Children's Hospital of Philadelphia
Episcopal Hospital

Graduate Hospital of the University
of Pennsylvania
Hahnemann University Hospital
Hospital of the University of Pennsylvania
Jeanes Hospital
Medical College of Pennsylvania
Hospital
Mercy Catholic Medical Center
Mt. Sinai—Daroff Division
Northeastern Hospital of Philadelphia
Pennsylvania Hospital
Temple University Hospital
Thomas Jefferson University Hospital

Pittsburgh
Allegheny General Hospital
Children's Hospital of Pittsburgh
Eye and Ear Hospital of Pittsburgh
Magee-Women's Hospital
Mercy Hospital of Pittsburgh
Presbyterian University Hospital
St. Francis General Hospital

Pottstown
Pottstown Memorial Medical Center

Pottsville
Pottsville Hospital and Warne Clinic

Quakerstown
Quakerstown Community Hospital

Reading
Community General Hospital
Reading Hospital and Medical Center
St. Joseph Hospital

Sayre
Robert Packer Hospital

Scranton
Mercy Hospital
Moses Taylor Hospital

Sellersville
Grand View Hospital

State College
Centre Community Hospital

West Chester
Chester County Hospital

Wilkes-Barre
Veterans Administration Medical
Center

Williamsport
Divine Providence Hospital
Williamsport Hospital

York
York Hospital

RHODE ISLAND

Newport
Naval Regional Center

Providence
Rhode Island Hospital

Warwick
Kent County Memorial Hospital

SOUTH CAROLINA

Aiken
Aiken Community Hospital

Anderson
Anderson Memorial Hospital

Charleston
Medical University of South Carolina Hospital

Columbia
Baptist Medical Center
Richland Memorial Hospital
William Jennings Bryan Doan Veterans Hospital

Florence
McLeod Regional Medical Center

Fort Jackson
Moncrief Army Hospital

Greenville
Greenville Hospital System

Greenwood
Self Memorial Hospital

Orangeburg
Orangeburg Regional Hospital

Spartanburg
Spartanburg General Hospital

SOUTH DAKOTA

Aberdeen
St. Luke's Hospital

Rapid City
Rapid City Regional Hospital

Sioux Falls
Sioux Valley Hospital

Watertown
Memorial Medical Center
St. Ann's Hospital

Yankton
Sacred Heart Hospital

TENNESSEE

Bristol
Bristol Memorial Hospital

Chattanooga
Erlanger Medical Center

Johnson City
Johnson City Medical Center Hospital

Kingsport
Holston Valley Hospital and Medical Center

Knoxville
East Tennessee Baptist Hospital
Fort Sanders Regional Medical Center
University of Tennessee Memorial Hospital

Memphis
Baptist Memorial Hospital
Methodist Hospital
Regional Medical Center

St. Francis Hospital
St. Jude Children's Research Hospital
University of Tennessee Medical Center

Millington
Naval Regional Medical Center

Mountain Home
Veterans Administration Medical Center

Nashville
George W. Hubbard Hospital of Meharry Medical College
Metropolitan Nashville General Hospital
Vanderbilt University Hospital

TEXAS

Amarillo
High Plains Baptist Hospital
Northwest Texas Hospital
St. Anthony's Hospital
Veterans Administration Medical Center

Beaumont
St. Elizabeth Hospital

Big Spring
Veterans Administration Medical Center

Carswell
USAF Regional Center

Corpus Christi
Memorial Medical Center
Naval Regional Medical Center
Spohn Hospital

Dallas
Baylor University Medical Center
Methodist Hospitals of Dallas
Parkland Memorial Hospital
Presbyterian Hospital of Dallas
St. Paul Hospital

El Paso
Providence Memorial Hospital
R.E. Thomason General Hospital
William Beaumont Army Medical Center

Fort Sam Houston
Brooke Army Medical Center

Galveston
University of Texas Medical Branch Hospitals

Harlingen
Valley Baptist Medical Center

Hereford
Deaf Smith General Hospital

Houston
Ami-Park Plaza Hospital
Ben Taub General Hospital
M.D. Anderson Hospital and Tumor Institute
St. Joseph Hospital

Lackland Air Force Base
Wilford Hall USAF Medical Center

Lubbock
Lubbock General Hospital
Highland Hospital
Methodist Hospital

McAllen
McAllen Methodist Hospital

Midland
Midland Memorial Hospital

Odessa
Medical Center Hospital

Plainview
Central Plains Regional Hospital

San Angelo
Angelo Community Hospital

San Antonio
Audie E. Murphy Memorial Veterans Hospital
Medical Center Hospital

Santa Rosa Medical Center
Southwest Texas Methodist Hospital

Temple
King's Daughters Hospital
Olin E. Teague Veterans Center
Scott and White Memorial Hospital

Waco
Hillcrest Baptist Hospital
Providence Hospital

Wharton
Gulf Coast Medical Center

UTAH
Murray
Cottonwood Hospital

Salt Lake City
Holy Cross Hospital
Latter-Day Saints Hospital
St. Mark's Hospital
University of Utah Hospital
Veterans Administration Medical Center

West Valley City
Pioneer Valley Hospital

VERMONT
Bennington
Southwestern Vermont Medical Center

Burlington
Medical Center Hospital of Vermont

Randolph
Gifford Memorial Hospital

Rutland
Rutland Regional Medical Center

VIRGINIA
Alexandria
Alexandria Hospital

Arlington
Arlington Hospital
Northern Virginia Doctors Hospital

Big Stone Gap
Lonesome Pine Hospital

Charlottesville
University of Virginia Hospital

Chesapeake
Chesapeake General Hospital

Danville
Memorial Hospital

Fairfax
Commonwealth Hospital

Falls Church
Fairfax Hospital

Fredricksburg
Mary Washington Hospital

Hampton
Veterans Administration Medical
   Center

Harrisonburg
Rockingham Memorial Hospital

Leesburg
Loudoun Memorial Hospital

Low Moor
Alleghany Regional Hospital

Lynchburg
General-Marshall Lodge Hospitals
Virginia Baptist Hospital

Manassas
Prince William Hospital

Martinsville
Memorial Hospital of Martinsville

Newport News
Riverside Hospital

Norfolk
DePaul Hospital
Norfolk General Hospital

Portsmouth
Maryview Hospital
Naval Regional Center
Portsmouth General Hospital

Richmond
Medical College of Virginia Hos-
   pitals
.Richmond Memorial Hospital
St. Mary's Hospital

Roanoke
Community Hospital of Roanoke
   Valley
Roanoke Memorial Hospital

Salem
Lewis-Gale Hospital
Veterans Administration Medical
   Center

Suffolk
Louise Obici Memorial Hospital

Virginia Beach
Virginia Beach General Hosptial

Winchester
Winchester Memorial Hospital

WASHINGTON

Aberdeen
Grays Harbor Community Hospital
St. Joseph Hospital

Anacortes
Island Hospital

Auburn
Auburn General Hospital

Bellevue
Overlake Memorial Hospital

Bellingham
St. Joseph Hospital
St. Luke's General Hospital

Bremerton
Harrison Memorial Hospital
Naval Regional Medical Center

Coupeville
Whidbey General Hospital

Everett
General Hospital of Everett
Providence Hospital

Kennewick
Kennewick General Hospital

Kirkland
Evergreen General Hospital

Longview
Monticello Medical Center
St. John's Hospital

Mount Vernon
Skagit Valley Hospital

Olympia
St. Peter Hospital

Pasco
Our Lady of Lourdes Hospital

Puyallup
Good Samaritan Hospital

Seattle
Children's Orthopedic Hospital and
    Medical Center
Group Health Coop Central Hos-
    pital
Highline Community Hospital
Providence Medical Center
Swedish Hospital Medical Center
Virginia Mason Hospital

Sedro Woolley
United General Hospital

Spokane
Deaconess Medical Center
Sacred Heart Medical Center

Tacoma
Madigan Army Medical Center
Tacoma General Hospital

Vancouver
Southwest Washington Hospitals

Walla Walla
St. Mary Community Hospital
Walla Walla General Hospital

Wenatchee
Wenatchee Valley Clinic

Yakima
St. Elizabeth Hospital
Yakima Valley Memorial Hospital

WEST VIRGINIA

Charleston
Charleston Area Medical Center

Clarksburg
Louis A. Johnson Veterans Admin-
    istration Medical Center

Huntington
St. Mary's Hospital
Veterans Administration Medical
    Center

Morgantown
West Virginia University Hospital

Parkersburg
Camden-Clark Memorial Hospital

Wheeling
Ohio Valley Medical Center
Wheeling Hospital

WISCONSIN

Appleton
Appleton Medical Center
St. Elizabeth Hospital

Cudahy
Trinity Memorial Hospital

Eau Claire
Luther Hospital
Sacred Heart Hospital

Fond du Lac
St. Agnes Hospital

Green Bay
St. Vincent Hospital

Janesville
Mercy Hospital

La Crosse
La Crosse Lutheran Hospital
St. Francis Hospital

Madison
Madison General Hospital

Marshfield
Marshfield Clinic/St. Joseph's Clinic

Milwaukee
Columbia Hospital
Good Samaritan Medical Center
Milwaukee County Medical Complex
Mount Sinai Medical Center
St. Francis Hospital
St. Joseph's Hospital
St. Luke's Hospital
St. Mary's Hospital
St. Michael's Hospital
Veterans Administraion Medical Center

Monroe
St. Clare Hospital

Oshkosh
Mercy Medical Center

Waukesha
Waukesha Memorial Hospital

Wausau
Wausau Hospital Center

West Allis
West Allis Memorial Hospital

WYOMING
Cheyenne
De Paul Hospital
Memorial Hospital of Laramie County

PUERTO RICO
Mayaguez
Mayaguez Medical Center

Ponce
Hospital Damas
Hospital Oncologica Andres

San Germán
Hospital de la Concepcion

San Juan
I. Gonzales Martinez Oncologic Hospital
University Hospital
Veterans Administration Medical Center

Where can I get articles on cancer subjects?

Articles which appear in the most popular nontechnical magazines and journals are listed in the *Readers' Guide to Periodical Literature* or in the *Public Affairs Information Service*. These are usually available in most public libraries. Look in the index under the subject you are interested in—or, if you know it, under the author's name.

Where can I find articles which are in health-science journals?

The *Index Medicus*, which is found in medical libraries, most university and college libraries, and some public libraries, lists articles appearing in over 2,400 health-sciences journals. The National Library of Medicine's MEDLARS program gives you access to CANCERLINE, a computerized database system which contains:

- CANCERLIT: 400,000 citations and abstracts of articles from technical literature since 1963 on all aspects of cancer.
- CANCEREXPRESS: A selective database of recent articles from 400 high-quality biomedical journals.
- CANCERPROJ: Summaries of over 20,000 ongoing cancer research projects federally and privately funded during the most recent 3 fiscal years; foreign and domestic studies also listed.
- CLINPROT: Small, highly specialized file. Primarily designed for the clinical oncologist engaged in development and testing of clinical protocols. Database is over 4,000 descriptions of clinical investigations of new agents. Includes patient-entry criteria, therapy regimens, special study parameters. These databases and PDQ (Physician Data Query) are programs of the National Cancer Institute.

What are the addresses of the public information offices of the various governmental institutions concerned with cancer or cancer-related subjects?

Office of Cancer Communications
National Cancer Institute
Building 31, Room 10 A 30
Bethesda, MD 20014
301-496-6631

(Information on National Cancer Institute programs—research and patient services, public information and education materials)

International Cancer Information Center
National Cancer Institute
Bethesda, MD 20205
301-496-7403

(CANCERLINE, PDQ, computerized databases)

Food and Drug Administration
Office of Consumer Affairs HFE-88
Room 16-63
5600 Fishers Lane
Rockville, MD 20857
301-443-3170

(Federal regulations on drugs, food additives, polyvinyl-chloride food containers, etc.)

Consumer Products Safety Commission
5401 Westbard Avenue
Washington, DC 20207
Toll-free: 800-638-CPSC

(Questions about potential hazards of commercial products)

Office of Information
Department of Labor
Occupational Safety and Health
    Administration
Washington, DC 20210

(Work-related hazards)

Public Information Center, PM-215
Environmental Protection Agency
401 M Street, S.W.
Washington, DC 20460

(Hazards in the environment, out-
    side of industry)

Office on Smoking and Health
Park Building, Room 1—10
5600 Fishers Lane
Rockville, MD 20857
301-443-5287

Industrial Union of Metal Trades
    Department of AFL-CIO
815 16th Street, N.W.
Washington, DC 20006

(Asbestos control, insurance mat-
    ters)

National Institute of Neurological
    and Communicative Disorders
    and Strokes
Office of Scientific and Health
    Reports
Building 31, Room 8A06
National Institutes of Health
Bethesda, MD 20205
301-496-5751

(Brain tumors)

References

AMERICAN CANCER SOCIETY. *A Cancer Source Book for Nurses.* American Cancer Society, 1985.
——*A Manual for Practitioners.* 1982.
——*Cancer Facts and Figures.* 1986.
BAKER, LYNN S. *You and Leukemia—A Day at a Time.* Rochester, Minn.: Mayo Comprehensive Cancer Center, 1976.
BEAHRS, O.H., AND MYERS, M.H., eds. *Manual for Staging of Cancer.* Philadelphia: J.B. Lippincott Co., 1983.
BELSKY, MARVIN S., AND GROSS, LEONARD. *How to Choose and Use Your Doctor.* Greenwich, Conn.: Fawcett Publications, 1975.
BUDOFF, P.W. *No More Menstrual Cramps and Other Good News.* New York: Penguin Books, 1983.
CAMERON, E., AND PAULING, L. *Cancer and Vitamin C.* Menlo Park, Calif.: Linus Pauling Institute of Science and Medicine, 1979.
COPE, OLIVER. *The Breast: Its Problems—Benign and Malignant and How to Deal with Them.* Boston: Houghton Mifflin, 1977.
COWLES, JANE. *Informed Consent.* New York: Coward, McCann and Geoghegan, 1976.
DE VITA, V.T., HELLMAN, S., AND ROSENBERG, S.A. *Cancer: Principles and Practice of Oncology.* Philadelphia: J.B. Lippincott Co., 1985.
——*Important Advances in Oncology,* 1986
EISENBERG, HOWARD, AND SEHNERT, KEITH W. *How to Be Your Own Doctor—Sometimes.* New York: Grosset and Dunlap, 1975.
FISCHER, D.S., AND MARSH, J.C., eds. *Cancer Therapy.* Boston: G.K. Hall, 1982.
FJERMEDAL, G. *Magic Bullets.* New York: Macmillan, 1984.
FREDERICKS, CARLTON. *Breast Cancer: A Nutritional Approach.* New York: Grosset and Dunlap, 1977.
FREESE, ARTHUR S., AND GLABMAN, SHELDON. *Your Kidneys, Their Care and Their Cure, A Modern Miracle of Medicine.* New York: E.P. Dutton, 1976.

924

HOLLAND, JAMES F., AND FREI, EMIL III. *Cancer Medicine*. Philadelphia: Lea and Febiger, 1983.

HOLVEY, DAVID N., ed. *The Merck Manual of Diagnosis and Therapy*. Rahway, N.J.: Merck, Sharp & Dohme Research Laboratories, 1982.

ISSELBACHER, K.J., ADAMS, R.D., BRAUNWALD, E., PETERSDORF, R., AND WILSON, J.D., eds. *Harrison's Principles of Internal Medicine*. New York: McGraw-Hill, 1980.

JOHNSON, B.L., AND GROSS, J. *Handbook of Oncology Nursing*. New York: Wiley & Sons, 1985.

JOHNSON, TIMOTHY G. *What You Should Know About Health Care Before You Call a Doctor*. New York: McGraw-Hill, 1975.

KNOBF, M.K., FISCHER, D.S., AND WELCH, D. *Cancer Chemotherapy Treatment and Care*. Boston: G.K. Hall, 1984.

KUBLER-ROSS, ELISABETH. *On Death and Dying*. New York: Macmillan, 1969.

——*Questions and Answers on Death and Dying*. New York: Macmillan, 1974.

KUSHNER, ROSE. *Alternatives*. Cambridge, Mass.: Kensington Press, 1984.

LAWS, PRISCILLA W. *X-Rays: More Harm Than Good?* Emmaus, Pa.: Rodale, 1977.

MELLUZZO, P.J., AND NEALON, E. *Living with Surgery*. Philadelphia: Saunders, 1981.

NATIONAL CANCER INSTITUTE. *What You Need to Know About Cancer—Site Pamphlets and Research Reports*. Bethesda, Md.: The National Cancer Institute, Department of Health, Education and Welfare, 1985–86

——*Breast Cancer Digest*. 1984.

——*Cancer Rates and Risks*. 1986.

——*Coping with Cancer—A Resource for Health Professionals*. 1980.

——*PDQ, Patient Education and State of the Art Statements*, 1986.

PEPPER, C.B. *We the Victors*. Garden City, N.Y.: Doubleday, 1985.

ROSENBAUM, E.H., AND ROSENBAUM, I.R. *Comprehensive Guide for Cancer Patients and Their Families*. Palo Alto, Calif.: Bull Publishing Company, 1980.

RUBIN, PHILIP, ed. *Clinical Oncology for Medical Students and Physicians*. Rochester, N.Y.: American Cancer Society, 1983.

SEAMAN, BARBARA, AND SEAMAN, GIDEON. *Women and the Crisis in Sex Hormones*. New York: Rawson, 1977.

SHIMKIN, MICHAEL B. *Science and Cancer*. New York: U.S. Department of Health, Education and Welfare, 1973.

TIME-LIFE BOOKS EDITORS. *Fighting Cancer*. Alexandria, Va.: Library of Health, Time-Life Books, 1981.

U.S. DEPARTMENT OF HEALTH, EDUCATION AND WELFARE. *Cancer Mortality in the United States*. Bethesda, Md.: Public Health Service, 1982.

In the process of reading and using this book, questions which are not included in it may come to your mind. The authors would be most pleased if you would share your thoughts with them.

Kindly send any comments to:

Eve Potts, Marion Morra
c/o Avon Books
1790 Broadway
New York, New York 10019

MARION MORRA is the Assistant Director of the Yale Comprehensive Cancer Center at the Yale University School of Medicine in New Haven, Connecticut. She is also Assistant Clinical Professor at the Yale School of Nursing, teaching graduate-level classes in communications and health marketing. Marion is widely published, having written articles and authored books for both the health professional and the public, with emphasis on health and especially on the field of cancer. She serves on several major national committees for the National Cancer Institute and the American Cancer Society.

EVE POTTS has been a medical writer for more than 30 years. Her expertise is in making difficult medical information easy to understand. She has been director of Advertising and Medical Education for Spencer, Incorporated, served as a medical writer and consultant to the Department of Health and Human Services, written medical monographs for drug companies and served as a writer and consultant for public relations and educational writer and consultant for public relations and educational material for a wide variety of medical institutions.

The two authors, who are sisters, have collaborated on two books: *Understanding Your Immune System* (Avon, 1986) and the first edition of *CHOICES* (1980). They live and work in Connecticut.

Index

ACS, see American Cancer Society
ACTA scans, 98
AFTER, Ask a friend to explain
Reconstruction Organization, 380
AIDS, 284, 451
ALL (Acute Lymphocytic Leukemia),
445, 714, 716-25
ANLL, Myelomonocytic leukemia,
445, 453, 449
ANLL, Acute nonlymphocytic
leukemia, 445
AZT, 285
Abdominal Cancer, types (chart), 502
Acid Phosphatase Test, in prostate
cancer, 613
Acoustic neuroma, 703
Actinomycin D, 221
Acupuncture, 751, 764
Acute crythroleukemia, 445
Acute granulocytic leukemia, 445
Acute lymphatic leukemia, 445
Acute lymphoblastic leukemia, 445
Acute lymphocytic leukemia (ALL),
445, 714, 716-25
Acute lymphocytic leukemia in
children, 710, 445
Acute myelocytic leukemia (AMOL),
445
Acute myelogenous leukemia, 445
Acute nonlymphocytic leukemia, 445
Acquired Immune Deficiency
Syndrome, 284, 451
Adenocarcinoma, 317
Adenoma, colon, 504

Adenoma, in lung, 391
Adenosis, DES exposure, 597-603
Adjuvant treatment, 116
Adoptive immunotherapy, 22
Adrenal glands, 673
Adrenalectomy, 610, 621
Adriamycin, 221
Adrucil, 219
Adult Leukemia, 446-69
Air-contrast, x-rays, 75
Alkeran, 218
Alkylating agents, 203
Alkylating Agents, charts, 216-18
Allopurinol, 460
Alpha particles, 277
Alvizatos, Dr. Hariton, 302
American Board of Anesthesiology,
140
American Board of Colon and Rectal
Surgery, 132
American Board of Neurological
Surgery, 133
American Board of Obstetrics and
Gynecology, 133
American Board of Ophthalmology,
134
American Board of Orthopedic
Surgery, 134
American Board of Otolaryngology,
134
American Board of Pathology, 102
American Board of Plastic Surgery,
132

American Board of Psychiatry and
  Neurology, 133
American Board of Radiology, 78, 164
American Board of Surgery, 131
American Board of Thoracic Surgery,
  132
American Board of Urology, 135
American Cancer Society, 833-34
  getting help, 834
  how to reach, 834-35
  interferon, 272
  listing by states, 835-38
  Reach to Recovery, 841
  services, 834
American College of Surgeons,
  approved cancer program, 23
American Group Practice Association,
  16
American Medical Directory, 13
American Red Cross, caring for
  patient at home, 803
Amethopteria, 220
Anal region, 503
Androgens, chemotherapy, 255
Anemia, chemotherapy, 243, 244
Anesthesia, 136-43
  dangers, of, 136
  doctor, 21-22
  how administered, 142
  questions to ask, 121
  types of, 136
  wearing off, 147-48
Anesthesiologist, 21-22, 140
  board certified, 140
  discussion with, 140
  questions to ask, 141-42
Anesthetist, 21-22, 139
Angiogram, 700
Antibiotics, chemotherapy drugs
  (charts), 216-231
Antibodies,
  monoclonal, 72, 266, 267, 268
Antigens, 266
Antimetabolites, 204
  chart of, 220
Anus, male ill., 612
Appetite, loss of, 774 (Also, see
  Eating)
Armpit temperature, 804
Arsenic, skin cancer, 418
Arteriogram, 76
Asbestosis, 394
Ascending colon, 503
Ask a Friend to Explain
  Reconstruction, 380

Aspiration biopsy, 102, 105
Aspiration, bone marrow, 109, 458
Aspiration curettage, 577
Aspirin, in pain treatment, 766-67
Astler-Coller method, 509
Astrocytoma, 695, 701
Attitude, 6-7
Autopsies, 814
Azidothymidine, 285

BCG, 267, 283
BCNU, 226
Bacillus Calmette Guerin, 283
Back rub, 807
Bag, bladder cancer, 527
Bahamas, clinic, 298
Baker, Lynn S, 725
Balance problems, see Symptoms
Baltimore Research Center, 884-85
Barium enema (B.E.), 75
Barium swallow, 76
Barium x-rays, 502
Basal cell, skin cancer, 419-20
Bed bath, 807-808
Bedsores, care and prevention, 806
Bedwetting, use of plastic bag,
  808-809
Bence-Jones protein, 488
Beneficient Euthanasia, 798
Benign tumors, 46
Best's Insurance Reports, 820
Bilateral orchiectomy, 620
Bilateral salpingo oopherectomy, 553,
  588
Biofeedback, 239, 752, 764, 766
Biological response modifiers, 266
Biopsy, 102-109
  aspiration, 102, 105
  bone marrow, 109
  doctor, 102-103
  endoscopic, 102
  excisional, 102, 104-105
  frozen section, 106
  incisional, 162, 165
  needle, 102, 106
  outpatient, 107
  permanent section, 107
  punch, 102
  reading, 103-104
  second opinion, 69
  total, 102
  wide bore needle, 106

Bischlorethyl nitrosourea, 226
Black cancer, malignant melanoma, 429-30
Bladder cancer, 518-29, 524 (chart)
 bag, 522
 depression, 529
 diagnosis, 520
 doctor, 19
 ileal conduit, ileal loop, 526
 incision, 526
 living with bag, 527
 metastasis, 519
 papillary, 519
 precautions before operation, 526
 recurrence, 520
 segmental resection, 525
 sexual relations, 529
 staging, 523
 stoma, 526
 symptoms, 518-19
 transurethral resection, fulguration, 524-25
 treatment, 523-24
Bladder Cancer Project, 527
Bladder tumors, benign, 519
Blasts, meaning of counts, 456
Bleeding, 564
Bleeding between periods, causes, 578
Bleomycin, 220
Bleeding, in mouth, 649
 premenopausal, 578
Blenoxane, 220
Blood-brain barrier, 707-708
Blood cells, in leukemia, 447
Blood, doctor, 18
Blood in rectum, 502
 in stool, 502
 tests, 70
 tests, chemotherapy, 241
 tests for diagnostic cancer, 70
 tests, Leukemia (chart), 455-56
 types, 143
Blood stool test, 73
Bloody urine, 502
 chemotherapy, 239
Blue Cross/Blue Shield, health policies, 822
Board Certification, 13
Board certified, see American Board of
Body shields for radiation, 168
Bone Cancer, children, 714-15, 729-32
 aspiration, 109, 458
 children, amputation, 731

children, tests, 710, 712
 doctor, 18, 134
 metastasis, 731
 replacement grafts, 731
Bone marrow biopsy, 109, 458-59
Bone marrow damage, chemotherapy, 241
Bone marrow depression, 242, 457
Bone marrow test, 88
Bone marrow, transplant, 466
Bone marrow trephine, 459
Bone scan, 92
Bone scan and breast cancer, 110
Bowel habits, change in, 508
Bowens Disease, 422
Brain, doctor, 19, 133
 scan, 93
 surgery, aftereffects, 707
 tumors, 693-708
 tumors, benign, 698-99
 tumors, children, 714, 731-32
 tumors, encapsulated, 698
 tumors, operations, 705-706
 tumors, metastatic, 695, 700, 704
 tumors, tests, 693
 tumors, treatment, 699-707
 tumors, types, 695
 benign tumors, 311
 biopsy, outpatient, 332
 charts, 304-306
 dimpling or puckering, 305
 examining, 316-17
 frozen section vs. regular biopsy, 333
 inverted nipples, 314
 lump, calling doctor, 321, 434
 lumps, how to check, 304-305, 316-20
 lumpy, 313-24
 nipple discharge, 314
 nipple retraction, 305, 314
 two step procedure, 332-33
 questions to ask doctor, 306, 309-10
 cancer, alternatives, 325
 cancer, biopsy, inpatient or outpatient, 332
 cancer, with control pills, 315-16
 cancer, bone scan, 110
 cancer, breast feeding, 315
 cancer, chemotherapy drugs used, 349
 cancer, diet, 315, 316
 cancer, fibrocystic disease, 313
 cancer, if not removed, 350

cancer, inflammatory, 342
cancer, high risk, 303-304
cancer, hospital care following
  mastectomy, 366
cancer, lymph node involvement,
  335
cancer, in men, 311
cancer, moveable tumors, 314-15
cancer, radiation, 309, 371, 736
cancer, radium implant, 341
cancer, second opinion, 321
cancer, staging, 340-41
cancer, surgical (excisional) biopsy,
  331
cancer, symptoms, 304
cancer, terms (chart), 337-41
cancer, tests, 308-309
cancer, transillumination, 329
cancer, treatment choices, 348-49
cancer, ultrasound use, 97
Breast cancer,
  immunotherapy, 373
Breast prosthesis, radiation
  treatments, 186
Breast, questions to ask yourself, 306
Breast reconstruction, 375-79
  after radiation, 378
  cost, 380
  doctor, 379-80
  long after mastectomy, 377
  questions to ask doctor, 375
Brompton cocktail, pain treatment,
  761
Bronchogram, lung cancer, 76, 386,
  398
Bronchoscopy, lung cancer, 86, 386,
  397
BSO, 278
Burton, Dr. Lawrence, 298
Burzynski, Dr. Stanislaw, 301
Busulfan, 216

CANCERLIT, 922
CANCERPROJ, 922
CAT scans, 98
CBC, 70
CCNU, 194
CDDP, 216
CEA, 72-73, 226, 507
CEA tests, diagnosis, 72
CIS, see Cancer Information Service
CLINPROT, 922
CML, treatment, 463-64

CLL, 462-63
CT Scan, 98, 392
  brain tumor diagnosis, 699
  how done, 98
  lung cancer, 398
  radiation dose, 101
  preparation for, 100
  uses, 101
Canada, National Cancer Institute,
  Cancer Society, 862
Cancer
  adrenocortical, 532
  choriocarcenoma, 585-86
  clinical cooperative groups, 31
Cancer, age, statistics, 52
  benign, 39-40
  breast, 303-80
  brain, 692-709
  cell, 38-39
  cervix, 550, 553, 563-86
  children, 710-42
  classifications, 47-48
  contagion, 54
  cure, 49
  differentiated, 43-44
  doctor, 19
  doubling time, 43
  dysplasia, 42
  fallopian tubes, 551, 586
  family risk, 53
  female reproductive organs, 547-48
    chart, 550-51
    doctor, 547-48
    new treatment, 547
  heredity, 52
  hormone dependent, 254-55
  in situ, 48
  insurance, 825
  invasive, 48
  localized, 48
  malignant, 41-42
  metastatic, 48
  number of cells, 43
  ovary, 551, 552, 586-93
  penis, 605, 630-35
  prostate, 605-623
  rate of growth, 43
  risk of second, 53-54
  slow growing vs. fast growing, 41
  size, in centimeters, 50
  smell, 54
  spinal cord, 692-94, 704-705
  spread, 51
  symptoms, 54

testicle, 606-610, 623-28
two-step, 44
types of, 46-48
undifferentiated, 42
uterine tubes, 551, 586
uterus, 550, 553, 563-84
vagina, 548, 550, 559-62
viruses, 45
vulva, 548, 550, 554-59
warning signs, 54
what it is, 38-58
womb, 548, 550, 576-82
Cancer articles, how to find, 921-22
Cancer Center, clinical, 23, 29-30
comprehensive, 23, 29-30
clinical, listed by states, 856-90
comprehensive, listed by states,
856-90
laboratory, 31
non-clinical, by states, 856-90
Cancer Information Service, 262,
831-32
Cancer physical, definition, 69
Cancer Society, see American Cancer
Society
Candlelighters, 725, 838
Carbon dioxide laser, 279
Cataracts, radiation, 185
Catheter in operations, 145
Carbohydrates, adding to diet, 777
Carcinoma, 47, 48
Carmustine, 226
Catheter, indwelling, 208
Caudal anesthesia, 138
Cecostomy, 512
CeeNU, 226
Cells, differentiated, 42
dysplasia, 42
normal vs. abnormal, 38
number of, 43
undifferentiated, 42
Cells, drug-resistant, 210
Centrifuge, continuous flow, 460
Cerebellum, 695-96, 697
Cerebral angiogram, 76
Cerebrum, 696, 697
Cervical cancer, 550, 553, 563-86
age, 565
cryosurgery, 574
conization, 571, 574
diagnosis, risks, 550, 564
eletrocoagulation, 573
in situ, 569
pregnancy, 574, 576

staging, 572
treatment, 429-74
Cervix, dysplasia, 569
function, 548
precancerous conditions, 569
Chayne-Stokes respiration, 813
Cheek, cancer of, 636, 639, 647, 656-57
Chemosurgery, 124
Chemotherapist, 21
Chemotherapy, 200-261
alcoholic beverages, 212-13
alkylating agents, 203
antibiotics, 220
antimetabolites, 204
blood cells, 241-42
blood counts, 241-42
bloody urine, 239-40
bone marrow damage, 241
brain tumors, 707
combination, 206
constipation, 252-53
costs, 260-61
curative, 203
definition, 201-202
dental work, 213
developments in, 206-207
diarrhea, 253
doctor, 21
doses, 206
drugs used (chart), 216-31
dry skin, 249
eating, 233
effectiveness, 211-12
estrogen receptor tests, 255
experimental, 21
fingernails, 250
flu shots, 254
flu symptoms, 250
frequency of treatments, 211
hair loss, 235
heartburn, 250
hormone side effects, 249
hormones, 204
how given (chart), 216-31
how works, 201-202
injection, pain, 207
insurance coverage, 261
investigational drugs, 258, 228-31
(chart)
wigs, 236-37
Phase III drugs, 258
pumps, 208-209
length of side effects, 215
leucovorin rescue, 253-54

loss of effectiveness, 210
malignant melanoma, 435
marijuana, 234
menstrual problems, 246-47
metallic taste, 250
methods, 205, 206
mouth sores, 240
National Cancer Institute
  investigational trials, 259
natural products, 204
nausea and vomiting, 235
  nerve and muscle problems, 246
  new drugs, 256
  nurse's role, 204
  personality changes, 250
  Phase I drugs, 257
  Phase II drugs, 257
  plant alkaloids, 220
  precautions for blood problems,
    243-44
  pregnancy, 247
  prescribing doctor, 204
  protocols, 260
  questions to ask, 201
  regional perfusion, 211
  randomized trials, 260
  serious side effects, 215
  sexual relations, 248-49, 246
  shingles, 254
  side effects (chart) 216-31
  skin cancer, 428
  skin rashes, 249
  skipping treatments, 212
  sunburn, 253
  testicular cancer, 627
  tired feelings, 241
  urine color, 239
  uses, 202
  vaccinations, 254
  vaginal infections, 247
  veins, 250
  weight gain, 252
  weight loss, 235
  working while taking, 212
  with other medicines, 213
Chest drainage equipment, 409
Chest surgeon, 132
Chicken pox in leukemia, 724
Childhood cancer, 709-42
  discussing with child, 738-39
  financial help, 740
  handling anger, 739
  telling others, 739-40
  tests, 710-12

questions to ask, 713
Chlorambucil, 216
Choice, treatment, 117
Cholesteatomas, 695, 702
Cholesystogram, 76
Choriocarcinoma, 585
Chronic granulocytic leukemia, 444
Chronic lymphocytic leukemia, 444
Chronic myelocytic leukemia, 444
Chronic myelogenous leukemia, 444
Chronic myelosis leukemia, 444
Cirrhosis of the liver, 538-39
Cis-diamminedichloroplatinum, 216
Cis-platinum, 216
Clinical cancer center, 23, 29
Clinical cancer centers, by states,
  856-860
Clinical center, National Institute of
  Health, 32
Clinical cooperative groups, 31
  chairmen, 861
  Europe, 862
  National Cancer Institute, 29
Clinical diagnostic staging, 56
Clinical trials, how conducted, 256-57
Clinics, Freeport, Bahamas, 298
CML, 444, 452 (Chronic myelocytic
  leukemia)
CLL, 444 (Chronic lymphocytic
  leukemia)
Cobalt-60, 192
Cobalt treatment, see Radiation
Cocktail, Brompton, 761
Coin lesion, 405
Cold knife conization, 552, 571, 574
Colloid goiter, 666
Colon, ascending, 503
Colon, doctor, 18, 19
Colon, 503
Colon-rectal cancer (chart), 502
  chemotherapy, 517
  digestion, 514
  groups studying, 516-517
  stages, 509
  surgeon, 132
  surgery, 508
Colostomy, 511-12
  bag, 515-16
  caring for, 515-16
  diet, 515
  double barrel, 512
  permanent, 512
  sexual relations, 516
  supplies, Medicare, 517

support groups, 516-17
temporary, 512
transverse-loop, 512
Cold spot, 93
Colposcope, 84, 570, 599
Colonoscopy, 502
Colposcopy, 559, 570, 571
Combination chemotherapy, 206
Committee on Pain Therapy and
    Acupuncture, 892
Complete blood count,
    chemotherapy, 241-42
Comprehensive cancer center, 23,
    29-30
    second opinion with, 68
    addresses, 853-56
Computerized tomography, 98-99
Concern for Dying, 798
Congenital tumors, of brain and
    spinal cord, 695, 700, 702
Conization, 550, 571-74
    colposcopy, 571
    pregnancy, 574
Consent forms, patients' rights, 37
Consolidation therapy, 458
Constipation, chemotherapy, 252-53
    eating to prevent, 782
Consultation, asking for, 68
    cost, 67
    medical school for, 66
    vs. referral, 68
    who pays, 67
    who treats, 67
Consumer inquiries, 922
Consumer Products Safety
    Commission, 922
Contagion, 54
Contraceptive pills, FDA warning on,
    593-94
Contrast films, x-rays, 75
Contributions, how to make, 814
Convulsions, see Symptoms
Coordination loss, see Symptoms
*Coping at Home with Cancer, for
    patients, by a parent,* 740
Coping when cancer spreads or
    comes back, 743-71
Coping with Diagnosis, 2-3
Cordotomy, percutaneous, for pain,
    752, 769, 770
Coronary angiogram, 76
Cortisone acetate, 223
Cosmegen, 221
Costs, chemotherapy, 260-61

of laetrile, 247
Cotrell, Nina, 740
Counter immunoelectrophoreses, test
    for prostate cancer, 614
Cramps, food suggestions, 777-78
Cranial nerves, 696
Craniopharyngiomas, 695, 702
Craniotomy, 705
Cryosurgery, 124
    after effects, 575
    cervical cancer, 574
    follow-up, 576
    menstruation, 576
    procedure, 575
    skin cancer, 427
    sexual relations, 575-76
    symptoms to report, 575
Curative treatment, 716
Cure, 49
Curette, in skin cancer, 427
Cyanide, 240
Cyclohexyl chloroethyl nitrosourea,
    226
Cyclophosphamide, 217
Cyclotron, 163, 276
Cyst, 40
Cyst, ovarian, 586-90
Cystectomy, 525
Cystic mastitis, 313
Cystoscopy, 502
Cytarabine, 218
Cystic teratoma, 702
Cystogram, 76, 502
Cystoscope, 84
Cystology, 88, 592
    kinds of tests, 88
Cytokines, 267, 273
Cytosar-U, 218
Cytosine arabinoside, 218
Cytoxan, 217

D & C, 576-77
DAT, 464
DEM, 278
DES, 223, 225, 571, 594-603
    cancer of the female reproductive
        system, 571, 594-603
    daughters, cancer, 571
    daughters, colposcopy, 571, 598-603
    daughters and doctor's findings, 596
    daughters, estrogens, 601
    daughters, examination, 597
    daughters' risk, 597-603
    daughters, treatment, 596-603

daughters, precaution for
  treatment, 601
drugs, list of, 594-95
mothers, estrogens, 601
mothers, mammograms, 601
mothers, precautions, 601
sons, 594-602
use today, 594
DTIC, 217
Dacarbazine, 217
Dacey, Norma, 830
Dactinomycin, 221
Daunomycin, 221
Daunorubicin, 221
Death, see also Dying
Death, decision not to prolong dying,
  798
Death, Dying and the Biological
  Revolution, Our Last Quest for
  Responsibility, 798
Deep breathing, after operation, 151
Delalutin, 225
Department of Labor Office of
  Information, 923
Depo-Provera, 225
Depression, bladder cancer, 529
  treatment worse than disease, 772
Dexamethasone, 223
Dermatologist, 18
Dermoids, 695, 702
Descending colon, 503
Diagnosis, biopsy, 102
  bone marrow test, 88
  bronchoscopy, 86
  clinical history and physical, 70
  complete blood count, 70-71
  colonoscopy, 86-87
  comprehensive cancer center vs,
    regular hospital, 29-30
  coping with, 2-5
  cytology, 88
  ECG, EKG, electrocardiogram, 73
  endoscopy, 84
  endometrial aspiration, 88
  esophagoscopy, 87
  facing, 1-2
  fluid tests, 88
  Hemocult, 73
  length of time for, 62
  lumbar puncture, 74
  Pap smear, 88, 89
  proctosigmoidoscopy, 86
  radioactive scans, 89
  SMA 12, 70

second opinion, 65
serum factors, 70
spinal tap, 74
sputum test, 88
tests, delaying surgery for, 62
tests, done over, 62
tests, high risks, 77
tests, kinds, 61-62
tests, questions to ask doctor, 59
tests, risks, 62
ultrasound, 94
urine analysis, 70
urine sediment test, 88
vaginal pool aspiration, 88
x-rays, 74-75
Diagnostic radiologist, 21, 164
Diagnostic tests, 59-111
Diarrhea, chemotherapy, 253
  eating suggestions, 781
  radiation treatment, 176, 187
Diet, see also Eating
  during radiation treatments, 182
Diethylstilbesterol, 223, 225, 571,
  594-603
Differential count, meaning, 463-64
Differentiated tumor, 42, 130
Digital rectal exam, 502-506
Dilation and curettage, 576-77
Dimpling or puckering of the breast,
  305
Directory, lawyer referral service, 829
Directory, medical specialist, 13, 15
Discussing cancer, dealing with anger,
  802
  group discussions, 787-88
  protecting others' feelings, 789
  protecting children from knowing,
    788
  telling child's teacher, 788
  with children, 739-40
  with relatives, friends, neighbors,
    787
Discussing death, with doctor, 796-97
Doctor, see also Surgeon
  anesthesiologist vs. anesthetist,
    21-22
  board certified, 73
  board eligible, 14
  brain, spinal cord, 694
  breast biopsy, 332
  breast cancer, 310
  breast reconstruction, 379
  childhood cancer, 712-13
  credentials, 12-13

dermatologist, 18
endocrinology, 18
family practice, 12
female reproductive organs, 547-48
GI, 18
gastrointestinal cancer, 18
groups, 18
hematology, 18
how to choose, 8-22
hospital affiliation, 9, 16
internist, 18
judging (chart), 9-12
leukemia, adult, 443
long cancer, 382
medical school teacher, 66
nephrology, 18
neurology, 18
ophthalmology, 19
orthopedic surgery, 19
oncology, 20
otoloryngologist, 18
pathologist, 19
plastic surgery, 19
pediatrician, 18
proctology, 19
psychiatrist, 18-19
pulmonary disease, 18
radiologist, 21
radiation specialist, 163-64
   skin cancer, 339
solo practice, 17
specialties, described, 18-19
surgeon, 19
specialist, 16
testicular cancer, 625
thoracic surgery, 19
therapeutic radiologist, 163
urology, 19
younger vs. older, 19
Donating your body, or parts, 830
Dosimetrist, 164
Doubling time, 43
Double barrel colostomy, 512
Double blind studies, 259
Dronabinol, 234
Drug-resistant cells, 210
Drug treatment, see Chemotherapy
Drugs, cancers used for (chart),
   216-32
chemotherapy (chart), 216-32
evaluation, 257
immunotherapy (chart), 226
investigational chemotherapy
   (chart), 228-32

National Cancer Institute
   Investigational trials, 259
pain treatment, 569
randomized trials, 260
Dry skin, chemotherapy, 249
Duke's method, 509
Dumping syndrome, 536
Duodenal ulcer vs. stomach ulcer, 534
Duodenoscopy, 87
Dying, 788-801, 811-15
autopsies, 814
books to read, 798-800
contribution in memory, 814
final stage, 813
Hospice, 799
helping patient die in comfort, 812
making decision where to die,
   798-99
signs of impending death, 813
when friends stop visiting, 797
when hospital wants to prolong
   life, 812
Dysphagia, 689
Dysplasia, 42, 569, 597

ECAT scan, 99
ECG, EKG, Electrocardiogram test,
   73
ENT, 18, 134
Ear nerve, cancer of, 703
Ear, nose and throat, doctor, 18, 134
Eating, 773-84
calorie information, 784
constipation, 782
cramps, 782
high carbohydrate, 777
high fat, 777
low fat foods, 778-79
mouth and throat sores, 779
protein, 783
radiation treatments, 179, 182
roughage, 782
to prevent diarrhea, 781
to prevent nausea and vomiting,
   778-78
ways to increase appetite, 775-76
weight loss, 777
Edema, mastectomy, 358
Effector cells, 267
Electric needle, in skin cancer, 428
Electrocautery biopsy, 427
Electrocoagulation, cervical cancer,
   573

Electrode implants, for pain control, 752, 763
Electroencephalogram, 699
 Electron volts (ev), 162
Electrosurgery, 123-24
Embryonal carcinoma, 625
Emission computerized axial tomograph, 99-100
Emotions, doctor, 18
Encore, mastectomy group, 839
Endoscopy, 84
Endocrine System, 673
Endocrinology, 18
Endometrial cancer, aspiration curettage, 577
Endometrial aspiration, 88
Endometrial aspirator, 577
Endometrial cancer, 548, 556, 576-84
 diagnosis, 576
 D&C, 576-77
 dilation and curettage, 576-77
 staging, 579
 treatment, 550, 579
Endometrial hyperplasia, 577-78
Endometriosis, 577
Endoscopic biopsy, 102
Endoxan, 217
Environmental Protection Agency, 923
Ependymoma, 695, 701
Epidermoid carcinoma, 385
Epidural anesthesia, 138
Epidural dorsal column stimulator, 752, 768
Epiglottis, 680
Epipodophyllotoxin, 229
Erythrocytes, meaning of counts, 456
Esophaegeal cancer, 688-91
Esophagectomy, 690
Esophagogastroduodenoscope, 84
Esophagoscopy, 689-90
Esophagus, cancer of, 636, 640, 688-91
 staging, 690
Estinyl, 225
Estrogen cream, face, 592
 vaginal, 592
Estrogen receptor test, 255
Estrogen, controversy over, 590-94
 FDA warnings, 593
 bone loss, 592
 chemotherapy, 285-86
 DES (list), 594-95
 length of use, 591
 oophorectomy, 590-94
 risk, 590-603

Ethmylestradiol, 225
Evaluation, of drugs, 257
Ewings Sarcoma, 714, 728-29
 groups studying, 652
 tests, 714, 728
Examination, by medical student, 28, 34
Excisional biopsy, 102, 104-105
Exercises, mastectomy, 355-56
Exfoliate cytology, 533
Experimental drugs, chemotherapy, 21
Experimental treatment, see also Investigational treatment
 informed consent, 118
 questions to ask, 293
Exploratory chest operation, 387, 407
External beam radiation, 154, 155
Eye, cataracts, and radiation, 185
 doctor, 19
 problems, see Symptoms
 surgeon, 134
 tumors, in children, 714, 733-36

F.A.C.S., 131
Face cream with estrogens, 592
Facing the diagnosis, 1-2
Fallopian tubes, cancer of, 551, 554, 586
 treatment of cancer, 586
Family practice, 18
Fat, adding high fat foods to diet, 777
Fear, of cancer recurring, 786
Feeling tired, radiation side effect, 179
Fees, 22
Fellow, American Board of Surgeons, 131
Female hormones, chemotherapy, 255
Female reproductive organs, doctor, 19
 cancer of, 547-603
 questions to ask your doctor before having operation, 547
 DES, 594-603
Fiber in diet, 782
Fibrocystic disease, 313
Fibroid tumors, 424
Fibroma, nasopharyngeal, 658
Fibromas, skin, 424
Finances, and doctor, 22
 help, 828

Fingernails (dark), chemotherapy, 250
5-Azacytidine, 228
5-Fluorouracil, 219
5-FU, 219
  in skin cancer, 428
Flu shots, chemotherapy, 254
Flu symptoms, chemotherapy, 250
Fluorouracil, 219
Fluid tests, 88
Fluoroscope, 81
Fluoxymesterone, 224
Food and Drugs Administration, (FDA), Bureau of Radiological Health, 172, 289
  clinical trials, 256-57
  estrogen prescription warnings, 593
  Office of Consumer Inquiries, 922
  oral contraceptive pill warning, 593-94
Foodpipe, see Esophagus
Foods, see Eating
Fullness, 502
Freezing, surgery, 124
Frozen section biopsy, 106-107, 333

GI, see also Gastrointestinal
GI series, 76
GI tract, doctor, 18
Gallium scan, 90, 94, 309
Gamma rays, see Radiation
Ganglion, 424
Gastrectomy, 536
Gastrointestinal cancer, 500-545
  doctors, 501
  high risk groups, 500
  new treatments, 503
  questions to ask, 501
  symptoms, 500
  chart, 502
  tests, 500-501
Gastroscopy, 87, 502
General anesthesia, 137
German Cancer Research Center, 301
Gershanovich, Dr. M.L., 300
Glioblastoma multiforme, 695, 701
Glioma, 700
Goiters, colloid, 666, nodular, 666
Gold, 192
Gold, Dr. Joseph, 300
Grafts, skin, doctor, 439
  skin, types of, 438-39
Granulocytes, meaning of counts, 456
Greek cancer cure, 302

Group insurance, 821
Group practice, 8, 16
Guaiac test, 507
Guilt feelings, 811, 814
Gums, cancer of, 637, 639, 647, 657
Gynecological cancer, see also Cancer, female reproductive organs
  ultrasound use, 97
Gynecological exam and douching, 567
Gynecological oncologist, 130
Gynecologist, 133

HMO, Health maintenance organizations, 17, 826
HN2, 217
Hair loss, chemotherapy, 235
Hair pieces, and chemotherapy, 237-38
Halotestin, 224
Halsted mastectomy, 339
Headaches, see Symptoms,
Head, cancer of, 635-91
  diagnostic tests, 639-40
  treatment, 639-41
  types, 639
Head and neck cancer, chart, 639-40
  doctor, type of, 635
  new treatments, cancer institute, 636
  questions to ask, 635
Health Insurance (chart), 815
  comparisons, 820-21
  Institute, 820
Health Maintenance Organization, 17, 826
Health services, how to find, 802
Health changes, see Symptoms
Heartburn, chemotherapy, 250
Heat treatments, 282
Heating pad, caution against use after radiation, 767
Hemangiomas, 423-24
Hematocrit, meaning of counts, 456
Hematology, 18
Hemimastectomy, 333
Hemocult, 507
  blood stool test, 73
Hemoglobin, meaning of counts, 456
Hemorrhoids, 507
Heredity, 53
Heroic measures, 812
Hexamethylmelamine, 230

High risk, diagnostic tests, 77
High spinal anesthesia, 131
Histiocytomas, 425
History, clinical, how taken, 69
Hodgkin's disease, 470-82
    alcoholic pain, 478
    in children, 714
    lymphocyte depletion, 476
    lymphocyte predominance, 476
    mixed cellularity, 476
    mononucleosis, 479
    nodular sclerosis, 476
    outlook, 480
    questions to ask, 472
    Reed-Sternberg cells, 477, 479
    removal of spleen, 470
    risk factors, 470
    staging of, 479, 480
    symptoms, 470, 477
    tests, 471-72
    treatment, 480-81
Home care, 798-814
Home Care, 803
Home care courses, American Red
    Cross, 803
Home care, applying sterile dressing,
    805-806
    bed bath, 807
    bedsores, 806
    calling doctor, 811
    creating restful atmosphere, 805
    giving back rub, 807
    giving medicines, 809
    giving a shower, 808
    hospital bed, 806
    incontinence, 808-809
    leg cramps, 806
    preventing bedsores, 806
    services available, 802-804
    setting up patient's room, 803-804
    shaving, 808
    taking temperatures, 804
    teeth and mouth care, 808
Home Health Agencies, directory of,
    803-804
Home health benefits, 816
Homemaker services, 785
Hormone dependent cancers, 254-55
Hormones, chemotherapy, 204
    chart, 223
    estrogen receptor tests, 255
    therapy, for thyroid cancer, 669-70
    treatment, side effects, 249
Hospice, 799, 839-40

Hospice Action, 800
Hospital, accredited, 23
    admittance on weekends, 36
    approved cancer program, 23
    big city vs. non profit private, 34
    care in teaching hospital, 34
    clinical cancer center, 23, 31, 856-96
    comprehensive cancer center, 23,
        853-56
    for profit, 24
    good vs. bad, 33
    government supported, 24
    how to choose, 23-37
    judging, 23
    location, 25
    medical school affiliation, 33
    not accredited, 24
    number of beds, 24
    nurses, 35
    proprietary, 24
    public, 24
    questions to ask before leaving, 122
    questions to ask when in, 121-22
    research projects, 28
    services, 25
    size and care, 34
    teaching, 34
    teaching vs. non teaching, 22, 28
    VA, 24
Hospital bed for use at home, 806
    internal radiation, 194
Hospital insurance, 815-27
Hospital, medication errors, 37
    records and patients' rights, 36
Hot spots, scans, 93
How to Avoid Probate, 830
HTLV, 45-46
HTLV-1, 451
Human investigation committee, 260
Human leukocyte interferon, 272
Hunger, lack of, 774-75 see also
        Eating
Hydatidiform mole, 585
Hydroxyprogesterone caproate, 225
Hyperkeratosis, 422
Hyperplasia, 569
    endometrial, 577
Hyperthermia, 263, 281-82, 283
    local, 282
    total body, 282
    where treatment being tested, 283
Hypnosis, as pain treatment, 234, 751,
        764, 765
Hypopharynx, cancer of, 640, 660

Hypophysectomy, 610, 622
  transphenoidal, 708
Hypoxic cells, 277
Hysterectomy, 550, 579-84
  aftereffects, 581-84
  diagnostic tests before, 581
  fibroid tumors, 580
  menstrual periods, 581
  operation, 579-80
  radiation treatment for, 584
  radical, 552
  and sexual relations, 581
  subtotal, 552
  supracervical, 552
  total, 552, 380-81
  vaginal, 552, 581
  weight gain, 584
Hysterogram, 76
Hysteroscope, 84

IAL, 840
ICRF-159, 231
I Can Cope, 840
Ileostomy, 512-13
Ileum, 512
Imidozole, 217
Immune system, 263-65
Immunology, 263
Immunotherapy, 263-64, 373, 886
  BCG, 283
  Bacillus Calmette Guerin, 283
  immune system, 263, 264-65
  questions to ask, 216
  skin cancer, 428, 436
Immunomodulatory agents, 267
Impaired speech, see Symptoms
Implants, artificial testicle, 632
Impotence
  prostate cancer, 617
  bladder cancer, 529
In situ, 48-49, 569
Incisional biopsy, 102, 104
Incision, mastectomy, care, 353-54
Incontinence, ways to deal with
  problem, 808-809
Index Medicus, 921
Induction therapy, 457-58
Indwelling catheter, 208
Infection, doctor, 18
Infection, vaginal, 247
Infectious diseases, 18
Information, finding cancer articles,
  921

Informed choice, surgery, 127
Informed consent, 118
Informed consent, chemotherapy
  drugs, 259
Inhalation anesthesia, 137
Insurance, 815-27
Insurance, cancer, 825
  chart, 815-17
Insurance coverage, chemotherapy,
  261
  for prosthesis, mastectomy, 365
Insurance group, 821
Insurance, health maintenance
  organization (HMO), 826
Insurance, mail order policies, 825-26
Insurance Policy chart, 816-17
Insurance, tax deductions, 826
  turned down claims, 826
Intercourse, see Sexual relations
Interferon, 266, 272, 285
Interleukin, 267, 268-69
Interleukin-2, 285
Internal radiation, see also Radiation
  treatment, internal
Internal radiation, 154, 191-99
  length of treatment, 193
  materials used, 192
  pain with, 196-97
  permanent implant, special
    precautions, 198
  precautions for radioactive iodine
    therapy, 198
  precautions following treatment,
    197
  radioactivity of person, 194
  removal of, 196
  special diets for, 196
  unsealed sources, 197
  visitor restrictions, 195, 199
International Association of
  Laryngectomees, 683, 688, 840
International Union Against Cancer,
  840
Interstitial implant, 192
Intestines, doctor, 18
Intracavity implant, 192-93
Intraoperative radiation therapy, 274
Intravenous anesthesia, 138
Intravenous feeding, and operations,
  145
Invasive cancer, 48
Intravenous pyelogram (IVP), 76
Investigational drugs, chemotherapy
  (chart), 228-32

Investigational treatments, 228-32, 258, 262-92, 293-97
  chemotherapy drugs, 228-32, 257-58
  difference between unproven and investigational, 294-95
  groups doing (listing), 641-79
  immunotherapy, 263-264
  informed consent, 118
  interferon, 272
  hyperthermia, 281-82
  standards for, 295-96
  testing, 295-96
  types of, 295
  questions to ask, 293-94
  vs. unproven methods, 296-97
  Vitamin C, 286
Iodine-131, 192
Irradiation, see Radiation
Irridium-192, 192
Irritated skin, radiation, 180

Janker Clinic, 301
Jaundice, 502
Joint Commission on Accreditation for Hospitals, 23, 24
Judging your attitude, 6-7
Judging your doctor, 8

Kahler's disease, 487
Kaposi's sarcoma, 285-86
Kelly, Orville E., 785, 841
Keratosis, 420
Kidney cancer, 502, 529-30, 713, 715, 735-36
  chart, 502
  diagnosis, 529
  in children, 713, 715, 716
  operation, 531
  symptoms, 530
  treatments, 532
Kidneys, doctors, 18
Kilovolts (Kev), 162
Kissing cancer patient, 54, 410
Kohl, Marvin, 798
Kubler, Ross, Elisabeth, 798

L-Pam, 218
Laetrile, 300
LAK cells, 268-69
Laminar-air flow units, 245
Laparotomy, 20, 542

Laparatomy, in lymphoma diagnosis, 474
Laparoscope, 84
Large cell carcinoma, 385
Large intestine, 503
Laryngectomee, 682
Laryngectomy, 677-80
  hospital procedures, 681
  partials, 680-81
  total, 681
Laryngoscopy, 679
Larynx, cancer of, 632, 640, 674-88, 455, 461
  non-malignant growths, 678
Laser therapy, 278-79
  carbon dioxide, 279
  Nd-YAG, 279
Lavamisole, 267
Lawyers, writing will, 829
Leg cramps, exercises for, 806
Lentigo maligna melanoma, 434
Leucovorin rescue, chemotherapy, 253-54
Leukemia, acute granulocytic, 445
  acute lymphatic, 445
  acue lymphoblastic, 445
  acute lymphocytic, 445
  acute myelocytic, 445
  acute myelogenous, 444
  adult T-cell, 444, 450
  adult, 446-70, (chart), 444-45
  adult, classifications, 449
  adult, kind of doctor, 446
  adult, questions to ask, 446
  ALL, 445, 449, 714, 716-25
  ANLL, 445, 449, 453
  blood cells, 447
  blood tests, meanings, 455
  bone marrow aspiration, 458
  bone marrow transplant, 466-69
  chicken pox exposure, 724
  childhood (chart), 445
  childhood information, 725
  childhood, length of treatment, 723
  childhood leukemia, 445
  childhood, relapse, 722
  childhood, remission, 723
  childhood, symptoms, 714, 719
  chronic granulocytic, 444
  chronic myelocytic, 444
  chronic myelogenous, 444
  chronic myelosis, 444
  CLL, 444, 450, 462
  CML, 444, 450, 452

consolidation therapy, 458
drugs, DAT, 464-65
drugs, VAPA, 464
drugs, VP, 464
erythroleukemia, 445
extramedullary, 443
hairy cell, 444, 450
immunotherapy, 461
induction herapy, 457-58
lymphoid, 445
maintenance therapy, 458
myelomonocytic, 445
new treatments, 443
promyelocytic, 444
  causes of, 451
  chemotherapy and, 451
  highest risks, 443, 451
  pre leukemia, 449
  smoldering leukemia, 449
  cats and, 452
  stages of, 453-54
spicules, 459
splenectomy, 460
symptoms, 443
treatment, 463-65, 461
trouble passing urine, 460
vaccinations, 721
Leukopheresis, 245, 460
Leukeran, 216
Leukocytes, meaning of counts, 456
Leukopenia, chemotherapy, 242
Leukoplakia, 422
  mouth, 648
  vagina, 559
  vulva, 555
Lienography, 76
Limited mastectomy, 338
Linear accelerator, 162
Lip, cancer of, 636, 639, 647, 651-53
Lip shave, 652
Lipoma, 423
Living Bank, donation of body or
  body parts, 830
Living will, 798
Liver, benign tumors, 538
  cirrhosis, 538-39
  doctor, 18
  function, 536-37
  ultrasound use in, 97
Liver metastases, 538
Liver cancer, 536-39
  (chart), 502
  diagnosis, 539
  symptoms, 538

  treatment, 538
Liver scan, 93, 502
Liver spots, 425
Livingston-Wheeler Clinic, 299-300
Livingston, Dr. Owen, 299
Livingston, Dr. Virginia Wheeler, 299
Lobectomy, 406, 670
Localized cancer, 48
Localized radiation, 158
Lomustine, 226
Lost Cord Clubs, 688
Lower pharynx, cancer of, 636, 639,
  659-60
Low spinal anesthesia, 138
Lumbar puncture, 74
Lumpectomy, 338, 343, 347
Lung, description, 383
  doctor, 18
  incision for removal, 407
  operation, 406
  cancer, 381-410
  cancer, asbestos, 394
  cancer, biopsy, 386, 399
  cancer, bronchogram, 386, 398
  cancer, bronchoscopy, 386, 397
  cancer, coin lesion, 405
  cancer, contagious, 410
  cancer, deciding against surgery,
    405, 407
  cancer, deflating lung, 387
  cancer, different kinds of, 385
  cancer, doctor, 382
  cancer, exploratory chest
    operation, 387, 407
  cancer, granuloma, 390
  cancer, high risk factors, 381-82
  cancer, industrial pollutants, 393-94
  cancer, mediastinoscopy, 386,
    399-400
  cancer, mesothelioma, 394-95
  cancer, metastases, 406
  cancer, metastatic workup, 387, 402
  cancer, new treatments, 383
  cancer, non-cancerous growths, 391
  cancer, operability, 392
  cancer, pulmonary function test,
    386, 399
  cancer, questions to ask doctor, 382
  cancer, radiation following surgery,
    401-402
  cancer, radiation prior to surgery,
    401
  cancer, Sputum cytology test, 386,
    396

cancer, stages, 403
cancer, surgery, when recommended, 402
cancer, symptoms, 382
cancer, tests, 395
cancer, tests (chart), 386-87
cancer, thorascoscopy, 387
cancer, thoracotomy, 387, 406
cancer, tomogram, 386, 398
cancer, when spread to chest wall, 402
Lung operation, arm and leg exercise, 409
chest drainage equipment, 409
coughing after, 408
shortness of breath, 410
Lung tumor, symptoms, 390, 392-93
benign, 391
result of spreading, 391
Lymph nodes, enlarged, 477
surgery, 345-46
Lymph system, role in body, 473
Lymphangiogram, 76, 474
Lymphangiography, 474
Lymphoid leukemia, 445, 449, 455, 461, 632, 646, 674-88, 714, 716-25
Lymphokines, 267, 273
Lymphokineactivated killer cells, 268-69
Lymphoma, 447-48, 470-89
children, 714
classifications, 476
diagnosis, 473
female patients, questions to ask, 472
importance of staging, 476
laparatomy, 474
male patients, questions to ask, 472
malignant, 473-87
outlook, 387
polycythemia vera, 489
pregnancy, 477
presenting as leukemia, 724
Sjorgren's Syndrome, 489
studies, 652
symptoms, 470
treatment, 474

MEDLARS, National Library of Medicine, 922
MEDLINE, 922
Macrobiotic diet, 297, 298
Macrophages, 267

Magnetic resonance imaging, 401
Maintenance therapy, 458
Major Medical insurance, 816, 820
Make Today Count, 785-86, 841
Male hormones, chemotherapy, 255
Male organs (chart), 605, 608-610
Male organs, studies, 607
surgeon, 134-35
Malignant lymphoma, 473-87
Malignant melanoma, 413, 429-30
kind of doctor, 434
metastasized, 434
staging, 436
Malignant tumors, 41-42
Mammogram, controversy over, 325
cost of, 328
preparation for, 327
radiation doses, 324-25
Mammography, 308, 321
ultra sound, 328
Mammogram, x-ray, 83
Mammoplasty, 341
Marinol, 234
Mastectomy, adjusting to loss, 368-69
back pads, 363
bathing suits, 366-67
breast reconstruction, 375
care of arm, 358
caring for incision, 353-54
estrogen receptor test, 372
exercising arm, 355-56
extended radical, 340
follow-up visits, 370
Halsted, 339
immunotherapy, 373
nipple reconstruction, 377
modified radical, 339, 347, 349
partial, 338
pregnancy, 373
prosthesis, 360-61
quadrant, 338
radical, 339, 341, 349
Reach to Recovery, 354
segmental, 343, 347
sexual relations, 366-67
simple, 339, 351
special bras, 362-63
subcutaneous, 341
supraradical, 340
swollen arms, 357
symptoms following operation, 359
terminology (chart), 337-41
wedge resection, 338
Mastectomy forms, covers, 363

Mastectomy scar, self-consciousness, 366-67
Mastectomy prosthesis, kinds, 363-64
Marijuana, with chemotherapy drugs, 234, 388
  in pain control, 762
Matulane, 227, 251
Maxillofacial prosthesis, 645
Maxillofacial prosthodontist, 645
Mayo Clinic, Vitamin C, 286, 718
MEA, 278
Mechlorethamine, 217
Mediastinoscopy, 386, 399-400
Mediastinotomy, 400
Medical expenses, deductive costs, 82
  state sales taxes, 827
  record keeping, 827
Medical DIRECTORY, analyzing information, 15
  using, 14
Medical Insurance, see Insurance
Medical School Outpatient Clinic, second opinion, 66
Medical oncologist, 21, 204
Medicines, keeping track of, 809
Medicaid, coverage, 822
Medicare, coverage, 822-23
Medicare, Plan A, 816, 820
Medicare, Plan B, 816, 820
Medroxyprogesterone acetate, 225
Medulla oblongata, (111), 696, 697
Medulloblastoma, 695, 701
Megace, 225
Megestrol acetate, 225
Megavoltage machine, see Radiation treatment
Megavolts (Mev), 162
Melanoma, diagnosing, second opinion, 434
  evaluation before treatment, 435
  lentigo maligna, 434
  malignant, 413, 429-30
  nodular, 434
  studies, 651
  superficial spreading, 434
  treatment, 435
Meningioma, 695, 700, 702
Melphalan, 218
Menstrual cycles, chemotherapy, 246-47
Mesothelioma, 394-95
Metallic taste, chemotherapy, 250
Metastases, tests for, 110
Metastases, bladder cancer, 519

Metastasis, brain cancer, 695, 700, 704
  lung, 391
Metastatic cancer, 48
Metastatic workup, 92
  lung cancer, 386, 402
Mets, 51, 391
Methosarb, 224
Methotrexate, 220, 253
Metropolitan Life Insurance Company, 804
Miscellaneous chemotherapy drugs, (chart), 225-27
Mithracin, 221
Mithramycin, 221
Mitomycin, 222
Mitotane, 226
Molds, for radiation, 169
Moles, 431
Monoclonal antibodies 72, 266, 267, 268
  melanoma, 436
Mononucleosis, 479
Morphine, in pain treatment, 761
Mouth sores, chemotherapy, 240
  eating suggestion, 779
MRI (magnetic resonance imaging), 99
Multi-specialty groups, 16
Muscle weakness, see Symptoms
Mustargon, 217
Mutamycin, 222
Myelogram, 705
Myeloma, 487
  studies, 652
Mycosis fungoides, 413, 414, 440
  studies, 652
  staging, 440-41
  treatment, 441
Myeloma, 47, 48, 76
  anemia, 488
  Bence-Jones protein, 488
  diagnosing, 487-88
  exercise, 488
  treatments, 488
Myomectomy, 552
Myleran, 216

Nasopharyngeal fibroma, 658
Nasopharynx, cancer of, 636, 639, 658-59
National Cancer Institute, 29, 30, 115
  Canada, 862-63
  clinical center admitting

procedure, 33
clinical centers, 29-30, 856-90
clinical cooperative groups, 31
clinical research groups, 31, 854-855
clinical treatment program, 31,
   854-855
comprehensive cancer centers,
   29-31, 854-56
finding cancer articles, 921
interferon, 272
investigational trials, 260
new drug tests, 256
non clinical centers, 31, 856-90
office of cancer communications,
   922
role in investigational treatments,
   295
studies, male ogans, 607
special studies for DES daughters,
   601
tests on Laetrile, 300
Vitamin C, 286
National Directory of Medicare
   Home Health Agencies, 804
National Hospice Organization, 800,
   839-40
National Institutes of Health Clinical
   Center, 32-33
National Institute of Health,
   admitting procedures, 33,
   668-674
   Clinical center, 33, 668-674
   payment, 31
Natural killer cells, 267
Natural products, chemotherapy, 204
   chart, 220-22
Nausea and vomiting, chemotherapy,
   233
   immunotherapy, 263-64
   radiation treatments, 172, 187
   use of marijuana, 234
Neck, cancer of, 635-69
   diagnostic test, 639-40
   radical dissection, 642-43, 650
   treatment, 639-40
   types, 639-40
Needle aspiration, breast cancer, 309
Needle biopsy, 102, 502, 667
Needle implant, 193
Neo-hombreol, 224
Nephrectomy, 531
Nephroblastoma, in children, 715, 736
Nephrology, 18
Nerve and muscle problems,

chemotherapy, 246
Nerve block anesthesia, 139
Nerve blocks, in pain treatment, 752
Nerve stimulation, transcutaneous,
   752, 768
Nerve root clipping, 753, 769
Nervous system, doctor, 18
Neuroblastoma,
   in children, 714, 731
Neurofibroma, 695
Neurology, 18
Neurological surgery, 19
Neurologist, 133
Neuroma, 695, 700, 702-703
Neurosurgeon, 133
Neutron beam, see Radiation
   treatment
Neutron-beam therapy, 275-76
Nevi, 431
New drugs, 256
New treatments, breast cancer, 310,
   311-312
   brain and spinal-cord cancer,
     692-707, 694
   cancer of female reproductive
     organs, National Cancer
     Institute, 547, 692-707, 853
   childhood cancer, 716
   gastrointestinal cancer, 503
   Hodgkin's disease, 473
   lung cancer, 383
   lymphomas, all types, 473
   non-Hodgkin's disease, 473
   rhabdomyosarcoma, 716
   skin cancer, 414, 648-74
   US regulations, 289-90
New Voice Club, 688
Nipple discharge, 305, 314
Nipple retraction, 305, 314
Nitrogen mustard, 217
Nolvadex, 227
Non clinical cancer centers, listed by
   states, 856-60
Non-Hodgkin's disease, 446, 470-89,
   714
   aggressive lymphoma, 483
   histocytic, 476
   in children, 714
   indolent lymphoma, 483
   mixed cell, 476
   multiple myeloma, 489
   poorly differentiated lymphocytic,
     476
   questions to ask, 472

tests, 471-72, 489
well differentiated lymphocytic, 476
Non-Hodgkin's lymphoma, doctor, 443
risk factors, 470
staging, 484-85
symptoms, 470
tests, 471-72
treatment, 486-89
Nose Cancer, 636, 639, 657-59
Nose, doctor, 18
Nuclear Medicine, American Board of, 90
Nuclear scans, 91
Nurses, aides, and assistants, 36
Nurses, chemotherapy, 22, 204
kinds in hospital, 35
licensed practical (LPN), 35, 36
National League of Nursing, 804
ostomy, 22
questions, 151-52
RN, 35
role, 22
visiting, 785
learning home care, 802-805
Nutrition, 773-84

Oat-cell carcinoma, 385
Obdurator, 645-46
Obstetrics, 19
Obstetrics and Gynecology, American Board of, 133
Occult stool test, 507
On Children and Death, 800
On Death and Dying, 798
Oncologist, gynecological, 20
Oncologist, medical, 21
radiation, 21
surgical, 120, 130
types of, 20-21
Oncology, 20
definition, 52
nurses, 22
Oncongenes, 44-45
Oreton, 224
Oncovin, 222
Oopherectomy, 552, 588
o,p¹-DDD, 226
Operating room, length of time in, 146-48
persons in, 146
Operation, see also Surgery

common problems, 149-50
deep breathing, 151
prepping, 145
procedures after, 148-49
procedures before, 144
questions to ask, 119-21, 122
soreness, 151
stitches out, 151
tests before, 143
Opthalmologist, 134
Opthalmology, 19
Ora-Testryl, 224
Oral cancer, 647-57
Orchiectomy, 610, 620-21, 627
Orchiectomy, bilateral, 610, 620-21
Oropharynx, cancer of, 636, 640, 654-60
Orthopedic surgeon, 19
Osteogenic sarcoma, 714, 729
Ostomy groups, 516-17
Ostomy nurse, 22
Ostomy Quarterly, 842
Ostomy, sexual relations, 516
Othovoltage machine, see Radiation treatment
Otolaryngologist, 18
Outpatient, ultrasound, 98
Ovarian cancer, 551, 553, 586-90, 649, 660
groups studying, 650
staging, 589
Ovarian cyst, 586-87
precautions before surgery, 586-90
treatment for, 590
Ovariectomy, 552, 590
Ovaries, removal of, 590

Pain, 148, 356-57, 751-63
advanced cancer, 751
aspirin use, 766-77
coping with, 751-63
describing to doctor, 754-55
drugs, after operation, 148
following mastectomy, 357-58
prescribing medication, 756-61
treatment of (chart), 751-52
relaxation exercise to relieve, 762-63
Palliative surgery, 123
Palliative treatment, 116-17
Pancreatic cancer, 387, 539-45, 853
chart, 502
cysts, 541

doctor, 18
metastasis, 542
operation, 542
risks, 543
symptoms, 540
tests, 541
treatment, 545
ultrasound use in, 97
Pancreaticoduodenectomy, 542
Pancytopenia, chemotherapy, 202
Papillary cancer of bladder, 519
Pap test, 429, 559, 564-69, 576, 578
accuracy, 89
after hysterectomy, 567
classes of, 567
diagnosis for uterine, ovarian,
fallopian tube cancer, 548, 566-69
douching, 567
first, 564
meaning of, 567
need for yearly, 564
preparation for, 567
uses, 89
uterine cancer, 578
Pap smears, see Pap test
Parathyroid gland, cancer of, 636,
673-74
Parenteral feeding, 810
Parents' Handbook on Leukemia, 725
Parosteal sarcoma, 730-31
Parotoid tumor, operation
procedures, 662
Parotoid gland, cancer of, 636, 639,
662-63
Particle beam radiation therapy, 275
Pathologist, 19, 102
Pathology report, second opinion, 69
Patient history, how taken, 69
Patient's rights, consent forms, 37
hospital records, 37
medication errors, 37
second opinion in, 68
x-rays, doses, 81-82
Payment, clinical cooperative groups,
31
PDL, repair inhibitors, 278
PDQ (Physician Data Query), 32, 290
Pediatrician, 18
Pediatric solid tumors, groups
studying, 6
Pelvic exenteration, 553
Penis, cancer of, 605, 630-33
metastasized, 633
Penumoencephalogram, 700

Percutaneous cordotomy, pain
treatment, 752, 770
Perineal prostatectomy, 608
Periods, see Menstrual
Permanent section biopsy, 107
Personality changes, see Symptoms
Petachiae, 243, 455
Phase I, II, III drugs, 257-58
Phenylalanine mustard, 218
Philadelphia chromosome, 452-53
Phlebitis, 409
Phosphorous 192
Photodynamic therapy, 280-81
Physical therapist, 784-85
Physician Data Query, 32, 290
Physicians, see Doctors
Piles, 507
Pill, the, and cancer, 593-94
Pi-meson, particles, see Radiation
treatment
Pituitary adenoma, 695, 700
Pituitary gland, 673, 708
removal in breast and prostate
cancer, 622, 708
Placenta, cancer of, 585
Plain films, x-rays, 75
Plant alkaloids (chart), 220-22
Plasmapheresis, 460
Plastic surgeon, 19, 132
Plastic surgery, head and neck
cancer, 644
Platelets, 448
Platelets, chemotherapy, 242, 243
meaning of counts, 457
Platinum, Cis, 216
Plummer-Vinson syndrome, 648
Pneumoencephalogram (PEG), 77
Pneumonectomy, 406
Polycythemia vera, 489
Polyp, 40
colon, 504
removal of, 504-505
Pons, 696
Postsurgical treatment—pathologic
staging, 55
Potassium, in diet, 782
Precancers, skin cancer, 420
Preclinical trials, new drugs, 256-57
Prednisolene, 223
Prednisone, 223
Pregnancy, after mastectomy, 373
after vulvectomy, 558
cervical cancer, 574
chemotherapy, 247

conization, 574
Pregnant women, cervical cancer in, 576
 DES type drugs used (list), 594-95
 radioactive scans, 94
Premenopausal bleeding and clotting, 578
Prepping for operation, 145
Prescriptions, meaning of abbreviations, 809-810
Preventive surgery, 123
Primary tumor, 51
Procarbazine, 251
Proctology, 19
Proctologist 132
Proctosigmoidoscopy, 84, 502, 506
Progesterone for bleeding, 578-79
Prognosis, 118
Prostate cancer, 604-23
 diagnosing, 606, 613
 groups studying, 622
 impotency, 617
 pituitary gland removal, 622
 questions to ask, 606
 staging, 616
 sterility in, 617
 symptoms, 605, 611, 613
 tests, 604
 treatment chart, 616
Prostate, removal, 609, 614
 tumors, 605, 611
Prostatectomy, 608-609, 614, 615
Prostatic Cancer Project, 64
Prosthodontist, maxillofacial, 645
Prosthesis, childhood bone cancer, 731
 head and neck reconstruction, 646
 mastectomy, see Mastectomy
Protein, adding to diet, 776
 needs, 783
Protocols, chemotherapy, 260
Proton particles, see Radiation treatment
Provera, 224
Psychiatrist, 18-19
Public information offices, 922-23
Pulmonary, see also Lung
Pulmonary angiogram, 76
Pulmonary function test, 386, 399
Punch biopsy, 102
Purinethol, 219
Pyelogram, intravenous, 76
Pyrimidine analogs, 278

Quality of survival, 118
Questions and Answers on Death and Dying, 800
Questions to ask, anesthesiologist, 121
 about chemotherapy, 201
 brain and spinal cord tumors, 693-94
 before investigational experimental treatment, 294
 breast reconstruction, 375
 childhood cancer, 713
 diagnosis, 60-61
 diagnostic tests, 60
 disability, surgical medical insurance, 818
 reproductive organs, 547
 following mastectomy, 352
 gastrointestinal cancer, 501
 head and neck cancers, 635
 Hodgkin's disease, 472
 immunotherapy, 262
 leukemia, adult, 446
 lung cancer, 382
 lymphoma, 472
 Non-Hodgkin's disease, 472
 prostate cancer, 606
 radiation, 153
 skin cancer, 412
 specialist, 65
 surgeon before operation, 119-21
 testicle, 607
 treatment, 112-13
 thyroid cancer, 663
 unproven treatments, 294
 when facing diagnosis, 60-61
 when in hospital, 121-22
 x-rays, 79

Radiation, adjuvant, 157
 amount in x-rays, 82
 and eye cataracts, 185
 brain tumors, 706
 choosing treatment center, 154
 curative, 156
 doses, mammogram, 322
 for relieving pain, 156
 internal, 154
 localized, 158
 malignant melanoma, 435
 oncologist, 21, 164
 palliative, 156
 primary, 156
 questions to ask, 153

types of (chart), 154
whole body, 158
Radiation physicist, 164
Radiation specialist, 145
Radiation therapist, 21
Radiation therapy nurse, 164
Radiation therapy technologist, 164
Radiation treatment, cause of thyroid
    tumors, 665
  diarrhea, 172, 187
  diet, 182
  doctors specializing in, 163-65
  dos and don'ts, 177-78
  doses, 165
  effects during, 171
  exposure, 171-72
  first appointment, 165
  feeling tired, 179
  followup, 189
  frequency, 169
  how done, 166
  how works, 157
  internal, 191
  machines used, 161
  marking of place, 166
  megavoltage machine, 162
  molds, 169
  most successful use, 157-58
  nausea and vomiting, 172, 187
  orthovoltage, 162
  particle beam, 163
  pregnant visitors, 172
  proton particles, 163
  radioactivity, 190-91
  safety, 168
  side effects (chart), 173-76
  side effects, 173-90
  special care after, 189
  sterility, 187
  superficial x-ray, 162
  supervoltage machine, 162
  swallowing difficulties, 183
  taking other medicine, 189
  tests, 170
  treatment plans, 169
  use of radioactive implants, 192
  when started, 159
Radical hysterectomy, 552
Radical neck dissection, 642-43, 650
  partial laryngectomy, 680
Radical surgery, 123
Radical vulvectomy, 553, 556
Radioactive iodine, 89
  special precautions, 198

Radioactive isotope, in cancer
    treatment, 192
Radioactive scans, diagnosis, 89
  substances, 89
Radiologist, 21
  board certification, 78
  diagnostic, 21
  diagnostic vs. therapeutic, 78-79
  therapeutic, 21
Radiology, see Radiation
Radio-resistant, 158
Radiosensitive, 158
Radiotherapist, 21, 163
Radiotherapy, see Radiation
Radium implant, 154
  for mastectomy, 341
  prostate, 609
  tongue cancer, 684
  vaginal cancer, 561
Radium needles, 192
Radium seeds, 192
Radium treatment, see Radiation
    treatment
Randomized trials, 260
Razoxane, 231
Razoxin, 231
Rads, definition, 82
Reach to Recovery, 354, 841
Reconstruction, breast, 377
Reconstructive surgery, head and
    neck cancer, 637
Recovery room, 147
Rectum, 504
  doctor, 18, 19
  female (ill.), 549
  male (ill.), 612
Rectal temperature, 804
Red blood cells, chemotherapy, 241
Red skin, radiation, 179-80
Reduction mammoplasty, 378
Reed-Sternberg cells, 477, 479
Referral, asking doctor for, 68
Referral vs. consultation, 68
Regional anesthesia, 137
Regional perfusion, 211
Regression, 49
Rehabilitation organizations, 828-29
Relaxation exercises, in pain
    treatment, 762-63
Rem, definition, 82
Remission, 49
  adult leukemia, 457
  childhood cancer, 722
  5 year, 49

Renal arteriography, 502
Reticulocytes, meaning of counts, 456
Reticuloedothelial cells, 441
Retinoblastoma, 714, 734-35
  tests, 714, 734
Retreatment, staging, 56
Retropubic prostatectomy, 608-609, 616
Rhabdomyosarcoma, 714, 736-38
  new treatments, 713, 716, 738
  tests, 712
Rhizotomy, 753, 770
Ribavirin, 285
RIL-2, 269
Risk factors, 50
  cancer of the vulva, 554
  gastrointestinal cancer, 500
Rubidomycin, 221

SMA-12, 70
Saddle block, 138
St. Jude Hospital, 725
Salivary glands, cancer of, 636, 639, 660-63
  treatment, 636, 660-63
Salpingectomy, 553
Sandwich technique, radiation, 159
Sarcoidosis, 390
Sarcoma, 47, 48
  osteogenic, in children, 714, 729-31
Sattilaro, Dr. Anthony, 297-98
Scans, CT, CAT, ACTA, 98, 392
  bones, 91-92
  brain, 93
  cold spot, 93
  gallium, 90
  hot spots, 93
  liver, 93
  pregnant women, 94
  radioactive diagnosis, 89
  thyroid, 93, 666
Scheef, Dr. Wolfgang, 301
Schiller's test, 550, 559
Seborrheic keratoses, 425
Sebaceous hyperplasia, 425
Second opinion, 69
  comprehensive cancer center, 68
  cost, 66
  diagnosis, 65
  different from first, 67
  how to find doctor for, 65
  how to get, 65

in hospital, 65
  medical school for, 66
  pathology report, 69
  research center, 68
  who pays, 67
Segmental resection, 338, 525
Seminoma, 625
Senile lentigo, 425
Serum factors, 70
Sex and the Male Ostomate, 516
Sex, Courtship and the Single Ostomate, 516
Sex, Pregnancy and the Female Ostomate, 516
Sexual changes, hormone treatments, 249
Sexual relations
  bladder cancer, 529
  chemotherapy, 246
  colostomy, 516
  cryosurgery, 575-76
  hysterectomy, 582
  ostomates, booklets available, 516-17
  ostomy, 516
  vaginal implant, 561
  vulvectomy, 558-59
  with cancer patient, 54
Sezary syndrome, 441
Shave, helping patient to, 808
Shingles, chemotherapy, 254
Shower, helping patient to, 808
Side effects, chemotherapy, 215, chart, 216-32
  radiation treatments, 173-89
  serious, chemotherapy, 215
Sigmoid colon, 503
Sigmoidoscopy, 502, 506
Simple vulvectomy, 553, 556
Sinus cancer, 636, 643, 657-59
6-MP, 219
6-Mercaptopurine, 219
6-Thioguanine, 220
Sjorgren's syndrome, 489
Skin cancer, 411-41
  actin keratosis, 413
  arsenic, 418
  basal cell, 413, 419
  blacks, 418
  Bowen's disease, 422
  chart, 413
  doctor, 18, 412
  fibroma, 424
  ganglion, 424

hemangiomas, 423-24
hyperkeratosis, 422
immunotherapy, 428
keratosis, 422
keratoaeanthoma, 422-23
leukoplakia, 422
lipoma, 423
malignant melanoma, 429
moles, 431
mycosis fungoides, 413, 414, 440
nevi, 431
new treatments, 413, 651
precancers, 420
protection against, 416
questions to ask, 412
recurrence, 428
removing growths, 426
risk factors, 411
sebaceous cysts, 424
skin graft, 438
squamous-cell, 413, 419
staging, 426
sweat glands, 423
symptoms, 412
tattoos, 425
tests, 412
treatment, 426-29
warts, 423
wens, 424
xeroderma, 423
Skin graft, 438
  doctor, 439
Skin tags, 425
Skin, wet, 181
Skull, doctor, 19
Small cell carcinoma, see Oat-cell
Small intestine, 503
Smell of cancer, 54
Smell, loss of, see Symptoms
Smoking, head and neck cancer, 641
Social security benefits, disability,
  824-25
Soft foods, 783
Soft palate, cancer of, 636, 639, 659
Specialist, how to find, 65
  who recommends, 65
  requirements for, 18
Speech therapy, 684
Spicules, 459
Spinal anesthesia, 138
Spinal cord, cancer of, 692-708
  tests, 693, 699-700
  doctor, 19
  types, 695

Spinal puncture, diagnosing spinal
  cord tumors, 705
Spinal tap, 73
Spleen, cancer of, 47
Spleen removal, 21, 470
Splenectomy, 21, 470
  in leukemia, 470
Spontaneous tumor regression,
  265-66
Sputum examinations lung cancer,
  387, 396
Sputum test, 88
Squamous cell carcinoma, 385
Squamous cell, skin cancer, 413, 419
Stage I disease, 48
Stages, bladder cancer, 524
  brain and spinal cord tumors,
    700-701
  cervical cancer, 573
  colon-rectal cancer, 515
  endometrial (uterine) cancer, 579
  Hodgkin's disease, 479
  kidney cancer, 530
  lung cancer, 403
  malignant melanoma, 436
  mycosis fungoides, 441
  ovarian cancer, 589
  skin cancer, 426
  stomach cancer, 535
  vaginal cancer, 560
  cancer of the vulva, 556
Staging, understanding, 55-58
Sterile dressing, 805-806
Sterility, chemotherapy, 246
  prostate cancer, 617
  radiation treatments, 187
Stitches, removal after operation, 151
Stolton, Jane Henry, R.N., 803
Stoma, 511
  bladder cancer, 527
  button, 685
  neck, 681
  neck, cleaning, 686
  precautions before operating, 513
Stomach cancer, 502, 533-36, 650
  (chart), 502
  diagnosis, 533
  dumping syndrome, 536
  operation, 534
  stages, 535
  symptoms, 533
  treatments, 533-34
Stomach, doctor, 18
  ulcers, 534

Stool-guaiac test, 507
Stools, dark, 502
Stopping treatment, 114
Streptozocin, 229
Subtotal hysterectomy, 552
Sunblock, 416
Sunburn, chemotherapy, 253
   medicines which cause, 417
   radiation, 180
Sunlamps, skin cancer, 416
Sunscreen, 416
Supervoltage machine, see Radiation
      treatment
Superficial spreading melanoma, 434
Superficial x-ray, see Radiation
      treatment
Supracervical hysterectomy, 552
Suprapubic prostatectomy, 608, 616
Supraradical mastectomy, 349
Surgeon, board certified, 131
Surgeon, brain, 132
   chest, 131
   choosing one, 135
   colon, rectal, 132
   ear, nose and throat, 134
   eye, 134
   general, 18, 131
   gynecologist, 133
   nervous system, 133
   neurological, 18
   obstetrics and gynecology, 19
   orthopedic, 19, 134
   otolaryngologist, 134
   plastic, 18, 132
   proctologist, 132
   qualifications, 131
   reconstructive, 644
   spinal cord, 133
   thoracic, 19, 132
   urologist, 134-35
Surgical biopsy, breast cancer, 309
Surgical conization, 552, 571, 574
Surgical insurance, 812, 819-20
Surgery, also see Operation
Surgery, 119-52
   American Board of, 131
   colon-rectal cancer for pain, 768-70
   cost of, 152
   danger of, 128
   day of week performed, 126
   decision to perform, 128
   delaying for tests, 62
   discussing with doctor, 125-26
   evaluation before, 128

how radical, 129
informed choice, 127
intravenous feedings, 128
operations overdone, 127-28
palliative, 123
preventative, 123
questions to ask, 119-21
radical, 123
recovery room, 147
safety, 123
specific, 123
types of (chart), 130
when tumor has spread, 129-30
when used, 122
Surgical evaluative staging, 56
Swallowing difficulties, radiation
      treatment, 174, 182
Swallowing, difficulty in, 689
Sweat gland cancer, 423
Symptoms, see also under specific
      types of cancer
   cancer, 55
   balance problems, in brain cancer,
      693, 698
   bone pain, 488
   brain cancer, 693, 696
   brain tumors, 696
   cancer of the vulva, 548, 555
   cervical cancer, 548, 563
   convulsions, in brain cancer, 693,
      698
   coordination loss, in brain cancer,
      692, 698
   drowsiness, in brain cancer, 693
   eye problems, in brain cancer, 693,
      698
   fever, low grade, 478
   gastrointestinal cancer, 500
   headaches, in brain cancer, 693,
      696
   hearing changes, in brain tumor,
      692, 698
   impaired speech, in brain tumor,
      692, 698
   itching, 478
   kidney cancer, 529
   lymph nodes, enlarged, 477
   muscle weakness, in brain tumor,
      692, 698
   night sweats, 478
   penis cancer, 630-31
   personality changes, in brain
      cancer, 692, 698
   personality changes,

chemotherapy, 250
smell, loss of, in brain tumor, 692,
    698
skin cancer, 441
spinal cord cancer, 692, 696
ureter tumors, 531
vomiting, in brain tumor, 692, 698
Synchrotron, 163
Sympathy, expressing, 815
Syringomas, 425

TUR, 472, 524-25, 616
Talking about cancer, 787-97, 800-802
Talking, after laryngectomy, 682
Tamoxifen, 226
Tattoos, 425
Technitium, 99m, 110
Teeth
    radiation, 185
Temperature, by mouth, 804
    rectal, 804
    under armpit, 804
Teratoma, 622, 695, 702
Teslac, 232
Testicle, cancer of, 604-610, 627-30
    artificial implant, 632
    biopsy, 627
    doctor, 625
    questions to ask, 607
    staging, 624
    (chart) treatment, 608
    undescended testicles, 624
Testicles, artificial implants, 632
Tests, CEA (carcinoembryonic
        antigen), 72
    CT, CAT, or ACTA scans, 98
    biopsies, 102
    bone marrow, 88, 106, 458
    breast cancer, 310
    bronchoscopy, 86
    cancer spread, 110
    childhood cancer, 710-12
    colonoscopy, 86-87
    colposcopy, 86
    complete blood counts, 70
    cytoscope, 86
    cytology, 88
    diagnostic, 59-111
    diodenoscopy, 87
    ECG, EKG, electrocardiogram, 73
    endometrial aspiration, 88
    endoscopy, 84
    escophagogastroduoenoscopy, 84

fluid, 88
gastrointestinal cancer, 501
gastroscopy, 87
hematocrit, 70
hemocult, 73
hemoglobin, 70
high risks, 76
hysterectomy, 85
laparoscopy, 85
lumbar puncture, 73
Pap smear, 88, 89
proctosigmoidoscopy, 86
radioactive scan, 89
risks, 63
serum factors, 70
SMA, 70
spinal tap, 73
sputum, 88
testicle cancer, 606
ultrasound, 94
urine analysis, 70
urine sediment, 88
vaginal pool aspiration, 88
white blood cell count (WBC), 70
x-ray exams, 74
Testolactone, 232
Testosterone proprionate, 232
Tetrahydrocannobinol, THC, in pain
        control, 762
THC, 234
Therapeutic radiologist, 163
Thermography, breast cancer, 310
Thio-TEPA, 218
Thioguanine, 220
Thomas, Danny, 725
Thoracentesis, lung, 387
Thoracic surgeon, 19, 132
Thoracoscopy, 387
Thoracotomy, 387, 406
3 diodeoxycytidine, 285
Throat, doctor, 18
Thrombocytophenia, 242, 457
Thymosins, 267, 273
Thyroid cancer, in children, 616
    cancer, 639, 662-70
    treatment, 669
    questions to ask, 663
    doctor, 17
Thyroid scan, 93, 666
Thyroidectomy, 670
Tired feeling, chemotherapy, 211
    internal radiation, 197
    suggestions for eating, 781

Timesaver for Health Insurance,
    820-21
TNF, 267, 269
TNM classification, 57
Tobacco, head and neck cancer, 641
Tomogram, 386, 398, 562
Tomography, 98
Tongue, cancer of, 636, 639, 647,
    653-56, 659
Tonsil, cancer of, 636, 639, 659
Topical anesthesia, 121
Torus palatinus, 648-49
Total biopsy, 102
Total hysterectomy, 522, 579-81
Total prostatectomy, 609, 614
Tracheal opening, 684-85
Tracheostomy, 644
Transcutaneous nerve stimulation,
    752, 768
Transillumination, 329-30
Transphenoidal hypophysectomy,
    708
Transurethral resection, 608, 616
    fulguration, 524
Transverse colon, 503
Transverse loop colostomy, 512
Treatment, adjuvant, 116
    brain tumors, 706-707
    curative, 116
    endometrial cancer, 548, 579
    general, 112-18
    how decided, 114
    measuring effectiveness of, 115
    of choice, 116
    palliative, 116
    prostate cancer, 605
    questions to ask, 112-13
    stopping, 104
    testicle cancer, 607
    types of, 112-13
    types of (chart), 113
Triethylenethio-phosphoramide, 218
Tumor necrosis factor, 267, 269
Tumors, 38-48
    benign, 40
    cyst, 40
    disseminated, 47
    doubling time, 43
    malignant, 41-42
    number of cells, 43
    polyps, 40
    primary, 51
    rate of growth, 43
    size, 43

    solid, 47
    spontaneous regression, 265-66
Two-step procedure, 44
    breast, 332-33
Tylectomy, 338

Ulcerative colitis, 506
Ulcers, 534
Ultrasound, 98
    costs, 98
Undescended testicles, 624
Undifferentiated cells, 42
Union Internationale Contre le
    Cancer, 840
United Ostomy Association, 842
Unproven methods of cancer
    treatment, 293-302
    questions to ask yourself, 293
Urinanalysis, 502
Urine color, chemotherapy, 239
Urine retention, 502
Urine sediment test, 88
Urine tests, 71
Urologist, 19, 134-35
Uterine cancer, 550, 563-84
Ureter, male, 612
Uterine cancer, see Servical cancer,
    endometrium
Uterus, hyperplasia, 569

VP 16-213, 229
Vaccinations, danger in leukemia, 725
Vagina, leukoplakia of, 559
Vaginal cancer, 550, 559-62
    diagnosis, 550, 559
    radium implant, 561
    sexual ralations, 562-63
    staging, 560
    treatments, 550, 560-61
Vaginal estrogen cream, 592
Vaginal hysterectomy, 552, 581
Vaginal infections, 247
Vaginal pool aspiration, 88
Vaginectomy, 553
Vas deferens, 612
Veatch, Robert M., 798
Vein darkening, chemotherapy,
    250-51
Velban, 222
Venogram, 77
Ventriculogram, 700

Veterans Administration, financial help, 828
Vinblastine, 222
Vincristine, 222
Viruses, 45
Visiting nurses, 785
Vitamin C, 286
Voice box, cancer of, 636, 674-79
Voice changes, 681
Vomiting, see Symptoms
Vulva, biopsy, 555
  cancer incidence, 558
Vulva cancer, staging, 556
Vulva, leukoplakia, 555
  operations, 555, 556
  symptoms, 550, 555
  treatment, 555, 557
Vulvectomy, and pregnancy, 558
  complications of, 558
  radical, 551, 556
  sexual relations, 558-59
  simple, 553, 556

WBC, meaning, 456
WR-2529, 278
WR-2923, 278
WR-638, 278
Warning signs, 54
Warts, 423
Weight gain, chemotherapy, 252
Weight, ways to gain, also see Eating, 777
Wens, 424
Wertheim's operation, 552
White blood cells, chemotherapy, 241
Whole body radiation, 158
Wide-bore needle biopsy, 106
Wigs, and chemotherapy drugs, 237-38
Will, writing a will, 929-30
Wills, donating your body, 830
Wills, lawyer referral services, 829
Wills, writing your own, 829-30
Wilms tumor, 652, 714, 735-36
  outlook, 736
  tests, 565, 712

X-ray, air contrast, 75
  arteriogram, 76
  barium enema, 75, 87-88
  bronchogram, 76
  cerebral angiogram, 76
  cholecystogram, 76
  computers, 74
  contrast films, 75
  cononary angiogram, 76
  cystogram, 76
  danger of, 79, 80
  diagnostic, 74
  diagnostic, where to get, 79
  difference in machines, 79
  doctor, 19
  fluoroscope, 81
  GI series, 76
  hysterogram, 77
  inspection of machines, 80
  intravenous pyelogram, 76
  lienography, 76
  lymphangiogram, 76
  mammogram, 83
  myelogram, 76
  ownership, 80-81
  plain films, 75
  pneumoencephalogram, 77
  pulmonary angiogram, 77
  rads per dose, 80, 82
  rem, 82
  role of radiologist, 78
  training of technicians, 79
  treatment, see Radiation
  venogram, 77
  vs. nuclear scans, 91
  when to have, 75, 79
  with dye, 76
Xeroderma, 423

Z dideoxcytidine, 285
Zoster immune globulin, ZIG, 724
Zoster immune plasma, ZIP, 724